Endoscopic Biopsy Interpretation

M. Priyanthi Kumarasinghe • Ian Brown
Editors

Endoscopic Biopsy Interpretation

A Practical Guide

Springer

Editors
M. Priyanthi Kumarasinghe
Department of Anatomical Pathology
PathWest Laboratory Medicine
QEII Medical Centre and University of Western Australia
Perth, WA
Australia

Ian Brown
Envoi Pathology
Kelvin Grove, QLD
Australia

ISBN 978-3-319-79116-6 ISBN 978-3-319-79117-3 (eBook)
https://doi.org/10.1007/978-3-319-79117-3

Library of Congress Control Number: 2018951925

Printed on acid-free paper

This Springer imprint is published by the registered company Springer Nature Switzerland AG.
The registered company address is: Gewerbestrasse 11, 6330 Cham, Switzerland

Dedicated to my parents Christie Dias Perera and Winifred Fernando who taught me the value of being educated and educating others.

M. Priyanthi Kumarasinghe

In loving memory of mother, Kay, who showed me the benefit of education and kindness.

Ian Brown

Preface

Biopsies and resection of the gastrointestinal tract are performed for a number of reasons. Firstly, for the investigation of a clinical symptom, common examples of which include abdominal pain, diarrhoea, nausea, vomiting and dyspepsia. Secondly, for the further investigation of an abnormal finding, examples of which include the investigation of anaemia, abnormal imaging of the gastrointestinal tract and investigation for a primary source of a malignancy of unknown origin. Thirdly, endoscopic biopsies are performed as a screening test for patients with known or potential inherited polyposis syndromes, positive family history of gastrointestinal tract malignancy, or a finding of positive faecal occult blood test. Fourthly, endoscopic biopsies are performed as a follow-up to previously diagnosed disease either to ensure adequate treatment, for example coeliac disease following gluten-free diet, or to screen for development of neoplasia such as in Barrett's oesophagus. Lastly, for the management of known pre-malignant or early malignant lesions of the upper and lower GI tracks including laterally spreading tumours of the colon and early oesophageal cancer in Barrett's oesophagus.

Over the past decade there have been numerous advances in endoscopic equipment and techniques with a much better understanding of endoscopic patterns for lesion characterisation and targeted biopsies. With these evolving techniques, there has also been a strong shift away from invasive surgical procedures towards minimally invasive endoscopic therapies. That being said, there is still a definite role for surgical management; however this is now mostly guided by the pathology reporting of resected specimens, which assist the clinician in determining nodal metastatic rates that mandate surgical resection so that now pathologists are not only integral in guiding diagnosis but also serve as a gatekeeper to more invasive therapies for patients.

For histopathologists the endoscopic appearance is the equivalent of the macroscopic assessment of the pathology. Hence a knowledge of the endoscopic finding provides important information useful to develop a final pathological diagnosis. Endoscopic findings can be broadly characterised as (1) normal appearance, (2) probable inflammation (mucosal hyperaemia, friability and oedema), (3) erosion or ulceration and (4) polyp/mucosal ridge/mass forming process. The clinical setting and site of occurrence and extent within the gastrointestinal tract provide additional information which helps narrow the potential differential diagnosis. Some conditions within the broad endoscopic patterns described above have additional characteristic endoscopic features and these are discussed further throughout the book.

An important aspect to the assessment of endoscopic biopsies is that adequate sampling has been undertaken. Guidelines for this are available and are continually being refined. The following table provides a summary of the minimal biopsy requirements required for histological assessment.

Site	Condition	Biopsy requirements
Oesophagus	Gastro-oesophageal reflux disease	Biopsies of irregular mucosa
	Barrett's oesophagus—no dysplasia	Quadrant biopsies for every 2 cm length of Barrett's mucosa
	Barrett's oesophagus—dysplasia	Quadratic biopsies for every 1 cm length of Barrett's mucosa. Targeted biopsies of abnormal mucosa
	Eosinophilic oesophagitis	At least two biopsies from mid-oesophagus and from lower oesophagus Targeted biopsies of abnormal mucosa
	Infectious oesophagitis	Targeted biopsies of abnormal mucosa or the edge of an ulcer
Stomach	Gastritis—standard	Updated Sydney Protocol: five biopsies: one from the antrum 2–3 cm from the pylorus lesser curvature, one from the antrum 2–3 cm from the pylorus greater curvature, one from the corpus 8 cm from the cardia lesser curvature, one from the corpus 8 cm from the cardia greater curvature, one from the angularis Targeted biopsies of any erosion, polyps, possible intestinal metaplasia, mass lesions
	Ulceration	Biopsies of base and edge
Small intestine	Possible coeliac disease	Five to six biopsies throughout the duodenum. Should include the duodenal bulb
Large intestine	Microscopic colitis	≥2 biopsies from right colon ≥2 biopsies from left colon
	Inflammatory bowel disease—screening for dysplasia	Pancolitis: four-quadrant biopsies every 10 cm from the cecum to the rectum, for a minimum total 33 biopsy samples OR Targeted biopsies performed with the aid of methylene blue chromoendoscopy

Table adapted from the Standards of Practice Committee of the American Society for Gastrointestinal Endoscopy (*GASTROINTESTINAL ENDOSCOPY* Vol. 78, No. 2: 2013)

Perth, Australia M. Priyanthi Kumarasinghe, MBBS, MD, FRCPA
Kelvin Grove, Australia Ian Brown, MBBS, BGEN, FRCPA

Contents

Editors and Contributors

Editors

M. Priyanthi Kumarasinghe, MBBS, MD, FRCPA Department of Anatomical Pathology, PathWest Laboratory Medicine, QEII Medical Centre and University of Western Australia, Perth, WA, Australia

Ian Brown, MBBS, BGEN, FRCPA Envoi Pathology, Kelvin Grove, QLD, Australia

Contributors

Mahsa S. Ahadi, MD, FRCPA Department of Anatomical Pathology, Royal North Shore Hospital, University of Sydney, St. Leonards, NSW, Australia

Benjamin M. Allanson, MBBS Department of Tissue Pathology and Diagnostic Oncology, Royal Prince Alfred Hospital and School of Pathology and Laboratory Medicine, Sydney, NSW, Australia

University of Western Australia, Perth, Australia

Anthony J. Gill, MD, FRCPA Cancer Diagnosis and Pathology Group, Kolling Institute of Medical Research, Royal North Shore Hospital, University of Sydney, St. Leonards, NSW, Australia

David G. Hewett, MBBS, MSc, PhD, FRACP Faculty of Medicine, University of Queensland, Brisbane, QLD, Australia

Department of Endoscopy, Queen Elizabeth II Jubilee Hospital, Brisbane, QLD, Australia

Ammar O. Kheir, MBBS, MRCP, FRACP Faculty of Medicine, University of Queensland, Brisbane, QLD, Australia

Department of Endoscopy, Queen Elizabeth II Jubilee Hospital, Brisbane, QLD, Australia

Gregory Y. Lauwers, MD Gastrointestinal Pathology Service, Department of Pathology, Moffitt Cancer Center, Tampa, FL, USA

Connull Leslie, MBBS (Hons), FRCPA Anatomical Pathology, PathWest Laboratory Medicine, QEII Medical Centre, Nedlands, WA, Australia

Gregory C. Miller, MBBS, FRCPA Envoi Pathology, Kelvin Grove, QLD, Australia

Faculty of Medicine, University of Queensland, Brisbane, QLD, Australia

Spiro C. Raftopoulos, MBBS, FRACP Interventional Endoscopist and Gastroenterologist, Department of Gastroenterology, Sir Charles Gairdner Hospital, Nedlands, WA, Australia

University of Western Australia, Perth, WA, Australia

Nicholas J. Tutticci, MBBS, FRACP Faculty of Medicine, University of Queensland, Brisbane, QLD, Australia

Department of Endoscopy, Queen Elizabeth II Jubilee Hospital, Brisbane, QLD, Australia

John R. Turchini, BMedSc, MBBS Department of Anatomical Pathology, Royal North Shore Hospital, The University of Sydney, St Leonards, NSW, Australia

Tetsuo Ushiku, MD, PhD Department of Pathology, The University of Tokyo, Tokyo, Japan

Part I

Introduction

Pathological Reaction Pattern Approach to Biopsies of the Gastrointestinal Tract: Oesophagus/Stomach/Small Intestine/Large Intestine

1

Ian Brown and M. Priyanthi Kumarasinghe

Contents

Histopathologists have two essential roles in assessing endoscopic biopsies in routine diagnostic practice: firstly, to distinguish a neoplastic condition from an inflammatory reaction pattern, and secondly, to determine the nature, or likely nature, of the neoplastic or inflammatory process. Since endoscopic biopsies only include the mucosa and superficial submucosa, transmural pathology cannot be appreciated. Emphasis is on the changes of the mucosa. An endoscopic biopsy devoid of mucosa is inadequate for assessment unless the tissue included is abnormal (e.g. ulcer tissue) or completely replaced by a neoplasm. Clinical and endoscopic information are often required to distinguish various aetiologies. A certain amount of digging or probing ("police work") is often required! This approach is expected from a modern gastrointestinal pathologist compared to the past

I. Brown (✉)
Envoi Pathology, Kelvin Grove, QLD, Australia
e-mail: ianbrown@envoi.com.au

M. P. Kumarasinghe
Department of Anatomical Pathology, PathWest Laboratory Medicine, QEII Medical Centre and University of Western Australia, Perth, WA, Australia
e-mail: priyanthi.kumarasinghe@health.wa.gov.au

M. P. Kumarasinghe, I. Brown (eds.), *Endoscopic Biopsy Interpretation*,
https://doi.org/10.1007/978-3-319-79117-3_1

where the role of a histopathologist was mostly restricted to morphological assessment only.

Distinction between a neoplastic and an inflammatory process is usually straightforward. However, determining the nature of the inflammation or neoplasm is more difficult and requires a structured systematic approach. A diverse group of aetiologies involve the mucosa resulting in a spectrum of inflammatory patterns. Inflammatory pattern that gives useful clues to aetiology could be a dominant pattern, a dominant pattern with sub-patterns or a "mixed pattern". Some site-specific special patterns may defy the common patterns; however, their unique appearance itself is often diagnostic.

The immunological basis of inflammatory conditions is such that only a limited number of patterns occur in the luminal gastrointestinal tract. Likewise, neoplasms correspond to a defined spectrum of lesions throughout the gut. This chapter presents a guide to diagnosis based on the appearance of the dominant pattern in the tissue sections. An aetiological differential diagnosis can be established or suggested from detail analysis of reactionary patterns. In some situations, a specific aetiology may be evident in the biopsy material, e.g. *Helicobacter* gastritis, while in other situations, further clinical history and additional investigations or response to therapy is required to establish a diagnosis, e.g. granulomatous inflammation. Another recent development is the use of endoscopic biopsies for biomarker and molecular testing. This chapter presents an introduction to basic inflammatory and neoplastic patterns and ancillary testing. Site-specific patterns with the clinical input and site-specific molecular testing will be elaborated within relevant chapters.

Part 1: Inflammatory Patterns

Acute Inflammatory Pattern

Acute pattern is defined by the presence of predominant neutrophilic infiltrate in the lamina propria and or epithelium ("activity"). More severe forms of acute injury are accompanied by erosions and ulceration. Inflammation may be focal or diffuse. There is minimal architectural disturbance or chronic inflammation (Box 1.1).

Box 1.1 Acute Inflammatory Pattern

- Predominant neutrophil infiltration
- Minimal architectural disturbance or chronic inflammation
- May be associated with erosion and ulceration
- May be focal or diffuse

Aetiology

- Infection
- Trauma—physical, chemical, temperature
- Immune mediated
- Toxins including medications
- Ischaemia

Chronic Inflammatory Pattern

This pattern is characterised by chronic mucosal inflammation composed of lymphocytes, plasma cells and eosinophils. Mucosal architecture is often disturbed. Lymphoid follicles and histiocytic can be seen. There is no neutrophilic component. Mucosal distortion manifests as irregular branching and loss or shortening of glands (failing to reach the muscularis mucosae of glands). Mucosal distortion may be accompanied by atrophy. Metaplastic pattern may be seen as a sub-pattern (e.g. pyloric, Paneth cell and intestinal metaplasia depending on the site) (Box 1.2).

Box 1.2 Chronic Inflammatory Pattern

- Chronic inflammation is dominant.
- Mucosal, glandular and surface architecture are often disturbed.
- Mucosal distortion may be accompanied by atrophy.
- Metaplastic and atrophic sub-patterns may be present and even dominate.

Aetiology

- Any cause of acute inflammation that persists
- Chronic infection
- Immune dysfunction disorders

Active Chronic Pattern

This pattern is characterised by a combination of features of acute and chronic inflammatory patterns representing chronic persistent and active injury.

Lymphocytic Pattern

Lymphocytic pattern is characterised by the presence of intraepithelial lymphocytes ("intraepithelial lymphocytosis"). Variable inflammation in the lamina propria usually accompanies a lymphocytosis. This is an increase in the number of normally present intraepithelial T lymphocytes in the luminal gastrointestinal tract. There may be associated mucosal architectural change, e.g. villous blunting in coeliac disease (Box 1.3).

Box 1.3 Lymphocytic Pattern
Intraepithelial lymphocytosis
Lamina propria lymphocytic infiltrate
Mucosal distortion +/−

A certain number of intraepithelial lymphocytes are required to reach the following threshold levels to be considered as abnormal: oesophagus ≥20/HPF, stomach ≥25/100 epithelial cells (surface and crypt), duodenum ≥30/100 epithelial cells and colon ≥10/100 epithelial cells. Atypical lymphocytic infiltrates should trigger consideration of a lymphoproliferative disorders. In the setting of immunosuppression, EBV infection may need to be ruled out.

Aetiology

- Coeliac disease
- Infection - virus, tropical sprue
- Medications - sartan family medications (olmesartan usually), immune modulatory medications, new biological agents
- Immune dysfunction disorders, e.g. common variable immunodeficiency, autoimmune enteropathy

Collagen Deposition Pattern

This pattern is characterised by the deposition of sub-epithelial collagen layer measuring ≥10 μm. Typically, there is lamina propria inflammation with surface epithelial damage. Collagenous gastritis, duodenitis and colitis are well established.

Deposition of collagen (type VI mainly with lesser amounts of types III and I) and tenascin in the subsurface epithelial zone to a thickness of ≥10 μm is seen. Collagen deposition is irregular at the lower border and has a tendency to entrap and dilate superficial lamina propria capillaries. Typically, there is accompanying lamina propria inflammation (Box 1.4).

Box 1.4 Collagen Deposition Pattern
- Deposition of sub-epithelial collagen layer measuring ≥10 μm
- Lamina propria inflammation
- Surface damage

Aetiology

- Coeliac disease
- Immune dysfunction disorders
- Medications, e.g. NSAIDs, sartan family medications

Histiocytic Infiltration Pattern

This pattern is characterised by an infiltration of the lamina propria by histiocytes. When these become ordered in closely associated groups, the term granuloma is appropriate.

Aetiology

- Xanthoma
- Malakoplakia
- Infections, e.g. Whipple, MAIC
- Lipid storage disorders
- Muciphages

Granulomatous Pattern

A granuloma is an organised collection of activated macrophages (or histiocytes) as opposed to diffuse histiocytic infiltration. Histiocytes in a granuloma are organised as a circumscribed collection with defined boundaries.

The two main types of granulomas noted in this spectrum of inflammation are foreign body type and immune type granulomas which are associated with a T cell-mediated immune response. The T cell-driven "typical" granulomatous pattern is characterised by aggregates of epithelioid histiocytes admixed with lymphocytes and plasma cells with and without multinucleated giant cells.

Unravelling granulomatous inflammation in the GI tract is a challenge to the pathologist and triggers considerable clinical interest. The most common clinical request is to differentiate infection (e.g. mycobacterial), Crohn's disease and sarcoidosis. However, there are many other causes that could mimic these commonly considered diagnoses both clinically and pathologically. A systematic and comprehensive approach is mandatory as some inciting causes are curable, while some others need long-term management.

A granulomatous response may be induced by a variety of infective and non-infective agents.

Aetiology

Infective causes:

- Systemic (TB, histoplasmosis, Whipple disease)
- GI-specific infections (*Salmonella*, *Yersinia*, *Campylobacter*, *Helicobacter*)
- Parasites—*Schistosoma*, *Enterobius*
- Venereal infections (syphilis, LGV)

Non-infective causes:

- Crohn's disease
- Medications (e.g. NSAID—diclofenac, biologic agents)
- Foreign material (talc, starch, barium, faecal material including pulse granuloma, gas–pneumatosis)
- Crypt/gland rupture-associated granuloma
- Sarcoidosis
- Inherited disorders—chronic granulomatous disease, Hermansky-Pudlak syndrome, Blau syndrome
- Diverticular disease-associated colitis
- Malignancy/neoplasm related
- Vasculitis (granulomatosis with polyangiitis, Churg-Strauss syndrome, Behcet's disease, giant cell arteritis)
- Common variable immunodeficiency (CVID)
- Cord colitis syndrome

Granulomas have the following morphologic types:

- Foreign body: multinucleate cells with eccentrically or haphazardly arranged nuclei admixed with histiocytes
- Epithelioid: single or multinucleate collections of histiocytes with abundant eosinophilic cytoplasm and "footprint"-like nuclei
  - Sarcoid type: epithelioid granuloma devoid of other inflammatory cells and often containing calcified bodies (Schaumann bodies and/or asteroid bodies)
  - Non-sarcoid type: epithelioid granulomas with other inflammatory cells +/− necrosis
- Necrotising: central zone of necrosis
  - Suppurative: necrosis with neutrophils
  - Caseous: necrosis devoid of any structure
  - Necrobiotic: eosinophilic degeneration of collagen with retention of some structure
- Granulomas accompanied by vasculitis: intense eosinophils and background necrosis

Some morphologic types of granulomas may reflect the underlying aetiology and may provide etiological clues. Diagnostic features such as foreign material, parasites, microbial organisms, and associated substances, e.g. mucin, and even subtle clues, e.g. specific secondary patterns of damage (e.g. vasculitis, brown pigment of chronic granulomatous disease), may be noted with vigilance. Additional levels are crucial to identify parasites and foreign substances. Special stains for microorganisms as well as other ancillary tests are invaluable to render an etiological diagnosis (Boxes 1.5 and 1.6).

Box 1.5 Morphologic Clues to Aetiology

- Foreign body type: look for foreign material and parasites.
- Sarcoid type: sarcoidosis, Crohn's disease and medication.

- Necrotising: exclude TB, *Yersinia* and fungal infection.
- Granuloma with background eosinophils: look for parasites and gas pockets (pneumatosis) and Churg-Strauss vasculitis.
- Granuloma with background necrosis: polyangiitis granulomatosis and intravascular fungal infection.
- Granuloma with background vasculitis: Behcet's, polyangiitis, Churg-Strauss, rarely Crohn disease and medications.

Box 1.6 Ancillary Studies on Paraffin-Embedded Tissue

- PAS/PASD—fungi
- ZN, Wade Fite—mycobacterial species
- PCR: TB, fungi and *Yersinia*

Additionally, and most importantly, the clinical setting should be always considered. Crucial information may be obtained by discussing the case with the referring clinician. Clinical investigations, e.g. stool culture, or serology, e.g. specific interferon gamma release (QuantiFERON-TB Gold), should be recommended when suspicion is high for infective organisms (Box 1.7).

Box 1.7 Clinical Clues

Significant past history—Crohn's disease, chronic granulomatous disease, CVID and vasculitis

Extra-intestinal disease—Crohn's disease, tuberculosis, sarcoidosis

History of immunosuppression—infective causes

Travel history/geographic location—potential exposure to parasitic and mycobacterial infection

Consumption of unpasteurised milk—mycobacterial infection

Medication history—recent introduction of a new medication

Sexual practices: anal intercourse and risk of lymphogranuloma venereum

Patient's age: young patients consider an inherited condition

Importantly it is emphasised that an isolated collection of histiocytes should not be regarded as granulomatous pattern although true granulomas should be searched for and excluded. Endoscopic biopsies pose an additional challenge due to artefacts that may mimic a granuloma (Box 1.8).

Box 1.8 Mimics

- Sclerotic germinal centres of a reactive lymphoid follicle
- Cross-cutting of the pericryptal fibroblast sheath
- Disrupted a rounded collection of smooth muscle of muscularis mucosa
- Hypertrophic ganglion cells translocated to the mucosa
- Clustered and rounded collections of endothelial cells
- Schwann cell hamartoma, perineurioma and elastofibroma

In some cases, despite extensive investigation, an identifiable cause may not be found, and the term *idiopathic granulomatous inflammation* is appropriate. Site-specific features will be discussed in the specific chapters.

Eosinophil Pattern

This pattern is defined by an abnormal eosinophil infiltrate in the mucosa and epithelium. Definitions vary depending on site. An eosinophil infiltrate of >30 or 40/HPF is generally regarded as abnormal. Importantly this is characteristically accompanied by any or all of the following: eosinophil infiltration of epithelium, eosinophilic crypt abscess formation, degranulation and infiltration of muscularis mucosae. Mucosal oedema may be prominent in some case, and architectural change such as villous blunting may be seen. Eosinophilic pattern may be accompanied by other defined patterns (i.e. granulomatous pattern) or may be a component of the "mixed pattern". Allergic phenomenon is commonly suspected, and allergen may or may not be demonstrated after clinicopathological correlation (Box 1.9).

Box 1.9 Eosinophil Pattern

- Abnormal eosinophil infiltrate in the mucosa and epithelium.
- Cut-offs for counts vary depending on site. In general >30/HPF is abnormal.
- Intraepithelial eosinophils, eosinophilic crypt abscess formation and degranulation and infiltration of muscularis mucosae may be seen.

Aetiology

- Hypereosinophilic syndrome
- Parasitic infection, e.g. *Enterobius*, Strongyloides, others
- Allergy—food: cow's milk, soy protein (allergic proctocolitis)
- Drugs—NSAIDs, Gold, L-tryptophan, carbamazepine, methotrexate, tacrolimus, azathioprine, rifampicin, clozapine
- Connective tissue disorders
- Vasculitis—Eosinophilic granulomatosis with polyangiitis (Churg-Strauss syndrome)
- Neoplasia—lymphoma, Langerhans cell histiocytosis, systemic mastocytosis, myeloid neoplasms
- Inflammatory fibroid polyp
- Inflammatory bowel disease
- Solid organ and bone marrow transplantation

Ischaemic Pattern

Mucosal injury pattern is best described by the changes in the glandular mucosa characterised by crypt/gland "whithering" and loss, hyaline change in lamina propria with or without collagen deposition and minimal inflammation. Increased apoptosis in epithelial cells, often early in the course and sometimes prominent enough to produce an apoptotic pattern, can be seen. Surface erosion and an inflammatory membrane may develop imparting pseudomembrane formation. If the blood flow is re-established, an acute pattern may supervene due to host inflammatory response.

Ischaemic change results from prolonged, transient or unresolved interruption to blood flow to a degree that is insufficient to maintain normal mucosal cell homeostasis (Box 1.10).

Box 1.10 Ischaemic Pattern

- Crypt/gland "whithering" and loss
- Hyaline change in lamina propria
- Minimal inflammation
- +/− erosion, ulceration and crypt apoptosis

Aetiology

- Vascular obstruction due to:
  - *External compression*
    - Adhesions
    - Volvulus
    - Incarceration in hernia sac
    - Iatrogenic, e.g. surgical ligation
  - *Vessel wall abnormality*
    - Atherosclerosis
    - Vasculitis–Polyarteritis nodosa, Churg-Strauss, Takayasu's arteritis, Wegener's granulomatosis, connective tissue disorder related, Behcet's disease
    - Radiotherapy-related intimal hyperplasia
    - Amyloidosis
    - Arterial dissection
    - Scleroderma
    - Fibromuscular hyperplasia
    - HUS/TTP thrombotic microangiopathies
  - *Vascular lumen abnormality*
    - Thrombosis
    - Hypercoagulable state, e.g. embolus
    - Thromboembolus
    - Cholesterol
    - Tumour
    - Foreign body

- Intestinal hypoperfusion
  - Hypovolemia
  - Cardiac failure
  - Excessive exercise
- Miscellaneous causes
  - Drugs
    Digoxin
    Cocaine
    NSAIDs
    Pseudoephedrine
    Vasopressor agents
    OCP/estrogenic compounds
  - Colonic luminal obstruction with back pressure
    Tumours
    Hirschsprung's disease
    Faecal impaction
  - Infection
  - Clostridium difficile
  - Shiga toxin-producing bacteria, e.g. *E. coli* (O157:H7)
  - Mucosal prolapse associated local vascular obstruction

Apoptotic Pattern

Typical primary apoptotic pattern is characterised by prominent epithelial apoptosis which may lead to loss or degeneration of glands or keratinocytes in glandular and squamous mucosa, respectively. Typically, there is minimal or no inflammation. Considering etiological factors, clinical information is invaluable (Box 1.11).

Box 1.11 Apoptotic Pattern
- Prominent epithelial apoptosis
- +/− loss or degeneration of glands or keratinocytes

Aetiology
- Drugs including chemotherapy and immune modulatory agents
- Immune dysfunction disorders—GVHD, CVID, thymoma-associated colitis, autoimmune enteropathy and HIV
- Non-HIV virus
- Sodium phosphate bowel preparation

Toxic Injury Pattern

Toxic injury pattern is characterised by crypt, gland or epithelial destruction with mixed acute, chronic and often eosinophil-rich inflammation in the lamina propria. This pattern may show a secondary apoptotic pattern. Often both the inflammatory intensity and extent of crypt injury are variable in degree between the biopsies taken at one site and also from different sites. This is an uncommon pattern whereby a particular mucosal insult leads to activation of several immune or inflammatory pathways leading to epithelial injury by apoptosis or inflammation (Box 1.12).

Box 1.12 Toxic Injury Pattern
- Crypt, gland or epithelial destruction
- Mixed acute, chronic and often eosinophil-rich inflammation in the lamina propria
- +/− apoptosis, sloughing

Aetiology
- Medications—biological/immune modulatory medications, chemotherapy, others
- Toxins—ingested
- Toxin—infection related

Metaplastic Pattern

Metaplasia is defined as replacement of one differentiated mucosa with another. Hence, this pattern is characterised by the presence of differentiated mucosa or elements that are not native to the site and essentially reflects chronic injury. Hence more often than not, it is accompanied by at least chronic inflammatory pattern and will be discussed in detail in subsequent chapters. Sometimes the only abnormality noted is "the mucosa that is unusual" for the site sampled. If clinical notes are not scrutinised, the pattern may be overlooked especially in the presence of other dominant patterns.

This pattern includes columnar-lined oesophagus with and without intestinal metaplasia, intestinal and pancreatic metaplasia of the gastric mucosa, pyloric gland metaplasia of gastric body mucosa, gastric metaplasia of the duodenum, pyloric metaplasia of the ileum and colon and Paneth cell metaplasia of the left colon (Box 1.13).

Box 1.13 Metaplastic Pattern

- Presence of differentiated mucosa or elements that are not native to the site
- ++/– chronic inflammation
- +/– other inflammatory patterns
- +/– epithelial neoplasia

Aetiology

- Any form of chronic injury

Mixed Injury Pattern

This pattern is characterised by the absence of a well-defined dominant pattern and may be a clue to medication-induced injury, somewhat similar to a common pattern seen in drug-induced liver injury (DILI).

Medications cause damage to the mucosa in three ways:

1. Iatrogenic injury produced by direct contact of the mucosa with medications
2. Immunological mediated injury
3. Vasculopathic mediated injury

A classic example of direct mucosa injury due to direct contact with oral medications is "pill oesophagitis".

Often there is some evidence of toxic injury pattern however it is given a separate designation to reflect the broader aetiology. Again, several immune pathways are activated, such that a dominant pattern is difficult to appreciate. Admixtures of any of the patterns described above may be seen. Mucosal injury associated with mycophenolate mofetil is a classic example of mixed pattern (Box 1.14).

Box 1.14 Mixed Injury Pattern

- No defined dominant pattern.
- Pill substances may be evident.
- Unique patterns are described.

Aetiology

- Medications, e.g. biologic agents—particularly immune modulators
- Crohn's disease
- Autoimmune enteropathy
- Other immune dysregulation disorders

Deposition Pattern

Endogenous or exogenous materials may accumulate in the mucosa in epithelial cells, stromal elements or both. Endogenous material may result from a local inflammatory process, a neoplastic disease or a genetic disorder. Therefore, other mucosal injury patterns are commonly associated with depositions. Deposits may be striking or subtle at low power. When subtle they can be overlooked due to the presence of a dominant inflammatory pattern. The colour and quality of the pigment may give clues to its aetiology.

Special Patterns

These are a diverse range of conditions with characteristic histopathological features that do not fit within the reaction patterns discussed above. Examples include sloughing oesophagitis and lichenoid pattern in the oesophagus; paediatric malabsorption disorders, such as tufting enteropathy and microvillus inclusion disease; and infections where the organism or its cellular response is evident in the tissue sections. Site-specific special patterns will be discussed in appropriate chapters.

Mucosal Prolapse Pattern

It is characterised histologically by smooth muscle proliferation and fibrosis in the lamina propria ("muscularisation") and glandular distortion, often with gland elongation and regenerative changes. The surface may become ulcerated. Sometimes a pseudomembrane may develop, and an ischaemic injury pattern may be superimposed. This is a change in the mucosal stroma and epithelium resulting from traction on the mucosa leading to it being pulled away from the deeper layers of the luminal wall. Mucosal prolapse pattern forming a polypoid lesion is well described in the large intestine (rectum commonly) and gastric antrum. Endoscopic appearance is often described as a polyp (Box 1.15).

Box 1.15 Mucosal Prolapse Pattern
- Muscularisation of lamina propria
- Hyperplastic and reactive mucosal glands/crypts
- +/− inflammatory cap and ischaemic changes

Aetiology
- Rectal prolapse
- Ostium of diverticulum
- Overlying/adjacent to a mass

Mucosal Vasculopathy

This is a group of conditions characterised by abnormality in the small vessels of the mucosa. In general, either the number of these vessels or their luminal diameter is increased. Abnormalities may be site specific, e.g. gastric antral vascular ectasia, or more generalised in nature, e.g. portal hypertension-related vasculopathy. Often the vasculopathy changes are subtle and masked by the dominant reactive pattern. A high index of clinical suspicion is required for confirmative diagnosis (Box 1.16).

Box 1.16 Mucosal Vasculopathy
- Vascular abnormality: the number of these vessels or their luminal diameter or wall thickness is increased.
- Background reactive pattern.
- +/− advanced damage: ischaemia and ulceration.

Aetiology
- Portal hypertension
- Angiodysplasia
- Radiotherapy
- Local vascular obstruction

Part 2: Neoplastic patterns

The approach to neoplasms and tumour-like processes of the gastrointestinal tract is to first assess the dominant make-up of the lesion in the biopsy tissue. Generally neoplasms are either composed of epithelial and rounded, epithelioid-like or spindle-shaped, mesenchymal-like cells. Rarely there are admixtures of these elements. Sometimes, there is no clear neoplastic process, and a tumour-like process such as a hamartoma, mucosal prolapse or inflammatory pseudopolyp needs to be considered. What follows is a diagnostic approach based on morphology. Each chapter of this textbook will consider the neoplasms and tumour-like processes relevant to the particular site using this general approach.

Normal Tissue at the Wrong Site (Heterotopia)

Three forms of heterotopia are encountered. These are **gastric** heterotopia containing specialised, acid-secreting epithelium **pancreatic** heterotopia which mostly contains only exocrine pancreatic elements and sebaceous gland heterotopia which is limited to the oesophagus.

Non-neoplastic Glandular Proliferations

Hamartomas
Hamartomas are benign tumour comprising a disorganised collection of tissue elements native to the site of occurrence. They may occur sporadically or as part of several tumour syndromes.

Table 1.1 Hamartoma tumour syndromes

Syndrome	Gene	Gastrointestinal findings	Other findings	Malignancy risk
Juvenile polyposis syndrome	SMAD4, BMPR1A	Multiple GI-polyps, inflamed stroma with gland dilatation	Epistaxis, telangiectasia	Colon, rectum and stomach 60%
PTEN hamartoma syndrome (mostly Cowden syndrome)	PTEN	Oesophageal glycogenic acanthosis, Hamartomatous polyps frequently containing adipose tissue and lymphoid follicles, Ganglioneuroma, lipoma and fibrolipoma of the colon, Inflammatory/hyperplastic polyps of the stomach, Colorectal adenoma	Trichilemmoma, skin hamartoma, macrocephaly, benign and malignant tumours of the breast, thyroid, endometrium	Breast (85%), thyroid and kidney (35%), endometrium (30%) and colon (10%)
Peutz-Jeghers syndrome	STK11 (LKB1)	Polyposis of the GI tract, small bowel (>90%), colon (25%) and stomach (25%) Arborising core of smooth muscle	Mucocutaneous melanosis, sex cord tumours with annular tubules (SCTAT) of ovary, adenoma malignum of the cervix, calcifying Sertoli cell tumours of the testes	80–95% Colorectal, gastric, pancreatic, breast and ovary
Hereditary mixed polyposis syndrome	(BMPR1A, GREM1)	Atypical polyposis with juvenile polyps, adenomas, hyperplastic polyps and inflammatory polyps of colon and rectum		Unknown

Sporadic hamartomas are usually solitary and have no increased risk for neoplasia. By contrast hamartoma tumour syndromes are generally associated with a constellation of findings and do represent a marker of risk for gastrointestinal and extra-gastrointestinal neoplasms including several malignancies. A summary of the common hamartoma tumour syndromes is outlined in Table 1.1.

Epithelial Proliferations with No Stromal Invasion

Epithelial neoplasms are the most commonly encountered in the gastrointestinal tract. Most are of glandular origin and retain their glandular pattern during neoplastic transformation. These glandular pattern lesions may be confined to a basement membrane (dysplasia or adenoma).

Dysplasia (Intraepithelial Neoplasia)

Abrupt transition with lack of surface maturation for all grades of dysplasia together with loss of nuclear polarity in higher grade lesions is considered as a feature highly characteristic for an intraepithelial neoplastic process. These changes are generally regarded as an unequivocal neoplastic change in the epithelium that is confined to the mucosa. The process may occur in flat mucosa or develop in the setting of a polypoidal glandular proliferation such as an adenoma or a hamartoma. Dysplasia is characterised by variable degrees of architectural and cytological abnormality. Cytological abnormalities reflect underlying genetic abnormality and include the following features—increase in size, irregular shape, increased nuclear/cytoplasmic ratio, nuclear crowding, hyperchromasia and the presence of nucleoli. Architectural features are irregular gland outline, variability in glandular size, gland crowding in glandular tissues and hyperplasia with parakeratosis in squamous tissue. Increased mitotic and apoptotic activity is also frequently present. Dysplasia is graded on the basis of the degree of cytological and architectural abnormality into low and high grade. Standard terminologies have been introduced to maintain consistency of interpretation and logical management. However, the neoplastic progression of normal to dysplasia and finally to invasive carcinoma is a biological continuum. Therefore, there are no strict cut-offs for this dichotomisation. As a result, standardised terminology systems based on a combination of cytoarchitectural features have been recommended to categorise epithelial dysplasia throughout the GIT. All such terminologies have been adopted from the system developed for dysplasia associated with inflammatory bowel disease in the twentieth century. Updates have been made considering site-specific issues and will be discussed appropriately later.

The term "atypical epithelium/changes" as a diagnostic category is not included in standard terminologies and strongly discouraged to avoid confusion. Atypia is often used by pathologists to describe the biological uncertainty based on the microscopic features but does not reflect the degree of uncertainty. The terms mild, moderate or severe atypia based on individual impression of a conglomerate of cytoarchitectural features can be ever so confusing. The term atypism is better suited to describe these morphological changes. Most standardised terminology system used throughout the GIT discourages the use of the term *atypia* as a diagnostic category.

High-grade dysplasia in squamous tissues represents a near to or complete full-thickness neoplastic transformation of the cells which is often best appreciated by the location of mitotic figures in the upper half of the epithelium. In glandular tissues, high-grade dysplasia is marked by architectural features of glandular crowding, branching or budding glands, cribriform and micropapillary or cystically dilated crypt patterns. The cytological indicators include loss of cell polarity, rounding up and enlargement of nuclei with irregularly thickened nuclear membranes and conspicuous nucleoli. Atypical mitotic figures may also be seen.

There is notable difference between Western and Japanese pathologists in the diagnosis of high-grade dysplasia and carcinoma. Many features described as high-grade dysplasia and most described above as suspicious for carcinoma are often diagnostic of carcinoma according to Japanese criteria.

Adenoma

Intestinal-Type Adenoma of Conventional Type

This lesion is most commonly encountered in the large intestine; it can also be seen in the stomach and small intestine. The lining epithelium resembles intestine mucosa and is composed of columnar cells with basically located nuclei and eosinophilic cytoplasm and interspersed goblet cells. Intestinal adenomas exhibit variable cytological and glandular abnormality. On the basis of architecture, they are further characterised as being tubular, tubulovillous or villous. Tubular adenomas are defined by the presence of more than 75% of tubular structures in the polyp. The villous component of a conventional adenoma is significant if comprising at least 25% of the polyp: if between 25% and 75% of the polyp, this is diagnostic of a tubulovillous adenoma; if >75% of the polyp, this is a villous adenoma. On the basis of cytoarchitectural abnormality, dysplasia can be graded as low or high grade. In low-grade dysplasia, gland architecture is regular, and the lining epithelium consists of pencillate columnar cells with abundant eosinophilic cytoplasm, small hyperchromatic columnar nuclei, interspersed goblet cells and an absence of atypical mitotic figures. In high-grade dysplasia, glandular architectural arrangement occurs characterised by close-packing glands and glands with papillary infolding, complex architecture with back-to-back configuration, complex budding and cribriform patterns. Often the nuclei are enlarged and variable in size with prominent nucleoli. Loss of polarity is an important feature, and atypical mitotic figures may be found.

A small percentage of intestinal adenomas arise in the setting of inherited syndrome such as familial adenomatous polyposis, MUTYH and Lynch syndrome. Clues to an inherited origin include young age at onset, multiple adenomas and multiple sites of involvement. Adenomas developing due to Lynch syndrome are typically high-grade and villous component.

Intestinal-Type Polyps of Serrated Type

Serrated polyps are characterised by the unique architectural pattern of epithelial infolding into the gland lumen creating a sawtooth ("serrated")-type appearance. Currently three types of serrated polyps are recognised—hyperplastic polyp, sessile serrated adenoma and traditional serrated adenoma. These are almost entirely restricted to the large intestine.

Gastric-Type Adenomas

These are most commonly found in the stomach, gastro-oesophageal junction region or proximal small intestine. The lesions may be pure or display an admixture of various patterns, usually a combination of pyloric gland and foveolar-type adenoma.

Pyloric Gland Adenoma

Pyloric gland adenoma is a neoplastic proliferation of cells with differentiation towards gastric pyloric gland cells. Most cases are sporadic, although recent studies suggest an increased prevalence in both Lynch syndrome and familial adenomatous polyposis.

In the absence of morphological dysplasia, pyloric gland adenoma is characterised by a proliferation of regular, tubular glands lined by cuboidal cells that have clear to eosinophilic cytoplasm and a round nucleus with generally small nucleolus. Development of morphological dysplasia is characterised by architectural irregularity, increase in cell size, increase in nuclear size and increased prominence of nucleoli. To date no well-established guidelines exist for separation of low- and high-grade dysplasia; however, cytoarchitectural features used above for intestinal dysplasia are commonly applied. Development of invasive carcinoma may be deceptive. A back-to-back gland pattern or infiltration by single tumour cells indicates malignancy.

Pyloric gland adenoma displays cytoplasmic expression of MUC6. Expression of MUC5ac may be found in cells near the luminal aspect of the tumour:

- Chief cell adenoma (see stomach chapter)
- Foveolar adenoma (see stomach chapter)

Adenomas of Special Type

These are benign tumours of specific anatomic glandular structures and therefore restricted to the site of the originating structure. Examples include Brunner gland adenoma (syn Brunneroma, Brunner gland hamartoma) and adenomas of the oesophageal submucosal glands.

Papilloma

This is a proliferation of squamous mucosa characterised by a papillary architecture with fibrovascular cores in the papillae. Koilocytotic atypia may be appreciated if HPV infection is the cause. Papilloma may also arise on the basis of local irritation, for example, due to acid reflux in the oesophagus.

Epithelial Proliferations with Stromal Invasion

Epithelial lesions may also appear to invade the stroma of the biopsy (usually, but not always, representing adenocarcinoma). Important clues to invasive growth include a desmoplastic stromal reaction and/or complexity and infiltrative patterns of the epithelium. Desmoplasia is a fibroblastic proliferation in response to a growing epithelial tumour. Often the fibroblasts sit in a myxoid background with minimal collagen deposition and with associated inflammatory reaction comprising lymphocytes and neutrophils. If the tumour is more slowly growing, the desmoplastic response may be more collagenous. Sometimes it may be keloidal. Submucosal invasive tumours in the large intestine almost always produce a desmoplastic stromal reaction; however well-differentiated adenocarcinoma and squamous cell carcinoma in the oesophagus and stomach may invade without a stromal reaction.

Occasionally epithelium may be misplaced into submucosa, particularly in a polypoidal tumour that has undergone torsion. This process is referred to as pseudoinvasion and needs to be separated from true invasion. The absence of a desmoplastic stromal reaction or irregular gland or tumour nest outlines helps exclude true invasion.

Table 1.2 Most commonly encountered forms of carcinoma

Carcinoma type	Morphological characteristics
Adenocarcinoma—intestinal type	Glandular or villoglandular arrangements; tumour cells are columnar with pencillate nuclei and eosinophilic cytoplasm; necrotic debris ("dirty necrosis") is common within gland lumina
Adenocarcinoma—gastric type (including pyloric gland type)	Complex cribriform or small gland pattern; tumour cells are cuboidal and have clear or lightly eosinophilic cytoplasm; necrosis uncommon
Mucinous adenocarcinoma	>50% mucinous
Signet-ring cell carcinoma	>50% signet-ring cell forms
Neuroendocrine carcinoma	Small cell type: diffuse or nested architecture; small-/intermediate-sized cells with high nucleus to cytoplasmic ratio, granular chromatin and inconspicuous nucleoli Large cell type: organoid, nested and/or trabecular architecture; large cells with vesicular nuclei and nucleoli Both: neuroendocrine immunohistochemistry positive
Squamous cell carcinoma	Differentiation varies; eosinophilic to basophilic appearance; keratinisation and evidence of desmosomes
Adenosquamous carcinoma	Mixed adenocarcinoma and squamous cell carcinoma elements
Medullary carcinoma	Solid growth in nested, organoid or trabecular patterns; tumour-infiltrating lymphocytes and peritumoural lymphoid infiltrate. Neuroendocrine immunohistochemistry negative
Undifferentiated carcinoma	No line of differentiation appreciable by morphology, mucin histochemical stains or immunohistochemistry
Mixed adenocarcinoma and neuroendocrine carcinoma (MANEC/MiNEN)	>30% component of conventional adenocarcinoma mixed with neuroendocrine neoplasia

Carcinoma

Epithelial proliferations invading the stroma represent carcinoma. In most cases a desmoplastic stromal reaction is present. In cases where invasion is restricted to the mucosa, the diagnosis of carcinoma will require the presence of a marked degree of glandular complexity, merging of glands, and punched out cribriform patterns. Intramucosal adenocarcinoma in the large intestine is designated as high-grade dysplasia because it does not exhibit malignant behaviour. Similarly, squamous cell carcinoma involving only the epithelium of the oesophagus is designated as high-grade dysplasia. In both these situations, the diagnosis of invasive carcinoma relies on the demonstration of submucosal invasion. Carcinoma of the gastrointestinal tract may exhibit a wide variety of types. The WHO classification for each type varies, and reference to this is required in each situation. Table 1.2 lists the most commonly encountered forms of carcinoma.

Most carcinoma arises in a sporadic setting; however it is always worth bearing in mind that in inherited or other predispositions to development of carcinoma may exist. The most common examples include familial adenomatous polyposis (FAP), Lynch syndrome, MUTYH associated polyposis, juvenile polyposis syndrome, Peutz-Jeghers syndrome, neurofibromatosis type 1, PTEN hamartoma tumour syndrome (Cowden syndrome), inflammatory bowel disease, chronic fistula and previous radiotherapy. The pre-existing in situ lesion, such as an adenoma, may be seen at the edge of the carcinoma.

Pseudoinvasion/Epithelial Inversion into the Submucosa

This is a common process in the gastrointestinal tract particularly with protuberant or pedunculated lesions that are prone to torsion or mechanical trauma. The process is almost exclusively seen when the lesion undergoing torsion is composed of glandular epithelium. Pseudoinvasion is most commonly encountered in conventional adenoma of the sigmoid colon. Peutz-Jeghers polyps also often display foci of pseudoinvasion.

Features that help separate pseudoinvasion from true malignant infiltration include the following:

- The epithelium extends through a narrow gap in muscularis mucosae rather than broad-based invasion.
- Rounded appearance to the focus.
- Rounded appearance of glands within the focus.
- Lamina propria surrounds the glands of the focus.
- There is a background of dense collagen but not true desmoplasia.
- Often marked hypertrophy of the muscularis mucosae.
- Haemosiderin deposition and red cell extravasation.
- Chronic inflammation.
- Extravasated mucin with either no epithelium present or epithelium confined to the edge. Note that neoplastic epithelium floating within the mucin pools is a concerning feature for invasive adenocarcinoma.

Metastasis (Foreign Appearance for Site)

Metastases may be epithelial or mesenchymal in origin. The former is more common and is mostly via a transcoelomic route; hence another site in the abdominal cavity is the usual primary site—gastrointestinal tract and female genital tract. Lobular carcinoma of the breast has a marked predilection to spread to serosal surfaces and thus may secondarily involve the luminal gastrointestinal tract, especially the stomach and rectum. Melanoma is the most common non-epithelial tumour to present as a metastasis.

Diffuse Round Cell (Epithelioid-Like) Pattern

As glandular epithelial neoplasms become less differentiated, they assume a diffuse architectural pattern with sparse or no glandular differentiation. Here the differential diagnosis broadens, and we are forced to consider non-glandular epithelial neoplasms, in particular squamous cell and neuroendocrine neoplasm, as well as a broad range of non-epithelial neoplasms such as lymphoma, melanoma and mesenchymal origin tumours. To help with this differential, we have found it useful to think in terms of the dominant cytoplasmic tincture of the tumour cells, blue cell, pink cell or clear cell, on the H&E stain. This generally narrows the diagnostic considerations. In most cases, morphological clues (discussed in the individual chapters) help to further narrow the possible diagnoses. If morphology does not provide any assistance with the differential diagnosis, then a broad initial screening panel of LCA, AE1/AE3 and S-100 should be employed to define a line of differentiation. Based on the morphological clues and/or initial immunoreaction pattern, further targeted stains can be performed to establish the final diagnosis. The tables below list the most common diagnoses for these various patterns and the immunochemical stain that best characterises the diagnosis.

Blue Cells

See Table 1.3.

Pink Cells

See Table 1.4.

Clear Cells

See Table 1.5.

Neuroendocrine Neoplasms (NENs)

Neuroendocrine neoplasms of the gastrointestinal tract occur at all sites. They are usually sporadic, but a significant number arise in an inherited setting, in particular MEN1 and neurofibromatosis type 1 syndromes. Histological features common to a well-differentiated neuroendocrine neoplasm or neuroendocrine carcinoma can be considered on the basis of architectural, cytomorphological and stromal patterns.

Table 1.3 Blue cells

Diagnosis	Preliminary immunohistochemical profile
Lymphoma	LCA, CD3 or CD20
Plasma cell tumours	CD138
Leukaemia	Myeloperoxidase, CD43
Carcinoma—adenocarcinoma	AE1/AE3 (mucin histochemical stain)
Neuroendocrine Neoplasms	AE1/AE3, neuroendocrine markers (chromogranin, synaptophysin and CD56)
Carcinoma—squamous cell (poorly differentiated "basaloid" pattern)	AE1/AE3, P63, p40, high molecular weight CK
Mastocytosis	CD117, CD25
Sarcoma—Ewing's/PNET	CD99
Metastasis	Variable pattern

Table 1.4 Pink cells

Diagnosis	Preliminary immunohistochemical profile
GIST	CD117, DOG1
Histiocytic tumours	CD68
Glomus tumour	SMA
Granular cell tumour	S-100, SOX10
Langerhans cell histiocytosis	S-100, CD1a
Epithelioid smooth muscle tumour	SMA, desmin, h-caldesmon
Carcinoma—squamous cell	P63, high molecular weight CK
Metastasis	Variable pattern

GIST = gastrointestinal stromal tumour; SMA

Architectural Patterns

Characteristic architectural patterns have been classified into four types by Soga and Tazawa [1].

Type A: the *insular solid* pattern composed of small- to medium-sized tumour nests. Seemingly solid patterns may result from close packing of trabeculae and ribbons; Type B, the *trabecular* pattern typified by cell ribbons in single or, occasionally, double or multiple layers; Type C, the *glandular* pattern, comprising glandular patterns with either true glandular lumen or pseudoglands showing a cellular rim surrounding a central vessel; and Type D, the *mixed* pattern. Tumours with complex architecture resulting from combinations of two or more of the patterns are also described.

Table 1.5 Clear cells

Diagnosis	Preliminary immunohistochemical profile
GIST	CD117, DOG1
Carcinoma—any	AE1/AE3
Histiocytic lesions (xanthoma)	CD68
Lymphoma	LCA
Mastocytosis	CD117, CD25
Langerhans cell histiocytosis	S-100, CD1a
Clear cell sarcoma	S-100, HMB45
PEComa	HMB45
Epithelioid smooth muscle tumour	SMA, desmin, h-caldesmon
Metastasis—clear cell renal cell carcinoma	CD10

GIST = gastrointestinal stromal tumour

Cellular Morphology

Neuroendocrine neoplasms (NENs) are divided into neuroendocrine tumours (NETs) and neuroendocrine carcinomas (NECs) based on well differentiated morphology of NETs compared to poorly differentiated morphology of NECs. Well-differentiated tumours (NETs) are characteristically composed of relatively uniform round cells with variable amounts of eosinophilic cytoplasm and central nuclei with granular ("salt and pepper") chromatin pattern. Poorly differentiated tumours (NECs) show more cytological variability and nuclear hyperchromasia and may be of small cell or large cell type.

Stroma

Typically there is a richly vascular fibrous stroma. Stromal elastosis may accompany ileal neuroendocrine tumours but is generally not evident in endoscopic biopsies. Psammomatous-type dystrophic calcification may occur with somatostatinoma, and amyloid deposition may be encountered in any functional tumour.

Well-differentiated lesions have a low mitotic activity, while poorly differentiated tumours have high mitotic rate, frequent apoptosis and foci of tumour necrosis.

Table 1.6 WHO (World Health Organisation) classification of small intestinal neuroendocrine neoplasms

	Well-differentiated endocrine tumour (benign behaviour)	Well-differentiated endocrine tumour (uncertain behaviour)	Well-differentiated endocrine carcinoma (low-grade malignant)	Poorly differentiated endocrine carcinoma (high-grade malignant)
Duodenum Jejunum Ileum	Mucosa Submucosa ≤10 mm No vascular invasion	Mucosa Submucosa >10 mm or vascular invasion	Well- to moderately differentiated Invasion to/ beyond muscularis propria or metastases	Small cell carcinoma

The WHO classification of neuroendocrine neoplasm is based on tumour site, tumour size, mitotic rate and proliferation index and the presence of angiolymphatic invasion (see Table 1.6) [2–4].

Neuroendocrine neoplasm will express cytokeratin and are reactive for at least two neuroendocrine markers. These include stains expressed in the following fashion:

1. Cytoplasm or cell membrane (neurone-specific enolase, NSE, PGP9.5 and neural cell adhesion molecule—NCAM, CD56)
2. Synapse-like microvesicle reaction—synaptophysin
3. Large dense-core vesicle reaction—chromogranin A, CD57

Specific hormone production in tumour cells (which does not necessarily correlate with release into the blood or with the production of a specific clinical syndrome) can also be detected by immunohistochemistry, e.g. insulin, gastrin, glucagon and somatostatin. However, this is not necessary for histological classification.

The pathology report for biopsy and endomucosal resection specimens of neuroendocrine neoplasm should include the following:

1. Tumour site (and clinical setting)
2. Diagnosis:
   (a) WHO 2017 classification (based on tumour grade—record mitotic count and Ki67 index) (see Table 1.6)
   (b) Common name—if clinical setting is known, e.g. “carcinoid”, gastrinoma
3. Tumour size (and depth/extent of invasion)
4. Angioinvasion (and perineural invasion)
5. Immunohistochemical results—neuroendocrine stains, Ki67 and specific hormone stains
6. Resection margin status (if endomucosal resection)

Lymphoma

Up to 25% of all extranodal lymphomas occurred in the gastrointestinal tract. B cell non-Hodgkin lymphoma is most common followed by T cell non-Hodgkin lymphoma with Hodgkin lymphoma being very rare. More than half of all gastrointestinal tract lymphomas arise in the stomach, approximately one quarter occur in the small intestine and 10% occur in the large intestine. However lymphomas account for only approximately 1% of malignancies in the large intestine, whereas they account for 1/3–1/2 of malignancies in the small intestine.

A predisposing or precipitating factor may be responsible for lymphoma development. Examples include *Helicobacter pylori* infection and gastric MALT lymphoma, coeliac disease and intestinal T cell lymphoma and immunosuppression and EBV-associated lymphoproliferative disorders.

It is important to recognise that most forms of lymphoma can occur in any site in the gastrointestinal tract; however in many circumstances, a particular tumour is more likely to be found at a particular site. Hence throughout this textbook, the form of lymphoma will be discussed in most detail at the site of which it most commonly occurs.

The morphological approach to lymphoma uses a combination of (1) tumour cell size (small or large), (2) growth pattern (follicular or diffuse) and (3) pattern of infiltration of the epithelium (e.g. lymphoepithelial lesions, intraepithelial invasion). The background clinical setting is also important (e.g. coeliac disease, *Helicobacter pylori* infection, HIV infection). Immunohistochemical stains are required to establish the tumour lineage (B cell, T cell or Hodgkin lymphoma) and to ultimately establish the lymphoma subtype. B cell lymphomas show expression of CD20 and/or CD79a. T cell lymphomas show expression of CD3, CD5 and CD43. Molecular investigation may also be helpful to either establish the diagnosis (flow cytometry of fresh tissue, T cell receptor gene rearrangement studies on paraffin-embedded material) or to provide a specific diagnosis (translocation FISH, e.g. cyclin D1).

An initial approach to a probable lymphoma, suggested by combination of morphology and/or positive staining for LCA, is to assess reaction for CD3 and CD20. Depending on the lineage, further stains can be performed as per the following tables.

Suggested B cell lymphoma panel: CD5, CD10, CD20 and BCL2 (optional depending on potential subtype) CD21 for follicular dendritic cells, CD79a, PAX5, CD23, cyclin D1, MUM-1, MYC and BCL6 (Table 1.7)

Suggested T cell/NK cell panel: CD3, CD5, CD4, CD8, CD56, CD103 and cytotoxic cell markers (TIA, granzyme, perforin—at least one) (Table 1.8) [5, 6]

Table 1.7 B cell lymphoma and plasma cell neoplasms: immunohistochemical and molecular features

	CD5	CD10	CD20	Others	BCL2	BCL6	Translocation
Follicular lymphoma	–	+	+	PAX5	+	+	IGH-BCL2 t(14;18)(q34q21)
MALT	–	–	+	CD43–/+			MALT 1 t(11;18) (q21;q21) in1/3
Immunoproliferative small intestinal disease (IPSID)	–	–	+	CD138 in plasmacytic cells; α-heavy chain; IgA+			
Mantle cell	+	–	+	Cyclin D1, IgD+, PAX5+, SOX11	+	–	CCND1-IGH t(11;14)(q13;q32)
B-CLL/small lymphocytic leukaemia	+	–	+	CD23+, CD43+	+	–	
Burkitt lymphoma	–	+	+	Ki-67 near 100%, EBV+	–	+	MYC t(8;14) (q24;q32)
Diffuse large B cell lymphoma	–	±	+	PAX5+, Ki67 <90%	±	±	MYC/BCL2/ BCL6±
Post-transplant lymphoproliferative disorder	–	+	+	EBV+, CD30, CD15± (in Reed-Sternberg-like cells)	+		
Lymphoplasmacytic lymphoma	–	±	+		+	–	CXCR4 (WHIM) somatic mutations
Extramedullary plasmacytoma	–	–	–	CD79a±, CD138+,	–	–	
Plasmablastic lymphoma	–	–	–	CD79a±, CD138+, MUM1+, EBV+	±	–	MYC±

Table 1.8 T cell lymphoma: immunohistochemical and molecular features

T cell lymphoma	Immunophenotype	T cell receptor
Enteropathy-associated T cell lymphoma	CD3+, CD5–, CD7+, CD4–, CD8– (occasional +), CD103+, cytotoxic T cell marker (TIA, granzyme, perforin) + and CD56– (rare +)	TCR αβ+
Monomorphic epitheliotropic T cell lymphoma	CD3+, CD5–, CD8+/–, CD56+/– and CD30– cytotoxic T cell markers (TIA1+/–, granzyme B+, perforin+/–)	TCR γ/δ+
Extranodal NK/T cell lymphoma, nasal type (ENKTL)	NK cell type: CD2+, cytoplasmic CD3+, CD5–, CD4–, CD8– and CD56+, with cytotoxic markers (TIA-1, perforin and/or granzyme B) T cell type: surface CD3+, CD5+, CD4+ or CD8+ or CD4–/CD8– Both EBV+	NK type: TCRαβ– and γδ– T cell type: TCRαβ or γδ+/–
Indolent T cell lymphoproliferative disease of the gastrointestinal tract	CD3+ T cells, CD4+ (cytotoxic markers –) > CD8+ (cytotoxic markers +) ≫ CD4–/CD8–	TCR αβ+ or γδ+
Intestinal T cell lymphoma of no specific type	CD3+, CD5+, CD4+ or CD8+ or CD4–/CD8–	TCR αβ+ or γδ+

Spindle Cell Pattern

The second major group of neoplasms are of mesenchymal origin and in the main assume a spindle or oval cell morphology. The majority of these encountered in gastrointestinal tract biopsies have a bland appearance of the tumour cells and generally behave in a benign fashion. Malignant counterparts are sometimes encountered and in general show larger tumour size, cytological atypia and obvious mitotic activity. As with the epithelial neoplasms, morphological clues generally narrow the differential diagnosis; however, immunohistochemistry is commonly required to determine the cell of origin. Among the mesenchymal tumours, adipose cell tumours and vascular lesions are generally distinctive enough to be separated on purely morphological grounds. While not necessary in every case, a suggested general immunohistochemical panel is SMA, desmin, S-100, EMA, CD117, CD31 and AE1/AE3. Additional stains can be added as required (Table 1.9).

Vascular Lesions

Vascular lesions may represent either true neoplasms, reactive proliferations or a prominent dilatation of a single or small group of vessels. Involved vessels may be lymphatic or blood bearing. The latter may involve arteries, arterioles, capillaries or veins. In general, lymphatic tumours are characterised by light eosinophilic staining proteinaceous material within the lumen. This may be accompanied by foamy histiocytes. Arteries and veins usually have red cells in the lumen and a smooth muscle layer in their walls. We have found it useful to classify vascular lesions in terms of whether they represent a dilatation of a vessel or whether there is a proliferation of vessels. Immunohistochemical stains that define vessels include CD34 and CD31. A D2-40 is useful to define lymphatic vessels. HHV8 expression confirms the diagnosis of Kaposi sarcoma.

1. Vessel dilation
   (a) Lymphatic—lymphangiectasia and lymphangioma

Table 1.9 Cell or origin, tumour type and preliminary immunohistochemical profile

Cell of origin	Tumour type	Preliminary immunohistochemical profile
Smooth muscle	Leiomyoma Leiomyosarcoma	SMA, desmin, h-caldesmon
Neural	Schwannoma, neurofibroma Granular cell tumour MPNST	S-100, SOX10, NFP
Perineural	Perineurioma "fibroblastic polyp"	EMA, claudin 1
Fibroblastic/ myofibroblastic	Inflammatory fibroid polyp Inflammatory myofibroblastic tumour, fibromatosis Solitary fibrous tumour	CD34, ALK-1, STAT-6, B-catenin
Vascular	Glomus tumour, angiosarcoma Kaposi sarcoma Haemangioma—capillary, juvenile, anastomosing	SMA CD31 HHV8
Adipose	Dedifferentiated liposarcoma	CD34, MDM2
Epithelial	Sarcomatoid carcinoma	AE1/AE3
Unknown	Synovial sarcoma, clear cell sarcoma, PEComa	EMA, AE1/AE3 HMB-45
Metastasis	Melanoma, sarcomatoid carcinoma, stromal tumour of the ovary/testis origin	AE1/AE3, S-100, other depending on morphology or clinical history
Other	Endometriosis Elastofibroma	Oestrogen Receptor, CD10

   (b) Venous—venous bleb
   (c) Capillary—ectasia
   (d) Calibre-persistent vessel
2. Vessel proliferation
   (a) Pyogenic granuloma
   (b) AV malformation
   (c) Portal hypertensive enteropathy (severe)
   (d) Angiodysplasia
   (e) Haemangioma
   (f) Kaposi sarcoma
   (g) Angiosarcoma

Adipose Tissue (Like)

Adipose tissue tumours (lipomas) are usually easily diagnosed by the presence of regularly sized cells that have clear cytoplasm, a small eccentric nucleus and a thin cell membrane. Lipomas are overwhelmingly benign when encountered in the intestine. Air insufflation may on occasion lead to multiple clear vacuolated spaces in the mucosa that can mimic lipoma. This process is known as pseudolipomatosis. The main clue is the variable size and small size of the clear spaces. A biopsy from an everted diverticulum (colon mainly) will also lead to adipose tissue in a mucosal biopsy.

Biphasic Pattern: Glandular and Stromal Proliferation

Occasionally, tumours are encountered that are composed of both epithelial and stromal mesenchymal elements. These may represent true neoplasms as listed below. One important exception is endometriosis which should always be considered in a female of reproductive age:

1. Synovial sarcoma
2. Gangliocytic paraganglioma
3. Endometriosis
4. Metastases:
   (a) Carcinosarcoma
   (b) Mesothelioma
   (c) Teratoma

Stromal Expansion with Stromal Inflammation

Some tumours show an apparent proliferation of stromal elements but also contain a prominent inflammatory process. Secondary inflammation occurring in or involving a mesenchymal tumour should be considered; however, in most cases, it is clear that no such neoplasm exists. Often the epithelial elements of the lesion are architecturally disturbed, with epithelial proliferation or gland dilatation. Potential causes for this pattern include:

- Mucosal prolapse
- Hamartomas:
  - Juvenile polyp
  - Cronkhite-Canada polyp
- Inflammatory pseudopolyp
- Inflammatory fibroid polyp
- Ulcer base/granulation tissue

Cystic Lesions

Many processes can present as a predominantly cystic lesion of the gastrointestinal tract. Despite this, cysts are uncommonly identified in mucosal biopsies because they typically develop deeper in the intestinal wall. Causes of cystic lesions encountered in mucosal biopsies are listed below:

- Unique to site, e.g. Brunner gland cyst
- Pneumatosis
- Cystic vascular lesions—lymphangiectasia and venous bleb
- Cystic change in a neoplasm
- Inflammatory/postinflammatory cystic epithelial proliferation (gastritis or colitis cystica profunda)
- Endometriosis

Tumour-Like Inflammatory Lesions

There exist a range of non-neoplastic primarily inflammatory disorders of the gastrointestinal tract that present as a mass lesion with the endoscopic appearance suggestive of a neoplastic process. Furthermore, reactive epithelial atypia or atypia in component stromal cells may add to the mimicry of a neoplasm. Pathologists need to be aware of this process in order to avoid over diagnosis of a neoplasm.

General examples:

- Mass-forming ischaemia
- Inflammatory polyp
- Exuberant granulation tissue in an ulcer base
- Endoscopic biopsies of tumours after neoadjuvant chemotherapy

Immunohistochemical and Molecular Biomarkers

Increasingly pathologists are required to apply specialised immunohistochemical stains or to undertake molecular analysis of tumour tissue. Broadly the reasons for this are (1) to establish the diagnosis and aid with subtyping of the tumour (e.g. EBV in situ hybridisation in gastric carcinoma), (2) to help define the tumour prognosis (e.g. mismatch repair studies in a colorectal mucinous tumour), (3) to identify an underlying genetic predisposition (e.g. mismatch repair studies in a colorectal carcinoma to identify potential Lynch syndrome) and (4) to determine the likely efficacy of targeted therapy (e.g. Her2 expression in gastric carcinoma and KRAS mutation status in colorectal carcinoma).

The immunohistochemical and molecular biomarkers will be discussed in more detail in the relevant chapters.

References

1. Soga J, Tazawa K. Pathologic analysis of carcinoids; histologic re-evaluation of 62 cases. Cancer. 1971;28:990–8.
2. Rindi G, Kloppel G, Alhman H, et al. TNM staging of foregut (neuro)endocrine tumours: a consensus proposal including a grading system. Virchows Arch. 2006;449:395–401.
3. Klöppel G, Couvelard A, Perren A, et al. ENETS consensus guidelines for the standards of care in neuroendocrine tumours: towards a standardized approach to the diagnosis of gastroenteropancreatic neuroendocrine tumours and their prognostic stratification. Neuroendocrinology. 2009;90:162–6.
4. Bosman FT, World Health Organization; International Agency for Research on Cancer. WHO classification of tumours of the digestive system. 4th ed. IARC Press: Lyon; 2010.
5. O'Malley DP, Goldstein NS, Banks PM. The recognition and classification of lymphoproliferative disorders of the gut. Hum Pathol. 2014;45(5):899–916.
6. Foukas PG, de Leval L. Recent advances in intestinal lymphoma. Histopathology. 2015;66:112–36.

Part II

Oesophagus

Oesophagus: Inflammatory Patterns

2

Mahsa S. Ahadi, Anthony J. Gill, John R. Turchini, Spiro C. Raftopoulos, and M. Priyanthi Kumarasinghe

Contents

M. S. Ahadi (✉)
Department of Anatomical Pathology, Royal North Shore Hospital, University of Sydney, St. Leonards, NSW, Australia

A. J. Gill
Cancer Diagnosis and Pathology Group, Kolling Institute of Medical Research, Royal North Shore Hospital, University of Sydney, St. Leonards, NSW, Australia

J. R. Turchini
Department of Anatomical Pathology, Royal North Shore Hospital, The University of Sydney, St Leonards, NSW, Australia

S. C. Raftopoulos
Interventional Endoscopist and Gastroenterologist, Department of Gastroenterology, Sir Charles Gairdner Hospital, Nedlands, WA, Australia

University of Western Australia, Perth, WA, Australia

M. P. Kumarasinghe
Department of Anatomical Pathology, PathWest Laboratory Medicine, QEII Medical Centre and University of Western Australia, Perth, WA, Australia
e-mail: priyanthi.kumarasinghe@health.wa.gov.au

Introduction to Upper GI Endoscopy

Upper gastrointestinal endoscopy (oesophagogastroduodenoscopy, OGD) is an endoscopic procedure that enables visualisation of the upper gastrointestinal tract from the oropharynx to the proximal 10–20 cm of the jejunum. There have been great advances in technology over the past decade with modern endoscopes now capable of high-resolution imaging coupled with the ability to interrogate identified abnormalities using a number of push-button technologies such as electronic chromoendoscopy (narrowband imaging, flexible spectral imaging, colour enhancement and i-scan) and digital and optical zoom magnification.

M. P. Kumarasinghe, I. Brown (eds.), *Endoscopic Biopsy Interpretation*,
https://doi.org/10.1007/978-3-319-79117-3_2

With the advent of such technologies, the endoscopist is now able to clearly target abnormal areas of concern for histologic diagnosis and further contribute to patient care by histologic staging and endoscopic treatment.

Histological findings subsequent to endoscopic procedures may have a significant impact on patient care with the endoscopist and pathologist playing an integral role in determining management options. This may include long-term surveillance or invasive surgical procedures.

There are many indications that may warrant upper gastrointestinal endoscopy. These can be divided into three broad groups: diagnosis, treatment and surveillance.

Persistent symptoms commonly result in referral for diagnostic endoscopy. Many symptoms can be non-specific; however, clear indications for upper gastrointestinal endoscopy include persistence of upper GI symptoms such as pain and nausea not responding to medical therapy or presence of alarm symptoms such as dysphagia, odynophagia, persistent vomiting and refractory reflux. In some cases, suspected diagnoses require histological confirmation such as the need for histological diagnosis of coeliac disease in a patient with positive coeliac serology.

Endoscopy is also widely used in management, and this is particularly true for patients presenting with known oesophageal, gastric or duodenal premalignant or early malignant lesions. This includes but is not limited to those patients with Barrett's oesophagus and dysplasia, early squamous cell dysplasia and gastric or duodenal adenomas. Many of these lesions are now amenable to resection using advanced endoscopic techniques such as endoscopic resection (ER) and endoscopic submucosal dissection (ESD). The pathologist plays an especially important role in this context with clear guidelines being published in respect to risk of lymph node involvement and need for further surgical management based on the histological assessment/staging of these specimens.

Lastly, there are a number of disorders where surveillance is required for detection of early neoplasia that would institute a change in management. One such example is Barrett's oesophagus where surveillance intervals and need for therapeutic interventions (ER, ESD, radio-frequency ablation) are strongly linked to the established histopathologic diagnosis and grade of dysplasia. Other similar conditions include duodenal polyposis in the context of familial adenomatous polyposis (FAP) where Spigelman stage (histologic and endoscopic scoring system) can mandate major surgery, as well as surveillance in known cases of squamous cell dysplasia and gastric intestinal metaplasia in select high-risk groups.

Ultimately, endoscopic evaluation of upper GI disorders has evolved into a complex and intertwined diagnostic and therapeutic intervention that in many instances relies heavily on accurate and appropriately reported histology which in many cases can have direct and significant impact on patient management and long-term outcome.

The most common non-neoplastic process of the oesophagus encountered in clinical practice is "oesophagitis". A common biopsy sample received in routine practice is one from the gastro-oesophageal junction (GOJ), gastro-oesophageal reflux disease (GORD) being the most common inflammatory disorder affecting the oesophagus in up to about 40% of the Western population. GORD develops when gastric contents, including gastric acid, pepsin and bile, reflux into the oesophagus and result in troublesome symptoms and/or complications. The injury leads to a diverse group of inflammatory responses which depends on the severity of reflux and host response. GOJ biopsies usually show squamous and columnar mucosa. Latter may represent gastric "cardia" or metaplastic columnar epithelium. Division of squamous and columnar mucosal changes in the GOJ is arbitrary. GOJ biopsies often show inflammation and reactive changes in both squamous and columnar mucosa (squamocolumnar injury pattern). Squamous mucosa, may show reflux-related changes (reflux pattern). Columnar mucosa in GOJ biopsies may be metaplastic oesophageal mucosa (metaplastic pattern).

Reflux-induced changes and the development of Barrett's oesophagus were recognised in the 1970s, after endoscopic biopsies became more widespread. Since then, a spectrum of inflammatory diseases of the oesophagus, well beyond pure reflux disease, have been described. A diverse group of aetiologies involve the native squamous mucosa, resulting in a spectrum of inflammatory patterns. The microscopic patterns are often nonspecific. Clinical and endoscopic information are often required to distinguish various aetiologies. As discussed in the previous chapter, a great deal of attention should be paid to clinical information to arrive at an aetiological diagnosis.

Oesophageal squamous mucosa shows some unique inflammatory patterns with similarities to inflammatory dermatoses. The common inflammatory patterns with both histological and clinical aetiological clues, diverse patterns that could be seen in association with some aetiologies such as reflux as well as unique patterns such as sloughing oesophagitis and skin disorders involving the oesophageal squamous mucosa, are discussed in this Chapter.

Inflammatory Patterns

Acute Oesophagitis Pattern (With/Without Erosion and Ulceration)

Acute oesophagitis pattern is characterised by intraepithelial neutrophils and oedema with or without erosion and/or ulceration.

Normally, the squamous mucosa of the oesophagus contains few or no inflammatory cells.

This pattern of injury, although non-specific, is most commonly caused by GORD, infections and medications. Malignancy, amyloidosis, radiation injury and vasculitis are also potential causes of acute oesophagitis, particularly if erosions and ulcerations are present. Corrosive substance ingestion causes coagulative necrosis and inflammatory patterns, which depend on the time of biopsies and the type of corrosives ingested. Active lesions are rarely biopsied [1–3].

Acute Oesophagitis Pattern: GORD

By far, the most common cause of acute ulcerative or erosive oesophagitis pattern is GORD (Fig. 2.1a, b). However, all cases of GORD do not necessarily show ulceration or erosion but usually show the "reflux pattern" of injury (see below). Clinical and endoscopic features should be considered before an acute oesophagitis pattern is determined to be related to GORD. Other curable aetiologies such as infections and medication-induced changes should be excluded even if there is clinical evidence of GORD. Double pathology is not uncommon in patients with GORD! Presence of "mixed pattern of injury" should alert the pathologists to the possibility of medication-related injury. In particular, if the clinical history indicates satisfactory reflux control, an alternative aetiology for ulceration should be considered [1–3].

Acute Oesophagitis Pattern: Infections

General features of acute inflammation pattern commonly associated with erosion and/or ulceration are noted in infections, similar to GORD.

An important point to be aware of is that although infections are usually associated with severe inflammation, severely immunocompromised individuals may not exhibit a robust inflammatory response. A compromised immune system is the most important risk factor for the development of infectious oesophagitis. HIV or AIDS patients and solid organ transplant patients are particularly at risk. Recent antibiotic use, corticosteroids, chemotherapy, radiation therapy, malignancies and in particular haematologic malignancies are additional risk factors that should be sought in the clinical history, if not already provided.

Fungal, viral and bacterial organisms may cause infective oesophagitis. The most common cause of infective oesophagitis is *Candida albicans*. *Candida glabrata* is also a consideration, particularly in hospitalised diabetic patients. Other fungal infections are rare but include *Histoplasma*, *Aspergillus*, *Blastomyces* and *Cryptococcus* [1–6].

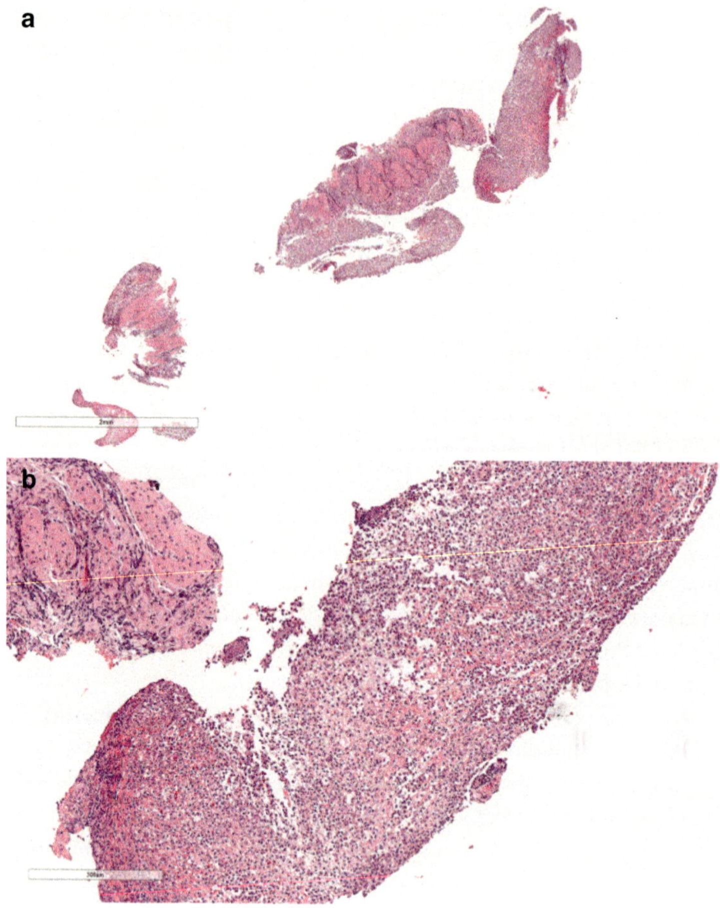

Fig. 2.1 Acute ulcerative oesophagitis pattern of GORD (**a**, **b**)

Candida Oesophagitis

A mixed inflammatory infiltrate of neutrophils, lymphocytes and eosinophils is noted, with and without erosion and ulceration and *Candida* organisms (Figs. 2.2a–d and 2.3a, b). Intraepithelial lymphocytes are evenly distributed in the epithelium with neutrophils often present in small, superficially located clusters ("a diagnostic clue") (Fig. 2.2c) and accompanied by parakeratosis (Fig. 2.2d). A prominent neutrophilic infiltrate, abscess formation, erosion/ulceration and necrosis can be seen in some immunosuppressed patients and fungi may invade to deeper levels of the oesophageal wall. Invasion of mucosal and submucosal blood vessels can be seen. Granulomas are occasionally present. However, as noted above, in immunocompromised patients, the associated inflammatory response may be minimal.

Patients typically present with dysphagia and odynophagia and may have concurrent oral thrush. At gastroscopy, characteristic multiple small white or yellow mucosal plaques can be visualised. If scraped away, an ulcerated mucosa may be revealed underneath. The plaques can become confluent in severe infections. In long-term and/or significant infections, granulation tissue and mucosal sloughing may also be seen.

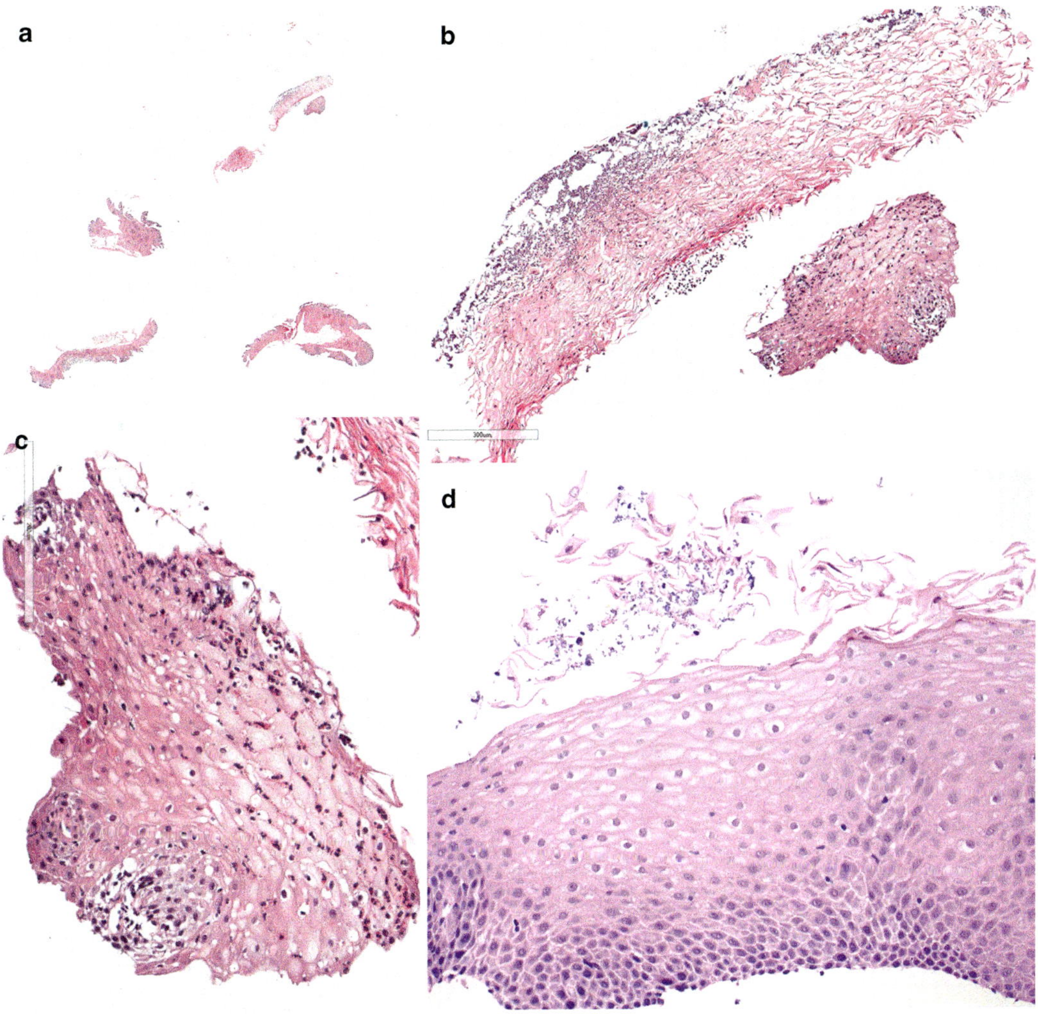

Fig. 2.2 Acute ulcerative or erosive oesophagitis pattern of *Candida*. (**a**) Oesophageal squamous mucosa. (**b**) *Candida* organisms within squamous debris. (**c**) Neutrophil clusters on the surface. (**d**) Parakeratosis

Since *Candida* species colonise the oesophagus in about one-fifth of healthy adults, histological confirmation of fungal invasion into tissue or ulcer slough is important. *Candida* can colonise preexisting ulcers or damaged mucosa of any aetiology, and the pathologist should consider the possibility of dual pathology. In addition, as several *Candida* species are commensal in the GI tract and oropharynx, yeast forms from the oropharynx can contaminate oesophageal specimens. The presence of a few yeast forms in the absence of an inflammatory infiltrate can be considered a contamination. In some patients, the *Candida* infection may be opportunistic, infecting areas of inflammation and ulceration resulting from other causes

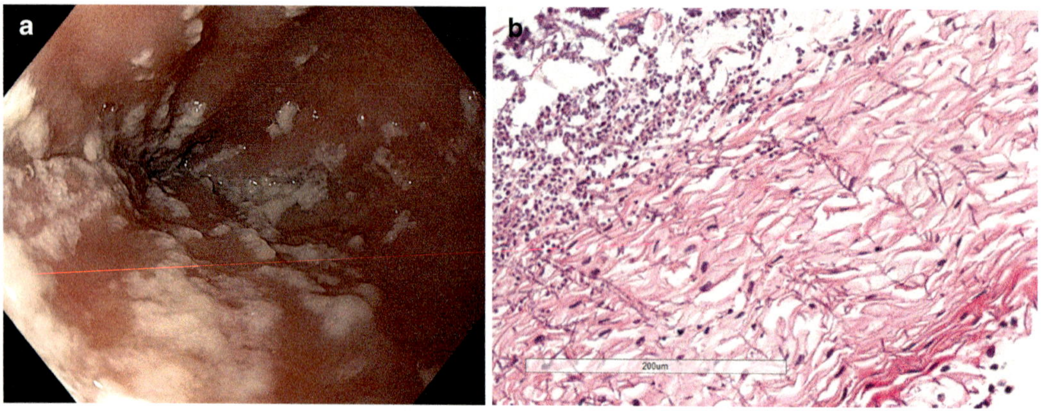

Fig. 2.3 Case 1—Oesophageal candidiasis. (**a**) A 72-year-old lady with past history of type 2 diabetes mellitus. Referred by general practitioner for evaluation of a 2-week history of odynophagia not responding to proton pump inhibitor therapy. Gastroscopy was performed revealing multiple white plaque-like lesions, along the length of the oesophagus consistent with oesophageal candidiasis, confirmed by biopsies (**b**)

(Boxes 2.1 and 2.2). Fungi exposed to antifungal therapy or ambient air may produce bizarre and unusual forms [2–6].

Box 2.1 *Candida* Oesophagitis

- Most common cause of infective oesophagitis
- Diagnostic clue: a mixed inflammatory infiltrate with evenly distributed intraepithelial lymphocytes and small, superficially-located neutrophil clusters accompanied by parakeratosis
- Commonly colonise the oesophagus in 1/5 of healthy people
- Dual pathology: Colonise pre-existing ulcers or damaged mucosa of any aetiology
- A few yeast forms: likely contaminants
- True *Candida* oesophagitis:
  - Pseudohyphae are present in contrast to yeast forms.
  - Invasion into tissue or ulcer slough.

Box 2.2 *Candida* Organisms

- A mixture of budding yeast forms, hyphae and pseudohyphae. *C. glabrata* only features tiny budding yeast forms similar to *Histoplasma*.
- Yeasts: have a diameter of 3–5 μm with refractile cell walls.
- Pseudohyphae: non-septate, sausage-like, arranged perpendicular to the long axes of keratinocytes in the superficial epithelium.
- Yeast forms: oval and more basophilic.
- Budding spores and pseudohyphae: look in squamous debris, ulcer slough and fibrinopurulent exudate.
- Periodic acid-Schiff or Grocott's methenamine silver stain highlights the fungi.

Acute Viral Oesophagitis

Viral oesophagitis, the second most common cause of infectious oesophagitis, mostly results in ulceration of the oesophagus. Herpes simplex virus (types 1 and 2) and cytomegalovirus are common causative agents in viral oesophagitis. Occasionally, human papillomavirus, varicella zoster virus and Epstein-Barr virus can be associated with oesophagitis [6, 8, 21].

Herpes simplex virus (HSV) Oesophagitis

Typically, with ulceration (Fig. 2.4a), the infected squamous cells of intact or denuded epithelium are degenerated and acantholytic and show hard,

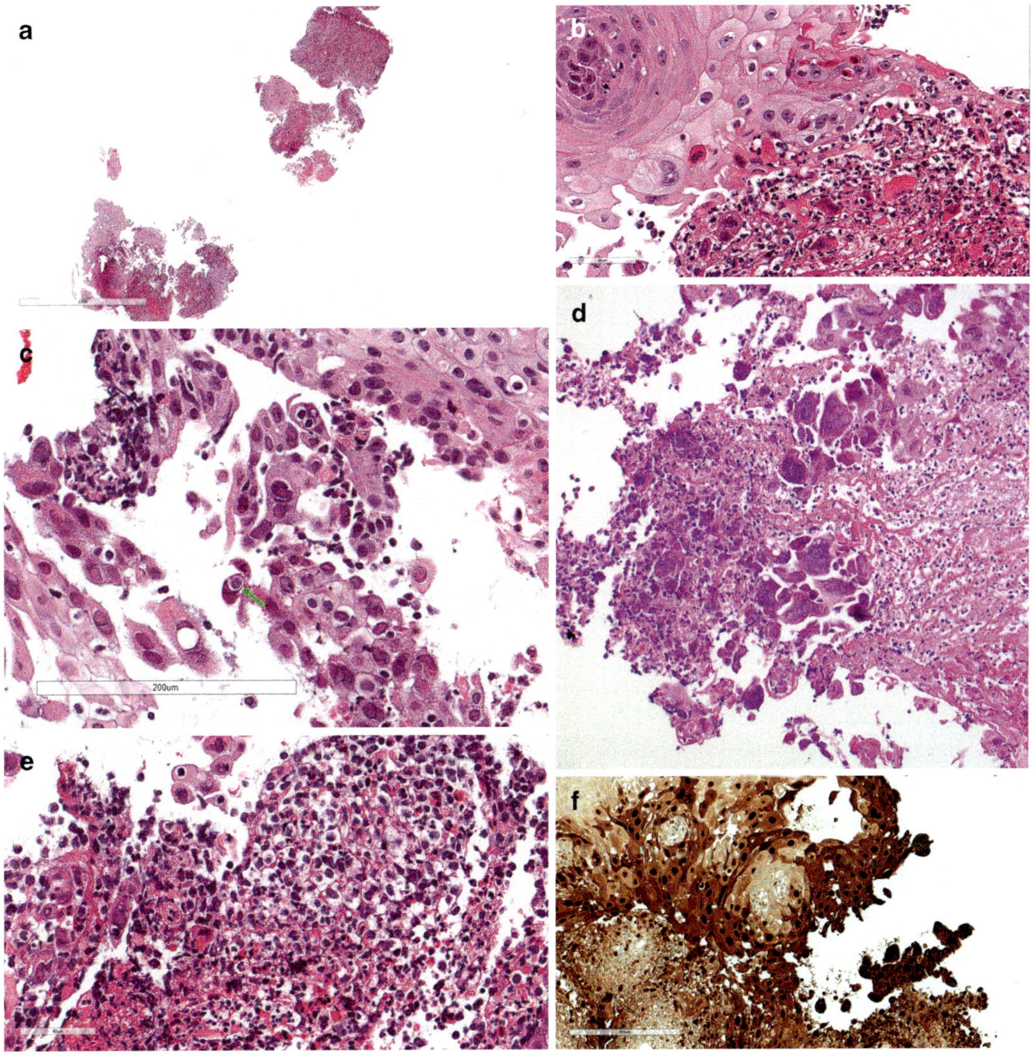

Fig. 2.4 Acute ulcerative or erosive oesophagitis pattern of HSV. (**a**) Marked ulceration with adjacent infected squamous mucosa. (**b**) Degenerated and infected squamous cells with hard, brightly eosinophilic cytoplasm. (**c**) Cowdry type A inclusions (arrow) and many Cowdry type B inclusions. (**d**) Multinucleate cells with dark smudgy nuclear inclusions. (**e**) Macrophage-rich infiltrate—a clue. (**f**) HSV IHC

brightly eosinophilic cytoplasm (Fig. 2.4b). Viral cytopathic effects are noted including multinucleation, moulding and typical intranuclear inclusions. These inclusions have a blue-grey colour and vary from those with a clear halo between them and the thickened nuclear membrane (Cowdry type A) (Fig. 2.4c) or homogenous and powdery inclusions that completely fill the nucleus (Cowdry type B) (Fig. 2.4c, d). The nuclear membranes of infected cells are often prominent and irregular. Multinucleate cells with dark smudgy nuclear inclusions are also present (Fig. 2.4d). These diagnostic inclusions are usually located at the edge of a vesicle or ulcer. If edge of the lesion is not sampled, the diagnosis may be missed.

Infection is associated with a mixed inflammatory infiltrate of intraepithelial neutrophils, eosinophils and lymphocytes, as well as a dense macrophage-rich infiltrate that can be a helpful diagnostic clue (Fig. 2.4e). These macrophages tend to form aggregates in endoscopic biopsy specimen, possibly due to the force of biopsy forceps. In some cases, these aggregates may get so large that the pathologist may worry about the possibility of a large cell lymphoma.

The infected squamous cells can be found closely adjacent to these macrophage aggregates, often with a small zone of intervening neutrophils.

Similar but smaller aggregates have been noted in the biopsies from cytomegalovirus oesophagitis, but not in *Candida* or GORD. Therefore, presence of these macrophages in a biopsy that does not contain diagnostic viral inclusions warrants additional studies (either deeper levels, immunohistochemistry (Fig. 2.4f), molecular testing if appropriate or repeat biopsy for viral studies). Concomitant infection by another microorganism such as *Candida*, cytomegalovirus or bacteria may occur, particularly in immunocompromised patients.

Patients with herpetic oesophagitis present with dysphagia and odynophagia. Chest pain, fever and bleeding may occur, and many have disseminated infection at the time of diagnosis which may be life-threatening, particularly in elderly and immunocompromised patients. In immunocompetent patients, herpetic infection is often self-limited. Unlike in *Candida*, where oral disease is present in the majority of patients, coexisting herpes labialis and oropharyngeal ulcers are only seen in about one-fourth of patients. Herpetic lesions predominantly occur in the middle to lower oesophagus, where they appear as multiple vesicles or punched-out ulcers with discrete edges (typically <2 cm). However, many patients have a non-specific erosive oesophagitis (Box 2.3) [3, 5–14].

Box 2.3 HSV Oesophagitis

Look at the edge of the ulcer for:

- Degenerate and acantholytic squamous cells with hard, brightly eosinophilic cytoplasm
- Viral cytopathic effects: multinucleation, moulding and typical intranuclear inclusions
- Mixed inflammatory infiltrate of intraepithelial neutrophils, eosinophils and lymphocytes
- Macrophage aggregates

Cytomegalovirus (CMV) oesophagitis

Inflammatory response can vary from minimal to deep ulceration with prominent granulation tissue and necrosis. The diagnostic features are seen in ulcer base tissue (in contrast to changes of squamous mucosa in HSV oesophagitis) as the squamous epithelium is rarely infected by CMV (Fig. 2.5). The characteristic viral inclusions are found deep within ulcer beds. Inclusions can be intranuclear or cytoplasmic, such as classic "owl eye" large intranuclear inclusions or granular, eosinophilic inclusions in the cytoplasm. Fully developed CMV intranuclear inclusions are single, large and deeply amphophilic with a pale rim of nuclear chromatin. These inclusions are seen on routine H&E preparations and found in endothelial and stromal cells and only rarely in epithelial cells.

Adjacent nuclei may be enlarged, appear smudged or have a "ground-glass" appearance but lack typical inclusions. Atypical intranuclear inclusions, described by Schwartz and Wilcox, are more subtle. These changes include the lack of halo around the inclusion, the presence of an enlarged perinuclear amphophilic zone in cells without inclusion and the presence of smudgy densely eosinophilic nuclei in smooth muscles. Atypical CMV inclusions are said to be particularly numerous in cases of AIDS.

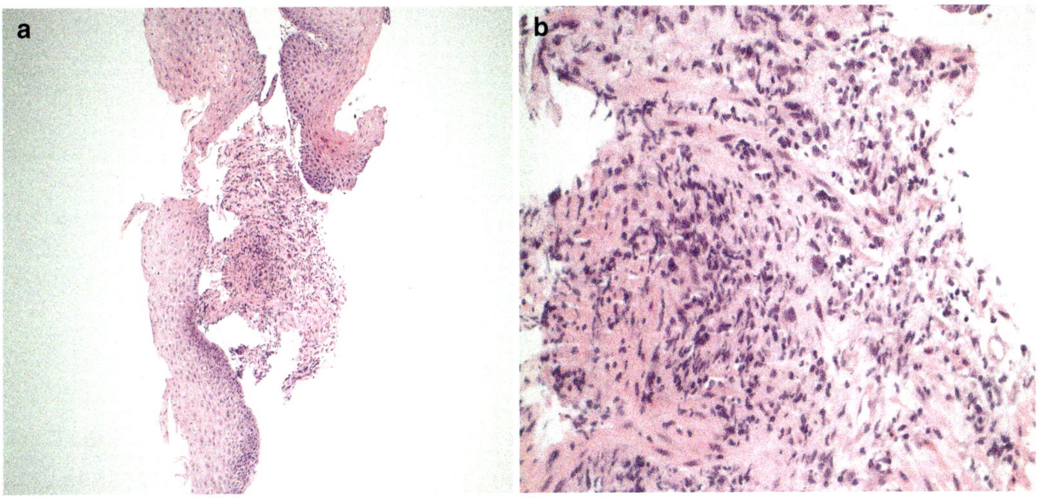

Fig. 2.5 Oesophageal squamous mucosa showing ulcer slough (**a**) and enlarged nuclei of stromal cells indicative of cytomegalovirus infection (**b**)

In cases suspicious for CMV oesophagitis, endoscopists should be educated to preferentially sample the ulcer bed.

CMV is another ubiquitous virus that similar to HSV, reactivates in the immunosuppressed patients. CMV-induced oesophagitis typically occurs in the immunosuppressed population and in particular AIDS and organ transplant patients, and in fact, CMV is the most common cause of ulcerative oesophagitis in the HIV-positive population. Rare cases of CMV oesophagitis have been reported in immunocompetent patients, especially in the elderly.

The clinical presentation of CMV oesophagitis is similar to those of HSV and *Candida*, but unlike HSV, CMV oesophagitis is typically accompanied by systemic CMV infection. Deep linear ulcers, solitary shallow ulcers, multiple ulcers, giant ulcers (>1 cm) and diffuse erosive oesophagitis have been described. Most lesions are located in the mid to distal oesophagus [3, 6, 7, 15–20].

HIV-Associated Oesophagitis

The ulcers are often located in the middle or distal oesophagus and are often deep and >1 cm in diameter. Other causes of ulceration in the immunocompromised setting should be excluded before the diagnosis of idiopathic HIV-associated oesophageal ulcer is made. A high incidence of oesophagitis and oesophageal ulcers is seen in AIDS patients. While many are due to combinations of HSV, CMV and/or candidiasis, in a proportion of these patients, giant oesophageal ulcers are present and no pathogens are identified. The HIV p24 core protein has been detected in ulcerated mucosa, suggesting that HIV is capable of producing ulcers in the absence of other pathogens, possibly via local immune dysregulation [6].

Bacterial Infections

Sheets of bacteria (best visualised on tissue Gram stain) are typically present with associated necrosis and mucosal erosion. Notably, inflammation may be scant or absent in neutropenic patients. The presence of dyskeratotic cells with many bacteria can be a tip-off that the biopsy came from the top of particularly necrotic squamous cell carcinoma. Gram-positive bacteria, including *Staphylococcus aureus*, *Staphylococcus epidermidis*, viridans streptococci and beta-haemolytic streptococci, are the most commonly implicated organisms

Clinically significant bacterial oesophagitis occurs almost exclusively in immunocompromised patients.

Secondary bacterial colonisation of areas of prior oesophageal injury is more common. Prior to the rare diagnosis of a primary bacterial oesophagitis, it is essential to confirm the presence of bacterial invasion of squamous mucosa or the deeper wall and exclude coexistent viral or fungal infection, neoplastic process or prior surgery [3, 6].

Mycobacterial Infection

Typical inflammatory pattern in Mycobacterial Infection is granulomatous. This infection is exceedingly rare in the oesophagus. Please refer to the granulomatous pattern for details.

Parasites

Parasitic infection of the oesophagus is very uncommon in developed countries but may occur in developing countries. Chagas disease is the most common parasitic infection of the oesophagus. Theoretically, parasites can cause eosinophilic oesophagitis pattern [6].

Epithelial and Stromal Atypia in Acute Ulcerative Pattern

Marked reactive changes in the epithelium as well as stroma of ulcer tissue can be alarming. Malignant lesions are often accompanied by ulceration. Clinical and endoscopic impression is invaluable to detect subtle and small areas of malignant cells. Deep levels and ancillary testing may be required (refer to the neoplastic patterns) (Box 2.4) [1].

Box 2.4 Acute Patterns with Ulceration and Erosion

- Expect variable degrees of inflammation ranging from lack of any significant inflammatory response to severe ulceration and necrosis.
- Exclude GORD (clinically), classically seen in the distal oesophagus.
- Always probe further for clinical history of medications, immunosuppressive conditions, chemotherapy, radiotherapy, recent antibiotic therapy or long-term corticosteroid use including inhaled corticosteroids.
- Look for secondary patterns and special patterns (medication, infective).
- Look for specific "diagnostic" features: organisms, viral inclusions, coloured deposits including medication-associated substances.
- Be mindful of double pathology.
- Examine deeper levels with/without ancillary tests.
- Ask for more if clinical diagnosis is crucial: preferential sampling.
- Do not miss malignancy.

Acute Oesophagitis Pattern: Medications

Medication-induced injury may also manifest as acute oesophagitis pattern with or without erosion and/or ulceration. A clue to medication-induced acute oesophagitis pattern is the presence of other patterns such as apoptotic, eosinophilic and lymphocytic patterns imparting a "mixed pattern" of injury that will be discussed later. Often evidence of toxic damage with ballooning of epithelial cells can be seen. In some cases, acute pattern is the dominant pattern with another pattern being less obvious. Morphological clues of medications such as pill fragments and crystal deposition may be visible within the tissue itself.

Medication-induced upper gastrointestinal tract injuries are probably fairly common, yet these injuries are rarely documented in pathology reports and will be discussed further as a special pattern of pill oesophagitis.

Active Chronic Oesophagitis Pattern

In biopsy samples, non-specific chronic inflammation is seen with a lymphocytic infiltrate into the lamina propria. Active chronic pattern is expanded by more descriptive patterns described in detail in this chapter with clinicopathological correlation. Typical active chronic

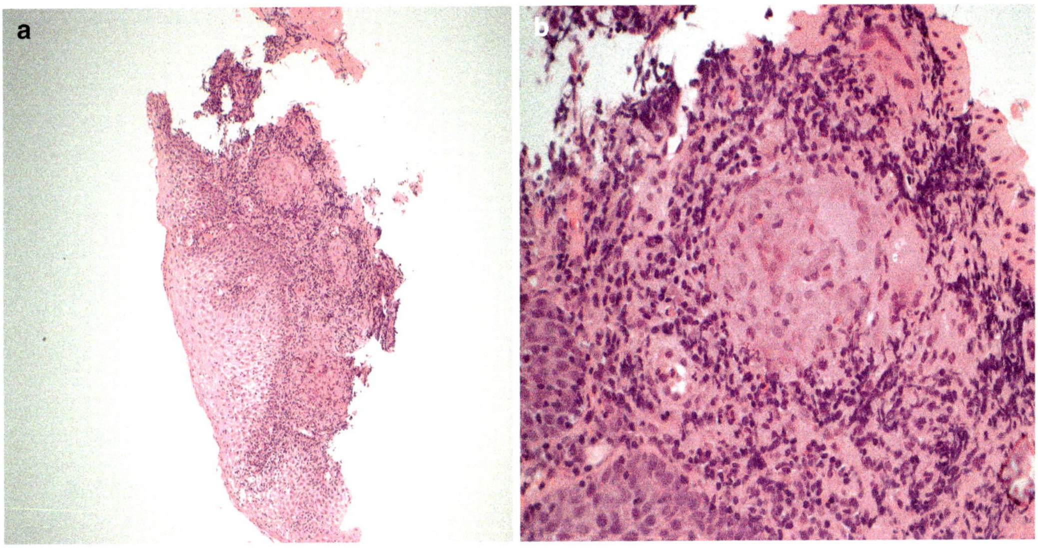

Fig. 2.6 Oesophageal squamous mucosa showing mucosa and submucosa with granuloma formation seen in Crohn's oesophagitis

inflammation pattern of the glandular mucosa in the tubular gut is not a specific pattern. Nondescript active chronic inflammation pattern outside the clinically and endoscopically defined setting of reflux, infection and medication injury, in particular in paediatric population, needs exclusion of Crohn's disease (CD).

Histologically, there are no definitive diagnostic features, and this is especially true for mucosal biopsies which do not reveal the transmural nature of the disease. Often non-specific inflammation is seen with a lymphocytic infiltrate within the lamina propria. CD is further discussed below.

Granulomatous Pattern

Chapter 1 details a general discussion on granulomatous pattern in endoscopic biopsies of the gastrointestinal tract. This pattern is relatively uncommon in the oesophagus.

Upper gastrointestinal manifestation of Crohn's disease and infections should be considered if this pattern is noted. Clinical correlation is therefore required.

Crohn's Disease

Although Crohn's disease (CD) is mainly identified in the lower gastrointestinal tract, oesophageal involvement is reported, accompanying CD in the rest of the gastrointestinal tract. Isolated oesophageal CD is extremely rare (Fig. 2.6). Oesophageal involvement is reported in 0.2–1.8% of adult CD patients and larger population of paediatric patients (as high as 42% of CD cases). The clinical presentation is non-specific and includes dysphagia, odynophagia, epigastric and chest pain and heartburn. Oesophageal CD usually occurs in the distal two-thirds of the oesophagus with aphthous ulcers and superficial erosions seen in most patients endoscopically. Cobblestoning, deep ulcerations and/or stricturing indicate more advanced disease [2, 3, 22–28].

Eosinophilic Pattern

This pattern is characterised by eosinophil-predominant intraepithelial inflammation often accompanied by basal cell hyperplasia and reactive changes (Figs. 2.7a, b and 2.8a–f).

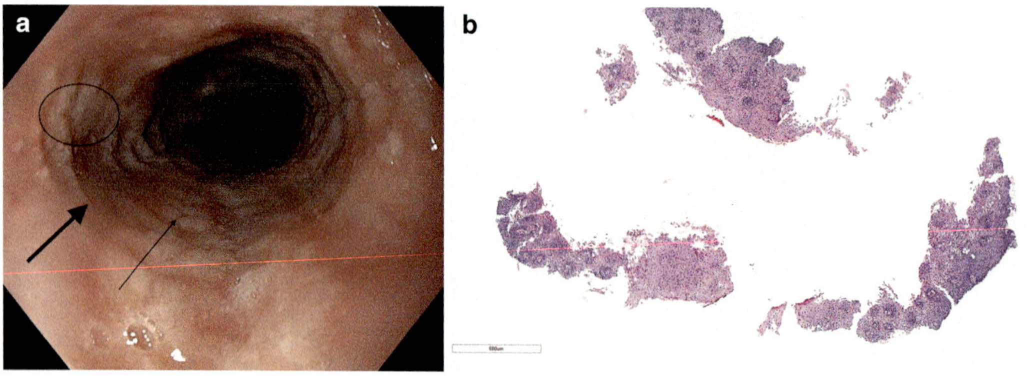

Fig. 2.7 Case 2—Eosinophilic oesophagitis. A 36-year-old man presenting with a 4-year history of dysphagia to solids and multiple episodes of food bolus obstruction relieved with self-induced vomiting. Past medical history also included asthma and a known history of allergies to shellfish. Gastroscopy revealed multiple rings (thick arrow), furrows (thin arrow) and white exudates (circle) consistent with a diagnosis of eosinophilic oesophagitis (**a**). Four biopsies were taken from the distal and mid-oesophagus for histologic confirmation (**b**)

Eosinophils often accompany many other inflammatory patterns. Eosinophilic oesophagitis (EO) pattern is reserved to describe the inflammation almost exclusively showing eosinophils. A variety of causes result in this pattern (Box 2.5).

Box 2.5 Aetiologies of Eosinophilic Pattern

- Gastro-oesophageal reflux disease
- Eosinophilic oesophagitis
- Medications
- Food allergy
- Systemic collagen vascular disorders
- Hypereosinophilic syndrome
- Infections: viral and fungal (no documented evidence of parasitic infections)
- Inflammatory bowel disease
- Neoplasia
- Post-procedure biopsies, e.g. following photodynamic therapy

Of all above, the two frequently queried diagnoses are gastro-oesophageal reflux disease and “eosinophilic oesophagitis” (EoE), also termed idiopathic eosinophilic oesophagitis. Although termed idiopathic, the classic EoE is believed to have an atopic/allergic basis. Other rarer causes are easily forgotten in the absence of clinical information.

Typically, EoE is a male predominant disorder, usually presenting in their 20s and 30s. Patients often have a long history of intermittent dysphagia to solids often associated with recurrent food bolus obstructions and retrosternal chest discomfort not responding to Proton pump inhibitor (PPI) therapy. Coexisting food allergies and other atopic diseases are common and present in up to 86% of patients.

Endoscopic appearances when present are highly specific for the diagnosis and include oesophageal rings, longitudinal furrows and white papules (representing eosinophilic crypt abscess). In up to 20% of patients, oesophageal strictures may be present and in some patients are significant enough not to permit passage of an adult gastroscope.

The diagnosis of EoE is essentially a clinicopathologic diagnosis, at the minimum requiring the triad of consistent clinical history, typical endoscopic findings and presence of >15 eosinophils/HPF (Fig. 2.8a).

Marked basal cell hyperplasia is invariably seen and is a useful clue to suspect the diagnosis at low power (Fig. 2.8b). Eosinophils in the surface layers (surface layering) (Fig. 2.8c), eosinophilic microabscesses (Fig. 2.8d) imparting a "moth-eaten" appearance (due to associated intercellular oedema and acantholysis), subepithelial sclerosis (Fig. 2.8e) and degranulation of eosinophils (Fig. 2.8f) are other important diagnostic features (Box 2.6).

Box 2.6 Classic EoE: The Triad

Clinical Setting:

- Male predominant disorder, typically presenting in 3rd and 4th decades of life.
- A long history of intermittent dysphagia to solids often associated with recurrent food bolus obstructions and retrosternal chest discomfort not responding to PPI therapy.
- Coexisting food allergies and other atopic illness are common.

Endoscopic Appearance:

- Oesophageal rings, longitudinal furrows and white papules (representing eosinophilic crypt abscess).
- Strictures may be present (20%) and in some patients is significant enough not to permit passage of an adult gastroscope.

Histologic Findings:

- Marked (>50%) basal cell hyperplasia
- A minimum of at least 15 eosinophils per HPF preferentially in proximal or mid-oesophagus; variable intensity and often patchy
- Degranulation of eosinophils (a clue but should not be counted)
- Eosinophils on the surface layers (surface layering)
- Eosinophilic microabscesses
- Subepithelial sclerosis

The disease should be isolated to the oesophagus. Earlier consensus guidelines required an 8-week trial of PPI to exclude so-called "PPI responsive EoE" as a separate entity; however, in recent years, it has been shown in adult patients achieving clinical and histological remission on PPI therapy that they are part of the same EoE continuum, rather than a separate entity based on responders and nonresponders to PPI therapy showing overlapping phenotypic, genetic and mechanistic features.

Increased eosinophils even exceeding the cut-off number (15/HPF or more) in the oesophagus are not specific to EoE. However, many cases frequently contain greater numbers of eosinophils, sometimes exceeding 250 eosinophils/HPF. Only eosinophils where the nucleus is seen should be counted avoiding inclusion of isolated granules due to degranulation (Fig. 2.8f). Collection of four or more eosinophils is regarded as an eosinophilic microabscess. They impart a "moth-eaten" appearance due to associated intercellular oedema and acantholysis.

Intraepithelial eosinophils (IEE) can be patchy. Therefore, examining multiple high-power fields (HPF) per biopsy specimen is also important. Current data supports the histologic cut-off point of 15 eos/HPF for diagnosis of eosinophilic oesophagitis. Other inflammatory cells such as lymphocytes and mast cells are often present but are not the dominant pattern. The number of mast cells can be significantly increased. Damage and sloughing of the surface squamous cells can also be seen.

Most of above mentioned features in isolation may be present in GORD, although marked basal cell hyperplasia out of proportion to reactive changes, excessive counts of IEEs, surface layering, eosinophilic microabscesses and subepithelial sclerosis are not features described in GORD. We believe that the presence of 15 or more eosinophils per HPF in proximal or mid-oesophagus compared to lower oesophagus or GOJ and lamina propria fibrosis is a major diagnostic clue to eosinophilic oesophagitis [29–42].

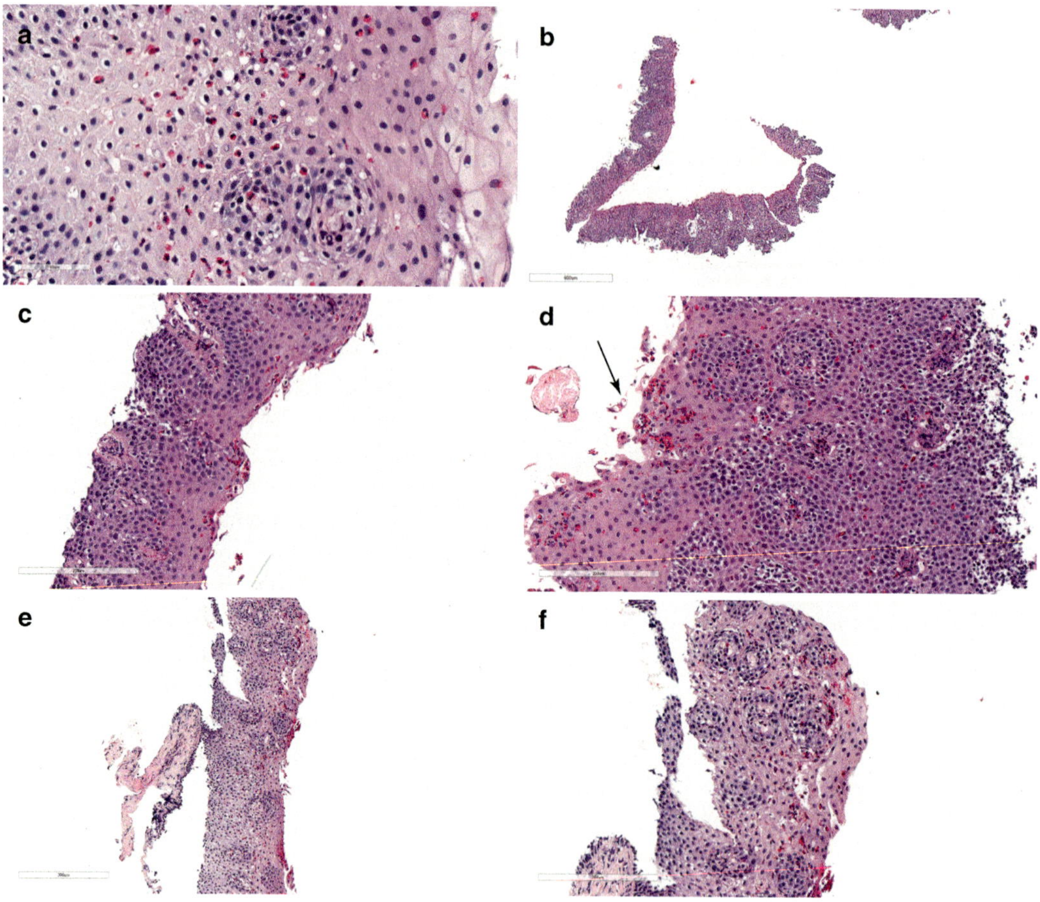

Fig. 2.8 Oesophageal squamous mucosa with numerous eosinophils seen in eosinophilic oesophagitis. (**a**) Increased intraepithelial eosinophils (>15 eosinophils/HPF). (**b**) Marked basal cell hyperplasia, easily appreciated on low power. (**c**) Surface layering. (**d**) Microabscesses (*arrow*). (**e**) Subepithelial sclerosis. (**f**) Degranulation of eosinophils

Lymphocytic Pattern

Lymphocytic oesophagitis is characterised by presence of an increased number of intraepithelial lymphocytes (Fig. 2.9a) with prominent peripapillary distribution (Fig. 2.9b) and associated spongiosis but without associated neutrophils or eosinophils (Box 2.7).

Box 2.7 Associated Diseases

- GORD
- Crohn's disease
- Mucosal irritants
- GVHD
- Lichen planus
- Infections
- Medications
- Post-ablation biopsies

Endoscopic appearance can mimic that of eosinophilic oesophagitis, with oesophageal rings present in over 50% of cases. Many cases, however, have normal mucosal findings or only minor changes including oesophagitis, erythema or nodularity.

"Lymphocytic oesophagitis" is best considered a reactionary pattern than an entity as diagnostic criteria are not defined, with the number of intraepithelial lymphocytes necessary to make the

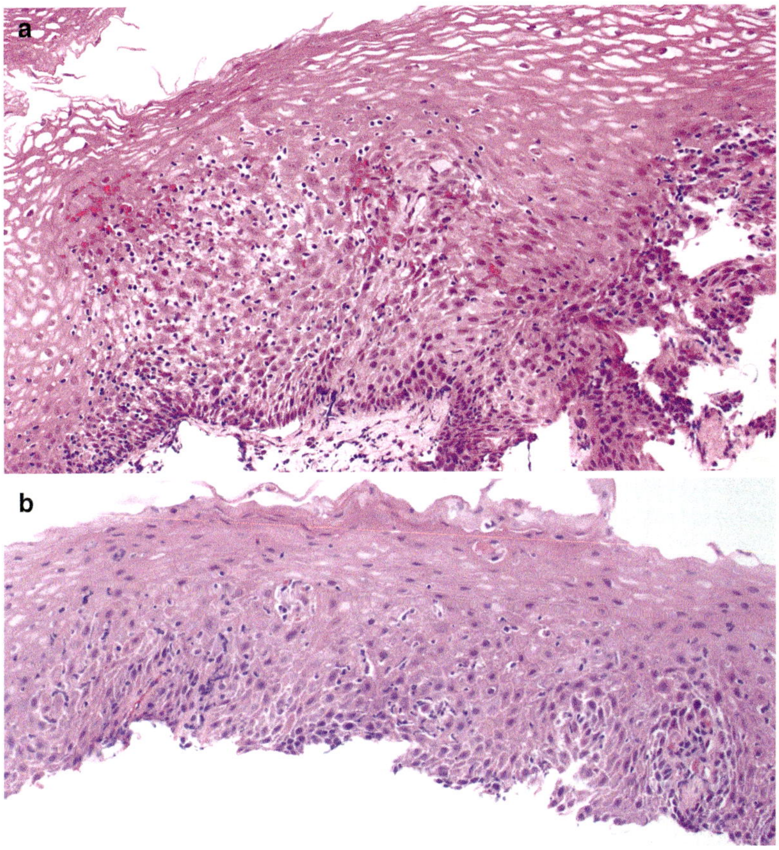

Fig. 2.9 Lymphocytic oesophagitis. (**a**) Intraepithelial lymphocytes. (**b**) Peripapillary distribution

diagnosis range from as low as 12 to 50 per HPF, suggested by different investigators. A clear association with lymphocytic gastritis and small intestinal lymphocytosis has not been established; although immune disorders including Crohn's disease can give rise to lymphocytic pattern throughout the gut mucosa [43–48].

Apoptotic Pattern

The histologic manifestations of GVHD (graft vs host disease) are usually found in the upper third of the oesophagus. Acute inflammation, erosions, ulcers and necrosis characterise acute GVHD, whereas in the chronic setting, there is desquamation of oesophageal mucosa and associated pauci-cellular submucosal fibrosis which may not be evident in biopsy samples.

Other causes of this pattern include medication-induced injury, in particular mycophenolate, and infections. CMV infection needs to be excluded by immunohistochemistry when apoptotic pattern is observed outside the setting of GVHD.

Although the gastrointestinal tract is a common site for GVHD, oesophageal involvement is uncommon. Clinical symptoms are non-specific and include dysphagia and chest pain [3, 49–51].

Mixed Pattern

This pattern is regarded as a red flag to hunt for pill substances in the biopsy and "quiz" the clinician for medication history, since medication-induced injury is the main culprit. In addition, a mixed pattern should also alert the pathologist to the possibility of double aetiology. Mixed pattern is characterised by a combination of acute and/or chronic injury pattern with sub-patterns (i.e. eosinophilic, deposition, apoptotic, vasculopathic) and is typical of medication-induced oesophagitis.

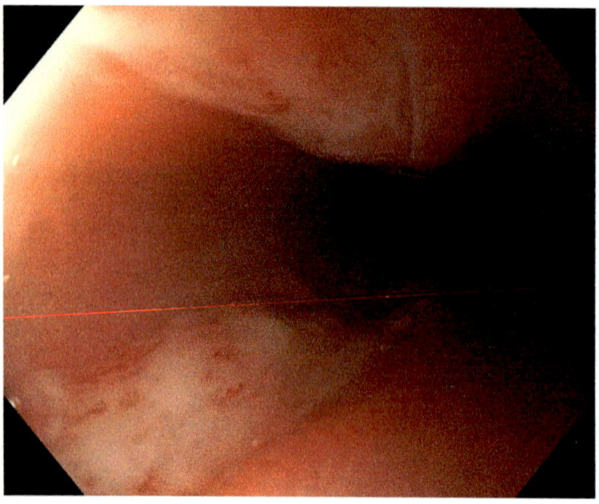

Fig. 2.10 Case 3–Pill oesophagitis. A 15-year-old lady with 2-week history of burning retrosternal chest pain and occasional radiation to the back. Recent USS and routine blood work were normal. Some recent improvement in symptoms, however, has ongoing postprandial retrosternal discomfort. Gastroscopy was done. Biopsies revealed mixed injury pattern

Medication-Induced Oesophagitis

While some medications produce characteristic histological patterns that guide the pathologists to identify the offending substance, most are largely indistinguishable from those of other drugs, GORD, infections and immune-mediated diseases (Fig. 2.10). "Pill-induced oesophagitis" (Fig. 2.11a) is the term used most commonly to describe medication-induced oesophageal injury. It is caused by direct contact of mucosa with medication and facilitation of mechanisms that eventually lead to disruption of the mucosal lining, rather than systemic toxicity or allergic reaction. The direct localised toxicity is generally caustic (acidic or alkaline) or hyperosmolar in nature. Other important factors such as medication contact time, pill coating and immediate versus sustained-release formulations also play a role. Altered anatomy (e.g. stricture) and motility disturbances are among other contributing factors. The most commonly reported agents include antibiotics (particularly doxycycline, tetracycline and clindamycin), NSAIDs, potassium chloride, iron supplements, ascorbic acid, bisphosphonates and resins. Tetracyclines are the most common type of antibiotic to cause pill oesophagitis, with doxycycline being the most frequent culprit.

Most patients are elderly and present with sudden onset odynophagia, retrosternal pain and dysphagia. Endoscopic findings include erythema, mucosal denudation, discrete ulcers or erosions and strictures. Remnants of the pill may also be seen. The usual sites of involvement are mid-oesophagus at the level of aortic arch, the level of an enlarged left atrium and the gastro-oesophageal junction.

Pill oesophagitis pattern is generally a non-specific oesophagitis pattern characterised by mucosal erosion, ulceration and associated fibroinflammatory exudate, and granulation tissue is usually seen (Fig. 2.11a). Although the main reason for obtaining biopsies may be to exclude a malignancy or infection, the presence of polarisable crystalline material or other specific histological findings may be an important clue to the diagnosis (Fig. 2.11b), but these are not present in all cases (Boxes 2.8 and 2.9) [54, 55, 60–62, 64].

Box 2.8 Pill Oesophagitis and mimics

Pill oesophagitis may simulate the endoscopic appearance of severe gastro-oesophageal reflux disease, although gastro-oesophageal reflux disease tends to present more insidiously.

- Pill oesophagitis that is limited to the narrowing of the mid-oesophagus is less likely to be confused with gastroesophageal reflux, which invariably involves the distal oesophagus.
- Biopsies from patients with gastro-oesophageal reflux disease reveal eosinophilic, rather than neutrophilic, inflammatory infiltrates, except in areas of erosion or ulcer.
- The identification of pill fragments should alert the pathologist to consider an element of drug-induced injury.

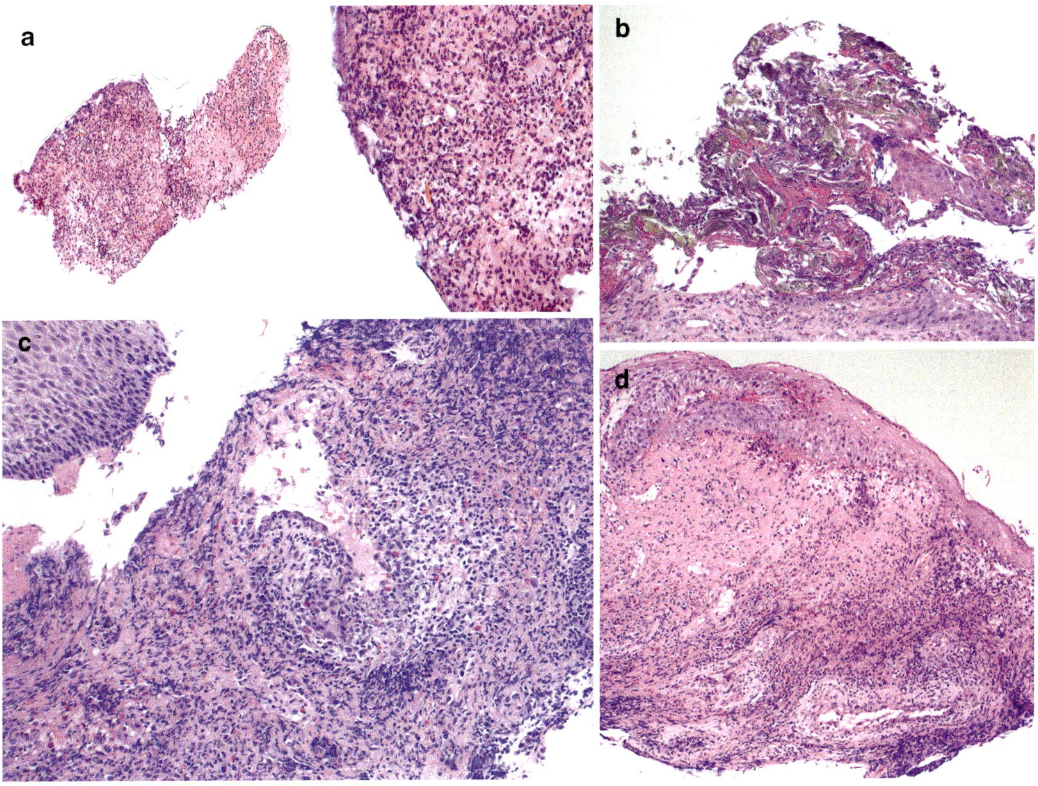

Fig. 2.11 Pill oesophagitis. (**a**) Ulcerated oesophageal mucosa. (**b**) Iron pill oesophagitis: brown-black crystalline material on ulcerated/injured surface. (**c**) Doxycycline effect. (**d**) Ulcerative oesophagitis with neutrophilic infiltrates as well as intraepithelial eosinophilia (alendronate)

- Viral infections, such as herpes and cytomegalovirus, also cause oesophageal ulcers and mimic pill oesophagitis, but tend to occur in immunosuppressed patients. Well-sampled viral ulcers often reveal characteristic inclusions.
- Always look for crystalline material in cases suspected for pill oesophagitis pattern and in all biopsies of oesophageal ulcers.

Box 2.9 Common Medications Causing Upper Gastrointestinal Tract Injury

- Non-steroidal anti-inflammatory drugs (NSAIDs)
- Antibiotics: tetracyclines including doxycycline
- Ferrous sulphate, potassium chloride, ascorbic acid, zidovudine
- Theophylline, quinidine, gluconate, alendronate (Fosamax)

- Taxanes (including Taxol)
- Resins: sodium polystyrene sulfonate in sorbitol (Kayexal, sevelamer)

Main patterns of medication-induced oesophagitis

Nonspecific mixed pattern, suggestive of medication/pill-induced injury (in the correct clinical context):

- Acute oesophagitis pattern with widespread spongiosis.
- Any admixture of intraepithelial eosinophils and/or lymphocytes with widespread spongiosis (especially when associated with neutrophilic pustules or erosion/ulceration).
- Any pattern of inflammation with associated pill fragments/crystalline material. Pill fragments are variably polarisable and refractile; some are bright pink with a periodic acid-Schiff special stain.
- Acute oesophagitis pattern in mid-oesophagus, in the absence of infective organisms.

Specific crystals +/− acute inflammation associated with resins

In most instances, Kayexalate produces a specific pill oesophagitis pattern which is easy to recognise in histological biopsies, and the finding of associated ischaemic or erosive GI tract disease merits a phone call to the clinician.

Specific Crystalline Patterns:

Iron pill oesophagitis (Fig. 2.11c): Luminal brown-black crystalline material adjacent to injured surface epithelium or admixed with luminal fibroinflammatory exudates. Confirmatory iron stains can be used to highlight iron deposition.

Doxycycline effect (Fig. 2.11d): Ulceration and a distinctive pattern of vascular injury with a pale perivascular, cell poor area ("halo") corresponding to an oedematous loose fibroblastic proliferation, perivascular inflammation consisting of lymphocytes, occasional plasma cells and variable numbers of eosinophils and neutrophils. There is vascular damage with prominent endothelial cell hyperplasia and an infiltration of the vessel wall by lymphocytes imparting "endothelialitis" pattern. A primary vasculitis needs to be differentiated. However, rarity of primary vasculitis in the oesophagus should be considered in the clinical setting of doxycycline ingestion, and this is indeed a unique pattern.

Mycophenolate mofetil (Cellcept, MMF) effect: Increased apoptosis to the extent that it may mimic graft-versus-host disease and variably active oesophagitis with focal erosion or ulceration is a common feature. Consider mycophenolate mofetil (Cellcept, MMF), a commonly used antimetabolite drug that is used for immunosuppression in the setting of organ transplantation. MMF-associated upper GI mucosal injury should not be used as an indicator for reducing drug when this drug is needed for the prevention of graft rejection.

Paclitaxel (Taxol)/colchicine effect: Epithelial necrosis and ulceration as well as ring-shaped arrested mitotic figures are commonly seen. Taxol is an antineoplastic agent that interferes with tubulin and inhibits its polymerisation into microtubules, which causes mitotic arrest, similar to colchicine. It can cause injury throughout the GI tract, but most commonly affects the oesophagus. Colchicine, used to treat gout, predominantly exerts its GI effects in the gastric antrum (see Chap. 4) and the duodenum. In the gastrointestinal tract, colchicine toxicity is associated with variable mucosal injury in the oesophagus, stomach and small intestine. Reduced epithelial cell layers, nuclear swelling and dyskeratosis have been described in the oesophagus. A characteristic finding is the presence of numerous mitoses arrested in metaphase. These may assume a characteristic "ring" pattern. The specific pathological changes caused by colchicine are usually limited to patients with renal failure (the population most susceptible to clinically significant colchicine toxicity). These changes should not be mistaken for high-grade dysplasia.

In contrast to colchicine-associated changes in nonneoplastic mucosa, the mitotic arrest mimicking high-grade dysplasia seen in GI tract specimens after taxane administration is not specific for toxicity but may also reflect taxane effect. It can be encountered in asymptomatic patients who have recently had medication. If these findings are seen histologically, they merit correlation with the clinical impression and should not be interpreted as toxicity in isolation (see Chap. 4).

Sloughing oesophagitis (oesophagitis dissecans superficialis) pattern (see below)

Sloughing oesophagitis/EDS is a distinctive pattern of injury that may be caused by different medications such as alendronate and CNS depressants, as well as other non-medication causes.

Specific Medications Causing "Pill Oesophagitis" Pattern

Potassium Chloride

Pill-induced oesophagitis was first described in a patient taking potassium chloride tablets. The toxicity is mainly due to the irritation by localised high salt concentrations. KCl injury should be considered in elderly patients with heart failure, who often require supplementation to counteract the effects of diuretics.

Bisphosphonates

Bisphosphonate injury is caused by a caustic alkaline effect on the mucosa. The most common offender is alendronate, whereas cases secondary to etidronate and pamidronate have been described only as case reports. Histologic findings include ulcerative oesophagitis with neutrophilic infiltrates as well as intraepithelial eosinophilia (Fig. 2.11e). The squamous epithelium appears reactive with enlarged and hyperchromatic nuclei. There also may be small intraepithelial vesicles. Clear, refractile, crystalline foreign material is often present in the fibroinflammatory exudate. Scattered multinucleated giant cells may associate with the crystals. Occasionally oesophageal strictures are present. We have seen an example of oesophagitis dissecans superficialis pattern with alendronate (Fosamax).

Tetracyclines

Tetracyclines, particularly doxycycline, are the most common antimicrobial agents to cause oesophagitis, accounting for up to 45% of cases. Histologic findings in tetracycline-induced ulcers reveal oedema of the squamous epithelium with dense neutrophil-rich infiltrates in the lower to middle regions of the mucosa. Vacuolar degeneration of the basal epithelial cells causes them to separate from the upper epithelial layers, creating an intramucosal cleft. The upper layers of squamous cells undergo coagulative necrosis and slough into the lumen.

Doxycycline

Doxycycline is an oral tetracycline antibiotic that has been associated with oesophageal and gastric ulceration. Recently, some vascular changes have been reported in association with doxycycline-related oesophageal ulcers, including vascular degeneration, prominent perivascular oedema and endothelialitis in the deeper vessels in the ulcer bed (Fig. 2.11d). Squamous epithelium with dense neutrophil-rich infiltrates in the lower to middle regions of the mucosa is seen. Vacuolar degeneration of the basal epithelial cells causes them to separate from the upper epithelial layers, creating an intramucosal cleft. The upper layers of squamous cells undergo coagulative necrosis and slough into the lumen ("doxycycline effect").

Nonsteroidal Anti-inflammatory Drugs (NSAIDs)

Nonsteroidal anti-inflammatory drug-induced ulcers are characteristically large, shallow, discrete, mid-oesophageal ulcers surrounded by normal mucosa. Patients on long-term NSAID therapy may have an endoscopically normal-appearing oesophagus, but histologically nonspecific oesophagitis may be seen. Alternatively, the oesophageal mucosa may appear inflamed, eroded or ulcerated. Patients also may develop reflux oesophagitis. Basal cell hyperplasia may not be present, because proliferation is inhibited by the prostaglandin inhibitors.

Iron

Iron-induced injury is typically limited to the upper GI tract, and within the oesophagus it can induce a chemical burn with erosive injury. Biopsies typically display luminal brown-black crystalline material adjacent to injured surface epithelium or admixed with luminal fibroinflammatory exudates (Fig. 2.11c). Confirmatory iron stains can be used to highlight iron deposition. Of note, sometimes exuberant proliferation of reactive fibroblasts and regenerative epithelial changes are seen near oesophageal ulcers that contain iron crystalline. These changes can be so striking as to raise the suspicion of a malignant process. This type of injury is seen in patients taking oral iron tablets who are usually older and with other risk factors for pill oesophagitis, such as polypharmacy, decreased saliva production and more time spent in the recumbent position.

Resins (Fig. 2.11f)

- Kayexalate (sodium polystyrene sulfonate) is a cation exchange resin used for management of hyperkalaemia upper gastrointestinal tract injury due to Kayexalate in sorbitol (erosive and ulcerative injury) and is uncommon, reversible and typically not associated with serious sequelae. The basophilic crystals have a "mosaic" pattern that can be appreciated on haematoxylin and eosin stain but is accentuated on acid-fast, PAS/alcian blue and Diff-Quik stains. It is useful to note that Kayexalate crystals are refractile but not polarisable. The crystals were either adherent to intact mucosa or admixed with exudates in 73% of patients with ulcers or erosions. Gastrointestinal bleeding was the most common indication for biopsy.
- Sevelamer is an anion exchange resin and phosphate binding agent used to treat hyperphosphatemia in renal failure. Although most of the specimens were colonic biopsies, oesophageal ulceration with crystals has also been reported. In contrast to Kayexalate, sevelamer crystals have curved cracks that resemble fish scales and often are two-toned with a yellow colour highlighted by pink linear accentuations. Sevelamer crystals are non-polarisable.
- Bile acid sequestrants: Cholestyramine is used to bind bile acids in patients who have bile salt-mediated diarrhoea, pruritus or hyperlipidaemia. Crystals can be seen in the GI biopsies from these patients, more often from the lower GI tract but occasionally from the upper GI tract. Bile acid sequestrant crystals are polygonal with variable eosinophilic colouration ranging from magenta to orange. They may have infrequent linear fractures but do not have the mosaic pattern or fish scale pattern of either Kayexalate or sevelamer. Bile acid sequestrants probably do not cause mucosal injury, but the crystals may cause confusion with other resins that may cause mucosal injury. Histologically, the crystalline structure of cholestyramine is similar to that of Kayexalate; however, the cholestyramine crystal has greater opacity, lacks a mosaic pattern and is usually red in colour on H&E. Another clue is that although both Kayexalate and cholestyramine crystals stain red with a periodic acid-Schiff stain, the former is also red with an acid-fast stain, whereas the latter is pink. Importantly, the effects of both sodium polystyrene sulfonate and cholestyramine seem to be reversible and are typically not associated with serious sequelae (Box 2.10 and Table 2.1).

Box 2.10 Differentiating Resin Crystals

- Kayexalate: purple to red with mosaic/fish scale pattern.
- Sevelamer: yellow with red lines and curved cracks (more resembles fish scale/roof shingles).
- Bile acid sequestrants: no mosaic pattern.

Endoscopic findings in drug-induced oesophageal injury generally suggest a chemical oesophagitis, with erosions or ulcerations and exudative

Table 2.1 Differentiating resin crystals

Resin crystal	Fish scale	H&E	Modified ZN
Kayexalate	Yes	Purple	Black
Sevelamer	Yes	Pink-yellow	Magenta
Bile acid sequestrates	No	Eosinophilic	Dull yellow

inflammation accompanied by thickening of the oesophageal wall. Strictures and circumferential wall thickening may simulate malignancy in some cases.

The triad of awareness of specific histological patterns, hunting for the presence of medication fragments and clinical data is the key. GI pathologists have to be familiar with clinical conditions that may increase a patient's susceptibility to potential medication-induced injury and actively look for direct or indirect evidence of related medications. The mixed pattern of injury secondary to medications can be divided into two main categories: medication-induced injury with non-specific patterns that require correlation with history and medication-induced injury with distinctive features associated with injury.

Sloughing oesophagitis/EDS is a distinctive pattern of injury that may be caused by different medications such as alendronate and CNS depressants, as well as other non-medication causes.

In addition to drugs, which are the main culprits in a mixed inflammation pattern, the possibility of infections and double pathology (a primary common pathology complicated by/associated with a secondary process such as infection or medication-related oesophagitis) needs to be considered and effectively excluded. For example, *Candida* oesophagitis can cause a lymphocytic pattern of inflammation with superficial microabscesses or erosion/ulceration (a mixed pattern) or secondary *Candida* oesophagitis can be seen in a background of GORD (e.g. acute oesophagitis accompanied by marked parakeratosis). Therefore, always look for medication-related changes and pathogenic organisms in a mixed pattern of inflammation (Boxes 2.11 and 2.12) [2, 3, 52–65].

Box 2.11 Medication-Induced Injury: Clinical Clues

- Conditions treated or associated with known offending medications
- Bedridden patients and patients with osteoporosis: bisphosphonate (Fosamax)
- Other diseases resulting in lodged pill substances in the oesophagus: Parkinson's disease, diabetes, oesophageal webs or other oesophageal structural abnormality
- Associated caustic injury when endoscopist reports a single ulcer surrounded by "clean-appearing" mucosa
- NSAID-induced injury in patients with multiple medical problems
- Patients on chemotherapy—Taxol
- New-generation medications—emerging
- Denial of medication intake but report consumption of healthy foods and supplements

Box 2.12 Medication-Induced Injury: Histological Clues

- "Diagnostic" patterns: Doxycycline, characteristic substances, e.g. resin.
- Mixed pattern of injury.
- Marked spongiosis.
- Lodged pill material.
  - When clinical clues are known or extracted!
  - When inflammatory pattern/s are otherwise difficult to explain.
- Be mindful of double pathology.

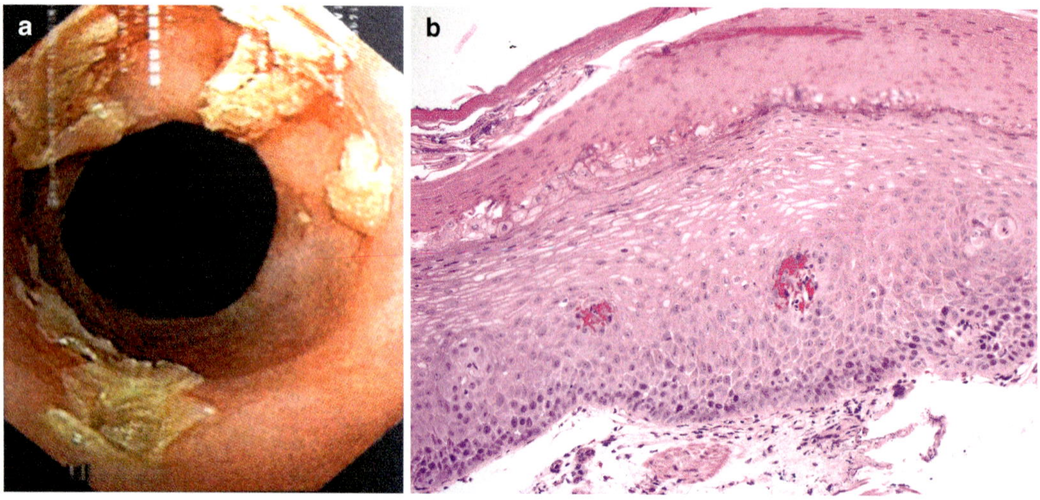

Fig. 2.12 Sloughing oesophagitis (oesophagitis dissecans superficialis). (**a**) Endoscopic appearance. (**b**) Oesophageal squamous mucosa with the "two-toned" appearance

Sloughing Oesophagitis (Oesophagitis Dissecans Superficialis)

Two-toned appearance of superficial necrotic eosinophilic squamous epithelium with underlying reactive mucosa, often with detached long strips of mucosa, is characteristic on low power (Fig. 2.12a, b). The superficial eosinophilic squamous cells may have flattened nuclei ("parakeratotic") or appear "mummified" due to coagulative necrosis. They also can show pyknotic to faded (ghost) nuclei and intense eosinophilic cytoplasm. The eosinophilic top layer of the squamous mucosa is often separated from the underlying intact squamous mucosa, and this sometimes creates a blister-like appearance. Most cases show some degree of detachment or splitting of the mucosa. Some cases at early stages have fluid-containing bullae or cysts with or without intraepithelial splitting above the basal layers. Vacuolisation of cytoplasm occurs progressing into fluid-filled cysts or bullae formation. Spongiosis is rare. The detached bottom layer attached to the lamina propria shows larger reactive nuclei. Inflammation is rarely seen and, if present, is often present at the junction between the necrotic epithelium and the underlying normal squamous mucosa. Ortho-parakeratosis and bacterial or fungal colonies are other accompanying features and patterns that may be noted. The inflammatory cell infiltrate is absent or sparse similar to entities such as corrosive oesophagitis, GVHD, scleroderma and some drug toxicities (Box 2.13).

Box 2.13 Sloughing Oesophagitis/Oesophagitis Dissecans Superficialis Pattern

- Microscopic appearance: a unique pattern in the oesophageal squamous mucosa.

  Characteristic: "two-toned look under low power".
- Top layer: total or partial detachment of superficial layer, intraepithelial splitting or at least a blister-like appearance with superficial eosinophilic squamous cells: parakeratotic cells, ghost-like/mummified cells.
- Bottom layer: mucosa shows larger reactive nuclei.

- Paucity of inflammation.

  Other Features:
- Bacterial overgrowth on the surface.
- Associated medications/toxins/injurious agents (known):

  Bisphosphonates, non-steroidal anti-inflammatory drugs (NSAIDs), potassium chloride, physical injury, hot beverages, caustic agents, alcohol, spicy foods, swallowing large amounts of food quickly.
- Associated conditions (known):

  Systemic diseases including coeliac disease, collagen vascular disorders and autoimmune bullous dermatoses.
- Endoscopic appearance: often classic with sloughing or peeling squamous mucosa.
- Differential diagnoses: artefactual trauma, dermatological bullous disorders, candidiasis, pill oesophagitis, corrosive oesophagitis, coeliac disease, invasive fungal infection.

The endoscopic findings are often classic and range from white patches of peeling oesophageal epithelium affecting the mid- to distal oesophagus to a dramatic appearance of diffuse sloughing of the entire oesophageal epithelium (Fig. 2.12b). An appearance of "filled with gift-wrap paper" has also been described. The mucosa underneath the peeled "membrane" is often unremarkable. These patients often present with non-specific clinical symptoms (e.g. cough, dysphagia, globus sensation, regurgitation, chest or epigastric pain, heartburn, nausea and vomiting) and the diagnosis is often not suspected until endoscopic examination.

Some authors consider oesophagitis dissecans superficialis (EDS) and sloughing oesophagitis (SE) as two different entities with overlapping endoscopic and histopathologic features. Currently the popular approach is to consider the spectrum as one disease since pathogenesis is ill defined.

This pattern of injury is believed to be due to direct contact injury and has been associated with use of multiple medications in debilitated patients. In some cases, a specific aetiology cannot be elucidated. A variety of medications, systemic diseases and conditions and physical injury have been associated with this pattern. Consumption of hot beverages, caustic agents, alcohol, spicy foods, swallowing large amounts of food quickly, repeated forceful vomiting, Mallory-Weiss syndrome, oesophageal sclerotherapy and nasogastric intubation, oesophageal strictures, severe infectious oesophagitis, renal failure and various autoimmune bullous dermatoses have also been associated with this pattern. Alternatively, oesophagitis dissecans superficialis may be idiopathic with no associated trauma or disease. Hence, exact mechanism of oesophageal injury remains unclear. Pathogenesis of EDS might be a result of direct insult to the oesophageal mucosa through physical, chemical, thermal or immunological mechanisms or associated with a topical or ischaemic injury.

Artefactual detachment of squamous epithelium in a normal oesophageal biopsy should be differentiated from sloughing oesophagitis. Here, there is no necrosis, inflammation or parakeratosis, and the epithelial splitting does not involve a specific level. If bullae and epithelial clefting is a prominent feature, skin disorders that can have similar oesophageal manifestations (such as Stevens-Johnson syndrome, pemphigus and bullous pemphigoid, which have been associated with bullous oesophagitis) must be excluded. Cases of sloughing oesophagitis show intraepithelial clefting, whereas pemphigus vulgaris, the most common vesiculobullous disorder that involves the oesophagus, shows suprabasilar bullous formation. Dermatitis herpetiformis presenting as EDS has been reported with coeliac disease, and the oesophageal histology featured papillary microabscesses. Chronic bullous disease can be ruled out by the absence of complement and immunoglobulin deposits by immunofluorescence, by the lack of corresponding cutaneous or oropharyngeal lesions and by a poor response to steroid therapy (Box 2.14).

Box 2.14 Traps and Clues

- Be aware of artefactual trauma.
- Pill oesophagitis: similar culprit (medications), most common in the middle or distal oesophagus and histologically may have necrotic squamous epithelium, but there is also spongiosis and inflammation (commonly mixed pattern of injury with eosinophils).
- Significant neutrophilic infiltration: superimposed infection and severe reflux must be ruled out.
- Marked bullae formation: exclude dermatological bullous disorders including DH (dermatitis herpetiformis) and coeliac disease.
- Consider other parakeratotic patterns.
- Endoscopic correlation is essential.

In spite of its sometimes dramatic presentation, EDS is a benign condition that resolves after discontinuation of the precipitating medications and treatment with proton pump inhibitors and/or corticosteroids without lasting oesophageal pathology. Although an association with medications, skin conditions, heavy smoking and physical trauma has been reported, the pathogenesis of EDS remains unexplained [2, 66–71].

Deposition Pattern

Endogenous or exogenous material may be noted in oesophageal biopsies. Oesophageal deposits occur in the lamina propria, and it is important to inspect the subepithelial tissue, even in small biopsy fragments. Dense subepithelial sclerosis (characteristically seen in EoE) can resemble amyloid, and special stains may be needed for the distinction. Presence of melanin pigment should alert the possibility of melanoma deposits. Deposits related to medications have been discussed in Chap. 2 and under mixed pattern and medication-related injury in this chapter. Endoscopic appearance and clinical background are invaluable.

Special Patterns

Reflux Pattern

A combination of basal cell hyperplasia, increased length of the papillae, intraepithelial inflammation, intercellular oedema (spongiosis), balloon cells and vascular changes in the squamous mucosa is the typical reflux pattern of injury (Figs. 2.13 and 2.14). Because the histologic features of GORD are not specific, a number of histologic features must be assessed before a presumptive diagnosis of reflux oesophagitis can be made.

Basal cell hyperplasia (Fig. 2.15a): Blue basal cells extending to >15% of the total epithelial thickness represent a reactive increase in the proliferative zone. Because individuals without GORD show mild epithelial hyperplasia 2–3 cm proximal to the lower oesophageal sphincter, this feature is not useful in diagnosing GORD if the biopsies are taken in the distal 3 cm. Basal cell hyperplasia is most easily appreciated when this layer exceeds 25% of the mucosal thickness.

- Also seen in eosinophilic oesophagitis, but biopsies are usually derived from the mid- and proximal oesophagus.
- Should be evaluated in a well-oriented area. In evaluating basal cell hyperplasia, areas close to papillae should be avoided. Location of the biopsies must also be considered; basal cell hyperplasia, elongation of the papillae and occasional eosinophils may be seen within 1–3 cm of the gastro-oesophageal junction, possibly as a result of physiologic reflux.

Papillary lengthening/elongation (Fig. 2.15b): Normally, papillae extend up to no further than 50% of the epithelial thickness. Extension of papillae into more than two-thirds of the mucosal thickness indicates reactive changes and generally papillae reaching the top half of the mucosal thickness is regarded as abnormal.

Intercellular oedema (Fig. 2.15c): Dilated intercellular spaces (DIS) or spongiosis may be the only histologic change seen in early or minimal GORD, defined as spaces larger than 2.5 μm, present diffusely in the basal and parabasal areas. Artefacts must be considered in the evaluation of DIS.

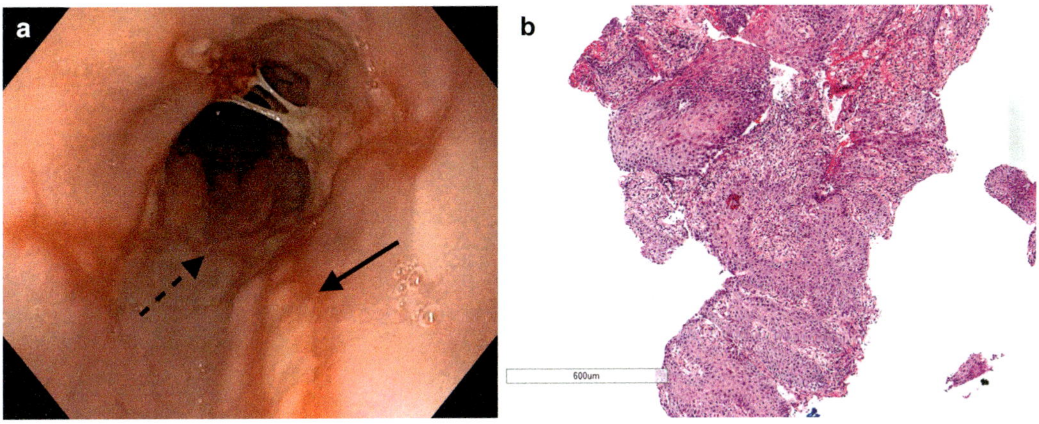

Fig. 2.13 Case 4—Reflux—Grade C. A 55-year-old lady referred for evaluation of a several month history of retrosternal burning. Gastroscopy was performed revealing mucosal breaks (solid arrow) bridging the tops of mucosal folds (dashed arrow—(**a**) involving <75%) circumference consistent with LA Grade C reflux oesophagitis. Biopsies were taken to exclude underlying dysplasia and showed ulcerative oesophagitis (**b**)

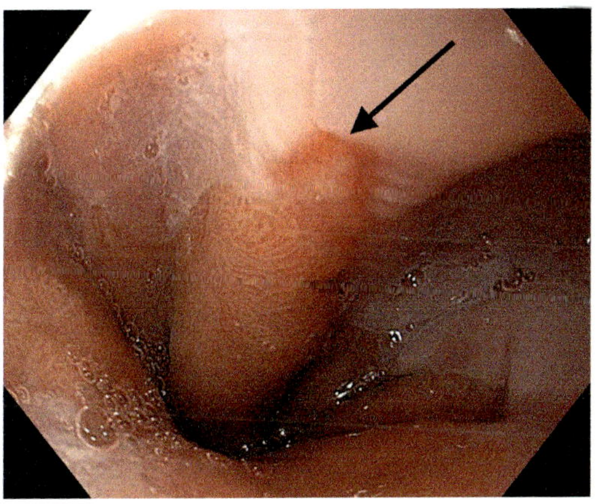

Fig. 2.14 Case 5—Reflux—Grade A. A 56-year-old man with long history of intermittent reflux-type symptoms. Referred for gastroscopy for further evaluation. Noted to have a single 2 mm linear erosion (arrow) consistent with mild (LA Grade A) reflux oesophagitis

Balloon cells: Swollen, pale, periodic acid-Schiff-negative cells with irregular pyknotic nuclei developing in the epithelial midzone are present in approximately two-thirds of GORD patients. Balloon cells develop in any damaged mucosa, but in the absence of other more characteristic features of GORD, they may be the only clue to chemical injury that has occurred.

Intraepithelial inflammation (Fig. 2.15d). Small numbers of lymphocytes, plasma cells and eosinophils typically populate the normal oesophageal lamina propria and their presence does not establish a diagnosis of oesophagitis.

- **Lymphocytes**: Lymphocytes are present in small numbers in normal mucosa, but are conspicuous and increased in number of patients with GORD. Intraepithelial lymphocytes have been referred to as "squiggle cells" or "cells with irregular nuclear contours" because of their curved nuclei that appear to fit between the epithelial cells. They have almost no visible cytoplasm. Intraepithelial lymphocytes are present associated with diverse aetiologies.
- **Eosinophils**: Intraepithelial eosinophils are considered characteristic but not sensitive or specific for reflux oesophagitis as they can be seen in other entities such as eosinophilic oesophagitis, hypereosinophilic syndrome, eosinophilic gastroenteritis, parasitic infections, fungal infections, recurrent vomiting, drug-induced injury, inflammatory bowel disease, allergic vasculitis and neoplasia. Intraepithelial eosinophils may be focal, necessitating a search for them on serial sections and on multiple levels.
- **Neutrophils**: Neutrophils, either in the squamous epithelium or in the lamina propria, serve as evidence for acute oesophagitis. Large collections of neutrophils suggest associated ulcer or erosion. The presence of neutrophils in an oesophageal biopsy especially should prompt a search for evidence of fungal or viral infection. Large numbers of neutrophils in the superficial epithelium should suggest the possibility of fungal superinfection and trigger special stains to rule out *Candida* organisms.

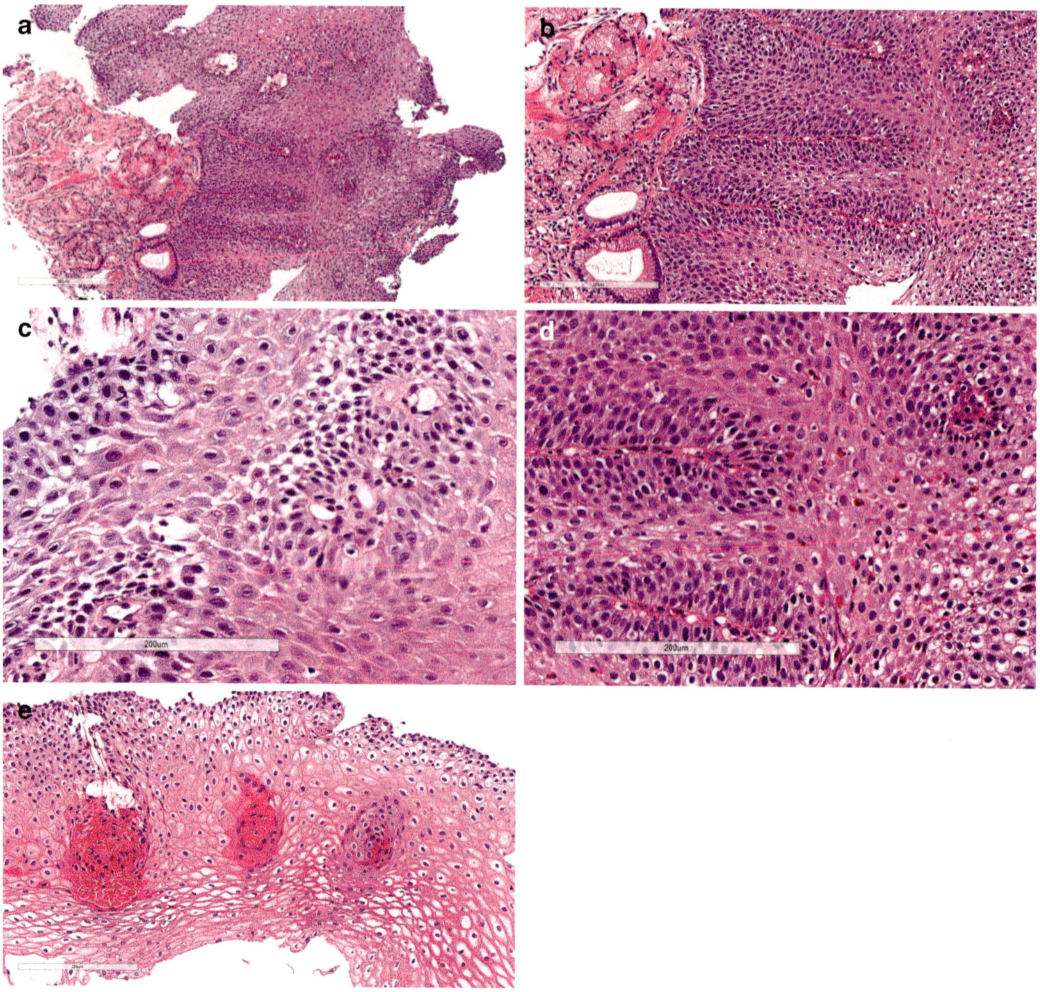

Fig. 2.15 Reflux pattern. (**a**) Basal cell hyperplasia. (**b**) Elongated papillae. (**c**) Intercellular oedema (spongiosis). (**d**) Intraepithelial inflammation. (**e**) Vascular lakes

Capillary ectasia (Fig. 2.15e): Dilated and congested venules located high in the elongated oesophageal papillae are a common finding in reflux oesophagitis, seen in up to 83% of affected patients. In contrast, this finding is present in only 10% of patients without GORD. Red cells often escape and form blood lakes. This change is often present in the absence of any inflammation and corresponds to the endoscopically identified red mucosal streaks.

Parakeratotic pattern may be seen in GORD as a sub-pattern (see below). In biopsies obtained from GOJ, columnar mucosa is often included with evidence of chronic inflammation ("squamocolumnar injury pattern", see below).

The endoscopic features vary with disease severity. Areas of erythema and longitudinal red streaks in the distal oesophagus are the first endoscopic abnormalities. In severe reflux, the oesophagus appears friable, diffusely reddened and haemorrhagic. Mucosal erosions and ulcerations result in "acute ulcerative pattern" in biopsies. Intramural thickening and strictures as well as metaplastic pattern (Barrett's oesophagus) ultimately develop as a response to chronic injury. Most erosions and ulcers occur distally, tapering off proximally. Inflammatory polyps may be present at the squamocolumnar junction. Strictures develop close to the gastro-oesophageal junction or immediately proximal to a hiatal hernia.

Histology, in comparison with clinical evaluation technique, has a relatively low sensitivity and specificity for GORD. GORD is represented in an endoscopic biopsy with a spectrum of inflammatory patterns with a significant overlap with other specific inflammatory diseases.

Biopsies are performed to confirm the presence of inflammation ("oesophagitis"), to determine its nature (e.g. peptic vs. drug-induced) and severity and to rule out coexisting pathology including neoplastic process. Oesophagitis can heal completely or it may progress onto any of the complications discussed below (Box 2.15).

Box 2.15 "Reflux Pattern" in Oesophageal/GOJ Biopsy

- Is characteristic of GORD in the lower/distal oesophageal biopsy.
- Is not specific for GORD: infection, eosinophilic oesophagitis, drug-induced injury and involvement by systemic diseases, such as progressive systemic sclerosis or Crohn's disease will show at least some of the features.
- Clinical context should be considered, otherwise reported as reflux pattern.
- Avoid overinterpretation of basal cell hyperplasia in cross-cut sections.
- Inflamed columnar-lined mucosa is often noted (squamocolumnar injury pattern): look for goblet cells (BO pattern) and even neoplasia (neoplastic pattern).
- Caution.
  - Severe reactive changes may mimic dysplasia.
  - The base of ulcers may contain bizarre cells that may mimic an invasive carcinoma (stromal cells may be weakly CK-positive!).

Reactive changes in biopsies from patients with GORD may appear so atypical that the differential diagnosis may also include malignancy. When extensive pseudoepitheliomatous hyperplasia is present, the question of an invasive carcinoma may also arise. Additionally, the base of ulcers may contain bizarre cells that may mimic an invasive carcinoma. Immunohistochemical stains using antibodies directed against endothelial and epithelial cells distinguish between the reparative reactions and malignancy. The presence of isolated cytokeratin-positive cells strongly suggests the presence of an invasive cancer, especially if these cells demonstrate significant nuclear atypia and lie within a desmoplastic stroma. However, it is important to note that reactive mesenchymal cells are sometimes cytokeratin immunoreactive [72–78].

Metaplastic Pattern

Columnar metaplasia (CM) of the oesophagus is always "gastric-type" mucosa and may have three morphologic types: gastric fundic-type (oxynto-cardiac) (Fig. 2.16a), gastric cardiac-type (transitional) (Fig. 2.16b), and intestinal-type mucosa (Fig. 2.16c). The latter is defined by the presence of interspersed goblet cells. Therefore, CM pattern may be of two major sub-patterns: intestinalised and non-intestinalised. Irrespective of subtypes and sub-patterns, CM is always a result of injury. CM of oesophagus is variably referred to as columnar-lined oesophagus (CLO) and columnar-lined mucosa (CLM) (Box 2.16).

Box 2.16 Three Types of Epithelium in CLM (and in BO)

- Gastric fundic-type (oxynto-cardiac).
- Gastric cardiac-type (transitional) mucosa
- "Intestinal type" characterised by the presence of interspersed goblet cells in either type of mucosa

Non-Intestinalised Metaplastic Pattern

This pattern of squamocolumnar injury pattern is characterised by the presence of inflamed squamous and columnar-lined mucosa in the same fragment in continuity or in separate fragments. GOJ biopsies characteristically show this pattern,

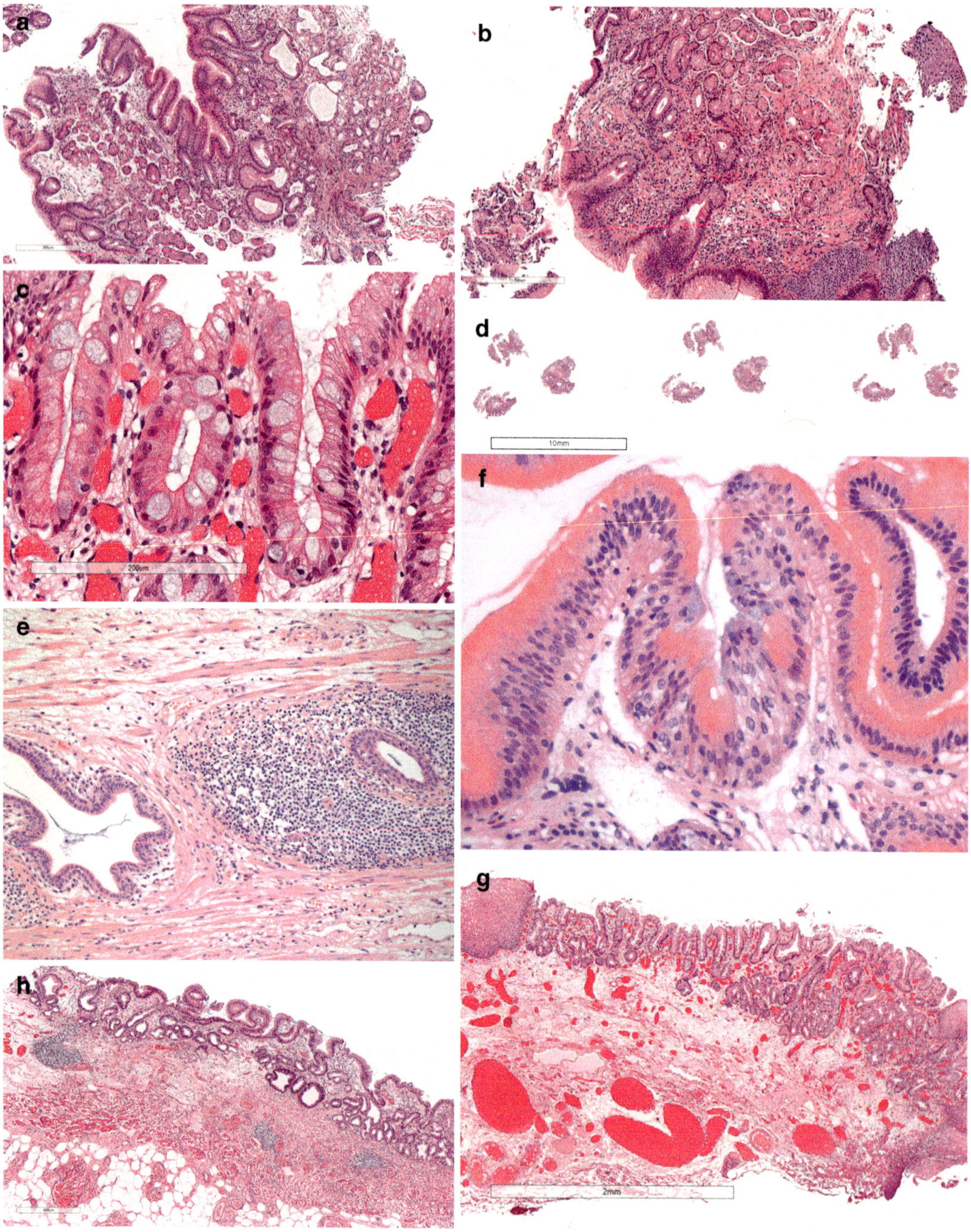

Fig. 2.16 Metaplastic patterns of columnar-lined mucosa. (**a**) CLM: gastric fundic-type/cardiac-oxyntic-type. (**b**) CLM: gastric cardiac-type. (**c**) CLM: IM (typical of BO). (**d**) Three fragments of CLM (H&E) with and without intestinal metaplasia (IM). (**e**) submucosal ducts—note squamous lining in one (native oesophageal structures). (**f**) Multilayering. (**g**) Duplicated MM of CLM in an EMR. (**h**) Duplicated MM of CLM in an EMR

in fact a common biopsy sample in routine GI pathology practice. However, this pattern can be seen in a biopsy obtained from any length of the tubular oesophagus. CLO is considered as evidence of Barrett's oesophagus (BO) in Europe and some parts of Asia (see discussion below).

When biopsies are labelled as GOJ, it is assumed that they are obtained from the GOJ or irregular Z-line. A range of secondary inflammatory patterns involving both squamous and columnar mucosa is the norm, the most common being a chronic inflammatory pattern. The inflammation is limited to the proximal gastric-type mucosa ("carditis") in the absence of similar changes in the remaining stomach unless there is a primary gastric pathology. Isolated "carditis" may be a more sensitive marker of GORD than inflammation involving the squamous mucosa, as suggested in pH monitoring studies.

Squamocolumnar injury pattern commonly seen in GOJ biopsies poses two fundamental questions as to origin of CLM; whether it represents proximal cardia or metaplastic oesophageal mucosa.

Cardia is believed to be a very short segment of proximal gastric mucosa ranging from 1 to 4 cm continuing as the body mucosa immediately after. Cardiac mucosa in the stomach is characterised by simple foveolar lining with underlying non-specialised antro-pyloric-type glands that continues with the specialised body-type mucosa. Reflux injury results in "chronic inflammatory pattern" signified by chronic inflammation and glandular distortion. This is impossible to differentiate from the damage that occurs in the gastric "cardia" and nearby body mucosa due to true inflammation of proximal cardia such as occurring with *H. pylori* infection. Obviously damaged proximal gastric mucosa can show any of the three types of morphology that could result from acid reflux to oesophageal squamous that transforms into metaplastic CLM.

Over time, various clues have been touted to help in the distinction. But these features have a very low sensitivity. Hence, metaplastic CLM of oesophagus and chronic inflammatory pattern of proximal gastric mucosa is virtually indistinguishable on microscopic examination of GOJ mucosa.

The concept can be made noncontroversial if endoscopic criteria are fool proof. Unfortunately, the junction between the cardiac-type mucosa and the squamous mucosa of the oesophagus is always irregular and may not exactly correlate with the functional gastro-oesophageal junction. This makes the distinction impossible both by endoscopic and microscopic examination.

The true existence of the cardia has been questionable. "Gastric cardia" is regarded as a manifestation of reflux and considered an abnormality by itself by some North American groups. The concept is an ongoing debate.

Intestinalised Metaplastic Pattern

This pattern is characterised by the presence of gastric-type columnar mucosa in "oesophageal" biopsies obtained from the oesophagus with goblet cells (intestinal metaplasia or IM) and indicates BO (see diagnostic criteria below) (Figs. 2.16c, d and 2.17a, b). BO is an acquired condition in response to gastro-oesophageal reflux, whereby the squamous mucosa is replaced by columnar mucosa.

There are two criteria to be fulfilled for a diagnosis of BO.

- Endoscopic: Extension of salmon-coloured mucosa into the tubular oesophagus extending ≥1 cm proximal to the gastro-oesophageal junction (GOJ)
- Histological: Confirmation of intestinal metaplasia in the endoscopic biopsy obtained from the above abnormal area (Box 2.17)

Box 2.17 Different Approaches to the Diagnosis of BO Across the Globe

- Presence of columnar-lined oesophagus alone with or without IM is adequate for a diagnosis of BO according to guidelines by the British Society of Gastroenterology (BSG). Similar guidelines are recommended by the Japanese Cancer Society.
- North American and Australian guidelines require the presence of IM for a diagnosis of BO.

In patients with suspected BO, at least eight random biopsies should be obtained to maximise the yield of IM on histology. In patients with short (1–2 cm) segments of suspected BO in whom eight biopsies may be unobtainable, at

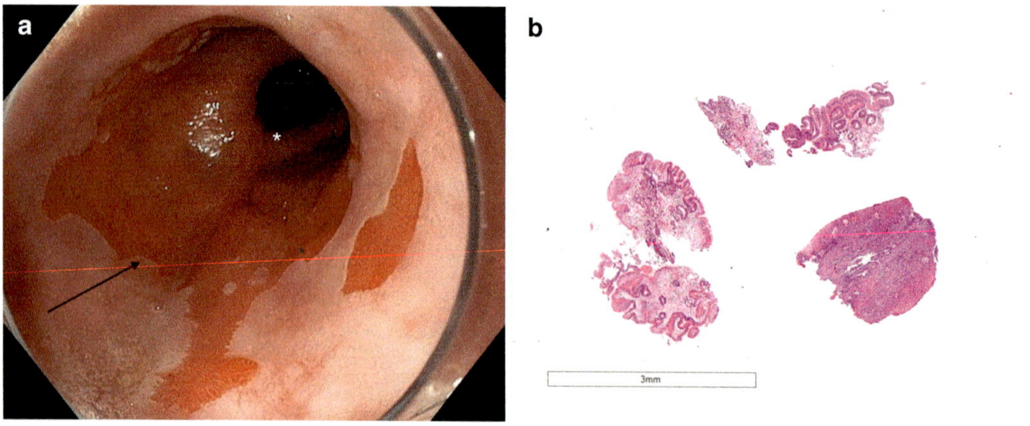

Fig. 2.17 CASE 6—Barrett's oesophagus. A 68-year-old man presenting for evaluation of a 10-year history of reflux symptoms. (**a**) Gastroscopy was performed which revealed displacement of the squamocolumnar junction (arrow) with a short segment of columnar-type mucosa extending 3 cm above the gastro-oesophageal junction (Asterix represents GOJ). (**b**) Four quadrant biopsies were taken at two levels to confirm the suspected diagnosis of Barrett's oesophagus. Biopsies showed metaplastic pattern with IM, confirming BO with no dysplasia

least four biopsies per centimetre of circumferential BO and one biopsy per centimetre in tongues of BO should be obtained.

Intestinal-type metaplastic mucosa is biologically unstable with the greatest risk of neoplastic progression through dysplasia to adenocarcinoma. Recent studies have demonstrated the presence of goblet cells in almost all early BO-related neoplastic lesions. The association of non-intestinalised metaplastic mucosa (i.e. CLM without goblet cells) with neoplastic progression is less well established. CLM without IM alone is not considered as an indication for surveillance according to current guidelines.

When a biopsy labelled GOJ shows goblet cells, a GI pathologist may feel obliged to comment further to decide whether GOJ biopsy contains IM of BO vs. IM of proximal stomach.

- Rely on endoscopic landmarks
- Exclude sampling from the hiatus hernia or cardia
- Record whether the biopsy samples are taken at the GOJ (irregular Z-line) or tubular oesophagus
- Differentiation: difficult on morphological grounds

Histological clues that may help in the distinction of metaplastic CLO from damaged proximal cardia can assist in differentiating IM in CLO from IM in damaged proximal stomach. Again, these features are not present in many GOJ biopsies and therefore are not sensitive. Pure organised normal fundic mucosa is almost always gastric fundic mucosa, but IM in such normal fundic mucosa is a very unusual finding.

Duplication of muscularis mucosae is common in BO. In endoscopic resection, this is a consistent finding (Fig. 2.16e–h). However, this is difficult to appreciate in most endoscopic biopsies due to lack of orientation and cross-cutting. Other helpful clues are patchy and therefore not reliable. Use of differential staining pattern of CK7 and CK20 in Barrett's epithelium compared to gastric cardia is also not specific enough to use as a reliable feature (Box 2.18).

Box 2.18 IM in CLO versus IM in Damaged Proximal Stomach

- IM in sub-squamous glands—favour IM in CLO (re-epithelialised oesophageal mucosa)
- IM in oesophageal ducts/submucosal glands (native oesophageal structures)—almost always IM in CLO (Fig. 2.11e)
- IM with multilayering—favours IM in CLO (Fig. 2.11f)
- IM in CLM with underlying duplicated MM—favours IM in CLO (Fig. 2.11h, g)

Presence of cardia is regarded as a manifestation of reflux and always abnormal by some North American groups. The presence of non-specialised gastric mucosa resembling the gastric cardia is increasingly being recognised as a quick adaptative mucosa to injury to glandular mucosa in the specialised mucosa of the stomach and well beyond the oesophagus and stomach. Therefore, the possibility of cardiac metaplasia of damaged gastric fundic mucosa still poses a problem. Therefore, currently it is accepted that the microscopic distinction of IM in CLO from IM in damaged proximal stomach is impossible.

When IM is noted in SC pattern in GOJ biopsies, a conclusion of "junctional mucosa with cardiac or oxyntic epithelium with intestinal metaplasia" or "columnar-lined mucosa with intestinal metaplasia and chronic inflammation" appears justifiable.

If endoscopic information is unavailable, a comment is desirable:

"The appearance would be in keeping with Barrett's disease if the biopsies have been obtained from the tubular oesophagus. Correlation with clinical and endoscopic findings is recommended".

Demonstration of IM/Goblet Cells

On H & E-stained slides, true goblet cells are rounded cells and show distended lightly haematoxylin-stained ("light blueish) vacuole and compressed basal nucleus with displacement of the cytoplasmic membranes of adjacent cells. They are usually randomly distributed throughout the mucosa (Fig. 2.18a). In contrast, its mimic, pseudogoblet cells, are distended gastric foveolar epithelial cells that are seen on the surface mainly and in a continuous manner. Cytoplasmic mucin is homogeneous and eosinophilic (Fig. 2.18b). Most of the time, a good H&E-stained section is all that is required to make the distinction. Experienced GI pathologists would hardly use alcian blue (AB) and alcian blue-PASD combination for the distinction. AB stain alone can be potentially confusing as non-goblet columnar cells can produce a blue hue (columnar blue cells) confounding the issue (Fig. 2.18c). Using the AB-PASD combination, pseudogoblet cells variably stain red/magenta/deep purple. True goblet cells stain bright purple (Fig. 2.18d). However, the intensity and shades of the colours can vary among laboratories. As previously discussed, a good H&E section assessed by an experienced GI pathologist using the features discussed is more reliable than relying on histochemical stains to differentiate a pseudogoblet cells from true goblet cells.

Ancillary stains including mucin proteins, CDX2 (Fig. 2.18e), Das-1, villin, Hep Par 1 and SOX9 have shown variable and at times, promising results. However, they are not recommended to be used in routine setting. Positive staining of epithelial cells of CLM with histochemical and immunohistochemical markers of intestinalisation (MUC2-positive cells) (Fig. 2.18f) has been proposed as evidence of "intestinalisation" before the appearance of the terminally differentiated goblet cells. However, this feature is not recommended as evidence of IM for a diagnosis of BO in routine practice so far.

Demonstration of IM:

- **A well-oriented and well-stained H&E slide is adequate.**
- True goblet cells: randomly distributed, rounded with distended light blueish vacuole, compressed basal nucleus, displacement of the cytoplasmic membranes of adjacent cells.
- Pseudogoblet cells: usually linear, homogeneous cytoplasmic mucin.
- IM is randomly distributed, most dense proximally.
- Additional levels may be required as IM is patchy.
- Use of ancillary stains: no added value in routine practice [79–92].

Lichenoid Pattern

This pattern is defined by presence of a band of inflammatory cells mostly comprising lymphocytes along the interface of epithelium and lamina propria with resultant basal cell degeneration (Fig. 2.19a–c). The epithelium may be atrophic or acanthotic or show a mixture of both patterns. Characteristic apoptotic and dyskeratotic squamous cells also known as "Civatte" bodies are seen scattered throughout the epithelium. Dyskeratotic squamous cells and basal cell degeneration differentiate this pattern from lym-

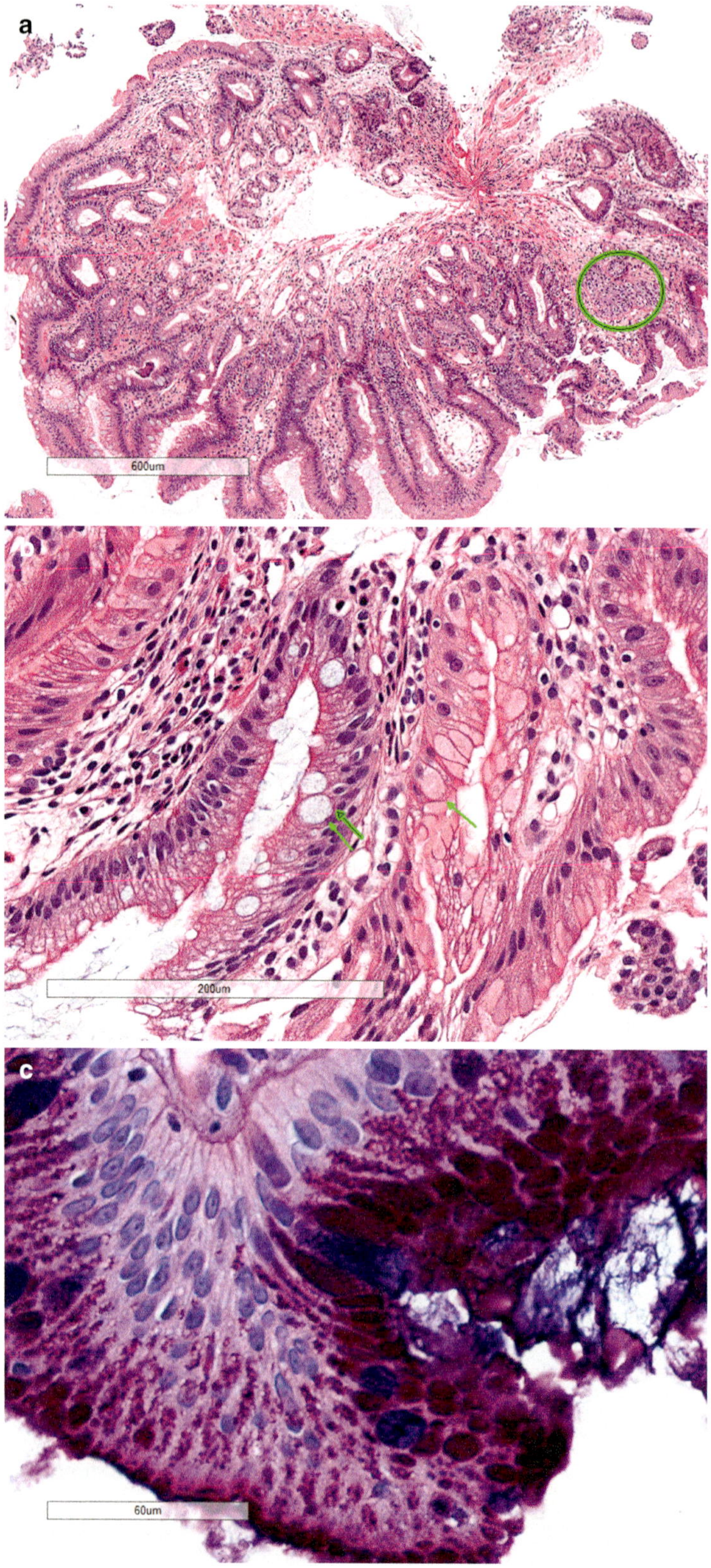

Fig. 2.18 Barrett's mucosa. (**a**) Interspersed goblet cells in the metaplastic CLM, note the squamous island (circle) (H&E). (**b**) Pseudogoblet cells with pink mucin—one arrow compared to true goblet cells—two arrows with blue mucin (H&E). (**c**) Pseudogoblet cells (PASD positive) and goblet cells (alcian blue positive). (**d**) IM-alcian blue-PASD. (**e**) CDX2 immunohistochemistry. (**f**) MUC2 immunohistochemistry

Fig. 2.18 (continued)

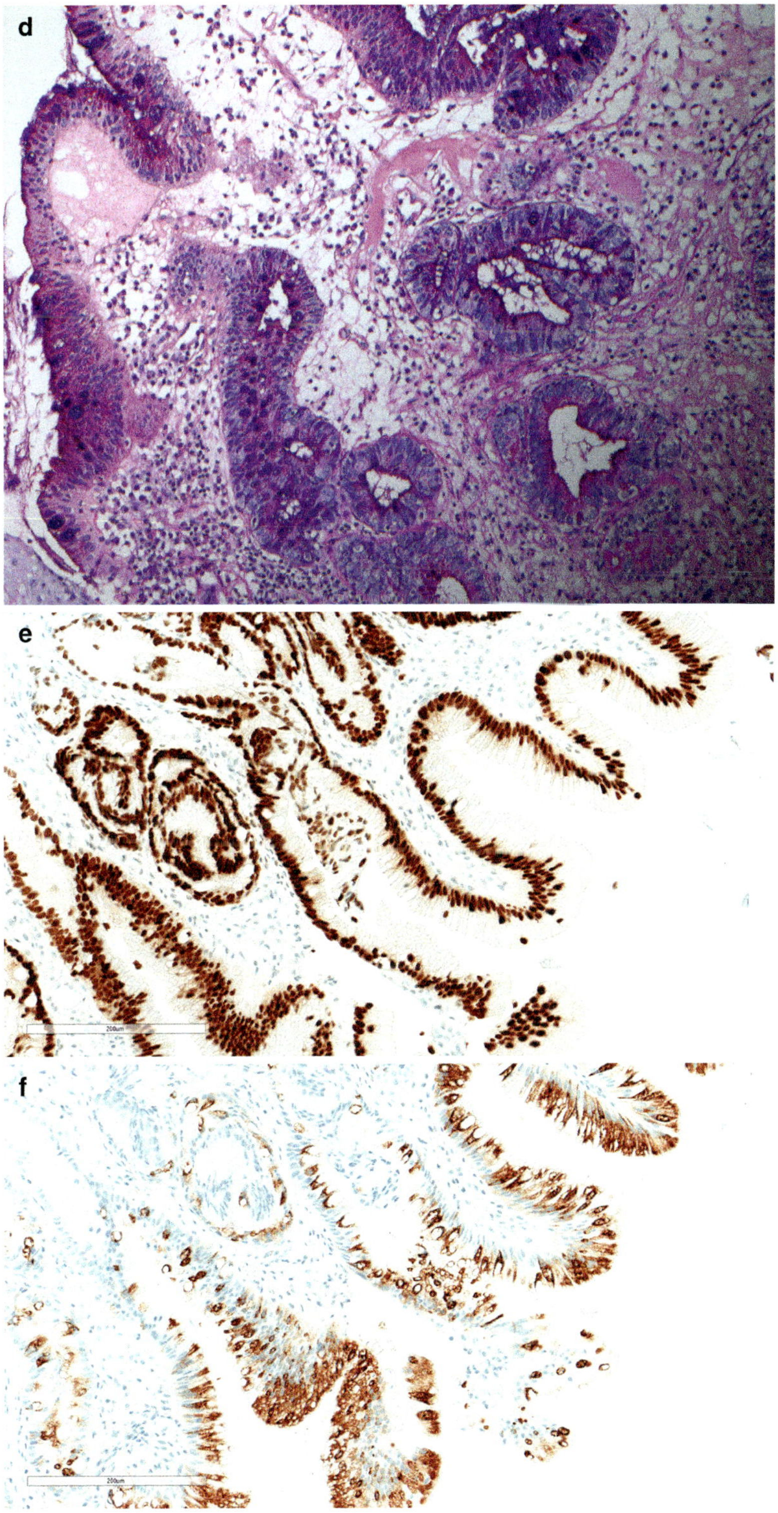

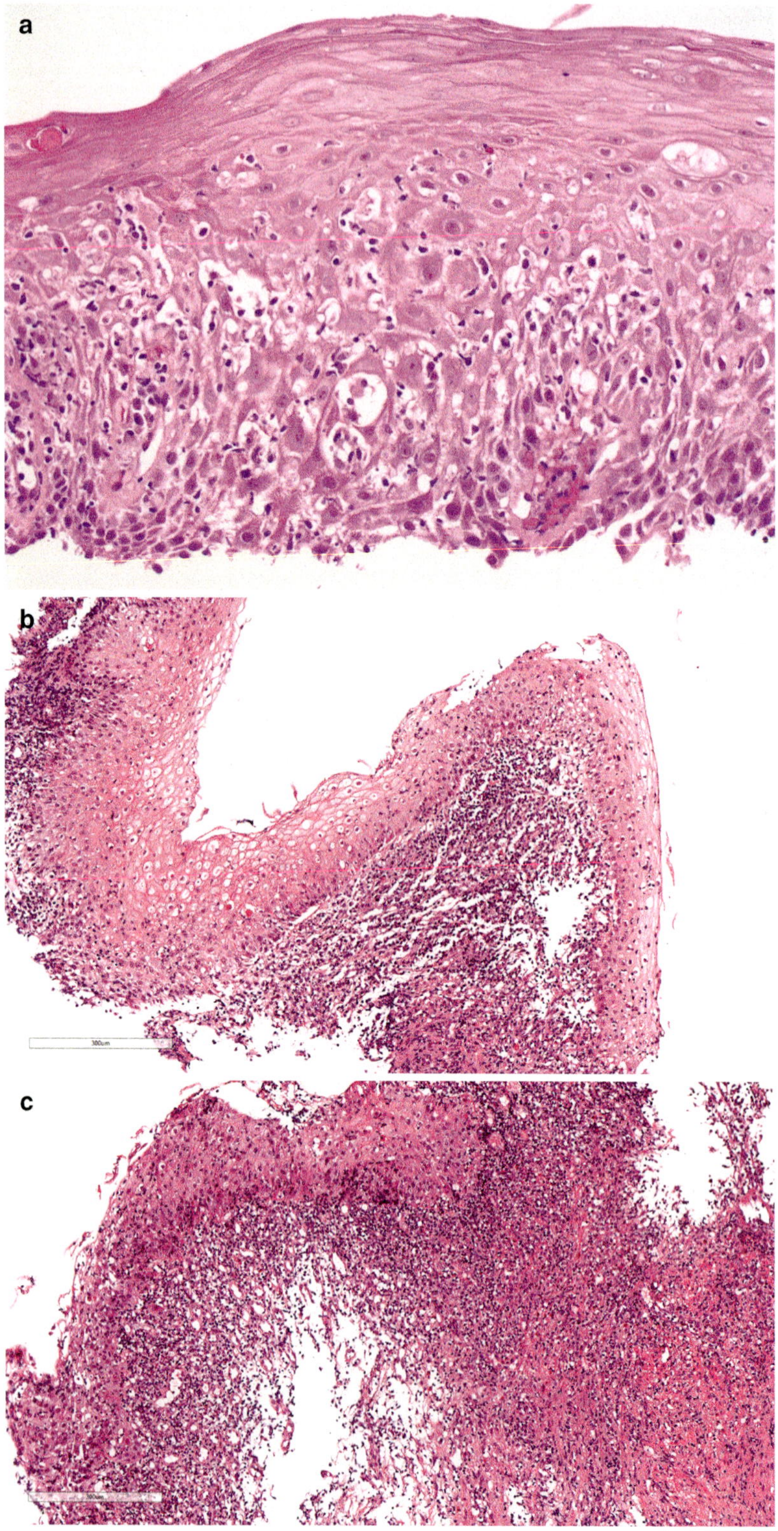

Fig. 2.19 Lichenoid pattern. (**a**) Characteristic apoptotic and dyskeratotic squamous cells of lichen planus. (**b**) Lichenoid pattern with partly atrophic squamous mucosa. (**c**) Lichenoid pattern with a heavy lymphocytic infiltrate in the lamina propria. (**d**) EBER-ISH positive cells in the lymphoid infiltrate in the case shown in (**c**) and (**d**)

d

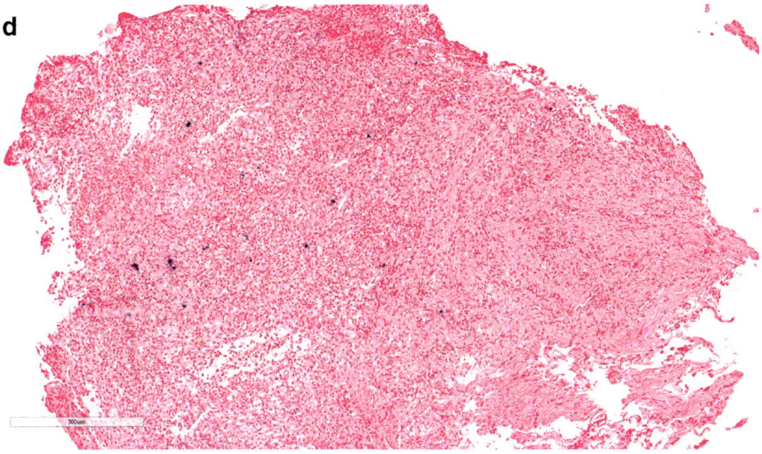

Fig. 2.19 (continued)

phocytic oesophagitis pattern. Lichenoid oesophagitis may appear to be an advanced lymphocytic inflammation-related damage beyond the lymphocytic oesophagitis pattern. There appears to be a strong correlation with Crohn's disease in children but not in adults.

A lichenoid oesophagitis pattern can be seen in association with the following conditions:

- Lichen planus oesophagitis (Fig. 2.19a).
- Rheumatologic conditions (rheumatoid arthritis, Raynaud's phenomenon, fibromyalgia, lupus and polymyalgia).
- Viral diseases (HIV, hepatitis B and hepatitis C), possibly EBV (Fig. 2.19d), and medications.
- Polypharmacy (in one study, 62% of patients with lichenoid oesophagitis were taking >3 medications including antihypertensives, antacids, levothyroxine, nonsteroidal anti-inflammatory drugs, steroids and mycophenolate).

The histologic features of oesophageal lichen planus differ from those in the skin. Cutaneous lichen planus is typically characterised by hypergranulosis, hyperkeratosis, acanthosis and "saw-tooth" elongation of the rete pegs. In comparison, the oesophageal epithelium, which normally lacks orthokeratosis or a granular layer, usually shows parakeratosis rather than orthohyperkeratosis and frequently lacks hypergranulosis. In addition, the oesophageal epithelium may be atrophic rather than acanthotic or it can show variable thinning and acanthosis. The histologic features of oesophageal lichen planus, therefore, more closely resemble those seen in oral rather than cutaneous disease.

Presence of a lichenoid pattern in oesophageal biopsies in the absence of previous or concurrent oral/cutaneous lichen planus and/or negative direct immunofluorescence is reported as lichenoid oesophagitis requiring further clinical and endoscopic correlation. The reason is being that histopathologic features of established oesophageal lichen planus and lichenoid oesophagitis are identical. Lichenoid pattern is the desirable term that is used once oesophageal lichen planus (LP) is excluded or when a diagnosis cannot be confirmed.

Medications such as gold, thiazides and antimalarials can induce lichen planus-like lesions and need to be excluded clinically.

Lichen Planus Oesophagitis

Lichen planus (LP) is an idiopathic papulosquamous eruption involving the skin, nails and mucosal surfaces. Mucosal lichen planus is predominantly a disease of middle-aged women. It can include lesions of the oral mucosa, pharynx and perineum but most commonly affects the oral mucosa (Fig. 2.19a–d).

Oesophageal LP most often affects the upper and middle thirds of the oesophagus. The characteristic endoscopic features of oesophageal LP include pseudomembranes, friable and inflamed mucosa, submucosal papules, lacy white plaques and erosions. In advanced disease, oesophageal strictures may form, mainly in the proximal oesophagus but also elsewhere in the oesophagus.

The histologic features of oesophageal lichen planus differ from those in the skin. Cutaneous lichen planus is typically characterised by hypergranulosis, hyperkeratosis, acanthosis and "sawtooth" elongation of the rete pegs. In comparison, the oesophageal epithelium, which normally lacks orthokeratosis or a granular layer, usually shows parakeratosis rather than orthohyperkeratosis and frequently lacks hypergranulosis. In addition, the oesophageal epithelium may be atrophic rather than acanthotic, or it can show variable thinning and acanthosis. The histologic features of oesophageal lichen planus, therefore, more closely resemble those seen in oral rather than cutaneous disease. The most characteristic finding in oesophageal lichen planus is a bandlike or lichenoid lymphocytic infiltrate involving the superficial lamina propria and basal epithelium. A predominance of mature T cells is present within the infiltrate, and these are associated with basal keratinocyte degeneration, often including characteristic Civatte bodies (which are necrotic keratinocytes with anucleate remnants) [2, 3, 93–96].

Squamous Proliferative Pattern

This pattern is characterised by various degrees of "proliferative" squamous mucosa. This pattern may look deceptively "normal" due to lack of inflammation in many occasions. Another deception is due to the nature of endoscopic biopsies in which orientation is a question. GI pathologists should pay attention to the endoscopic appearance and such information should be provided with the biopsy for accurate analysis.

Glycogenic Acanthosis

Multiple fragments of squamous epithelium may look deceptively "normal" due to lack of nuclear atypia and under low power in some lesions but may represent an endoscopically targeted lesion that appears as a white plaque, commonly in the distal oesophagus. Distended keratinocytes with intracytoplasmic glycogen of glycogenic acanthosis can be best appreciated if normal mucosa is also included in the biopsy (Fig. 2.20). PASD stain will highlight the pale colour of the keratinocytes with digested glycogen against normal keratinocytes in the background (two-toned appearance). These same cells with H&E will show pale pink cytoplasm with frosted glass texture. The basal layer is uninvolved. Diffuse glycogenic acanthosis can mimic candidiasis endoscopically and is considered a fairly specific manifestation of PTEN hamartoma syndrome. Endoscopic appearance may also suggest leukoplakia and lichenoid pattern of injury.

Squamous Papilloma

Squamous papilloma is another deceptive squamous proliferation (Fig. 2.21a, b). Papillomatous nature may be obvious in some biopsies with tongue-like but bland squamous proliferation, while in others, papillomatous nature may not be obvious. Endoscopic correlation is the key. Most oesophageal squamous papillomas are not related

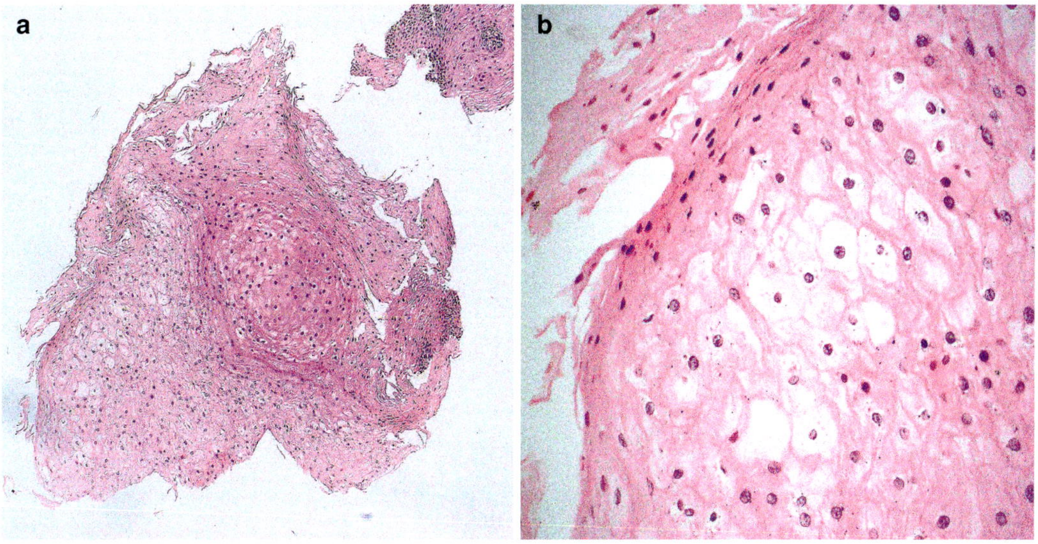

Fig. 2.20 Glycogenic acanthosis

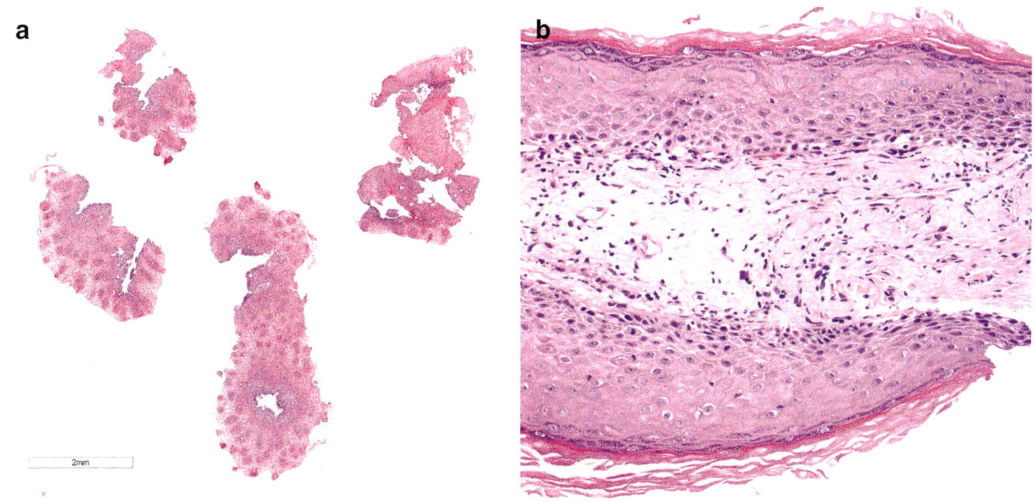

Fig. 2.21 (**a**, **b**) Squamous papilloma

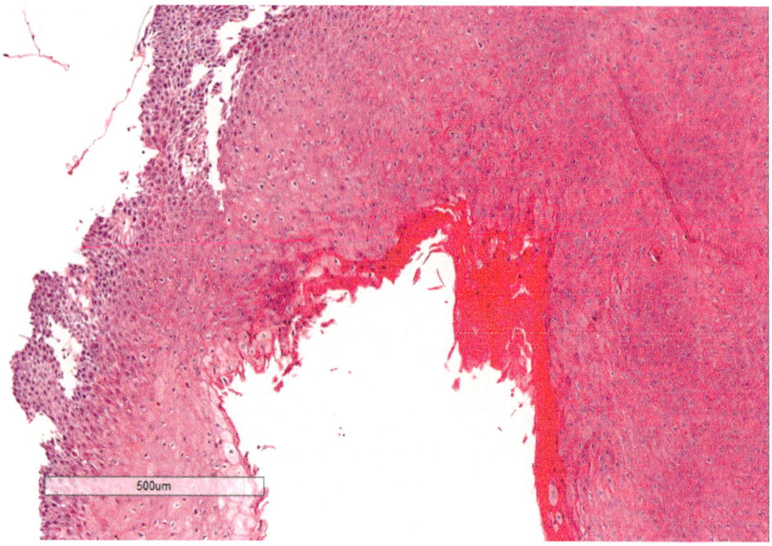

Fig. 2.22 Parakeratotic pattern

to HPV infection and viral cytopathic effect is rare. Currently HPV testing is not required once a squamous papilloma is diagnosed.

Epidermoid Metaplasia

These proliferations are difficult to identify in biopsies and microscopic features have been characterised in resections. Hence, they are regarded as flag bearers of squamous cell carcinoma (SCC). In resections, the lesions appear sharply demarcated from the adjacent normal mucosa and show squamous hyperplasia, basal expansion, acanthosis and a prominent granular layer with hyperorthokeratosis. Some consider these lesions to be a form of mature dysplasia [97, 98].

Parakeratotic Pattern

Presence of brightly eosinophilic surface squamous cells with abnormally retained nuclei characterises this pattern (Fig. 2.22). The colour itself is eye-catching as you start looking at the biopsies. Normal oesophageal mucosa is non-keratinising, and the parakeratotic pattern signifies injury. Other dominant patterns often accompany this pattern. However, parakeratotic pattern may present as the dominant pattern.

Parakeratotic pattern is seen in GORD, *Candida* oesophagitis, epidermoid metaplasia and sloughing oesophagitis as a sub-pattern.

Repair Pattern

Hyperplastic squamous epithelial fragments often show intraepithelial inflammation along with nuclear features such as nuclear enlargement, nucleoli and mitoses that may mimic neoplastic epithelium along with basal cell hyperplasia especially with severe reactive changes. However, these changes are largely confined to the basal layers, are non-abrupt and show gradual transition to normal mucosa. Basal layer maintains regular papillary elongations in contrast to irregular and fused basal projections in neoplastic mucosa. Medications and in particular chemotherapeutic agents as well as radiation can produce severe nuclear abnormalities; however, mucosa tends to be more atrophic and thinned out in the latter. These subtle features and clinical information are important clues to avoid overdiagnosis of neoplasia. Reactive hyperplastic squamous changes are common next to ulcerations/erosion. Step sections are often necessary.

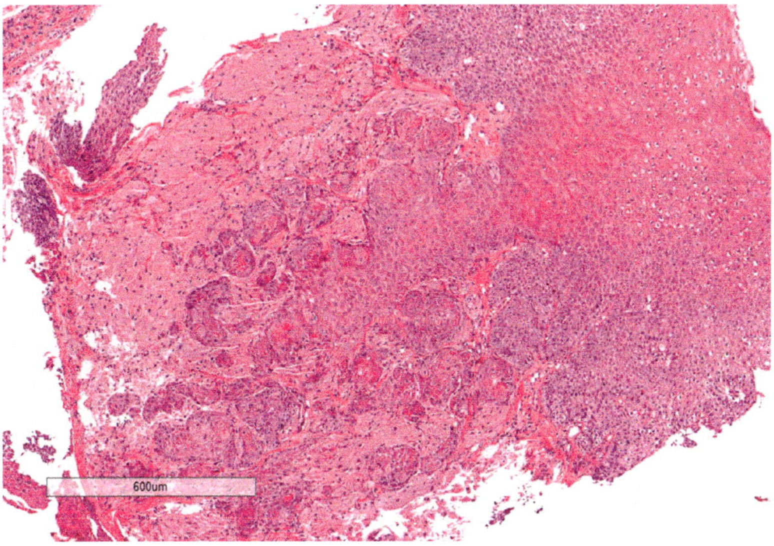

Fig. 2.23 Pseudoepitheliomatous hyperplasia: note underlying granular cell tumour

P16 immunostain may help as it sometimes delineates deceptively bland dysplasia (see neoplastic patterns). Ulcer base tissue with plump stromal cells and endothelium mimicking neoplasia is described earlier.

Pseudoepitheliomatous Hyperplasia

Hyperplastic squamous epithelium overlying a granular cell tumour is a recognised pitfall; in fact it may be misdiagnosed as SCC (see neoplastic patterns) (Fig. 2.23) (Box 2.19).

Box 2.19 When Biopsies of a Targeted Lesion that May Appear Nonneoplastic

Consider.

- Glycogenic acanthosis (GA)
- Squamous papilloma
- Epidermoid metaplasia
- Deceptive squamous dysplasia (differentiated)

Look for

- Parakeratotic pattern

Bizarre Stromal Reaction

Bizarre stromal reactions that may be present in an endoscopic biopsy may pose diagnostic difficulties with overdiagnosis of a malignancy (Fig. 2.24a–d). Endoscopically, patients may have a polypoid lesion. Microscopically, there are atypical cells associated with overlying squamous mucosa that show reactive changes generally with ulceration or erosion. Atypical cells could be stellate, spindle or epithelioid. They are not arranged in a specific pattern. The cells can show marked pleomorphism with large nuclei and nucleoli, raising concern for malignancy. Mitoses are scattered and abnormal forms have not been reported. Markers specific for malignancies such as lymphoma, melanoma, carcinoma and sarcoma are negative (see Chap. 3). Vimentin is often positive. Proliferation index is low. The case illustrated here was also negative for ALK1, CMV and EBER-ISH. Clinicopathological correlation and follow-up are prudent [99–101].

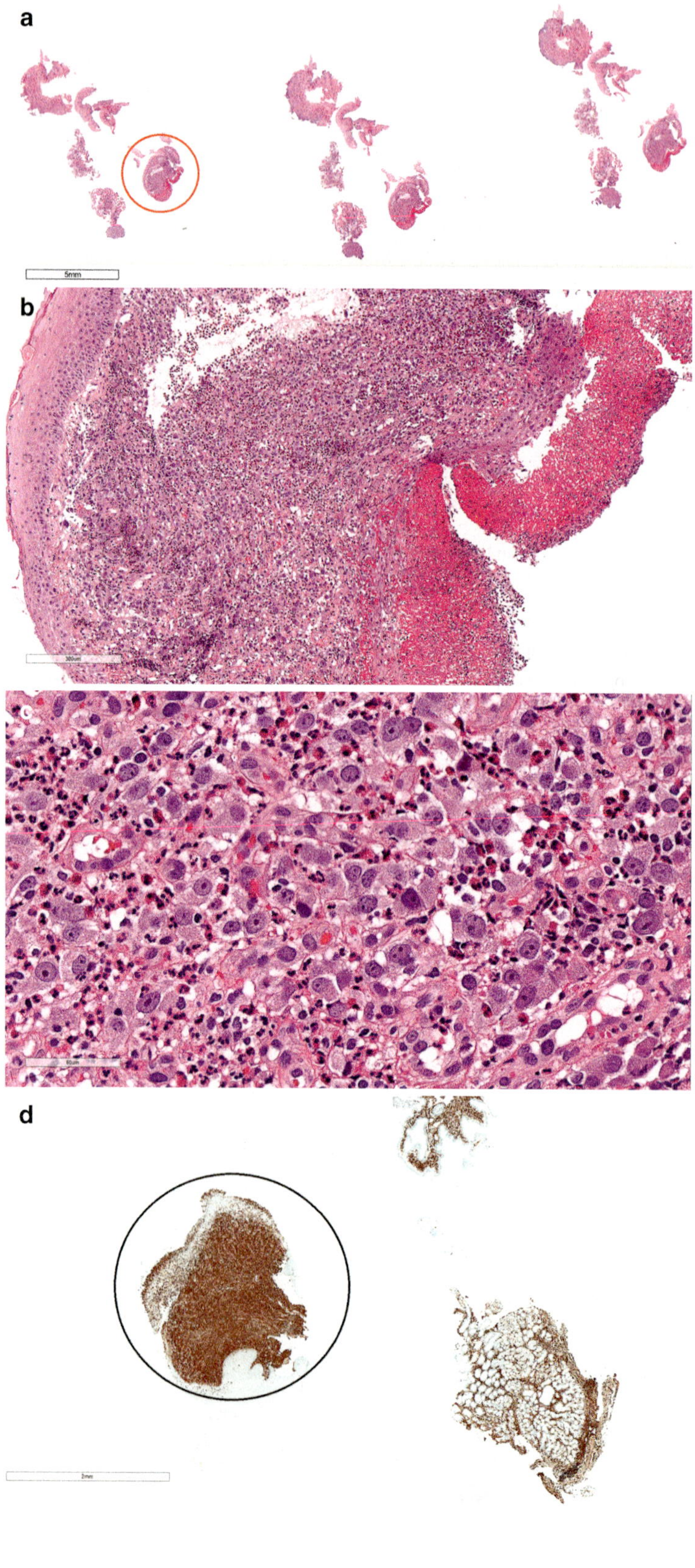

Fig. 2.24 (**a**–**d**) Bizarre stromal reaction. (**a**) Multiple fragments of oesophageal mucosa with one ulcerated fragment. (**b**) Ulceration and underlying stromal inflammation and "atypia". (**c**) Note large bizarre "epithelioid" cells. (**d**) Strong vimentin positivity. The biopsy was negative for an extended panel of immunohistochemical stains including cytokeratins,melanoma and lymphoid markers (not illustrated)

References

1. Noffsinger AE. Update on esophagitis: controversial and underdiagnosed causes. Arch Pathol Lab Med. 2009;133(7):1087–95.
2. Grin A, et al. Esophagitis: old histologic concepts and new thoughts. Arch Pathol Lab Med. 2015;139(6):723–9.
3. Almashat SJ, Duan L, Goldsmith JD. Non-reflux esophagitis: a review of inflammatory diseases of the esophagus exclusive of reflux esophagitis. In Seminars in diagnostic pathology 2014, 31(2): 89–99. WB Saunders, Philadelphia, PA.
4. Sutton FM, Graham DY, Goodgame RW. Infectious esophagitis. Gastrointest Endosc Clin N Am. 1994;4(4):713–29.
5. Choi JH, Lee CG, Lim YJ, Kang HW, Lim CY, Choi JS. Prevalence and risk factors of esophageal candidiasis in healthy individuals: a single center experience in Korea. Yonsei Med J. 2013;54(1):160–5.
6. Greenson JK. Infections of the esophagus. Am J Surg Pathol. 2002;7(1):19–26.
7. Greenson JK, Beschorner WE, Boitnott JK, Yardley JH. Prominent mononuclear cell infiltrate is characteristic of herpes esophagitis. Hum Pathol. 1991;22(6):541–9.
8. Canalejo E, Durán FG, Cabello N, Martínez JG. Herpes esophagitis in healthy adults and adolescents: report of 3 cases and review of the literature. Medicine. 2010,89(4):204 10.
9. Itoh T, Takahashi T, Kusaka K, Kawaura K, Nakagawa Y, Yamakawa JI, Kanda T. Herpes simplex esophagitis from 1307 autopsy cases. J Gastroenterol Hepatol. 2003;18(12):1407–11.
10. Zimmermann D, Criblez DH, Dellon ES, Bussmann C, Pfeifer D, Froh M, Straumann A. Acute herpes simplex viral esophagitis occurring in 5 immunocompetent individuals with eosinophilic esophagitis. ACG Case Rep J. 2016;3(3):165.
11. Wishingrad M. Sexually transmitted esophagitis: primary herpes simplex virus type 2 infection in a healthy man. Gastrointest Endosc. 1999;50(6):845–6.
12. Kato S, Yamamoto R, Yoshimitsu S, et al. Herpes simplex esophagitis in the immunocompetent host. Dis Esophagus. 2005;18:340.
13. Marinho AV, Bonfim VM, de Alencar LR, Pinto SA, de Araújo Filho JA. Herpetic esophagitis in immunocompetent medical student. Case Rep Infect Dis. 2014;2014:930459.
14. Kadayakkara DK, Candelaria A, Kwak YE, Loeser C. Herpes simplex virus-2 esophagitis in a young immunocompetent adult. Case Rep Gastroint Med. 2016;2016:7603484.
15. Cowdry EV. The problem of intranuclear inclusions in virus diseases. Arch Pathol. 1934;18:527–42.
16. Ranjan P, Gupta V, Goyal M, Dhawan S, Gupta P, Kumar M, Sachdeva M. Cytomegalovirus infection in gastrointestinal tract: a case series of three patients and review of literature. J Digest Endosc. 2015;6(3):133.
17. Wang H, Kuo C, Lin W, et al. The clinical characteristics and manifestations of cytomegalovirus esophagitis. Dis Esophagus. 2016;29:392.
18. Schwartz DA, Wilcox CM. Atypical cytomegalovirus inclusions in gastrointestinal biopsy specimens from patients with the acquired immunodeficiency syndrome: diagnostic role of in situ nucleic acid hybridization. Hum Pathol. 1992;23(9):1019–26.
19. Bonetti R. Luca, et al. Cytomegalovirus infection of the upper gastrointestinal tract: a clinical and pathological study of 30 cases. Scand J Gastroenterol. 2011;46(10):1228–35.
20. Greenson JK. Macrophage aggregates in cytomegalovirus esophagitis. Hum Pathol. 1997;28(3):375–8.
21. Pape M, Mandraveli K, Sidiropoulos I, Koliouskas D, Alexiou-Daniel S, Frantzidou F. Unusual Epstein-Barr esophageal infection in an immunocompetent patient: a case report. J Med Case Reports. 2009;3(1):7314.
22. Rudolph I, Goldstein F, DiMarino AJ. Crohn's disease of the esophagus: three cases and a literature review. Canadian J Gastroenterol Hepatol. 2001;15(2):117–22.
23. Naranjo-Rodríguez A, Solórzano-Peck G, López-Rubio F, Calañas-Continente A, Gálvez-Calderón C, González-Galilea A, Hervás-Molina A. Isolated oesophageal involvement of Crohn's disease. Eur J Gastroenterol Hepatol. 2003;15(10):1123–6.
24. Geboes K, Janssens J, Rutgeerts P, Vantrappen G. Crohn's disease of the esophagus. J Clin Gastroenterol. 1986;8:31.
25. Decker GA, Loftus EV, Pasha TM, Tremaine WJ, Sandborn WJ. Crohn's disease of the esophagus: clinical features and outcomes. Inflamm Bowel Dis. 2001;7(2):113–9.
26. Mashako MN, Cezard JP, Navarro J, Mougenot JF, Sonsino E, Gargouri A, Maherzi A. Crohn's disease lesions in the upper gastrointestinal tract: correlation between clinical, radiological, endoscopic, and histological features in adolescents and children. J Pediatr Gastroenterol Nutr. 1989;8(4):442–6.
27. De Felice KM, Katzka DA, Raffals LE. Crohn's disease of the esophagus: clinical features and treatment outcomes in the biologic era. Inflamm Bowel Dis. 2015;21(9):2106–13.
28. Pantanowitz L, Gelrud A, Apstein M, Nasser I. Crohn's disease of the esophagus. Ear Nose Throat J. 2004;83:420–2.
29. Roy-Ghanta S, Larosa DF, Katzka DA. Atopic characteristics of adult patients with eosinophilic esophagitis. Clin Gastroenterol Hepatol. 2008;6(5):531–5.
30. Kim HP, Vance RB, Shaheen NJ, Dellon ES. The prevalence and diagnostic utility of endoscopic fea-

tures of eosinophilic esophagitis: a meta-analysis. Clin Gastroenterol Hepatol. 2012;10(9):988–96.
31. Liacouras CA, Furuta GT, Hirano I, Atkins D, Attwood SE, Bonis PA, Burks AW, Chehade M, Collins MH, Dellon ES, Dohil R. Eosinophilic esophagitis: updated consensus recommendations for children and adults. J Allergy Clin Immunol. 2011;128(1):3–20.
32. Yantiss RK. Eosinophils in the GI tract: how many is too many and what do they mean? Mod Pathol. 2015;28:S7–21.
33. Lee S, de Boer WB, Naran A, Leslie C, Raftopoulous S, Ee H, Kumarasinghe MP. More than just counting eosinophils: proximal oesophageal involvement and subepithelial sclerosis are major diagnostic criteria for eosinophilic oesophagitis. J Clin Pathol. 2010;63(7):644–7.
34. Dellon ES, Speck O, Woodward K, Covey S, Rusin S, Shaheen NJ, Woosley JT. Distribution and variability of esophageal eosinophilia in patients undergoing upper endoscopy. Mod Pathol. 2015;28(3):383–90.
35. Dellon ES, Gonsalves N, Hirano I, Furuta GT, Liacouras CA, Katzka DA. ACG clinical guideline: evidenced based approach to the diagnosis and management of esophageal eosinophilia and eosinophilic esophagitis (EoE). Am J Gastroenterol. 2013;108(5):679–92.
36. Attwood SE, Smyrk TC, Demeester TR, Jones JB. Esophageal eosinophilia with dysphagia. Dig Dis Sci. 1993;38(1):109–16.
37. Davis BP, Rothenberg ME. Mechanisms of disease of eosinophilic esophagitis. Annu Rev Pathol. 2016;11:365–93.
38. García-Compeán D, González JA, García CA, Gutiérrez JP, Quintana OB, Rodríguez GG, Ruiz MA, de León Valdez D, Quintana JO, Garza HJ. Prevalence of eosinophilic esophagitis in patients with refractory gastroesophageal reflux disease symptoms: a prospective study. Dig Liver Dis. 2011;43(3):204–8.
39. Kapel RC, Miller JK, Torres C, Aksoy S, Lash R, Katzka DA. Eosinophilic esophagitis: a prevalent disease in the United States that affects all age groups. Gastroenterology. 2008;134(5):1316–21.
40. Sherrill JD, Rothenberg ME. Genetic dissection of eosinophilic esophagitis provides insight into disease pathogenesis and treatment strategies. J Allergy Clin Immunol. 2011;128(1):23–32.
41. Hirano I, Moy N, Heckman MG, Thomas CS, Gonsalves N, Achem SR. Endoscopic assessment of the oesophageal features of eosinophilic oesophagitis: validation of a novel classification and grading system. Gut. 2013;62(4):489–95.
42. Lucendo AJ, Molina-Infante J, Arias Á, von Arnim U, Bredenoord AJ, Bussmann C, Amil Dias J, Bove M, González-Cervera J, Larsson H, Miehlke S. Guidelines on eosinophilic esophagitis: evidence-based statements and recommendations for diagnosis and management in children and adults. United European Gastroenterol J. 2017;5(3):335–58.
43. Rubio CA, Sjödahl K, Lagergren J. Lymphocytic esophagitis. Am J Clin Pathol. 2006;125(3):432–7.
44. Cohen S, Saxena A, Waljee A, Piraka C, Purdy J, Appelman H, McKenna B, Elmunzer BJ, Singal AG. Lymphocytic esophagitis: a diagnosis of increasing frequency. J Clin Gastroenterol. 2012;46(10):828.
45. Conner JR, Sanchez CA, Reid BJ, Vaughan TL, Blount PL, Wang HH, Odze RD, Srivastava A. Lymphocytic esophagitis in Barrett's esophagus: correlation with patient symptoms and risk factors. In: Laboratory investigation, vol. 94. New York, NY: Nature Publishing Group; 2014. p. 169A–70A.
46. Ebach DR, Vanderheyden AD, Ellison JM, Jensen CS. Lymphocytic esophagitis: a possible manifestation of pediatric upper gastrointestinal Crohn's disease. Inflamm Bowel Dis. 2011;17(1):45–9.
47. Sutton L, Heintz D, Patel A, Weinberg A. Lymphocytic esophagitis in children. Inflamm Bowel Dis. 2014;20:1324.
48. Kissiedu J, Thota PN, Gohel T, Lopez R, Gordon IO. Post-ablation lymphocytic esophagitis in Barrett esophagus with high grade dysplasia or intramucosal carcinoma. Mod Pathol. 2016;29:599.
49. Filipovich AH, Weisdorf D, Pavletic S, Socie G, Wingard JR, Lee SJ, Martin P, Chien J, Przepiorka D, Couriel D, Cowen EW. National Institutes of Health consensus development project on criteria for clinical trials in chronic graft-versus-host disease: I. Diagnosis and staging working group report. Biol Blood Marrow Transplant. 2005;11(12):945–56.
50. Shulman HM, Kleiner D, Lee SJ, Morton T, Pavletic SZ, Farmer E, Moresi JM, Greenson J, Janin A, Martin PJ, McDonald G. Histopathologic diagnosis of chronic graft-versus-host disease: National Institutes of Health consensus development project on criteria for clinical trials in chronic graft-versus-host disease: II. Pathology working group report. Biol Blood Marrow Transplant. 2006;12(1):31–47.
51. Parfitt JR, Jayakumar S, Driman DK. Mycophenolate mofetil-related gastrointestinal mucosal injury: variable injury patterns, including graft-versus-host disease-like changes. Am J Surg Pathol. 2008;32(9):1367–72.
52. Panarelli NC. Drug-induced injury in the gastrointestinal tract. In Seminars in diagnostic pathology 2014, 31(2):165–175. WB Saunders, Philadelphia, PA.
53. Chen Z, Scudiere JR, Montgomery E. Medication-induced upper gastrointestinal tract injury. J Clin Pathol. 2009;62(2):113–9.
54. Misdraji J. Drug-induced pathology of the upper gastrointestinal tract. Diagn Histopathol. 2008;14(9):411–8.
55. Seminerio J, et al. Medication-associated lesions of the GI tract. Gastrointest Endosc. 2014;79(1):140–50.
56. Boyce HW Jr. Drug-induced esophageal damage: diseases of medical progress. Gastrointest Endosc. 1998;47:547–50.

57. Shih AR, et al. Drug-induced pathology of the upper gastrointestinal tract. Diagn Histopathol. 2017;23(2):84–95.
58. Daniels JA, et al. Gastrointestinal tract epithelial changes associated with taxanes: marker of drug toxicity versus effect. Am J Surg Pathol. 2008;32(3):473–7.
59. Abraham SC, Cruz-Correa M, Lee LA, Yardley JH, Wu TT. Alendronate-associated esophageal injury: pathologic and endoscopic features. Mod Pathol. 1999;12(12):1152–7.
60. Nagano Y, Matsui H, Shimokawa O, et al. Bisphosphonate-induced gastrointestinal mucosal injury is mediated by mitochondrial superoxide production and lipid peroxidation. J Clin Biochem Nutr. 2012;51:196–203.
61. Abraham SC, Bhagavan BS, Lee LA, Rashid A, Wu TT. Upper gastrointestinal tract injury in patients receiving kayexalate (sodium polystyrene sulfonate) in sorbitol: clinical, endoscopic, and histopathologic findings. Am J Surg Pathol. 2001;25(5):637–44.
62. Xiao SY, Zhao L, Hart J, Semrad CE. Doxycycline-induced gastric and esophageal mucosal injuries with vascular degeneration. Am J Surg Pathol. 2013;37(7):1115–6.
63. Brown IS, Bettington M. Doxycycline induced oesophagitis: five cases highlighting a distinctive pattern of injury. Pathology. 2017;49(1):90–2.
64. Banisaeed N, Truding RM, Chang CH. Tetracycline-induced spongiotic esophagitis: a new endoscopic and histopathologic finding. Gastrointest Endosc. 2003;58(2):292–4.
65. Swanson BJ, Limketkai BN, Liu TC, et al. Sevelamer crystals in the gastrointestinal tract (GIT): a new entity associated with mucosal injury. Am J Surg Pathol. 2013;37:1686e93.
66. Purdy JK, Appelman HD, McKenna BJ. Sloughing esophagitis is associated with chronic debilitation and medications that injure the esophageal mucosa. Mod Pathol. 2012;25(5):767–75.
67. Carmack SW, Vemulapalli R, Spechler SJ, Genta RM. Esophagitis dissecans superficialis ("sloughing esophagitis"): a clinicopathologic study of 12 cases. Am J Surg Pathol. 2009;33(12):1789–94.
68. Ma C, Limketkai BN, Montgomery EA. Recently highlighted non-neoplastic pathologic entities of the upper GI tract and their clinical significance. Gastrointest Endosc. 2014;80(6):960–9.
69. Patil R, Sunkara T, Ona MA, Gaduputi V, Reddy M. Fungal esophagitis presenting with esophagitis dissecans superficialis: cause or concurrence? A diagnostic conundrum. Gastroenterol Res. 2016;9(6):108.
70. Hart PA, Romano RC, Moreira RK, Ravi K, Sweetser S. Esophagitis dissecans superficialis: clinical, endoscopic, and histologic features. Dig Dis Sci. 2015;60(7):2049–57.
71. De S, Williams G. Esophagitis dissecans superficialis: a case report and literature review. Can J Gastroenterol. 2013;27(10):563.
72. Dent J, Brun J, Fendrick AM, Fennerty MB, Janssens J, Kahrilas PJ, Lauritsen K, Reynolds JC, Shaw M, Talley NJ. An evidence-based appraisal of reflux disease management—the Genval Workshop Report. Gut. 1998;44(suppl 2):S1–6.
73. Mattox HE, Richter JE. Prolonged ambulatory esophageal pH monitoring in the evaluation of gastroesophageal reflux disease. Am J Med. 1990;89(3):345–56.
74. Vantrappen G, Janssens J. Gastro-oesophageal reflux disease, an important cause of angina-like chest pain. Scand J Gastroenterol Suppl. 1988;168:73–9.
75. Sontag SJ. Gastroesophageal reflux and asthma. Am J Med. 1997;103:84S–90S.
76. Fiocca R, Mastracci L, Riddell R, Takubo K, Vieth M, Yerian L, Sharma P, Fernström P, Ruth M. Development of consensus guidelines for the histologic recognition of microscopic esophagitis in patients with gastroesophageal reflux disease: the Esohisto project. Hum Pathol. 2010;41(2):223–31.
77. Krugmann J, Neumann H, Vieth M, Armstrong D. What is the role of endoscopy and oesophageal biopsies in the management of GERD? Best Pract Res Clin Gastroenterol. 2013;27(3):373–85.
78. Winter HS, Madara JL, Stafford RJ, Grand RJ, Quinlan JE, Goldman H. Intraepithelial eosinophils: a new diagnostic criterion for reflux esophagitis. Gastroenterology. 1982;83(4):818–23.
79. Srivastava A, Appelman H, Goldsmith JD, Davison JM, Hart J, Krasinskas AM. The Use of Ancillary Stains in the Diagnosis of Barrett Esophagus and Barrett Esophagus–associated Dysplasia Recommendations From the Rodger C. Haggitt Gastrointestinal Pathology Society. Am J Surg Pathol. 2017;41:e8–e21.
80. Younes M, Ertan A, Ergun G, et al. Goblet cell mimickers in esophageal biopsies are not associated with an increased risk for dysplasia. Arch Pathol Lab Med. 2007;131:571–5.
81. Smith J, et al. Intestinal metaplasia is present in most if not all patients who have undergone endoscopic mucosal resection for esophageal adenocarcinoma. Am J Surg Pathol. 2016;40:537–43.
82. Allanson BM, Bonavita J, Mirzai B, Khor TS, Raftopoulos SC, de Boer WB, Brown IS, Kumarasinghe MP. Early Barrett esophagus-related neoplasia in segments 1 cm or longer is always associated with intestinal metaplasia. Mod Pathol. 2017;30:1170. https://doi.org/10.1038/modpathol.2017.36.
83. Paull A, Trier J, Dalton D, et al. The histologic spectrum of Barrett's esophagus. N Engl J Med. 1976;295:476–80.
84. Chandrasoma PT, Der R, Dalton P, et al. Distribution and significance of epithelial types in columnar-lined esophagus. Am J Surg Pathol. 2001;25:1188–93.
85. Bhat S, Coleman HG, Yousef F, et al. Risk of malignant progression in Barrett's Esophagus patients:

results from a large population-based study. J Natl Cancer Inst. 2011;103:1049–57.
86. Hvid-Jensen F, Pedersen L, Drewes AM, et al. Incidence of Adenocarcinoma among Patients with Barrett's Esophagus. N Engl J Med. 2011;365: 1375.
87. Bansal A, McGregor DH, Anand O, et al. Presence or absence of intestinal metaplasia but not its burden is associated with prevalent high-grade dysplasia and cancer in Barrett's esophagus. Dis Esophagus. 2014;27(8):751–6.
88. Spechler SJ, Sharma P, Souza RF, et al. American gastroenterological association medical position statement on the management of Barrett's esophagus. Gastroenterology. 2011;140:1084–91.
89. Shaheen NJ, Falk GW, Iyer PG, et al. ACG clinical guideline: diagnosis and management of Barrett's esophagus. Am J Gastroenterol. 2015;108:1238–49.
90. Fitzgerald RC, di Pietro M, Ragunath K, Ang Y, Kang JY, Watson P, Trudgill N, Patel P, Kaye PV, Sanders S, O'donovan M. British Society of Gastroenterology guidelines on the diagnosis and management of Barrett's oesophagus. Gut. 2014;63(1):7–42.
91. Whiteman DC, Appleyard M, Bahin FF, Bobryshev YV, Bourke MJ, Brown I, Chung A, Clouston A, Dickins E, Emery J, Eslick GD. Australian clinical practice guidelines for the diagnosis and management of Barrett's esophagus and early esophageal adenocarcinoma. J Gastroenterol Hepatol. 2015;30(5):804–20.
92. Oberg S, Johansson J, Wenner J, et al. Endoscopic surveillance of columnar-lined esophagus: frequency of intestinal metaplasia detection and impact of antireflux surgery. Ann Surg. 2001;234:619–26.
93. Salaria SN, et al. Lichenoid esophagitis: clinicopathologic overlap with established esophageal lichen planus. Am J Surg Pathol. 2013;37(12):1889–94.
94. Ma C, Limketkai BN, Montgomery EA. Recently highlighted non-neoplastic pathologic entities of the upper GI tract and their clinical significance. Gastrointest Endosc. 2014;80(6):960–9.
95. Katzka DA, Smyrk TC, Bruce AJ, et al. Variations in presentations of esophageal involvement in lichen planus. Clin Gastroenterol Hepatol. 2010;8:777–82.
96. Chandan VS, Murray JA, Abraham SC. Esophageal lichen planus. Arch Pathol Lab Med. 2008;132(6):1026–9.
97. Cottreau J, Gruchy S, Kamionek M, Lauwers GY, Arnason T. Prevalence of oesophageal epidermoid metaplasia in 1048 consecutive patients and 58 patients with squamous neoplasms. Histopathology. 2016;68:988.
98. Singhi AD, Arnold CA, Crowder CD, Lam-Himlin DM, Voltaggio L, Montgomery EA. Esophageal leukoplakia or epidermoid metaplasia: a clinicopathological study of 18 patients. Mod Pathol. 2014;27(1):38–43.
99. Dhungel BM, De Petris G. Bizarre stromal cells in the esophagus: report of 2 cases and literature review. Int J Surg Pathol. 2013;21:368–72.
100. Simonetta Piana MD. Riccardo Valli, Roberto Igino Sacchero, Bizarre Stromal Cells in the Esophagus. A New Case. Int J Surg Pathol. 2014;22(4):383–4.
101. Gill P, Piris J, Warren BF. Bizarre stromal cells in the esophagus. Histopathology. 2003;42:88–90.

Oesophagus: Neoplastic Patterns and Mimics

3

M. Priyanthi Kumarasinghe,
Benjamin M. Allanson, Spiro C. Raftopoulos,
and Gregory Y. Lauwers

Contents

M. P. Kumarasinghe (✉)
Department of Anatomical Pathology, PathWest Laboratory Medicine, QEII Medical Centre and University of Western Australia, Perth, WA, Australia
e-mail: priyanthi.kumarasinghe@health.wa.gov.au

B. M. Allanson
Department of Tissue Pathology and Diagnostic Oncology, Royal Prince Alfred Hospital and School of Pathology and Laboratory Medicine, Sydney, NSW, Australia

University of Western Australia, Perth, Australia

S. C. Raftopoulos
Interventional Endoscopist and Gastroenterologist, Department of Gastroenterology, Sir Charles Gairdner Hospital, Nedlands, WA, Australia

University of Western Australia, Perth, WA, Australia

G. Y. Lauwers
Gastrointestinal Pathology Service, Department of Pathology, Moffitt Cancer Center, Tampa, FL, USA

Similar to the rest of the tubular gut, the most common neoplastic pattern encountered in an oesophageal biopsy is the epithelial pattern as epithelial neoplasms are the most common tumours. The two main subtypes of carcinomas are squamous cell carcinoma, which is more common in the developing world, and oesophageal adenocarcinoma, which is more common in the developed world. Primary neuroendocrine neoplasms are uncommon. Lymphomas are exceedingly rare. Mesenchymal tumours are uncommon of which leiomyomas are the most common. Oesophagus is the most common site for intramural leiomyomas

M. P. Kumarasinghe, I. Brown (eds.), *Endoscopic Biopsy Interpretation*,
https://doi.org/10.1007/978-3-319-79117-3_3

of the tubular gut. Gastrointestinal stromal tumours are uncommon in the oesophagus. Granular cell tumours are rare tumours of the tubular gut, but the oesophagus is the most common site. Endoscopic biopsies targeting subepithelial mesenchymal lesions are not often representative unless special techniques such as tunnel biopsies or Endoscopic Ultra Sound-guided (EUS) Fine Needle Aspirations are performed, highlighting the importance of clinicopathologic correlation. Epithelial neoplasia is the most frequently encountered and, is most often the cause of diagnostic dilemmas in day-to-day reporting. Therefore, the epithelial patterns are discussed in more detail in this chapter and the others with less emphasis.

Often there is a high index of clinical and endoscopic suspicion for oesophageal neoplasms. However, gastroenterologists also identify apparent polypoid/nodular lesions and plaques that require histopathologic confirmation to confirm or exclude neoplasia. Finally, intraepithelial lesions of both squamous and glandular origin can be subtle on endoscopic examination.

It has also been shown in past studies that missed cancers occur in higher frequencies where another abnormality is detected, such as reflux changes, and no biopsies have been taken [1]. It is for this reason that many would now perform random biopsies from areas of apparent benign disease, to exclude unsuspected neoplasia.

Macroscopic appearance has been strongly linked into depth of invasion with Paris 0-I, 0-IIc/III highly predictive of submucosal invasive cancer versus Paris 0-IIa, IIb, and IIc more consistent with intramucosal cancer [2]. Therefore, ideally when lesions are targeted for biopsy, the endoscopist should provide the pathologist the macroscopy of the lesion as characterised by the Paris classification, the location as measured in centimetres from the teeth, and the position in a clockface orientation with the scope in a neutral position.

Epithelial Pattern with No Stromal Invasion

Intraepithelial lesions are commonly known as dysplasia or intraepithelial neoplasia (IEN). The two most common neoplastic epithelial patterns in the oesophagus represent squamous and glandular lesions. The distinction of the two types of epithelia in endoscopic biopsies is often not difficult. Therefore, as it happens in practice, the focus and further details are discussed under the squamous and glandular pattern.

The common challenges are distinguishing neoplastic from nonneoplastic lesions and differentiating those neoplastic lesions with stromal invasion (invasive carcinomas) from those without stromal invasion (dysplasia also known as intraepithelial neoplasia). Grading of intraepithelial lesions is required in an endoscopic biopsy. Biomarker testing may be indicated in invasive carcinomas.

Biopsies obtained from an endoscopically visible/targeted lesion may show deceptively bland appearance or be obviously abnormal. Endoscopic appearance is vital, and there are a number of pathological entities to consider at microscopic examination. A nodular/polypoid lesion with a clinical query of a neoplasm can co-exist with non neoplastic inflammatory conditions. Nonneoplastic entities are discussed in the preceding section. Irrespective of the type of epithelium dysplastic (intraepithelial neoplastic) lesions of the oesophageal mucosa shows abrupt transition from normal to abnormal that is a very useful feature in the distinction from inflammatory/reactive conditions.

Squamous Pattern with Atypia and No Invasion (Dysplastic/Intraepithelial neoplastic Pattern)

Squamo-proliferative pattern with cytological atypia featuring abrupt transition between dysplastic and non-dysplastic mucosa seen under low power signifies this pattern (Fig. 3.1).

Along with atypia the epithelium is usually thickened and proliferative. The basal layer is invariably involved. Neoplastic squamous pattern will show squamous atypia of varying degrees. Abnormal keratinocytes and parakeratosis are often seen, and corresponding endoscopic description may be the presence of a white plaque or a patch. Dysplastic cells are usually enlarged and show large rounded nuclei with higher N/C ratio, membrane irregularity, hyperchromasia, prominent nucleoli, and increased mitoses including abnormal forms (Figs. 3.1, 3.2, and 3.3). Dyskeratotic cells with intense eosinophilia are also noted. Low-grade intraepithelial lesions (IELs) can be difficult to diagnose, whereas high-grade IELs and nonkeratinising dysplasia are less problematic. Biopsy fragments that show dysplastic squamous patterns need to be appreciated with clues that may lead to a correct diagnosis after endoscopic correlation. Some patterns show subtle microscopic changes.

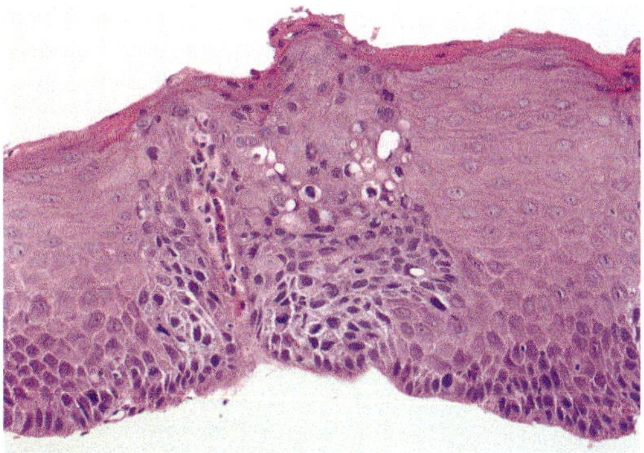

Fig. 3.1 Abrupt transition of dysplastic and non-dysplastic squamous epithelium

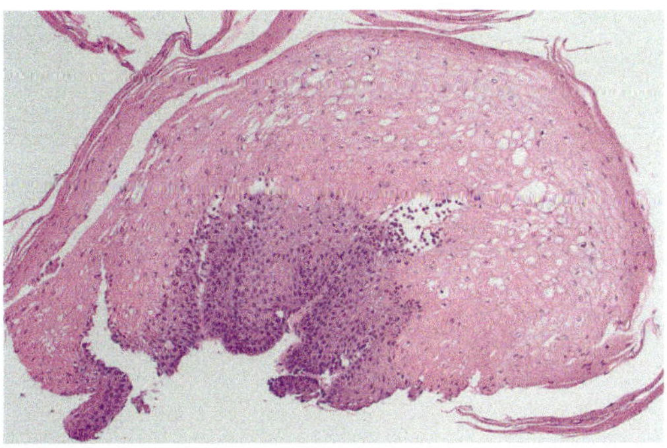

Fig. 3.2 Low-grade squamous dysplasia: dysplastic cells confined to the lower half of the stratified epithelium

Patients are often asymptomatic and lesions are identified when they undergo endoscopic examination for other reasons. Even so sometimes endoscopic changes can be subtle and easily missed.

Differential diagnosis of low-grade IELs includes nonneoplastic entities that result in the squamo-proliferative pattern such as squamous papilloma, "epidermoid metaplasia" [3, 4], reactive and repair changes, and "pseudoepitheliomatous hyperplasia". Intense eosinophilic cytoplasm of the "parakeratotic pattern" (see Chap. 3, Part 1) of inflammatory lesions can raise concern for dysplasia as they mimic dyskeratotic squamous cells that are often noted in squamous dysplasia (Box 3.1) [5].

Grading

Once confirmed, squamous dysplasia is graded into two tiers: low and high grade. Low-grade dysplasia shows neoplastic cells confined to the lower ½ (Fig. 3.2), whereas involvement of >50% of the thickness is considered high grade (Figs. 3.1 and 3.3a, b). The former three-tiered system (mild, moderate, and severe) is discouraged, similar to the approach in grading of epithelial dysplasias of the rest of the tubular gut.

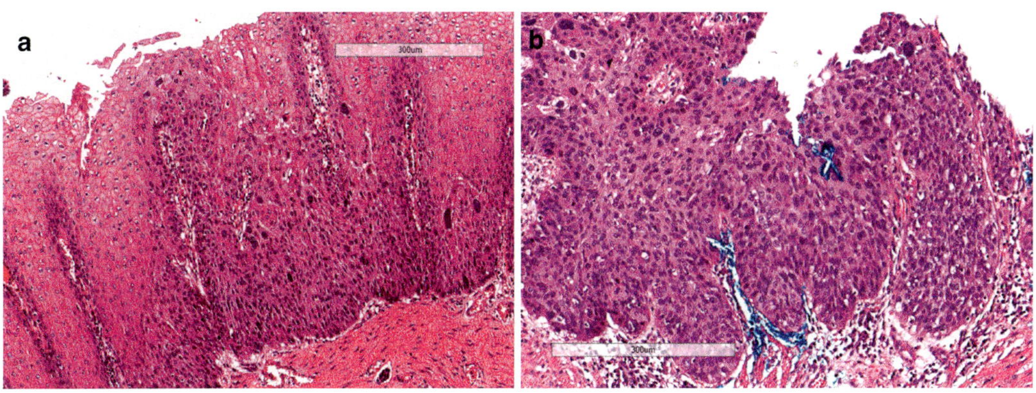

Fig. 3.3 High-grade dysplasia: dysplastic cells (a) involving more than half the thickness or (b) full thickness of the stratified epithelium

Carcinoma in situ may be regarded as a severe form high-grade intraepithelial neoplasia (Fig. 3.4a–c and 3.3b).

Box 3.1 Squamous-Proliferative Pattern

Exclude

- Pseudoepitheliomatous hyperplasia
- Repair-related basal hyperplasia
- Glycogenic acanthosis (GA)
- Squamous papilloma
- Epidermoid metaplasia

If genuine squamous dysplasia is confirmed

- Grade (low grade <50%, high grade >50% of thickness)

Exclude

- Invasion ("invasive pattern"): step levels are often needed

Pay attention to

- Clinical history and endoscopic features

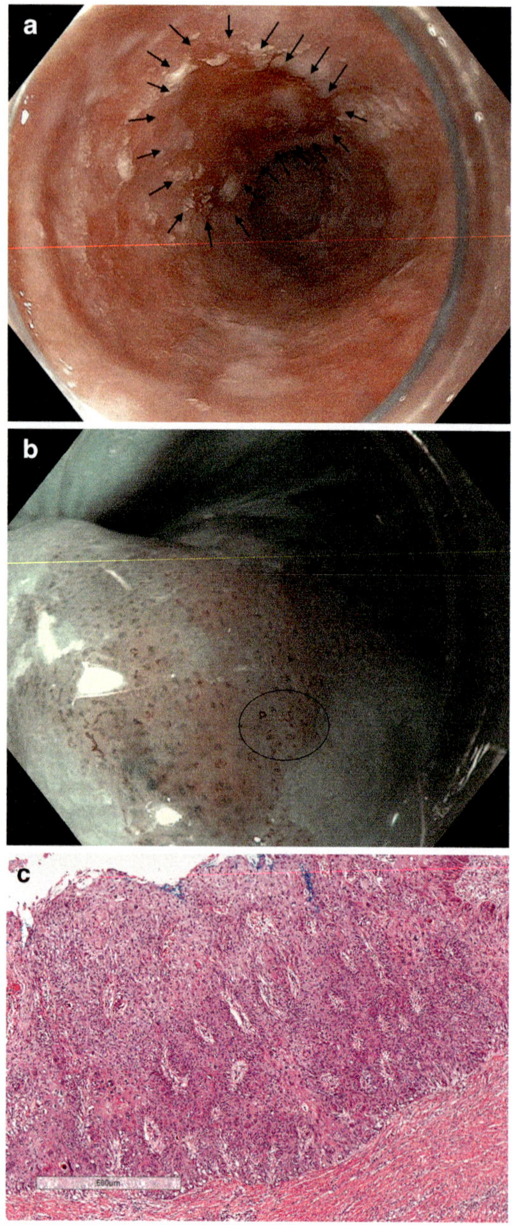

Fig. 3.4 Case 1: High-grade squamous dysplasia/intraepithelial neoplasia (carcinoma in-situ). A 75-year-old man was referred for evaluation of reflux symptoms and intermittent dysphagia to solids. At gastroscopy, at 35 cm from the teeth, in the 9 o'clock position, there was an area of mucosal irregularity which appeared as a red patch on white light endoscopy (WL image—arrows demarcate lesion) (**a**). On closer inspection with narrowband imaging and zoom magnification (NBI image—circle shows area of Type IV/V1 IPCL) (**b**), there was presence of dilated and irregular intrapapillary capillary loops (IPCL Type IV/V-1) consistent with likely high-grade dysplasia or carcinoma in situ. This entire area was resected via EMR and sent for histology that confirmed high-grade squamous dysplasia/intraepithelial neoplasia (carcinoma in situ) (**c**)

Squamous Pattern with Invasion [6, 7]

The straightforward diagnostic pattern (Fig. 3.5) shows irregular sheets and tongues of neoplastic squamous epithelium with dysplastic cytonuclear changes described above (high N/C ratio, membrane irregularity, hyperchromasia, prominent nucleoli, increased mitoses including abnormal forms and dyskeratotic cells with intense eosinophilia) and desmoplasia. Squamous pearls are easily seen in well-differentiated squamous cell carcinomas. It should be noted that intraepithelial lesions rarely form keratin pearls and their presence in a biopsy with the neoplastic pattern should alert invasion. Necrosis is often noted with invasive pattern but could also be present in biopsies of ulcerated intraepithelial lesions without invasion.

Superficially, invasive well-differentiated squamous cell carcinomas may not elicit a

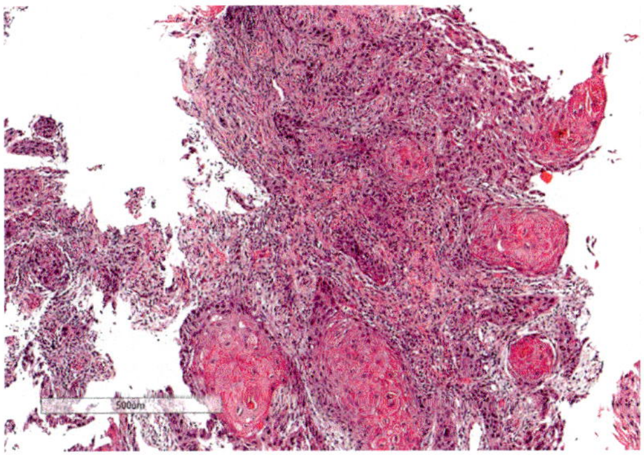

Fig. 3.5 Squamous dysplasia pattern with invasion: sheets and tongues of neoplastic squamous cells featuring keratin pearls with surrounding desmoplasia, characteristic of invasion

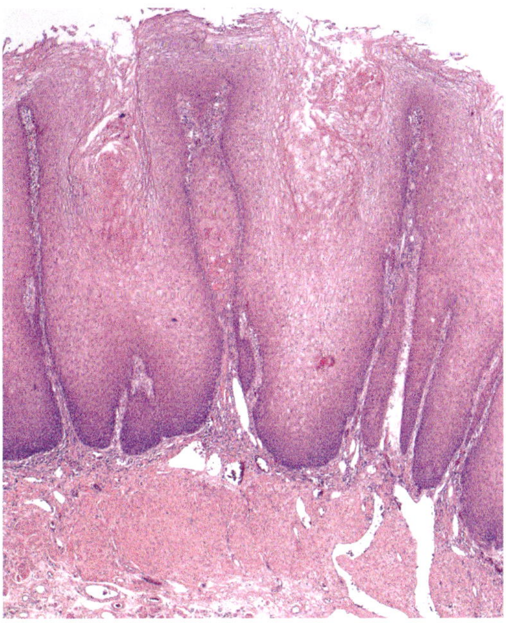

Fig. 3.6 Squamo-proliferative pattern without a stromal reaction pattern of very well-differentiated squamous cell carcinoma

stromal reaction and therefore can be a great diagnostic challenge in some cases (Fig. 3.6). Examination of repeated biopsies and endoscopic correlation is often required for a diagnosis. Even so, sometimes the diagnosis can only be suspected. Endoscopic appearance in these lesions is of great value to consider this possibility when stromal reaction is lacking, coupled with deceptive bland nuclear cytology. Squamo-proliferative pattern should alert further investigations and repeat biopsy that may show typical invasive pattern.

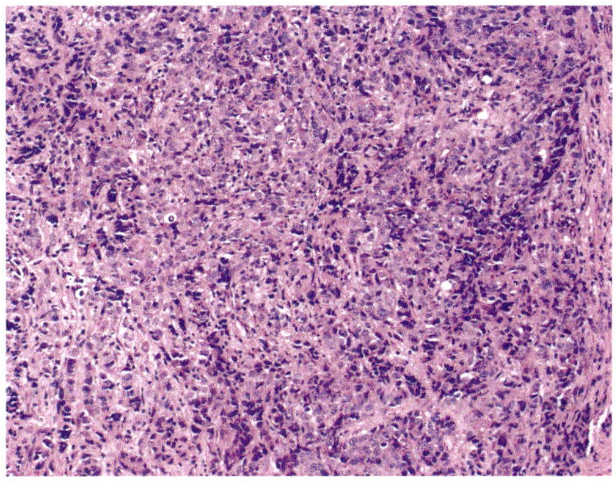

Fig. 3.7 "Blue cell pattern" of poorly differentiated carcinoma showing strands of malignant cells with high N/C ratio and many mitotic figures, lacking keratinisation

High-grade squamous carcinomas show clusters or sheets of basaloid malignant cells ("blue cell pattern"—Fig. 3.7), infiltration by single cells or strands of malignant cells and lack of evidence of keratinisation. Squamous and even epithelial origin may be difficult to be appreciated in "undifferentiated invasive patterns" without ancillary stains. Squamous components may not be included in the biopsy posing more diagnostic challenges (Fig. 3.8a). P63 and p40 immunohistochemical stains are helpful to confirm the squamous origin (Fig. 3.8a–d). An extended panel of immunohistochemical stains may be required to exclude rarer tumours presenting with a blue cell pattern (see table 1.3 in chapter 1).

Pitfalls

Inflammatory Reactive Changes

Nonneoplastic inflammatory patterns with severe reactive changes mimic invasive and noninvasive squamous lesions. Repair changes can produce nucleomegaly, hyperchromasia, prominent nucleoli, increased mitoses, and dyskeratotic looking cells with intense eosinophilia. Presence of the nonneoplastic sub patterns may give helpful clues that the lesions are not neoplastic. Clinical history, in particular use of medications

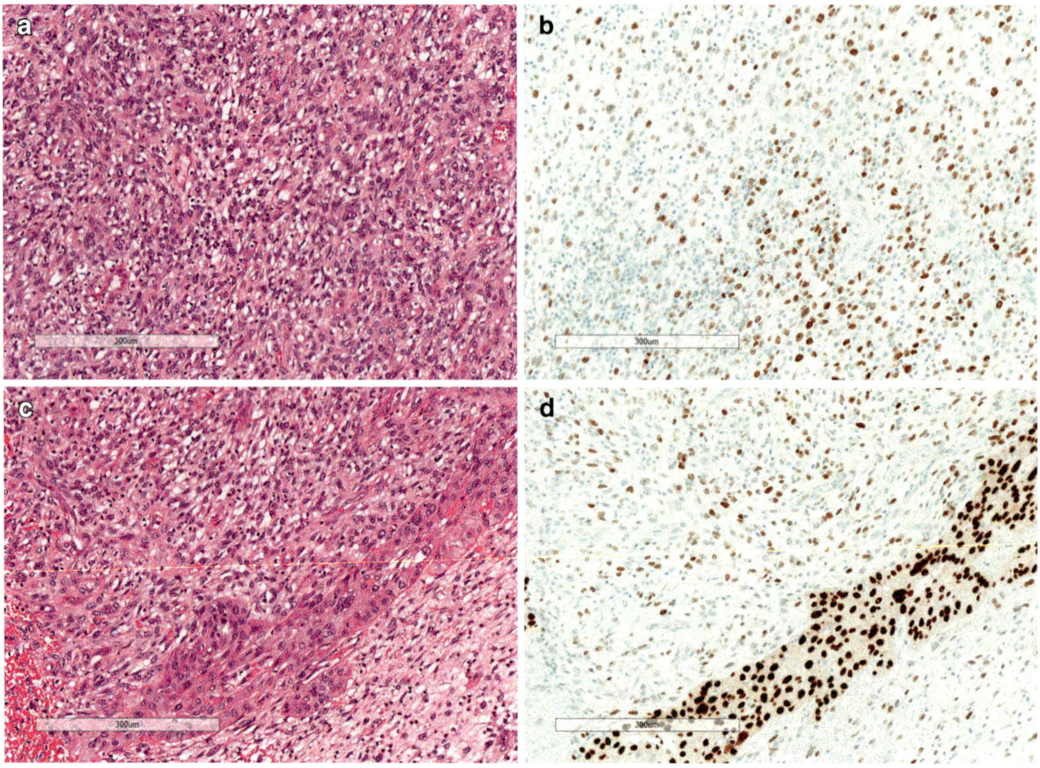

Fig. 3.8 (**a**) Undifferentiated pattern of squamous carcinoma (**b**) with moderate to weak p63 positivity (**c**) undifferentiated and differentiated patterns of squamous carcinoma side by side (**d**) with weak p63 positivity in the undifferentiated component compared to strong positivity in the differentiated component

and a setting of infective conditions as well as endoscopic appearance, should be correlated.

Spindle and Undifferentiated Patterns (Fig. 3.9)

In an oesophageal biopsy, spindle cell pattern warrants excluding a spindle cell (sarcomatoid) carcinoma before a diagnosis of a rarer mesenchymal tumour is made, even when a squamous component is not observed. Often a variety of cytokeratins are required for confirmation as cytokeratin expression can be very patchy. Squamous markers (e.g. p40 and p63) are often positive but may be weak and patchy [8].

Very Well-Differentiated Squamous Cell Carcinoma

Endoscopic correlation is of utmost importance in confirming these lesions as malignant. Neoplastic squamous cells may appear very bland and near "normal looking" in a biopsy while endoscopy shows an obvious mass lesion. Squamoproliferative pattern, even though bland, of an endoscopically suspicious lesion should alert further investigations and repeat biopsy that may show the typical invasive pattern in other areas of the lesion subsequently.

Ancillary Testing

Markers of neoplastic nature:

Aberrant p53 expression and p16 positivity have been demonstrated in the neoplastic squamous mucosa with variable results. Interpretation of p53 expression in proliferative squamous epithelium is difficult. Furthermore, p16 positivity should not be regarded as a surrogate marker for HPV infection in the setting of oesophageal squamous neoplasia. They are not recommended as reliable markers.

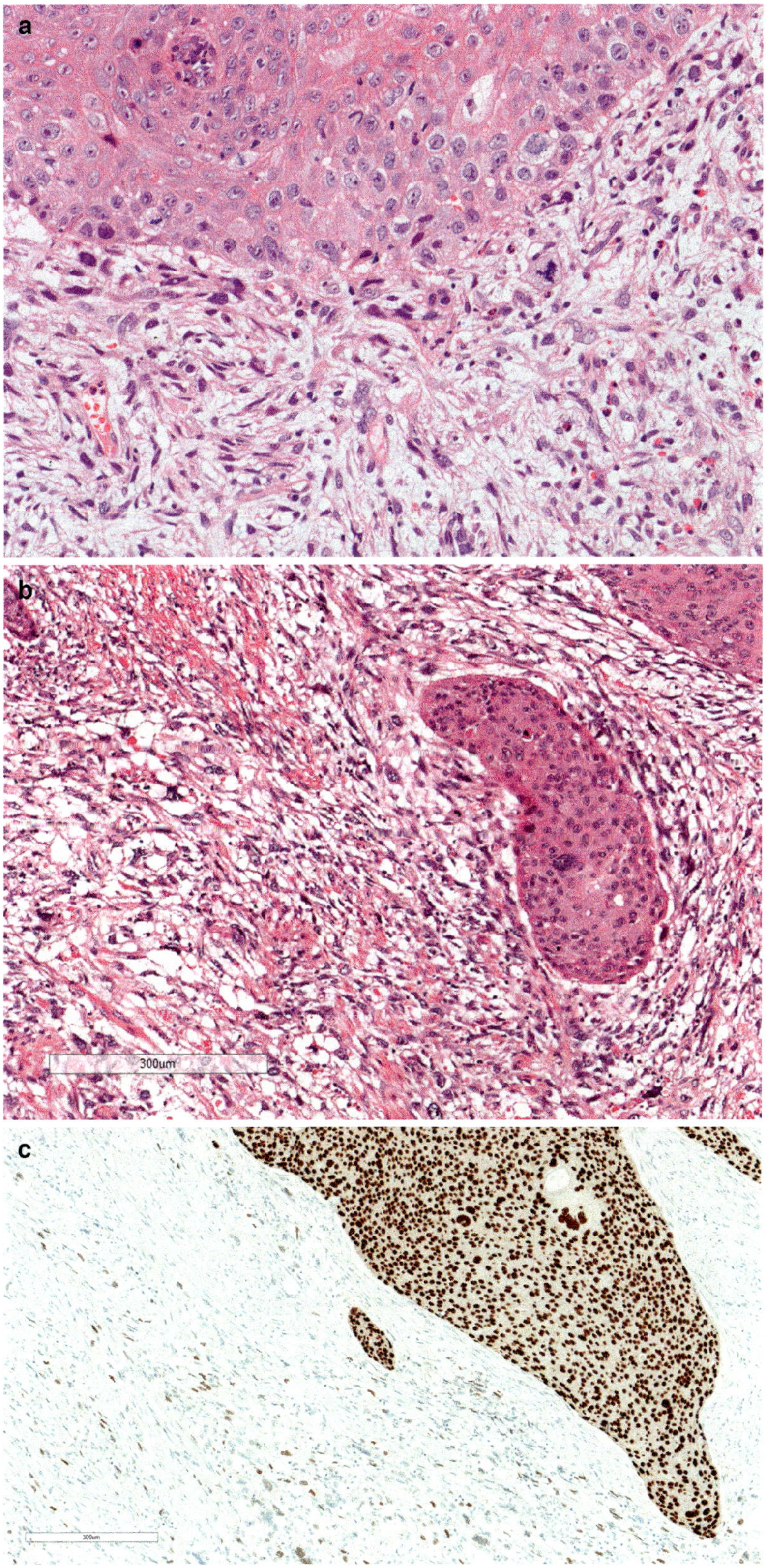

Fig. 3.9 "Spindle cell pattern": (a and b) note the spindle cell components next to differentiated squamous components. (**c**) Weak and patchy p63 positivity in spindle cell areas compared to strong positivity in differentiated squamous components

Markers of squamous origin:

Immunohistochemical features that favour squamous origin (employed mostly to confirm squamous origin in undifferentiated malignancies) are positivity for CK5/6, p63, and p40 as well as lineage markers such as CDX2 (adenocarcinomas of gastrointestinal origin), TTF-1 (lung and thyroid), and PAX8 (thyroid and renal) that show a negative result. P63 alone can be positive in non-squamous malignancies; p40 is more specific [8].

Glandular Pattern with No Invasion and No Atypia

When an endoscopic biopsy presents proliferated glandular mucosa, the most important step is to exclude glandular neoplasms, and the most common setting of glandular neoplasia in the oesophagus is Barrett oesophagus (BO). However, uncommon nonneoplastic glandular proliferations occur in the oesophagus (see under non neoplastic patterns).

When a glandular proliferation pattern without atypia is noted in an endoscopic biopsy, the immediate concern should be to refer to the site of biopsy and the endoscopic appearance.

Most of these glandular proliferations represent heterotopias that could show gastric, sebaceous, and pancreatic differentiation.

Gastric heterotopia (cervical inlet patch) consists of a discrete area resembling gastric mucosa. Typically, it occurs in the proximal oesophagus, usually 3-cm distal to the cricopharyngeus and can range in size from 2 to 45 mm. They present as isolated patches but can be multiple and circumferential in some cases. Mostly these are an incidental findings with no symptoms; however, in a small subset of patients, they can be secretory in nature and result in ulceration, stricturing with dysphagia, globus sensation, chronic cough, and laryngopharyngeal reflux. Biopsies reveal corpus or fundic-type gastric mucosa with parietal cells capable of secreting acid (Fig. 3.10).

The sebaceous pattern is accompanied by parakeratotic debris and represents heterotopic seba-

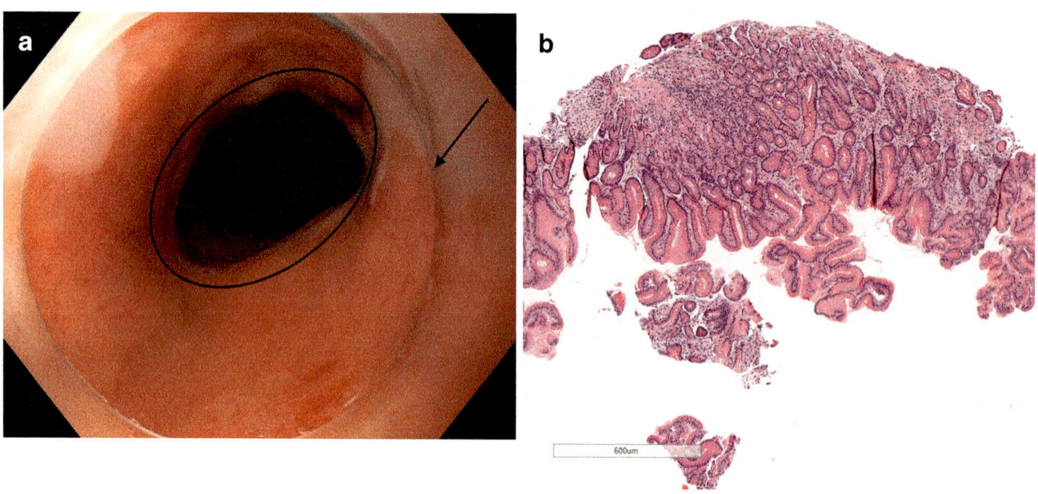

Fig. 3.10 Case 2: Gastric heterotopia (cervical inlet patch). An 83-year-old lady with 10-year history of intermittent dysphagia to solids. Gastroscopy was performed and revealed an almost circumferential salmon-coloured mucosa. (**a**) arrow demarcates squamous-gastric heterotopia demarcation with moderate-grade benign appearing stricture (oval) at the distal extent consistent with an inlet patch and possible secretory function although no overt ulceration noted. Biopsies were taken. Histology showed fragments of columnar-lined gastric-type mucosa with a mixture of nonspecialised and specialised glands and no intestinal metaplasia or dysplasia. Appearance was consistent with the cervical inlet patch/gastric heterotopia in the given clinical setting (**b**)

ceous rests (Fig. 3.11a–c). Endoscopically, they appear as yellow plaques or nodules frequently occurring in clusters. They are mostly an incidental finding and the size ranges from 1 to 20 mm in diameter. Their clinical relevance is uncertain with no malignant transformation reported in the literature, suggesting a favourable prognosis.

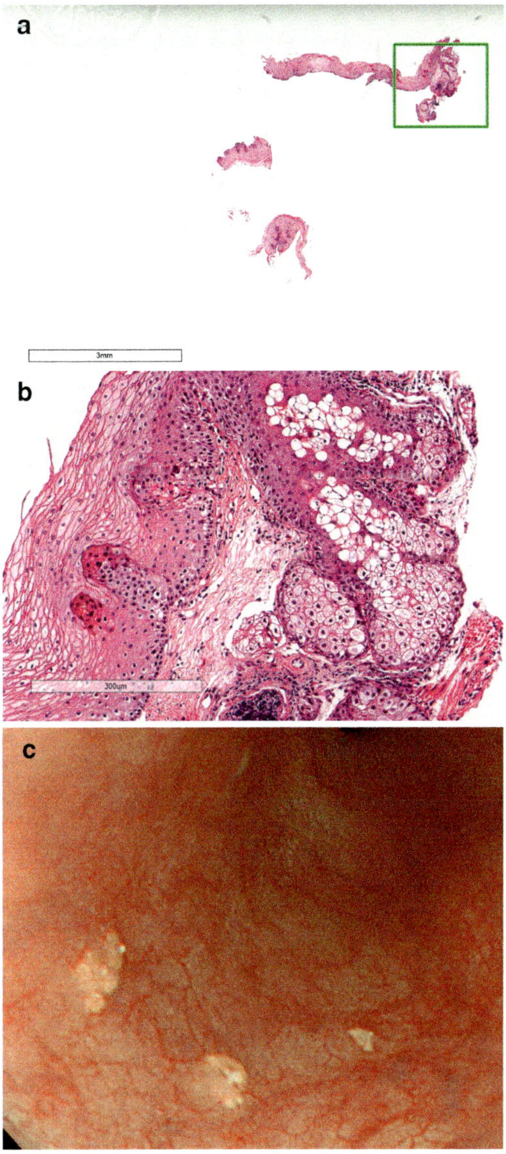

Fig. 3.11 (**a**) Heterotopic sebaceous rests with overlying squamous mucosa, note one of three abnormal fragments (boxed on low power). (**b**) Obvious sebaceous nature on high power. (**c**) Several irregular yellowish lesions on the surface of the squamous mucosa are noted

Pancreatic heterotopia, also known as "pancreatic acinar metaplasia" contains only exocrine pancreatic elements. These foci are commonly seen in the GOJ, reported in up to 24%. In one study it appears to be an incidental finding and in most cases there is no clinical significance (Fig. 3.12) [9].

Epithelial proliferation without atypia can represent hyperplastic and polypoid reactive changes of the columnar lined oesophagus (CLO) or "cardia". Endoscopic correlation is required to establish the nature of the proliferation. Active inflammation in such epithelial proliferations should prompt search for *Helicobacter* organisms.

Glandular Pattern with Atypia but No Invasion (Dysplastic/Intraepithelial Neoplastic Pattern)

Epithelial atypia that shows abrupt transition with lack of surface maturation is often diagnostic in all grades of dysplasia. Loss of nuclear polarity is characteristic of high-grade dysplasia.

Neoplastic glandular pattern in the oesophagus is mostly related to Barrett's-associated neoplasia. Biopsies of such lesions can be encountered irrespective of a history of BO and the clinical circumstances. Despite endoscopic surveillance, the majority of oesophageal adenocarcinomas are diagnosed in patients that have no prior diagnosis of BO. This is especially seen in subepithelial neoplastic foci that can be associated with surface squamous reepithelialisation of pre-existing Barrett's segments. However clinical suspicion is very helpful to escalate vigilance by pathologists to perform multiple step levels, even to the extent of exhausting the entire block, and review of indeterminate findings by a second GI pathologist.

Appreciating the neoplastic glandular mucosa of the oesophagus is an essential requirement of pathologists in the Western world where Barrett's oesophagus is common. At the same time, pathologists practising in countries where Barrett's oesophagus is uncommon should be attuned to the diagnostic neoplastic pattern, even though they encountered these lesions less frequently.

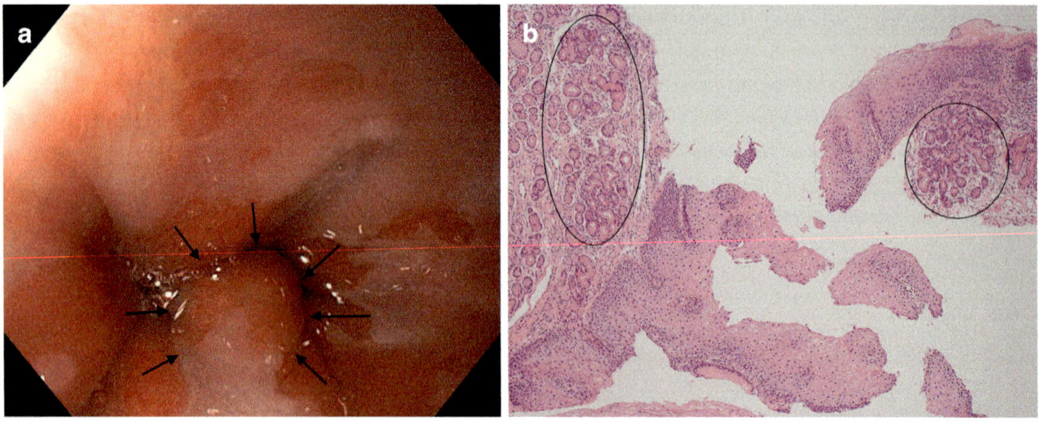

Fig. 3.12 Case 3: Pancreatic heterotopia/acinar metaplasia. A 69-year-old man with 10-year history of reflux symptoms was referred for gastroscopy. Minor reflux changes were noted at the gastroesophageal junction with nodular area seen at 6 o'clock. Appearance was not consistent with intestinal metaplasia (a). Biopsies were taken for further evaluation and showed pancreatic heterotopia (**b**)

At low power, the dysplastic pattern is characterised by the presence of epithelium that appears basophilic due to hyperchromatic nuclei of crowded cells compared to the uninvolved areas. The combination of abrupt transition with lack of surface maturation, and crowding and architectural abnormality of glands coupled with cytological atypia is characteristic, and often diagnostic.

Frequently, absence (or decrease) of goblet cells with mucin depletion is seen compared to the adjacent columnar mucosa. Basophilia alone is characteristic but not diagnostic, as reactive changes of CLO can mimic basophilia of the neoplastic pattern. Less frequently, dysplastic epithelium may have a lighter and a clear appearance (as in foveolar dysplasia, see below) or appear villiform with excessive mucin secretion ("hypermucinous" look).

The "dysplastic" pattern should prompt excluding reactive changes ("atypia") by careful systematic examination of the architectural and cytological features (table 3.2). Clinical and endoscopic correlation is very helpful as discussed below. In our experience p53 immunohistochemistry is very helpful in confirming a dysplastic process, as recommended by some learned societies although the experience has been variable. Further details are discussed later in the chapter under ancillary studies.

Box 3.2 Glandular proliferation pattern - Dysplastic sub pattern.

- At low-power, epithelium looks basophilic.
- Abrupt transition with lack of surface maturation and crowding with architectural abnormality of glands: often diagnostic.

Other clues:

- Absence (or marked decrease) of goblet cells and mucin depletion
- Clear (foveolar) and "hypermucinous and villiform" look

Once considered dysplastic:

- Grade the dysplasia.

If difficult to grade:

- Consider and exclude unusual reactive patterns and metastatic carcinoma or cancerisation of mucosa before confirming dysplasia.

Endoscopic Features

Multiple studies have shown that the random biopsy protocol has low sensitivity for the detection of early neoplastic changes in BO and has low adherence among endoscopists. When confirmed histologically, the current standard of care for BO surveillance involves careful inspection using high-resolution white light endoscopy and targeted evaluation of any focal lesions using advanced imaging techniques such as narrow band imaging and magnification. Targeted biopsies should be taken from any suspicious areas, with lesions described as per the Paris classification and location as a distance in centimetres from the teeth with clockface orientation. Flat Barrett's should have random four-quadrant biopsies every 2 cm in non-dysplastic BO segments, and every 1 cm if there is suspicion or history of dysplasia as per the Seattle protocol [10–13].

Currently most early invasive adenocarcinomas are managed endoscopically without the need for oesophagectomy; however, in some cases, further adjuvant therapies such as salvage surgery or chemotherapy and radiotherapy are required and dependent on the incident risk of nodal metastasis which is determined based on the histologic staging as per STOLTE or AJCC [12, 13].

Diagnosis and Grading of Glandular Dysplasia [12–28]

Once the epithelial proliferative pattern is considered dysplastic, grading is essential. Due to its relevance to further management and surveillance of dysplastic and invasive lesions originating in Barrett's mucosa, recommendations have been made to standardise the terminology (Table 3.1). The term "atypical epithelium/atypical changes" as a diagnostic category is not included in standard terminology and strongly discouraged, to avoid confusion. However, the term atypia (atypism) is often used by pathologists to describe the morphological features that express deviation from the normal patterns (due to "uncertainty") in the microscopic description. Most standardised terminology systems do not recommend the term "atypia" as a diagnostic category.

The currently used terminology has been adopted from the system originally developed for dysplasia associated with inflammatory bowel disease with modifications [14]. There is hardly any single feature that would make the absolute distinction of dysplastic lesions from reactive

Table 3.1 Standard terminology

Vienna	IBD****	WHO (2010)	Modifications
Negative for dysplasia/neoplasia	Negative for dysplasia	Negative for dysplasia	
Indefinite for dysplasia/neoplasia	Indefinite for dysplasia	Indefinite for dysplasia/ neoplasia	Indefinite: specify further
Noninvasive low-grade neoplasia (adenoma/dysplasia)	Low-grade dysplasia	Intraepithelial neoplasia (IEN)—low grade	
Noninvasive high-grade neoplasia (adenoma/dysplasia)	High-grade dysplasia	Intraepithelial neoplasia (IEN)—high grade	
High-grade adenoma/dysplasia		IEN (high grade)	
Noninvasive carcinoma (carcinoma in situ)		IEN (carcinoma in situ)	
Suspicious of invasive adenocarcinoma			HGD, suspicious of adenocarcinoma
Invasive neoplasia	Adenocarcinoma*	Adenocarcinoma	
Intramucosal carcinoma	Intramucosal	Intramucosal	Intramucosal adenocarcinoma
Submucosal carcinoma or beyond	Invasive adenocarcinoma	Invasive adenocarcinoma	Submucosal invasive adenocarcinoma

IEN = Intraepithelial neoplasia
****IBD = inflammatory Bowel Disease Dysplasia Morphology Study Group

Table 3.2 Epithelial alterations

	Negative	Indefinite	LGD	HGD	Carcinoma
Cytology					
High N/C ratio	–/+	+/–	+	++	++
Nuclear polarity	Maintained	Generally maintained, occasionally lost	Maintained	Lost ++	Lost ++/ rarely maintained
Abrupt change on surface	None	None (change may be diffuse)	+	+	+/–
Surface maturation	Maintained	+/reduced	–	–	–
Mitoses	–/+	–/+/++	+	++	++
Atypical mitoses	–	–	+/–	+	+
Full-thickness nuclear stratification	–	Pseudostratification	–	++	++
Atypical mitoses	–	–	+/–	+	+
Full-thickness nuclear stratification	–	Pseudostratification	–	++	++
Reduced goblet cells +/– dystrophic goblet cells	–	–/+/++	+	++	++
Hyperchromasia	+/–	+/–	+	++	++
Prominent nucleoli	–	–/+/++	–	+/–	+/–
Multiple nucleoli	–	–/+	–/+	–/+	+/–
Nuclear irregularity	+/–	+/–	+	++	+/++/+++
Nuclear pleomorphism	–	–/+/++	–	++	+
Architecture					
Villiform surface	–	–	–	+/–	+/–
Crypt budding and branching	–	–/+	+/–	++	++
Crowded/back-to-back glands	–	+/–	+/–	++	++
Irregular crypts	+/–	–/+	+/–	+/++	+/++/+++
Intraluminal bridges/papillae	–	–	–	+	+
Lamina propria between glands	++	+	+/Reduced	Reduced/-	Almost or totally absent
Intraglandular necrosis, angulated, and never-ending glands, single cells	–	–	–	–/+	+++
Desmoplasia	–	–	–	–	+ Submucosal invasive

"atypia". However, epithelial alterations in terms of architecture and cytology gradually accumulate from low- to high-grade dysplasia (Table 3.2). The neoplastic progression of BO from metaplastic columnar-lined mucosa (CLM) to dysplasia and finally to invasive carcinoma is a biological continuum. There is significant inter- and intra-observer variation in the diagnosis and grading of dysplasia [15–18]. Therefore, worldwide guidelines recommend double reporting, with at least one expert GI pathologist, and/or review of diagnosis and grading of dysplasia when considering long term follow-up and therapeutic implications [10–13, 19].

Low-Grade Dysplastic Pattern

The diagnosis of low-grade dysplasia can be difficult with overlapping cytoarchitectural feature of reactive change [20–22]. For this reason, the categories of indefinite (see below) and low-grade dysplasia may be managed in a similar manner although this practice may change in the future.

When the biopsy contains both abnormal and normal epithelium, or if a different biopsy from the same patient contains abnormal epithelium, helpful clues about the change can be obtained by comparing the nuclear features in the areas in question with those in the unaffected areas. The atypical nuclei of dysplastic epithelium extend onto the luminal mucosal surface, so both the surface and the underlying glands display nuclei that are much larger and hyperchromatic than the nuclei in unaffected epithelium (see crypt dysplasia later).

Two major sub patterns are observed within the low-grade dysplastic pattern and signify the two phenotypes of abnormal epithelium in neoplastic BO.

The first pattern is characterised by glands lined by cells with crowded, stratified, penicillate, hyperchromatic nuclei that extend onto the mucosal surface. This pattern generally correlates with the "intestinal" phenotype of dysplasia (Fig. 3.13a). This pattern is often categorised as low-grade dysplasia without much difficulty but depending on the degree of cytologic atypism, and in inflammatory background, some cases are categorised as indefinite for dysplasia. p53 immunostain is often helpful [10, 17, 23, 24].

The second pattern consists of cuboidal or short columnar cells on the mucosal surface with atypical nuclei (larger, hyperchromatic, irregular compared to those that are normal next door) that are basal with minimal or no stratification. This type is generally regarded as "gastric/gastric foveolar/nonadenomatous/non intestinal" (Fig. 3.13b) [18, 25–27]. This phenotype of dysplasia may be overlooked at low power due to the deceptively bland appearance and difficult to distinguish from the reactive metaplastic gastric

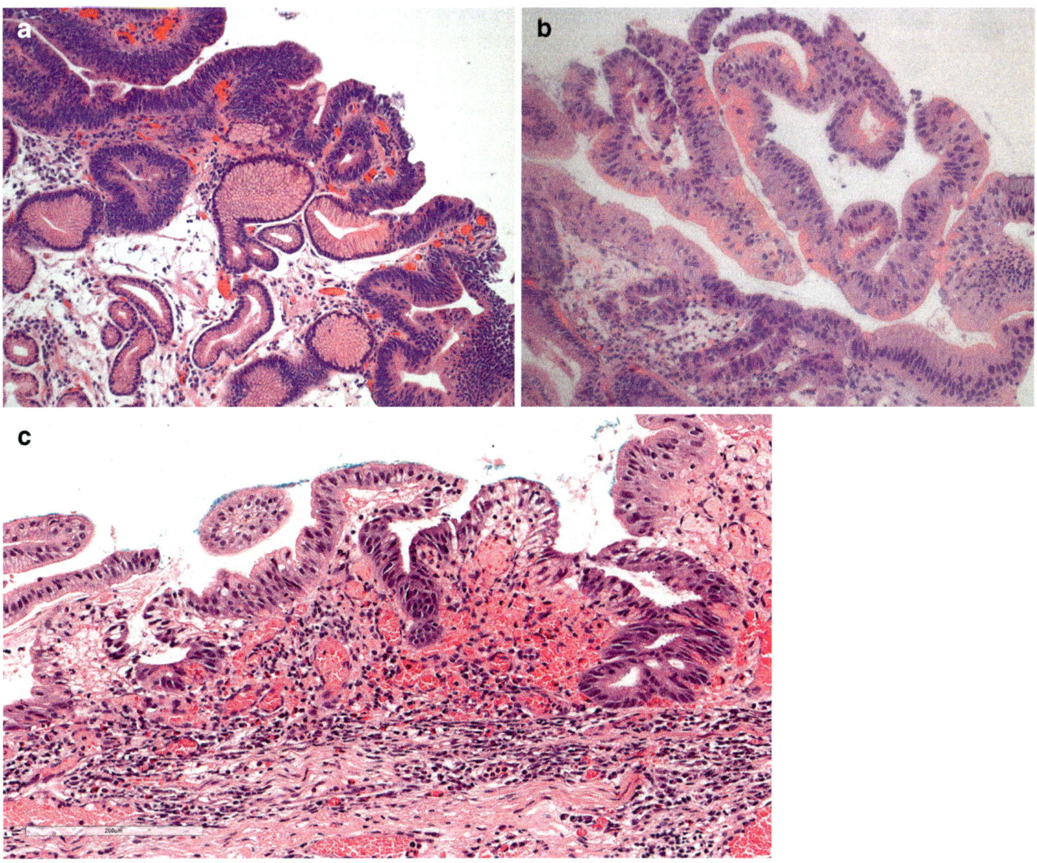

Fig. 3.13 (**a**) Low-grade dysplasia (intestinal phenotype): note loss of surface maturation and focal abrupt change. (**b**) Low-grade dysplasia (gastric foveolar phenotype): note cuboidal to columnar cells with clear to lightly eosinophilic cytoplasm and apical mucin reminiscent of foveolar epithelium. The nuclei are round to oval, some with discernable nucleoli, often considered to be a difficult diagnosis. (**c**) Patchy reactive changes notable on the surface: a mimic of low-grade dysplasia (there was no aberrant p53 expression)

foveolar-type epithelium of BO. Goblet cells are lacking or severely depleted. An important feature to distinguish this dysplastic pattern is full-thickness involvement of the entire mucosa as opposed to patchy reactive changes notable on the surface (Figs. 3.13c). This feature defies the general concept of surface involvement (top heavy pattern) of the dysplastic epithelium as occurs in large intestinal adenomas. Confirmation of dysplasia in this pattern can be extremely challenging, and often the atypism is categorised as "features indefinite for dysplasia" (see Box 3.3).

Box 3.3 Low-Grade Dysplastic Pattern

Pattern 1: "Intestinal" phenotype

- Columnar cells with crowded, stratified, pencillate, and hyperchromatic nuclei
- No surface maturation of the mucosa

Pattern 2: "Gastric/non-intestinal phenotype"

- Cuboidal to low-columnar cells with nuclear atypism (larger, darker, irregular) but basally located.
- Minimal or no stratification.
- Often lacks goblet cells.
- Overlooked at low power.
- Difficult to distinguish from metaplastic gastric foveolar epithelium of BO.
- Full thickness changes in dysplasia vs. more prominent surface changes in reactive atypia are helpful.

High-Grade Dysplastic Pattern (Fig. 3.14 to 3.19)

High-grade pattern is characterised by increasing architectural complexity with glandular crowding and high-end nuclear abnormalities (Table 3.2), prominent nuclear atypia, and loss of nuclear polarity together with characteristic features of any grade of dysplasia (lack of appreciable surface maturation and abrupt transition when appreciable). Loss of nuclear polarity is a more reliable feature considered to represent high-grade dysplasia compared to low-grade dysplasia. The basement membranes of individual glands appear to remain intact in contrast to the invasive pattern. Some features may raise the possibility of focal and subtle intramucosal carcinoma (Fig. 3.15e, f and see below).

Similar to LGD pattern, two types of high-grade dysplastic patterns (sub patterns) are encountered.

The first pattern shows glands lined by multilayered (Figs 3.14 and 3.16a–g), stratified epithelium with loss of polarity of nuclei that show high-end abnormalities. This pattern is generally regarded as adenomatous/intestinal dysplasia and akin to intestinal phenotype (Figs. 3.14 and 3.16a–g).

The second pattern shows glands lined by mostly a single layer of frequently cuboidal epithelium with high-end nuclear abnormalities (Table 3.2) and conspicuously eosinophilic cytoplasm. Nuclear stratification is not a consistent feature. Nuclei may be basal. Nuclear enlargement is a key to the diagnosis, and size is generally 3–4 times the size of lymphocyte. Nucleoli are conspicuous. This pattern is referred variably as non-adenomatous, gastric, and gastric foveolar type and may be lumped as "non-intestinal"-type dysplasia. This pattern is more common than pure intestinal phenotype dysplasia in the setting of Barrett's neoplasia (Fig. 3.15a–g).

However, the most common pattern noted in Barrett's setting is a mixture of the two "divergent differentiation" and is referred to as mixed or hybrid pattern with a mixture of both types of glands (Fig. 3.17) [28]. Dysplastic glands may be buried in subepithelial tissue ("buried glands") lined by the overlying re-epithelialised squamous mucosa (Fig. 3.18a). Invasion of neoplastic glands into the overlying squamous mucosa may signify the presence of intramucosal carcinoma (Fig. 3.18b).

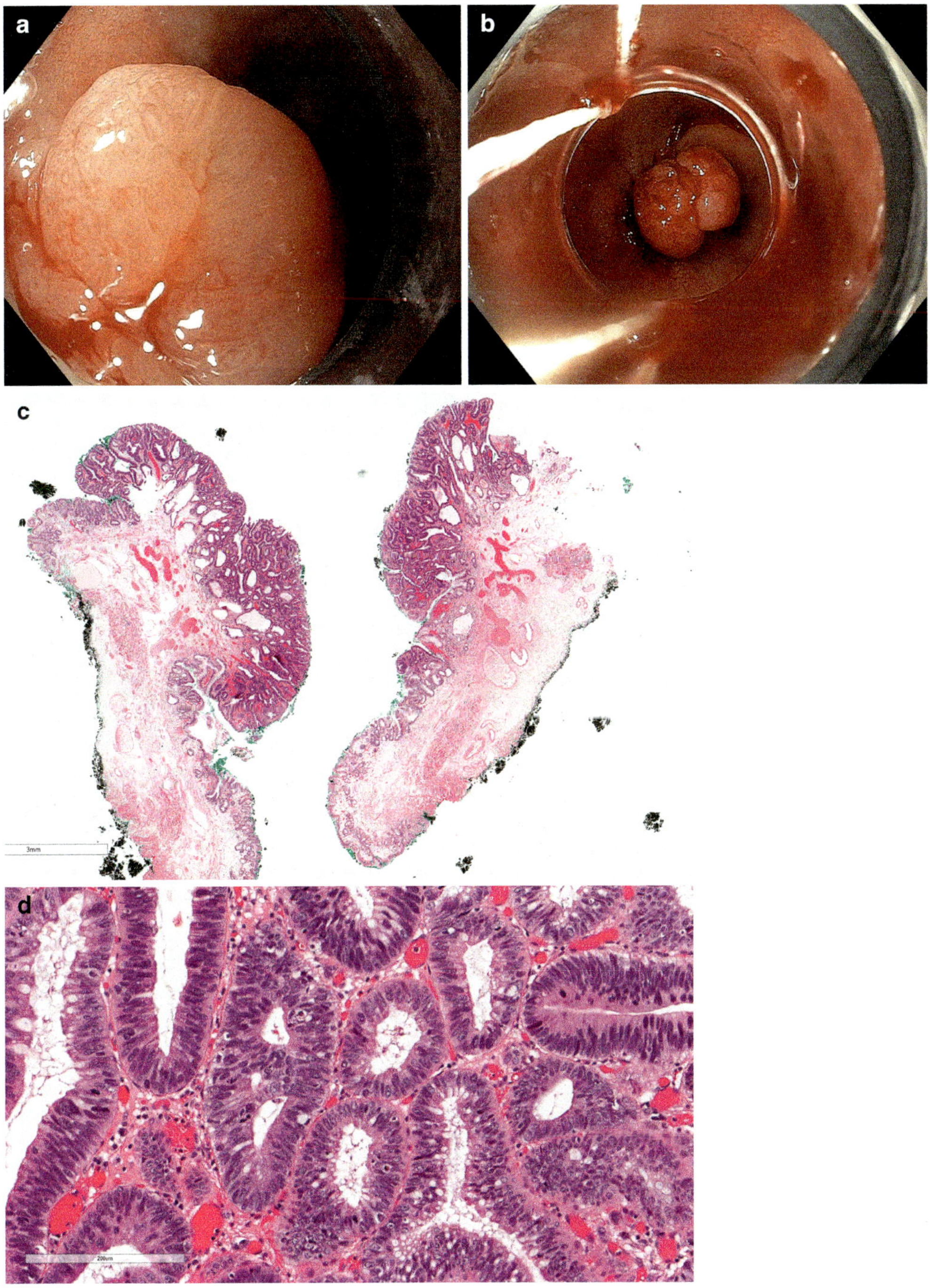

Fig. 3.14 Case 4: High-grade dysplasia/intraepithelial neoplasia in BO. A 74-year-old lady with known Barrett's oesophagus was referred for further evaluation and management of an oesophageal polyp reported as an adenoma with high-grade dysplasia by a community non-GI pathologist. On review by an expert GI pathologist, it was revised to nodular Barrett with high-grade dysplasia. The patient underwent gastroscopy with an 8-mm polyp (Paris 0-IIa) noted at 28 cm 11 o'clock position in a long segment of otherwise flat Barrett's oesophagus (C11M12). (a). The lesion was resected via EMR (b) pinned and sent for histology that confirmed polypoid intestinal-type dysplasia associated with BO (c, d)

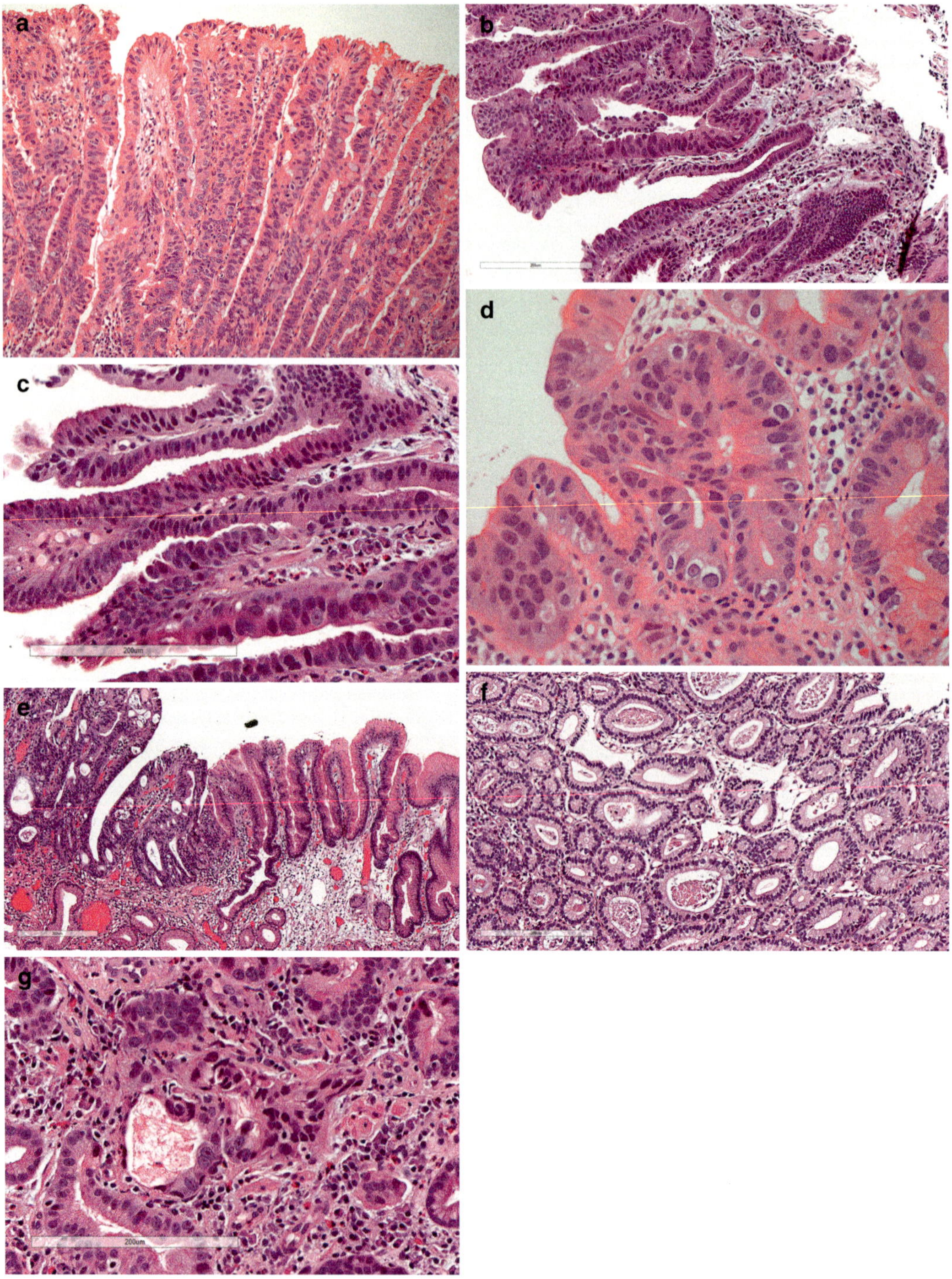

Fig. 3.15 a) High-grade dysplasia (gastric phenotype): Lack of surface maturation, crowded and almost complex glandular architecture and loss of nuclear polarity and marked cytological atypia. (b) High-grade dysplasia (gastric phenotype). Note increasing glandular crowding towards the upper half with high-grade nuclear abnormalities. (c) Obvious loss of nuclear polarity in the lower half of high-grade dysplasia compared to the upper half that shows areas of lesser degree of nuclear abnormality but would be still consistent with high-grade dysplasia. (d) High-grade dysplasia (gastric phenotype): Marked nuclear enlargement 3–4 times the size of a lymphocyte. (e) Abrupt transition from normal to abnormal. In this case high-grade dysplasia is obvious. The highly complex and cribriform pattern is suggestive of intramucosal carcinoma (IMC confirmed on EMR). (f) High-grade dysplasia with features raising the possibility of lace work pattern (IMC confirmed on EMR). (g) High-grade dysplasia with features highly suspicious of lamina propria invasion (IMC confirmed on EMR)

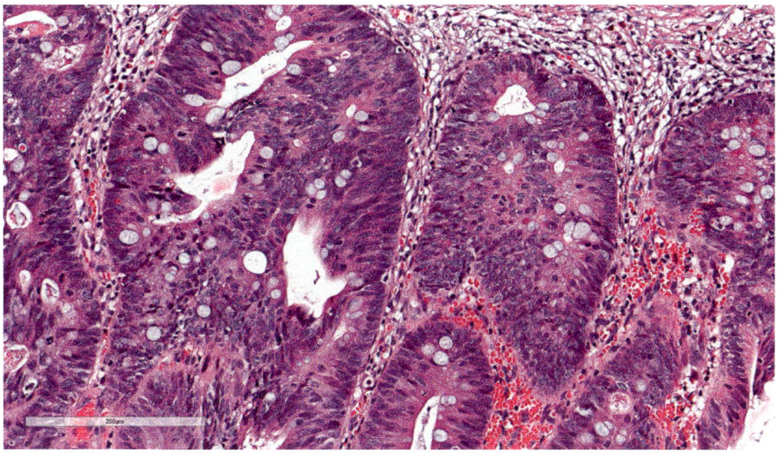

Fig. 3.16 High-grade dysplasia (intestinal phenotype): high-grade cytoarchitectural abnormality and loss of nuclear polarity. Note the glands lined by columnar cells with crowded, stratified, pencillate, hyperchromatic nuclei, and resemblance to traditional colorectal neoplasia (IMC on EMR)

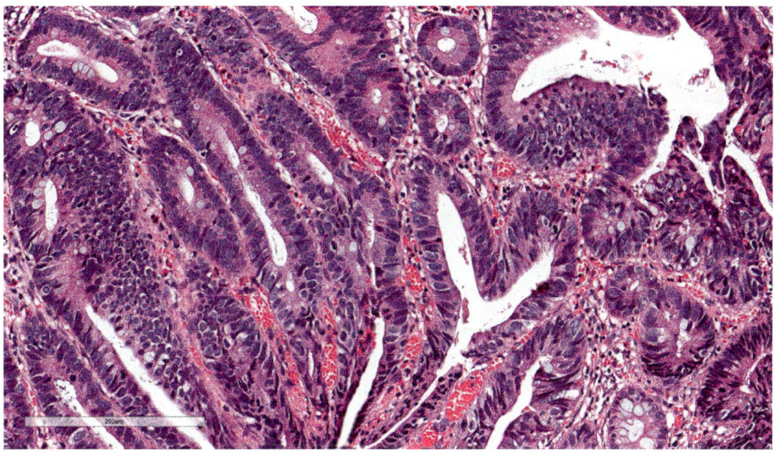

Fig. 3.17 Mixed phenotype of high-grade dysplasia (mixed intestinal and non-intestinal patterns/ divergent differentiation)

The different patterns noted in the dysplastic Barrett's mucosa may be related to possible different pathways of the neoplastic progression. These patterns have been variably referred to as gastric, intestinal, gastric foveolar, adenomatous, and non-adenomatous dysplasia over time by various authors. Markers that characterise different phenotypes and pathways have been again described (Fig. 3.19a, b) [25, 28]. They include mucin immunohistochemistry, CDX2 (so-called intestinal marker), CD10 (a marker of small intestinal differentiation), Das-1, villin, Hep Par 1 (CPS1), and SOX9 (Table 3.3). These markers show different expression profiles in the above mentioned patterns, but differential expression is not perfect. There is significant overlap of cytoarchitectural features and expression of these markers in different patterns and phenotypes. In particular, CDX2 expression does not differentiate between "intestinal" and "non-intestinal" phenotypes (Figure 3.19). As stated, more commonly mixed or hybrid patterns are observed. Importantly there is no proven clinical significance of these specific patterns thus so far, and even more importantly, pure patterns are rare. It is not universally recommended to report the phenotype in endoscopic biopsies in routine practice. Currently, there is not enough strong scientific evidence to accept these different patterns as entities. Furthermore, there are no widely accepted, robust criteria for the distinction between the two phenotypes. However, for practical purposes it is important that GI pathologists recognise these different patterns to avoid under and over diagnosis and inaccurate grading of BO-related dysplasia. Considering

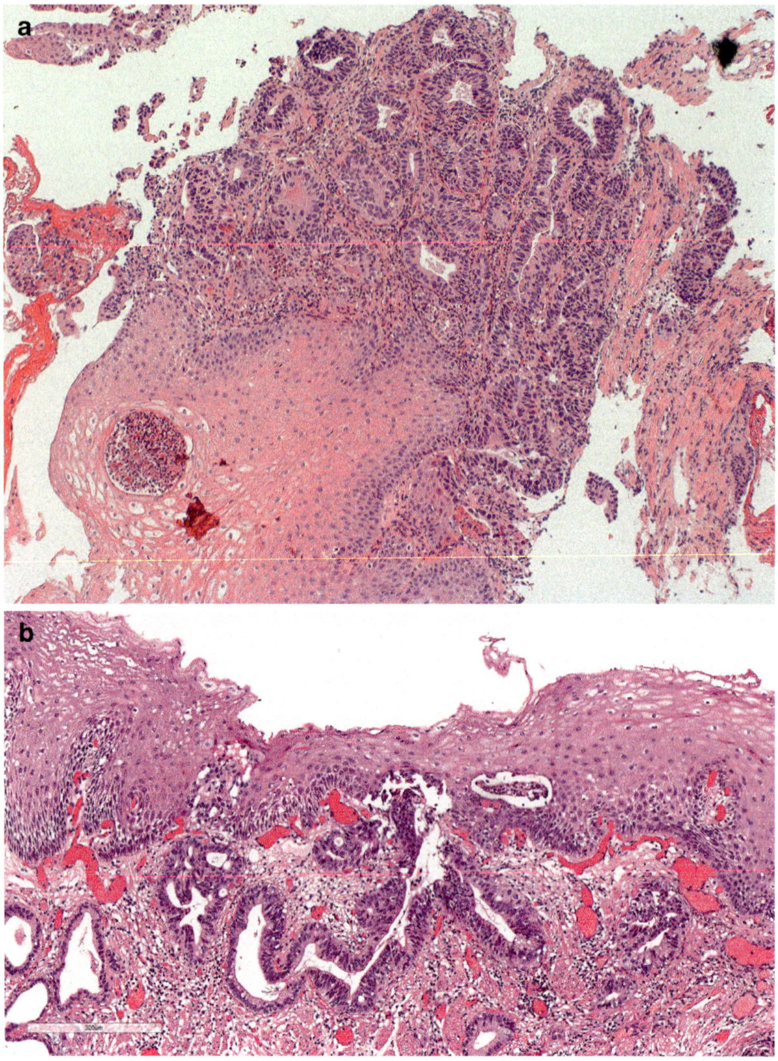

Fig. 3.18 (**a**) High-grade dysplasia in "buried glands" with overlying squamous mucosa. (**b**) High-grade dysplasia in "buried glands" with possible "invasion" of the overlying squamous mucosa

these issues, it is not surprising that one of the most common GI consultations in upper GI pathology is confirmation and grading of IEN/dysplasia. Most learned societies therefore advocate double reporting or second review of most BO-related neoplastic lesions before management decisions are taken.

Even less well-recognised and characterised patterns are pyloric and serrated patterns. The occurrence of these phenotypic sub patterns is extremely rare.

Historically oesophageal adenoma was a term used to describe polypoid dysplasia of "intestinal" phenotype. It is now widely accepted that these lesions almost exclusively arise in Barrett oesophagus and likely represent a nodular or polypoid form of dysplasia rather than an isolated polypoid adenoma, and therefore the term is best avoided in the Barrett's setting (Figs. 3.14 and 3.20). When present in the Barrett's setting, they are interpreted and managed along the same principals of assessing and managing BO-related neoplasia.

True adenomas can rarely originate from native oesophageal submucosal glands in the absence of Barrett's oesophagus and have also been seen in familial adenomatous polyposis syndrome. Due to their rarity, there is limited experience to guide management. However, in

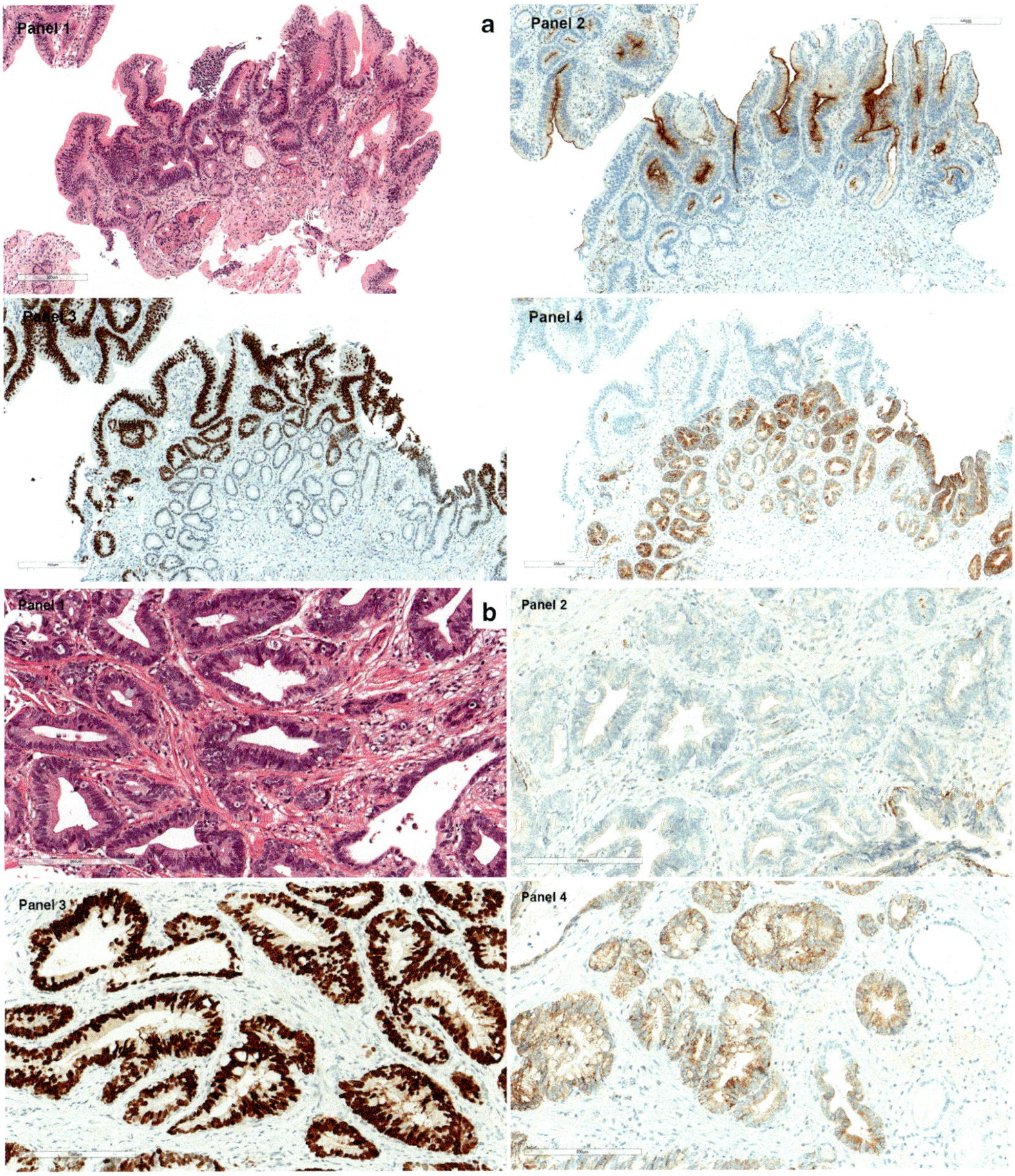

Fig. 3.19 (**a**) Panel 1: Intestinal type low-grade dysplasia—(H&E), Panel 2: CD10-positive luminal border, Panel 3: CDX2-positve, Panel 4: MUC5AC-negative in surface dysplasia compared to MUC5AC positive non-dysplastic gland in CLM (bottom half of mucosa). (**b**) Panel 1: Gastric-type high-grade dysplasia—(H&E), Panel 2: CD10-negative, Panel 3: CDX2-positive, Panel 4: MUC5AC-positive

general they are managed as per isolated colonic adenomas with snare resection for smaller lesions and endoscopic mucosal resection for larger lesions.

Diagnosis of dysplasia remains the gold standard for predicting risk of neoplastic progression in BO that depends on the degree of dysplasia (Boxes 3.4, 3.5, 3.6).

Table 3.3 Sub patterns

	Sub pattern 1: Intestinal ("adenomatous")	Sub pattern 2 Non-intestinal ("non-adenomatous", "gastric", "gastric foveolar")
MUC 2	+	–
MUC5AC	+/–	+++
MUC6	–	+/-
CDX2	+++	+++
CD10	+++ (luminal)	––
Villin	+++	+/–
DAS1	+++	++

Crypt Dysplastic Pattern

This pattern is characterised by nuclear abnormalities consistent with dysplasia; in particular high-end nuclear features are noted without obvious involvement of the surface epithelium.

Crypt dysplastic pattern (Fig. 3.21a, b) is problematic diagnosis in endoscopic biopsies and has taken its own course since its introduction [15, 29]. These changes are best appreciated in resections and EMR specimens adjacent to

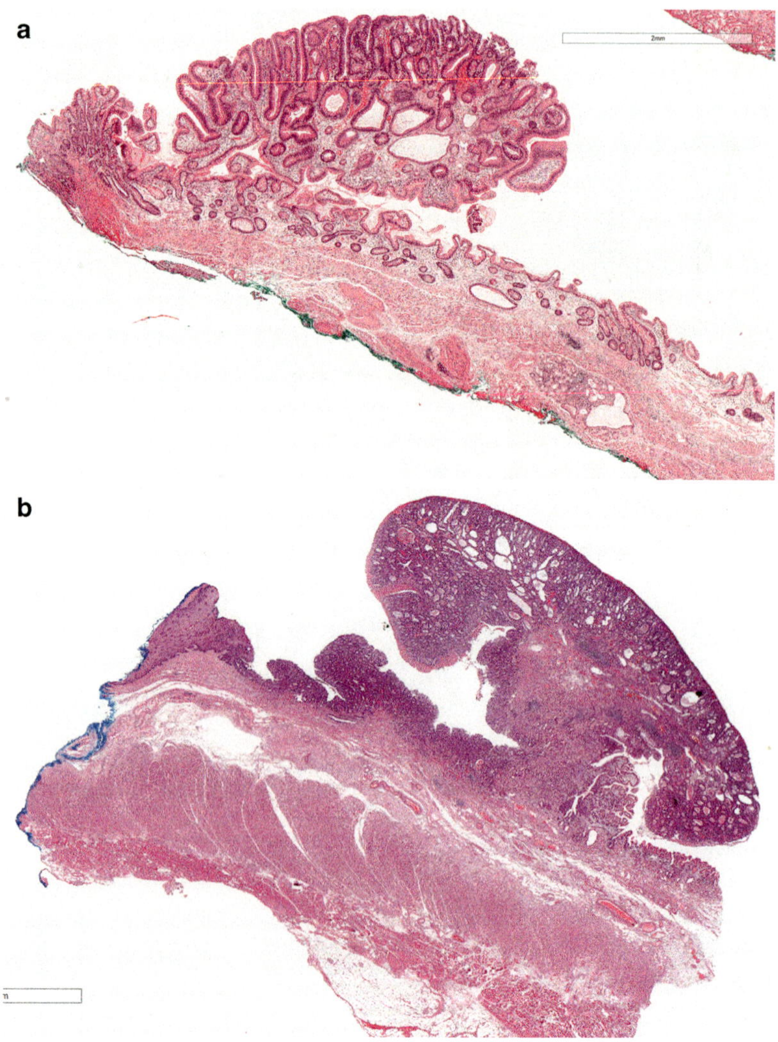

Fig. 3.20 (**a**) Nodular or polypoid type low-grade dysplasia in an EMR. (**b**) Nodular or polypoid type high-grade dysplasia with areas of IMC in a resection

Box 3.4 High-Grade Dysplastic Pattern

- Lack of surface maturation and abrupt change
- Marked cytological atypia
- Complex glandular architecture alterations
- Marked loss of nuclear polarity: a reliable criterion to differentiate from LGD**

**In the HG pattern without nuclear stratification, this feature may not be very useful.

Box 3.5 Phenotypic Sub Patterns with in the Dysplastic Pattern

- Phenotype sub patterns occur both within the low-grade and high-grade dysplastic patterns.
- Two basic patterns appear to be intestinal ("adenomatous") and non-intestinal ("non-adenomatous", "gastric", and "gastric foveolar").
- More often than not the phenotypic pattern is a hybrid (mixed).

Clinical relevance and the biology are not fully established.

definite dysplasia/carcinoma. Furthermore, molecular studies have found similar alterations in crypt dysplasia when compared with traditional dysplasia supporting the true existence of a biological entity. Supporting these assertions, some cases are confirmed to have more convincing surface involvement in step levels, and others harbour genuine dysplasia in other areas. However, longitudinal data on the progression of crypt-limited dysplasia as an isolated finding are unavailable. Confounding these issues, basal metaplastic glandular atypia ("baseline atypia") can closely mimic crypt dysplasia. When the changes approach beyond baseline atypia, a diagnosis of "features indefinite for dysplasia" is acceptable (Box 3.7).

Box 3.6 High-Grade Dysplastic Sub Pattern

Pattern 1 (intestinal):

- Crowded and complex glandular architecture
- Glands lined by columnar cells with crowded, stratified, pencillate, hyperchromatic nuclei
- Loss of polarity
- No surface maturation

Pattern 2 (Non-intestinal/foveolar like):

- Crowded tubular glands with retained architecture without marked complexity
- Glands lined by cuboidal cells cytologic atypia, characterised by nuclear hyperchromasia and enlargement with irregularity and prominent nucleoli, without nuclear stratification
- Often lacks nuclear stratification compared to Pattern 1
- Cells on the mucosal surface with dysplastic nuclei (large, dark, irregular) but they may be basal

Box 3.7 Crypt Dysplasia

- Nuclear abnormalities, even high-end, with or without architectural changes not involving the surface.
- Most common adjacent to definite dysplasia/carcinoma in EMRs and resections.
- Diagnosis on endoscopic biopsies is challenging.
- Basal metaplastic glandular atypia ("baseline atypia") is more common than crypt dysplasia.
- Should not be diagnosed on nuclear stratification and hyperchromasia alone (blue look).
- When in doubt, the category "indefinite for dysplasia" is desirable.

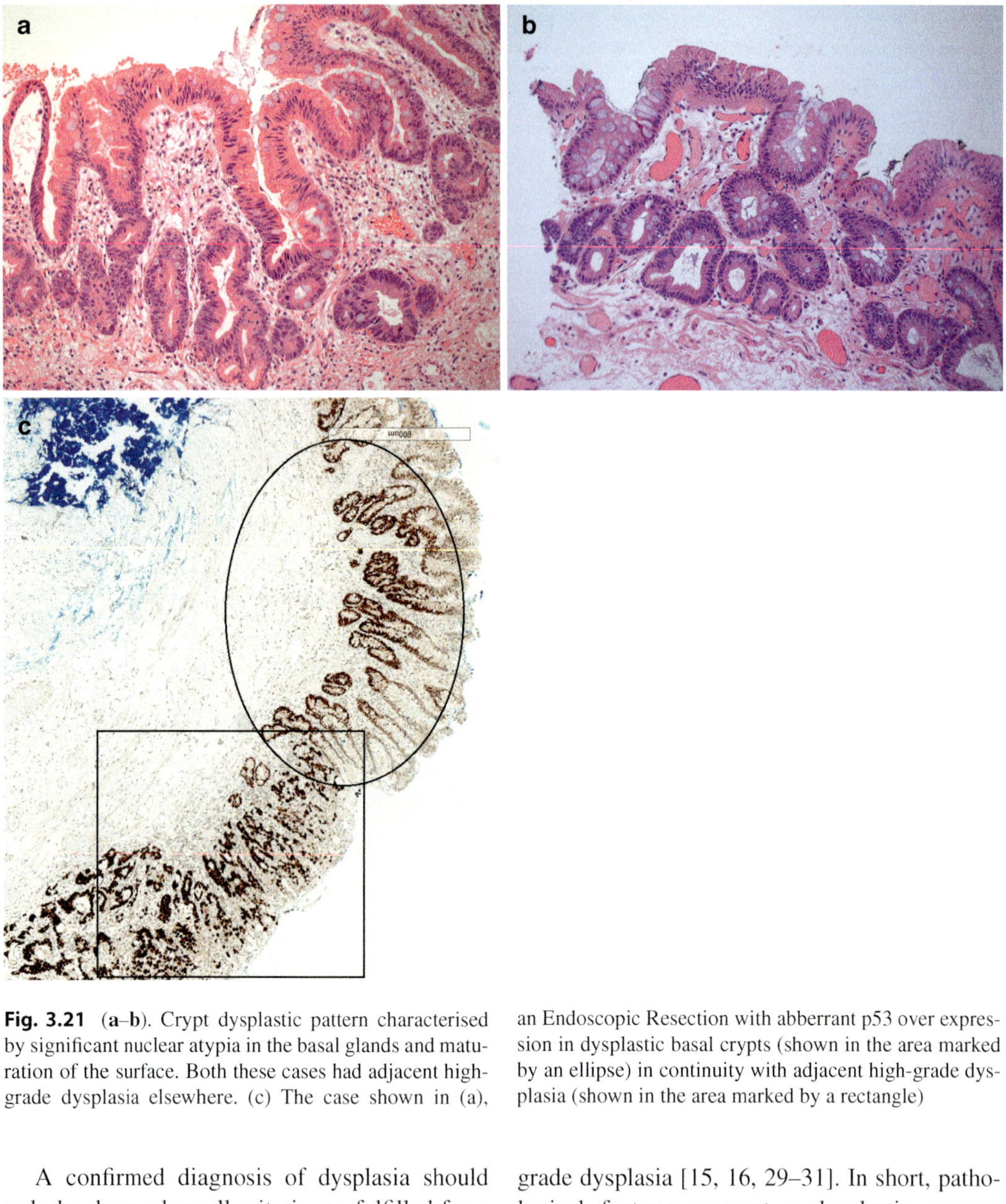

Fig. 3.21 (**a**–**b**). Crypt dysplastic pattern characterised by significant nuclear atypia in the basal glands and maturation of the surface. Both these cases had adjacent high-grade dysplasia elsewhere. (c) The case shown in (a), an Endoscopic Resection with abberrant p53 over expression in dysplastic basal crypts (shown in the area marked by an ellipse) in continuity with adjacent high-grade dysplasia (shown in the area marked by a rectangle)

A confirmed diagnosis of dysplasia should only be done when all criteria are fulfilled for a diagnosis of crypt dysplasia, in particular when high-end abnormalities are present. Immunostaining confirming abberrant p53 expression is very useful.

Epithelial Changes Indefinite for Dysplasia

This pattern is characterised by epithelial changes that do not fulfil criterial of either low- or high-grade dysplasia [15, 16, 29–31]. In short, pathological features suggest a dysplastic process without fulfilling the criteria of dysplasia of any grade (Fig. 3.22a–e).

The two most common settings in which this category is used are in the background ulceration or active inflammation (Fig. 3.22a and 3.24) and when the possibility of crypt dysplasia is strongly considered (Fig. 3.21a, b).

Technical issues such as poor preservation, staining, sectioning, and crosscutting also result in indefinite diagnoses (Fig. 3.23). As much as possible, such information should be communi-

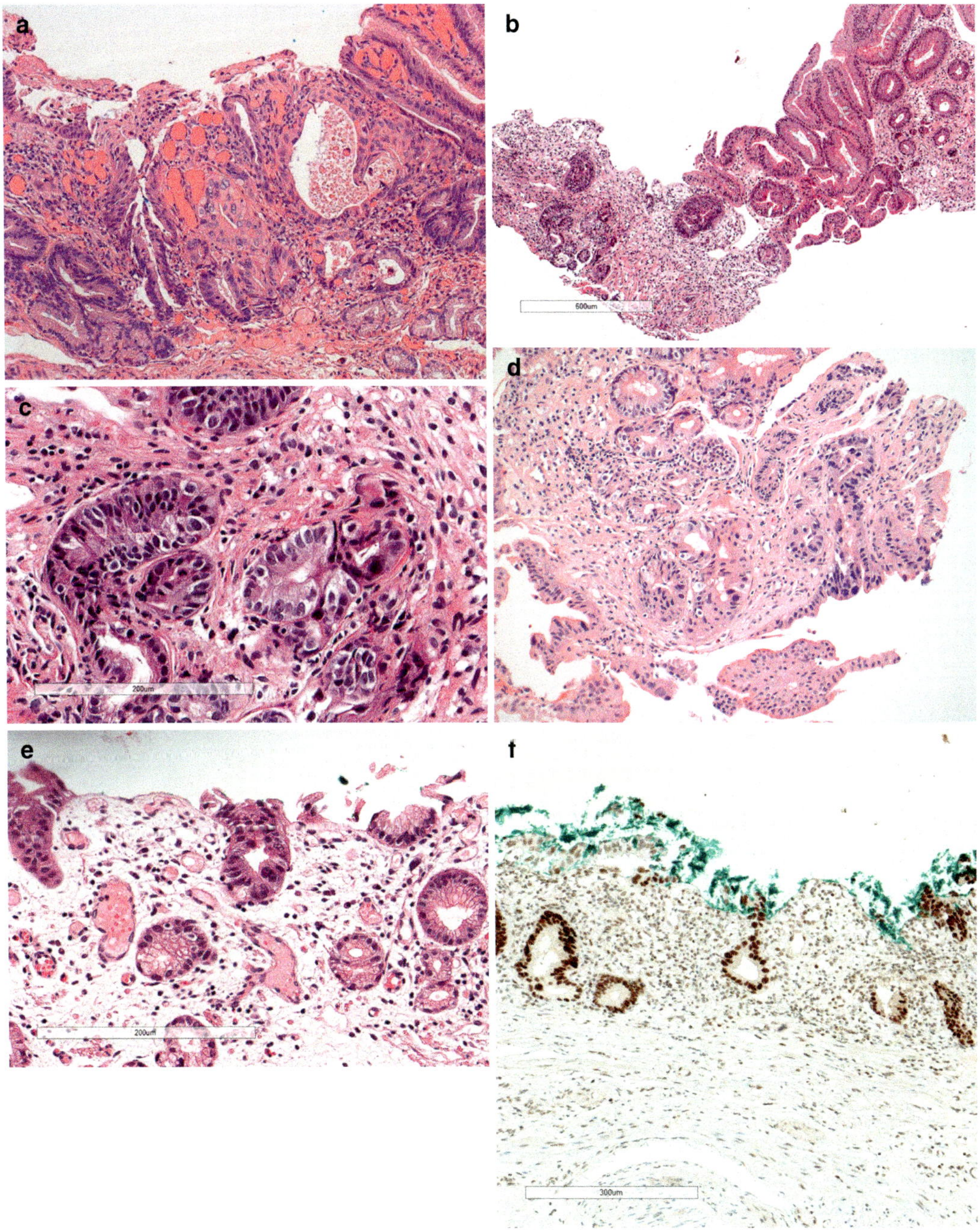

Fig. 3.22 (**a**) Patchy nuclear crowding within part of crypts with surface erosion ("dysplasia-like atypia"), also had adjacent ulceration (not shown): diagnosed as "indefinite for high-grade dysplasia"; on follow-up, there was no dysplasia. Note the retention of apical mucin cap in most cells. (**b**) Indefinite for high-grade dysplasia: Crushed parts of the biopsy featuring a few glands with high-grade nuclear changes. Repeat biopsies and EMR confirmed dysplasia in this case. (**c**) Indefinite for high-grade dysplasia: Isolated glands with atypical smudgy nuclei in a biopsy considered as indefinite for high-grade dysplasia", confirmed to have high-grade dysplasia on repeat biopsies and subsequent EMR. (**d**) Isolated glands and focal surface change with high-grade nuclear abnormalities considered as "indefinite for dysplasia" upgraded to high-grade dysplasia after consultation (subsequent EMR confirmed focal high-grade dysplasia). (**e**) Isolated foci on the surface with high-grade nuclear abnormalities that may be called "Indefinite for high-grade dysplasia" in a biopsy (confirmed HGD on EMR). (**f**) aberrant p53 staining (overexpression) in the case shown in (**e**)

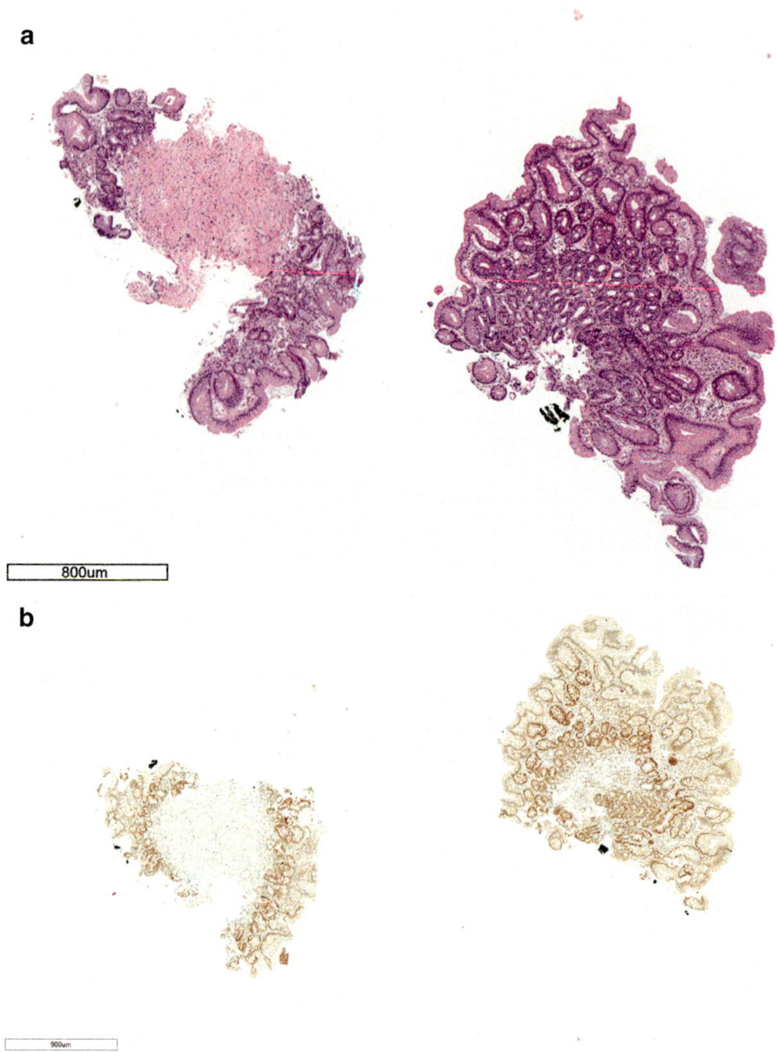

Fig. 3.23 (a). The biopsy fragment on the right-hand field shows exaggerated basal atypia due to tangential cutting whereas the one in the left is BO without dysplasia. (b). Normal p53 expression

cated in the report. The presence of isolated foci of "dysplastic" changes may be challenging (Fig. 3.22d, e)

Diffuse nuclear abnormalities, rather than abrupt change, the presence of too many normal mitoses, maintenance of the basal orientation of nuclei, and the diffuse "basophilic toxic" look of the cytoplasm are notable in reactive epithelia; therefore require caution before a definite dysplastic diagnosis is rendered. Indefinite for dysplasia category is justifiable in this situation with a comment on the possibility that all these changes may be reactive.

Dysplastic epithelium tends to show a range of variable nuclear abnormalities (Table 3.2) and look different compared to the adjacent epithelium in contrast to more uniform changes noted in reactive epithelium including in the neighbouring cells. A feature that is commonly seen in non-dysplastic epithelium is the retention of the apical mucin cap (Box 3.8 and Fig. 3.22a).

A frequent GI consultation is a case that shows exaggerated "atypia" of basal metaplastic glands with surface maturation (in excess of what is regarded as "negative for dysplasia"). Often the reason is a tangentially cut biopsy (Fig. 3.23). In short of cytoarchitectural features described previously, such cases should be considered nonneoplastic.

Box 3.8 Management of BO-Associated Dysplasia

- Negative for dysplasia—repeat surveillance gastroscopy in 3–5 years (four-quadrant biopsies every 2 cm).
- Positive for dysplasia.
  - Low-grade—EMR for nodular dysplasia, repeat surveillance gastroscopy in 6–12 months (four-quadrant biopsies every 1 cm) or consider ablative therapy for flat dysplasia.
  - High-grade—for ablative therapy of flat dysplasia and EMR of nodular dysplasia.
- Epithelial alterations indefinite for dysplasia—review by expert GI pathologist, high-dose PPI for 6 months and then repeat surveillance gastroscopy

Another situation for epithelial atypism to be considered indefinite is when high-end nuclear abnormalities are noted without high-end architectural changes and vice versa. Sometimes, an isolated gland shows severe nuclear abnormalities of either phenotype, particularly at the periphery of an ulceration (either active or healed). In these situations, high-grade dysplastic pattern may be suspected but cannot be confirmed as occasional severe reactive changes may show such abnormalities. Indefinite for dysplasia with a comment on the inability to exclude a high-grade dysplasia is reasonable (fig 3.22 b-e). The category of "indefinite for dysplasia" in the Barrett' setting is heterogeneous. Therefore, "indefinite for dysplasia" category should not be regarded as mere epithelial change that straddles reactive changes and low-grade dysplasia only.

Mimics of Dysplasia

Ulcer/Erosion with Marked Active Inflammation

Extreme cytological abnormalities without architectural changes can result from injury to the metaplastic CLO or adjacent squamous mucosa. Active inflammation may cause nuclear changes that mimic high-grade dysplasia. One should be cautious when numerous neutrophils infiltrate the overlying epithelium; however, the degree of inflammation is important to note. Barrett oesophagus with genuine high-grade dysplasia may be associated with a few neutrophils in the overlying epithelium, and the nuclear changes are so dramatic that the diagnosis of high-grade dysplasia can be made confidently. However if numerous intraepithelial neutrophils or an adjacent ulcer is present, category of "indefinite for dysplasia" is appropriate. Chronic inflammatory cells do not cause the type of nuclear abnormalities associated with active inflammation.

Active inflammation and ulceration occurs in non-neoplastic injury to oesophageal mucosa resulting in marked reactive changes. In the presence of such a clinical setting of possible injury with and without other pathological clues (e.g. pill substances), caution should be exercised. Patients with BO often have severe reflux associated with inflammation and ulceration, in particular those presenting for the first time, and their biopsies can be cytologically "atypical".

Metaplastic Glands with Overlying or Adjacent Squamous Epithelium (Fig. 3.24a)

Metaplastic columnar epithelium adjacent to squamous mucosa is dynamic, and the few glands immediately adjacent a squamous island display nuclear atypia even extending to the surface. A diagnosis of dysplasia should not be made on this appearance. Use of proton pump inhibitors may cause proximal migration of the squamo-columnar junction. With healing, squamous islands may develop within the Barrett's segment. In both situations, glandular mucosa may persist with overlying squamous epithelium ("buried glands"). Both dysplasia and adenocarcinoma may develop within these "buried" glands as illustrated before (Fig. 3.18a, b). Criterion of surface maturation cannot be used in this situation to confirm dysplasia. At endoscopy, reepithelialised squamous mucosa may look normal to the endoscopist, and buried glands may not be biopsied confounding the problem.

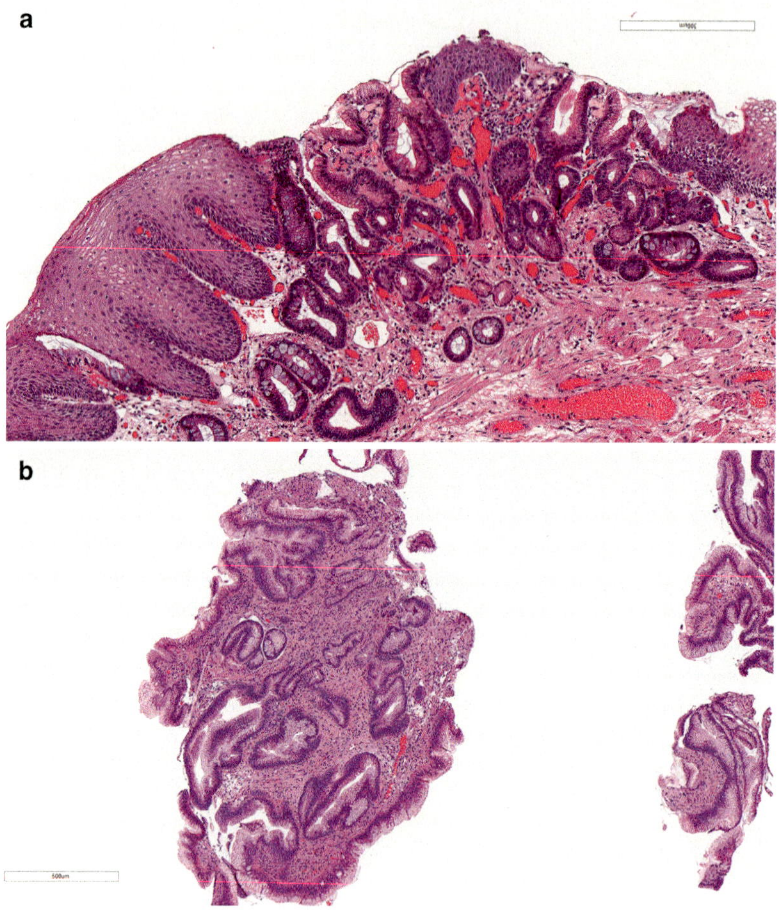

Fig. 3.24 (**a**) Metaplastic columnar epithelium in continuity and adjacent to squamous epithelium that may look "atypical". (**b**) Reactive gastric cardiac mucosa displays nuclear atypia, and misinterpreted as "low-grade dysplastic" epithelium

Reactive Gastric Cardiac Mucosa (Fig. 3.24b)

Reactive gastric cardiac mucosa displays nuclear atypia that may be misinterpreted as dysplastic metaplastic epithelium. The absence of goblet cells may be an important clue that the biopsy is gastric "cardiac", but it must be remembered that in biopsies of the dysplastic epithelium of BO, goblet cells may not be seen. True dysplastic epithelium lacking goblet cells will display greater nuclear atypia and glandular crowding than the reactive gastric cardiac epithelium.

Detached Fragments of Atypical Epithelium

Detached fragments of Barrett's mucosa often show atypical features, most likely due to mechanical trauma. Nuclear atypia could be severe raising the possibility of HGD. A confirmatory diagnosis of dysplasia should not be made on these features alone (Boxes 3.9 and 3.10).

Ancillary Testing

P53 Immunohistochemistry

Overexpression (Fig. 3.25a) and loss (Fig. 3.25b) of p53 protein by immunohistochemistry is recognised as an abnormal pattern that occurs in neoplastic glandular mucosa (both dysplasia and carcinoma) of the oesophagus [10, 17, 23, 24]. Majority of p53 mutations lead to stabilisation of mutated and inactive p53 protein in the nucleus (overexpression). Some mutations result in failed

Box 3.9 Indefinite for Dysplasia

Settings in which the category may be used

- Reactive changes vs. dysplasia.
  - Active inflammation, ulceration—could be either. **
  - Cytology abnormal but not the architecture—could be either.
  - Surface maturation in spite of basal atypia—favour reactive. ***
  - Diffuse change rather than abrupt—favour reactive.
  - Too many normal mitoses—think of a vigorous reactive process.
  - Basophilic toxic look of the cytoplasm—favour reactive.
  - Retention of apical mucin cap—favour reactive.
- Possible true crypt dysplasia.
- Confounding technical issues.
  - Poor preservation
  - Poor staining and sectioning
  - Poor orientation and cross cutting
- It is desirable to state the degree of uncertainty by raising the possibility of reactive changes, low-grade dysplasia, or high-grade dysplasia whenever possible.

**See stromal invasive pattern and HGD
***See crypt dysplasia pattern

Box 3.10 Be Cautious of a Diagnosis of Dysplasia

In the presence of

- Ulcer/erosion with marked active inflammation
- Reactive gastric cardiac type mucosa in biopsies of GOJ in BO
- Metaplastic columnar epithelium adjacent to a squamous island
- Detached fragments of atypical epithelium

translation of the mutant protein with loss of p53 immunostaining, when compared with normal wild-type background (Fig. 3.25b) that is now recognised as an abnormal pattern. Low background wild-type p53 expression is often seen in nuclei of stromal cells, nonneoplastic columnar mucosa and basal layers of squamous mucosa, which is a useful baseline to differentiate the aberrant patterns typical of dysplasia. There is no proven value of p53 immunostain to differentiate low and high grade dysplasia, and dysplastic lesions from invasive carcinoma so far.

Interpretation of p53 immunostaining can be problematic and poorly reproducible subject to variation in methodology, antibody clones used, and interobserver variation in interpretation. Notwithstanding this, some pathologists find staining for p53 of use, especially in distinguishing between atypical reactive proliferation (indefinite for dysplasia) and true dysplasia. Therefore, the experience is variable, and it is probably due to lack of guidance to interpretation and lack of standardisation of techniques.

According to some authorities addition of p53 immunostain to histopathological assessment improves the reproducibility of a diagnosis of dysplasia in Barrett's oesophagus, and should be considered as an adjunct to routine clinical diagnosis [10]. We find aberrant p53 expression to be a very useful tool to confirm dysplasia in difficult cases. It should be noted that p53 nuclear expression is seen in normal epithelia therefore, is not an "all or none" stain. It is the overexpression or loss that should be considered aberrant. Low background wild-type p53 expression is often seen in nuclei of lamina proprial cells, normal columnar mucosa (especially in the proliferative compartment) and basal layers of squamous mucosa. This normal expression is a very useful internal control when a satisfactorily validated p53 immunostain is used in diagnostic practice.

Others

Others such as Ki-67, AMACR positivity, loss of SOX2, and IMP3 have shown variable results and are not recommended in routine practice. [21, 24]. Molecular biomarkers to approach issues of BO and neoplasia are not well established [32–34].

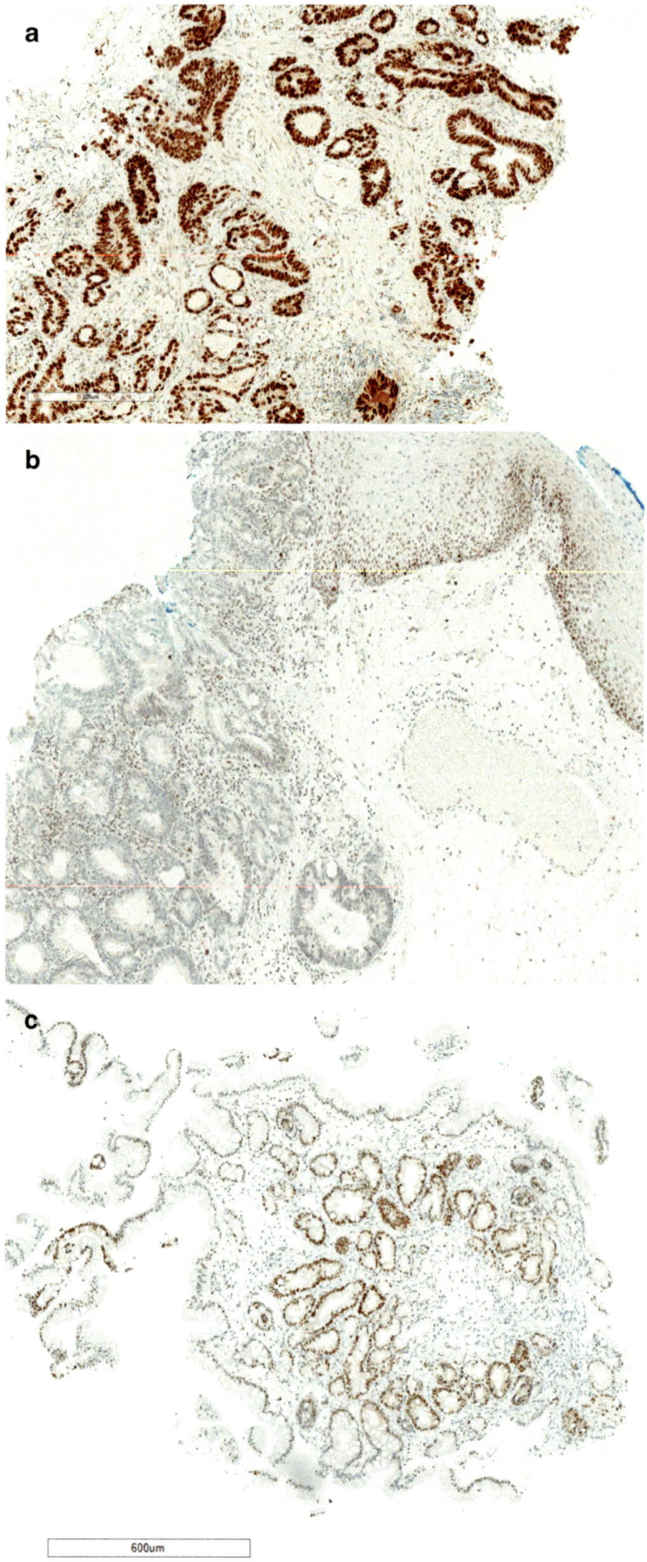

Fig. 3.25 (**a**) p53 overexpression in neoplastic epithelium (**b**) loss of p53 protein in neoplastic epithelium with retained normal expression in the stroma and basal layers of squamous mucosa. (**c**) Normal expression of p53 characterised by patchy moderate to weak nuclear staining mostly seen in the proliferative zone

Glandular Pattern with Atypia and Invasion

Similar to other sites of the tubular gut stromal invasive pattern is characterised by a desmoplastic stromal reaction and increasing complexity of the associated neoplastic epithelium. However, a desmoplastic stromal reaction may not be present in early invasive adenocarcinomas ("intramucosal carcinoma").

Two patterns of invasive epithelial patterns can be presented in an endoscopic biopsy. One without and the other is with a desmoplastic reaction.

The greatest challenges for a GI pathologist when encountered with the possible invasive pattern without a desmoplastic reaction is to differentiate severe reactive changes that mimic neoplasia as described and illustrated previously. Once reactive changes are excluded the second challenge is to differentiate early invasive pattern from non-invasive high-grade dysplastic pattern (Box 3.11).

Box 3.11 Neoplastic Pattern with Invasion

Points to ponder:

- Is this real invasive malignancy?
- Is it HGD only?
- Is there a stromal reaction?
- Is there true desmoplasia?

Both HGD and IMC are currently treated with endoscopic techniques. The third challenge is to exclude submucosal invasion that characterise higher stage lesions that often require oesophagogastrectomy or other adjuvant therapies [35, 36]. As the three situations are linked to different approaches to management, needless to state the first situation where accurate distinction of an invasive malignancy from severe reactive conditions is the most critical. The distinction of intraepithelial lesions, early invasive carcinomas, and invasive carcinomas that invade submucosa and beyond is not such a challenge in surgical resections in which the layers of the oesophageal wall are well delineated. The accuracy for differentiating these critical stages of neoplastic progression is better in endoscopic resection specimens compared to endoscopic biopsies, and comparable to surgical resections [36–40].

Interpretation of these lesions in endoscopic resections (ER) is beyond the scope of this book, and readers are advised to refer to dedicated protocols and literature on this [37, 38].

Invasive Pattern without Desmoplasia/Stromal Reaction (Invasive Pattern 1) (Fig. 3.26a–e)

This pattern signifies early invasive carcinoma amenable to endoscopic resection as a curative and staging modality and therefore has important implications for management. This diagnosis is challenging and subject to considerable interobserver variability.

Currently, microscopic features in endoscopic biopsies that have predicted adenocarcinoma in subsequent resection specimens, described in a limited number of studies are used to suspect or diagnose early invasive carcinomas in biopsies [41–43].

These include:

- Highly complex dysplastic glands ("HGD") with a cribriform growth pattern.
- Single cytologically abnormal cells in the lamina propria (one or more).
- Abortive glands in the lamina propria.
- Angulated glands.
- Never-ending, sheet-like, or "anastomosing/lacework" gland pattern.
- Glandular budding.
- Three or more dilated glands with intraluminal debris.
- Ulcerated HGD.
- HGD with neutrophilic infiltration.
- Spread of neoplastic glands into the adjacent or overlying squamous mucosa. ("pagetoid spread").

Of above features the presence of highly complex dysplastic glands with a cribriform growth pattern, single-cell infiltration, abortive and angulated glands, never-ending, sheet-like, or

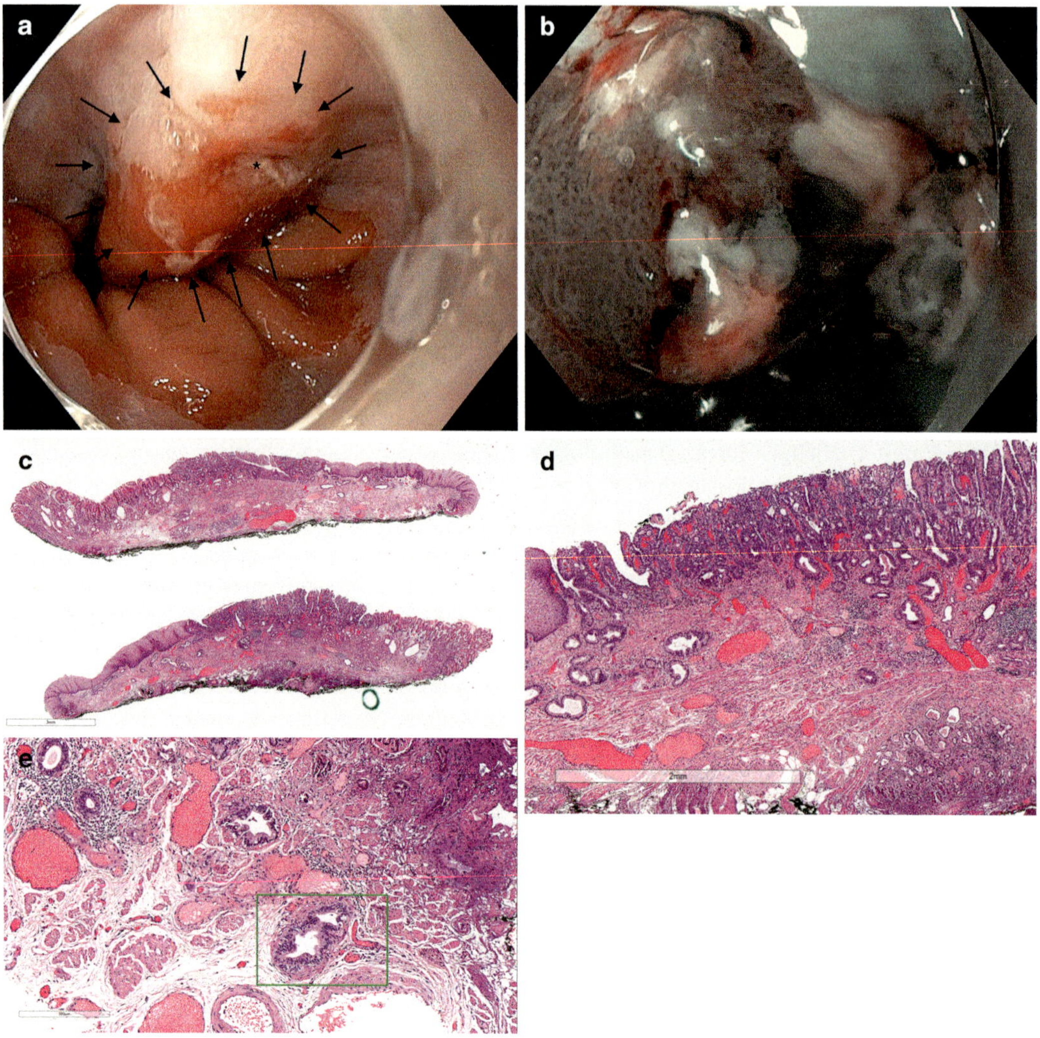

Fig. 3.26 Case 5: A 58-year-old man with past history of short segment Barrett's oesophagus (C0M2). Recent surveillance gastroscopy performed by a community gastroenterologist revealed a nodular area with biopsies reporting HGD. The patient was referred for further endoscopic management. Gastroscopy revealed an ulcerated polyp (Paris 0-Is and 0-III) (see image, Asterix showing 0-III, arrow highlighting polyp) (**a**) within the short segment of BO. The vascular pattern assessed with NBI zoom magnification revealed markedly distorted vascular pattern and morphology consistent with likely submucosal invasive cancer (**b**). This was resected, pinned, and sent for histology. Endoscopic Mucosa Resection (EMR) showed HGD, IMC, (**c**, **d**), and deeper invasion into superficial submucosa (SM Invasion) as seen areas marked by a box (**e**)

"lacework" gland pattern are characteristic of IMC (Fig. 3.27a–f).

Presence of an endoscopic lesion in a patient with BO is a vital piece of information that prompts the GI pathologist to perform series of step levels to the point of exhausting the block as the "invasive pattern" may be focal.

The term "intramucosal carcinoma" is applied to the earliest stage of invasive carcinomas, i.e. lesions that invade through the basement membrane and infiltrate the lamina propria and muscularis mucosa but not the submucosa (Figs. 3.28 and 3.29). The superficial nature of mucosal biopsies obviously limits the ability to

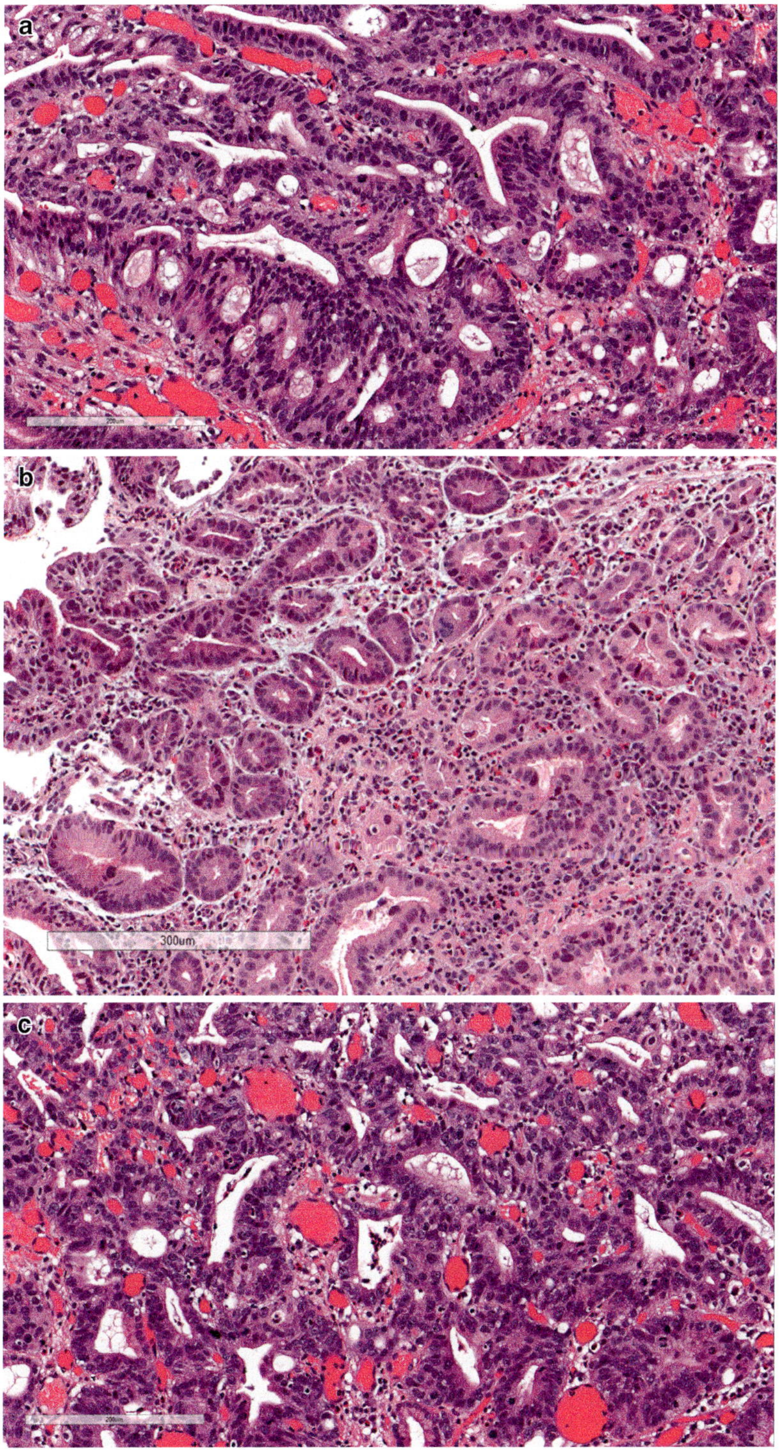

Fig. 3.27 Features of invasive pattern with no stromal reaction (IMC). (**a**) cribriform growth; (**b**) infiltration of lamina propria by single cells and by small groups (**c**) abortive and angulated glands; (**d**) "never-ending"; (**e**) sheet-like/lacework growth of neoplastic cells and many glands with intraluminal debris, (**f**) focal IMC with adjacent normal mucosa

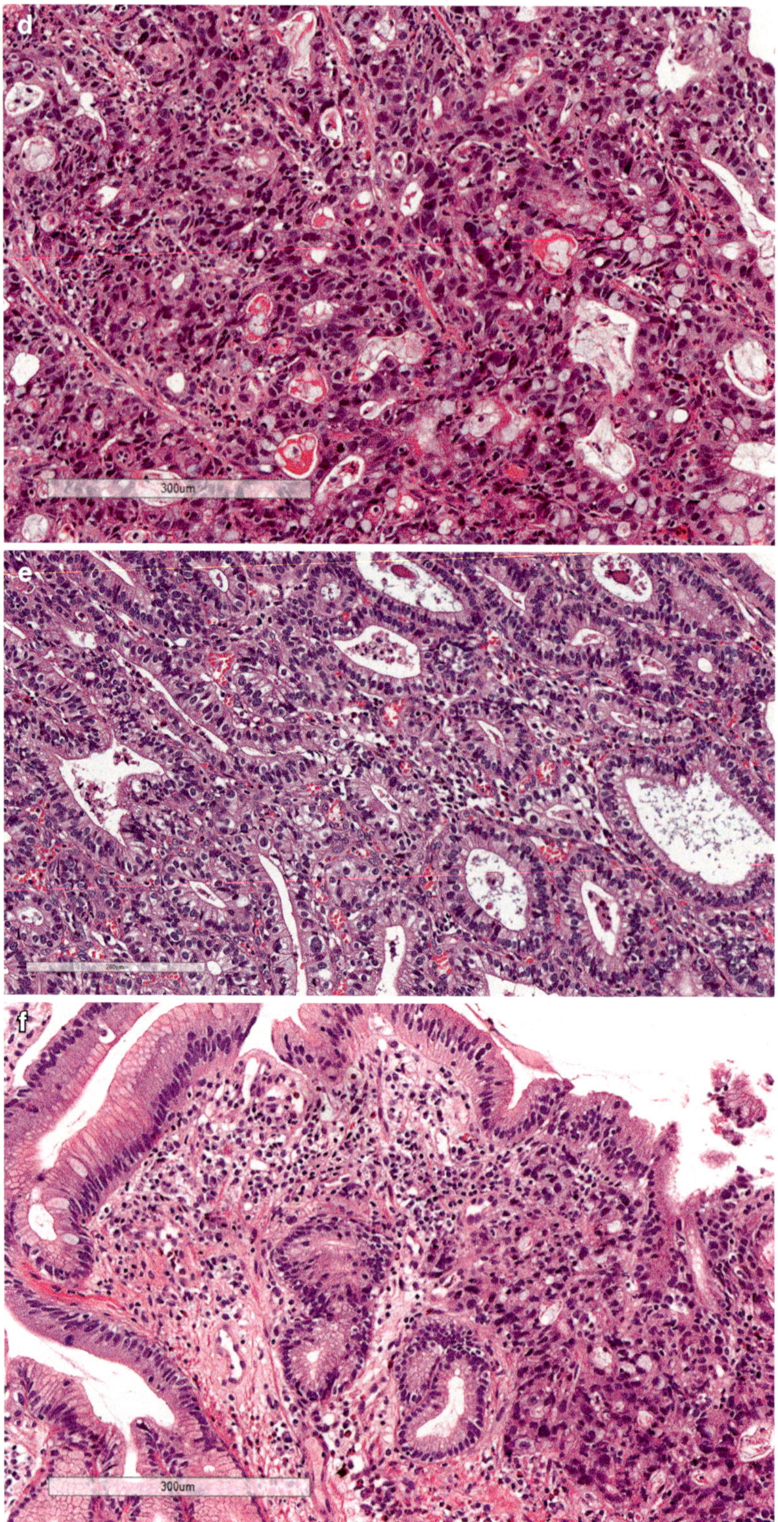

Fig. 3.27 (continued)

distinguish such lesions from deeply invasive carcinomas and high-grade dysplasia.

The pattern based on a combination of above microscopic features with an endoscopic lesion has a high predictive value for diagnosis of early invasion. We report such biopsies as "features of" or "features suspicious of" intramucosal carcinoma. The accuracy of such diagnoses should be validated in centres where endoscopic resections are performed routinely by comparing the features of endoscopic biopsies with subsequent ERs.

There is a notable difference between Western and Japanese pathologists in the diagnosis of high-grade dysplasia and carcinoma. Many features described as high-grade dysplasia and most described above as suspicious for carcinoma are often diagnostic of carcinoma according to Japanese criteria.

Pitfalls

Duplication of Muscularis Mucosa (dMM) (Figs. 3.28 and 3.29)

Duplication of muscularis mucosa is invariably seen in BO although it is not often appreciated. This phenomenon has not been given its due prominence considering its presence in most endoscopic biopsies of neoplastic and non-neoplastic BO and, resulting diagnostic problems [45–47]. The exact reason for this change is

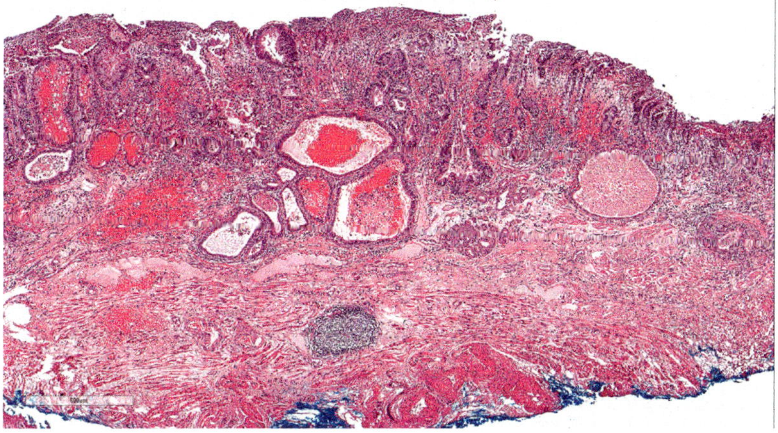

Fig. 3.28 EMR specimen with IMC: note invasive carcinoma infiltrating the lamina propria and inner layers of duplicated muscularis mucosa with no desmoplastic reaction

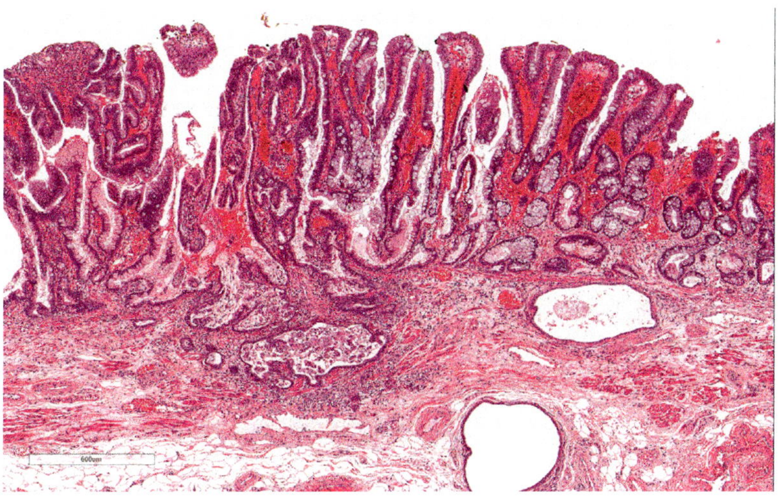

Fig. 3.29 EMR specimen with IMC: note invasive carcinoma infiltrating the lamina propria and deeper layers

not clearly defined although it could be a stromal metaplastic phenomenon or a response of injury. Split muscle fibres can be seen in endoscopic biopsies that are tangentially cut with both non-dysplastic and dysplastic mucosal glands appearing to be invading muscularis mucosae. Moreover, there is frequent in-growth of smooth muscle fibres into the lamina propria, similar to muscularisation that is seen in mucosal prolapse elsewhere in the tubular gut. These changes can result in dilatation of adjacent glands, and the combination of features can mimic well-differentiated invasive carcinoma.

Therefore, the significance of the changes related to dMM and its influence in determination of the presence or absence of invasion and assessment of depth of invasion should be appreciated. Accurate assessment of depth of invasion is more relevant in endoscopic resections. Additionally duplicated muscularis mucosae can appear as thick bundles of the muscle in endoscopic biopsies and raise concern about the possibility of presence of muscularis propria (thereby the possibility of perforation at endoscopy!) by the uninitiated pathologist.

Rare Subtypes of Glandular Neoplasms

Rare subtypes of glandular neoplasms may present in endoscopic biopsies posing additional challenges. Dilated invasive glands may appear deceptively benign (Fig. 3.30a, b).

Colonisation of Submucosal and Deep Mucosal Glands

Dysplasia can colonise submucosal and deep mucosal glands, and mimic invasive carcinoma. A desmoplastic reaction, necrosis, and gland destruction will be lacking in those biopsies. Lobular configuration of deep submucosal glands will be retained (Box 3.12).

Box 3.12 Pitfalls of the Early Invasive Pattern

- Colonised deep mucosal and submucosal glands by dysplasia
  - May mimic invasive carcinoma
- Duplication and splitting of muscularis mucosa
  - Tangential cut with interspersed dysplastic glands may mimic invasion.
  - Mucosal gland surrounded by duplicated smooth muscle fibres in lamina propria may mimic invasive carcinoma.
- Rare deceptive sub-patterns, e.g. dilated gland pattern of carcinoma
  - May appear bland and deceptively benign

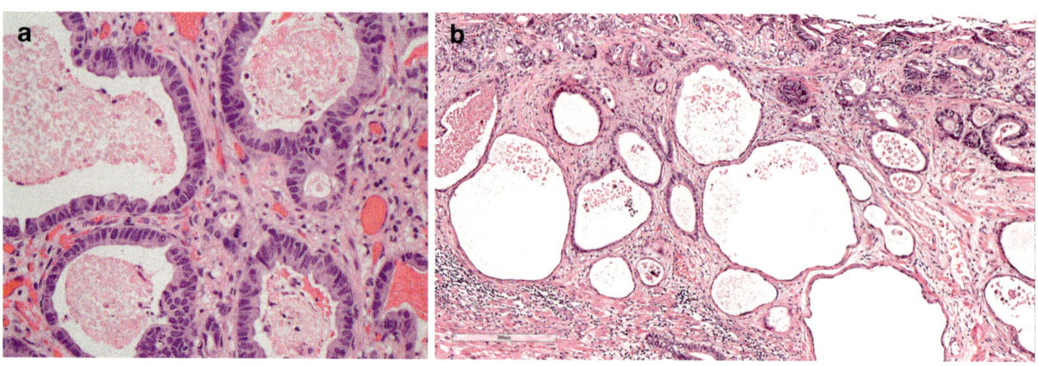

Fig. 3.30 (**a**, **b**) Invasive carcinoma: Dilated gland pattern

Invasive Pattern with Desmoplasia/ Stromal Reaction (Invasive Pattern 2)

All or some of the above features with a stromal reaction featuring desmoplastic and/or fibromyxoid stroma generally signifies the presence of carcinomas invading the submucosa and beyond (Fig. 3.31a–d). Typical invasive adenocarcinomas may be accompanied by tumour necrosis.

The endoscopic appearance of visible lesions (as per the Paris classification) can provide clues to the possibility of underlying submucosal invasion. Awareness of such details can prompt the pathologist to perform further levels as invasion may not be immediately apparent on initial levels. Submucosal infiltration in BOE neoplasia is more often encountered in protruding and depressed lesions (type 0-Is and 0-IIc).

The distinction between intramucosal and submucosal invasion is clinically important as the risk of lymph node (LN) metastasis increases and different management strategies employed [36, 40, 47].

Although the presence of IMC is almost always associated with a visible lesion, abnormalities can be subtle and overlooked by less experienced endoscopists. The first indication of a problem may be flagged by the pathologist finding dysplasia or suspecting invasive cancer on a biopsy, either targeted from a visible abnormality or from among systematic four-quadrant biopsy specimens.

When the invasive pattern with stromal reaction is obvious, it is important to exclude mimics of adenocarcinomas and other rarer epithelial malignancies. Involvement of the oesophagus by proximal cardiac adenocarcinomas is not uncommon (see Chapter 5). Proximal gastric adenocarcinomas are morphologically indistinguishable from oesophageal adenocarcinomas. Phenotypic sub patterns are identical. However, there are significant aetiological, geographic, ethnic, gender and molecular differences between the two, and such differences may be backed by clinical and endoscopic features as well as coexisting gastric pathology and absence of Barrett mucosa.

The diagnosis of a poorly differentiated adenocarcinoma (Figs. 3.32 and 3.33) needs exclusion of other poorly differentiated malignancies.

Histologic subtypes and patterns of oesophageal adenocarcinomas are described by the WHO and the major subtypes are generally comparable throughout the tubular gut (table 1.2 in chapter 1).

Non-epithelial invasive patterns are rarely encountered in an oesophageal biopsy. These follow the patterns similar to those described in the introduction (chapter1). Basic approach to diagnosis of these rarer patterns is similar to the rest of the tubular gut.

Patterns Important in Oesophageal Setting

Blue Cell Pattern

This pattern consists of sheets of malignant cells with overall blue colour to the cancer on low power (Figs. 3.33, 3.34, 3.35). This is due to the presence of crowded malignant cells with high nuclear-cytoplasmic ratio with large dark, often hyperchromatic nuclei with scant cytoplasm. Generally, the blue cell pattern represents poorly differentiated squamous or adenocarcinoma and high-grade neuroendocrine carcinomas (Figs. 3.33, 3.34, 3.35) [8]. Brisk mitotic activity with abnormal forms, necrosis, and apoptosis commonly accompany the blue cell pattern. Rare lymphomas, poorly differentiated mesenchymal tumours and metastases (i.e. melanoma) need to be excluded by an extended panel of immunohistochemical stains (Tables 1.3 to 1.5 in chapter 1).

Pink Cell Pattern

Granular cell tumours (GCT) occur rarely in the gastrointestinal tract, and most commonly in the oesophagus, which is involved in up to 65% of all cases that occur in the GI tract [48]. The typical endoscopic appearance is that of a sessile, yellowish-white subepithelial polyp, which feels firm to the blunt probe (table 3.3).

Diagnosis is most often made with pinch biopsies. However, if tunnel biopsies are not

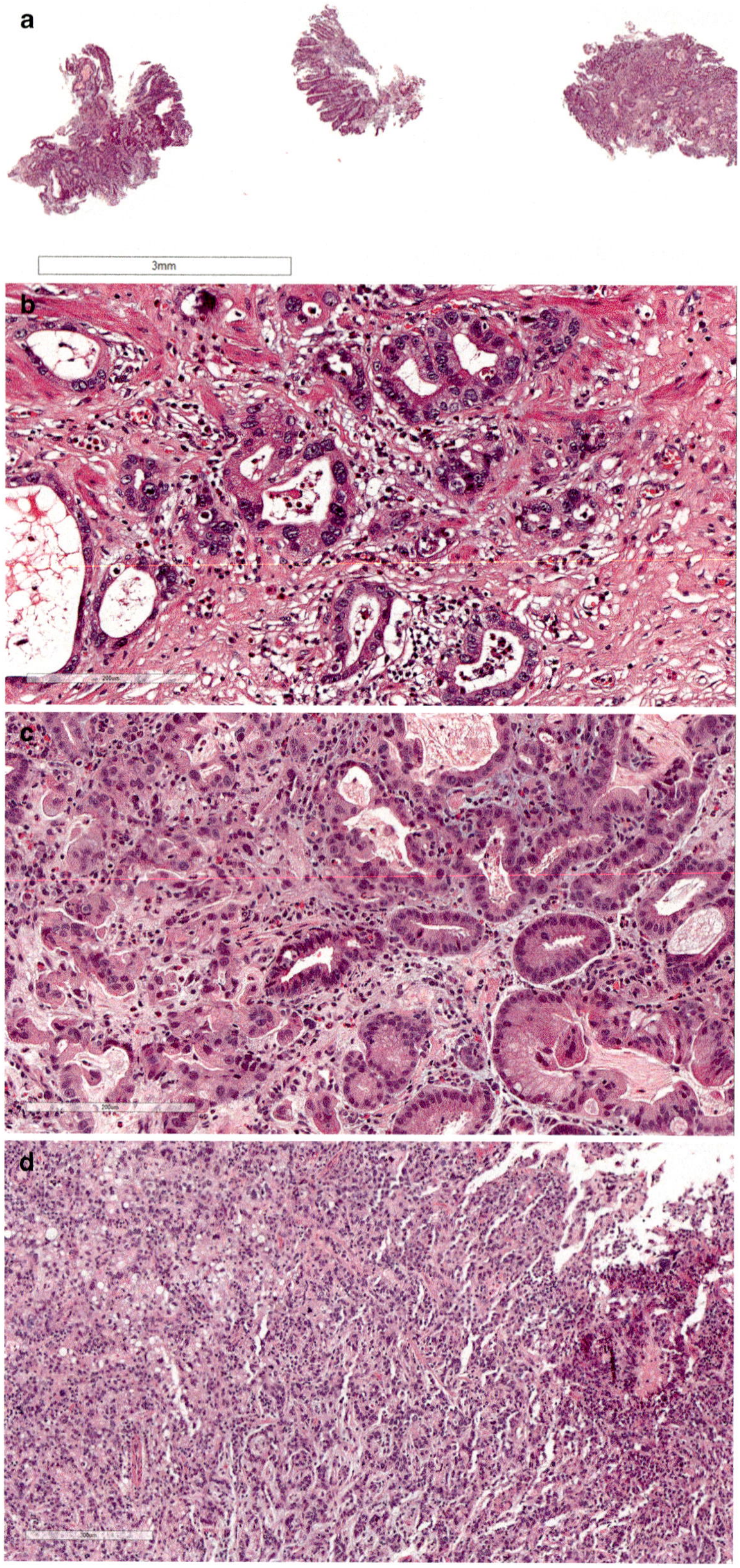

Fig. 3.31 (**a**) Invasive pattern with a stromal reaction: scanning power. (**b**) Invasive pattern with stromal reaction: malignant glands infiltrating desmoplastic stroma. (**c**) Invasive pattern with stromal reaction: malignant glands surrounded by fibromyxoid stroma. (**d**) Invasive pattern with stromal reaction: strands of malignant cells infiltrating fibromyxoid stroma

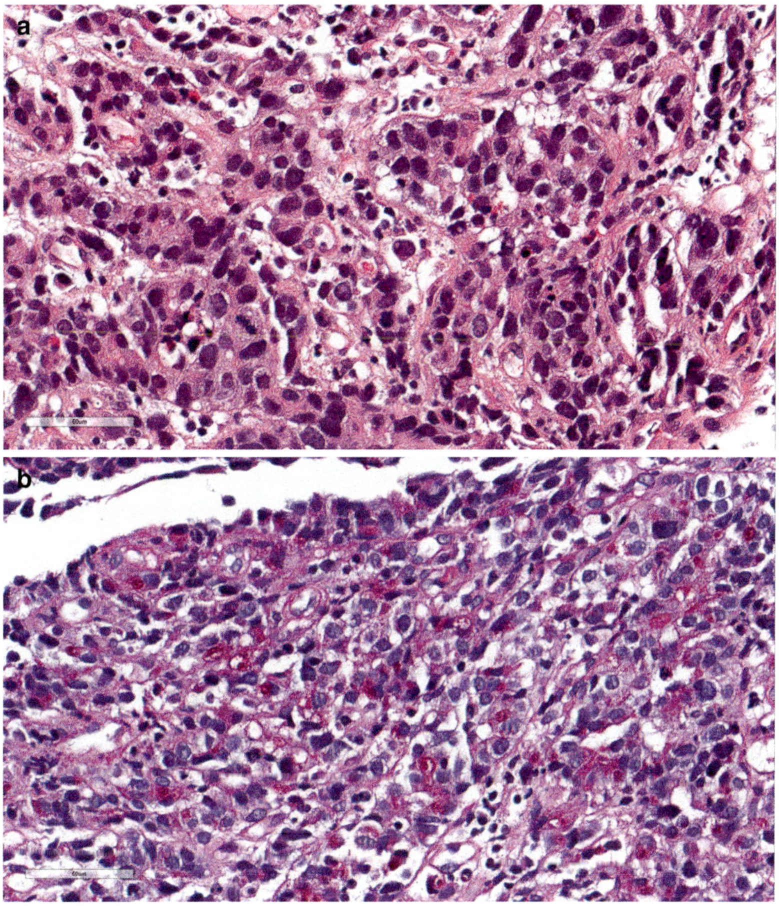

Fig. 3.32 (**a**) Poorly differentiated adenocarcinoma with mucin production demonstrated by PASD stain (**b**)

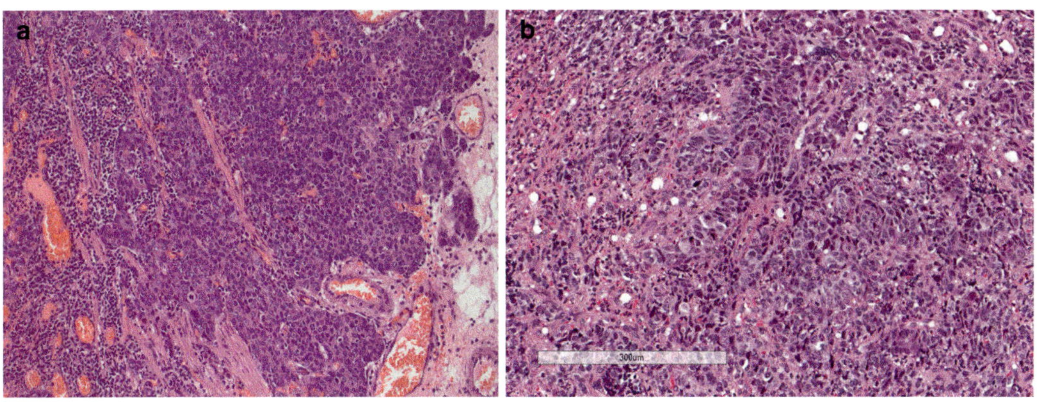

Fig. 3.33 (**a**, **b**) Poorly differentiated adenocarcinoma (Blue cell pattern), originating in BO

performed, an endoscopic biopsy may only show surface epithelial changes that may present as a deceptive squamo-proliferative lesion without the underlying lesion being sampled. Therefore, the reported endoscopic appearance should alert the pathologist to perform additional levels and appropriate ancillary tests for a diagnosis (Fig. 3.37a–d).

Squamo-proliferative pattern with atypia is often seen, and is a common pitfall. Concern

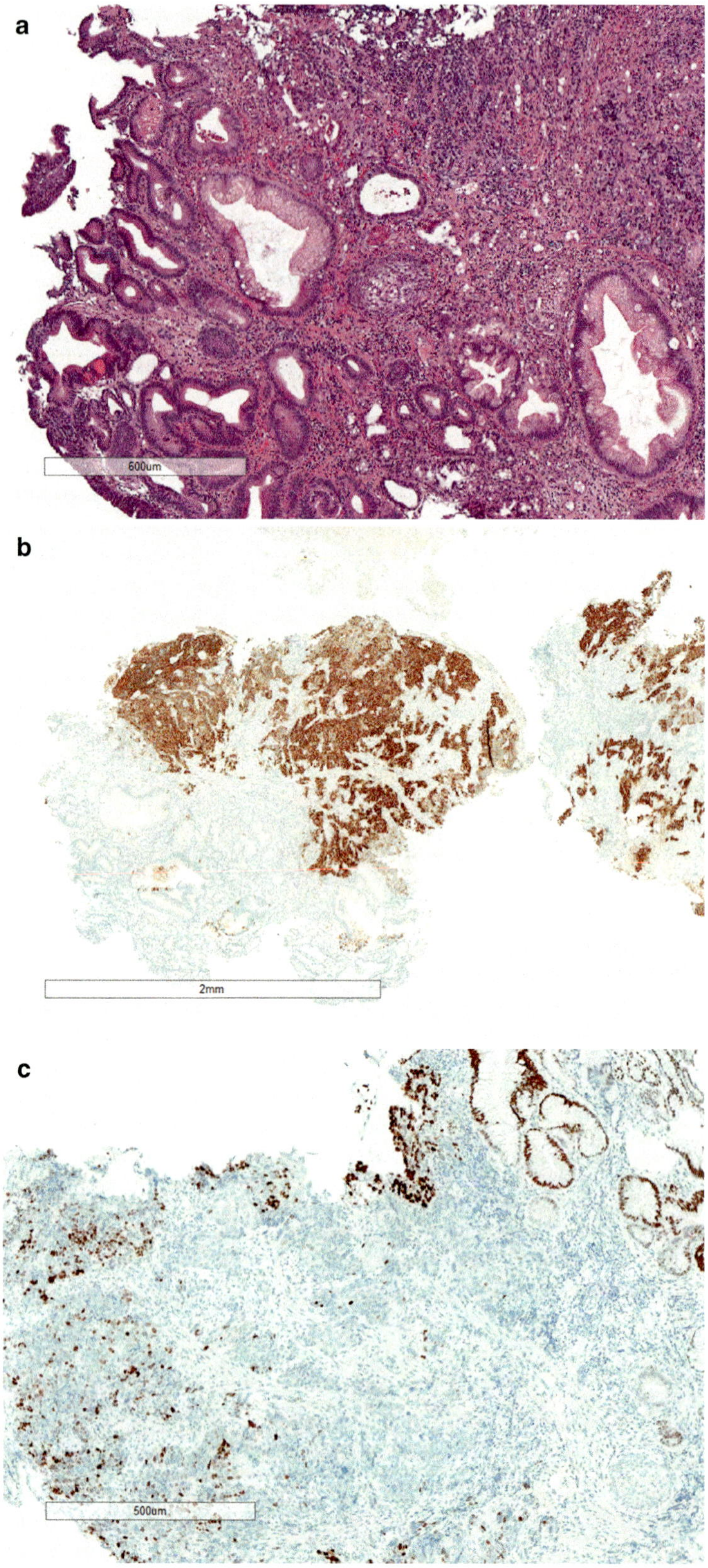

Fig. 3.34 (**a**) Poorly differentiated adenocarcinoma with neuroendocrine differentiation. Note adjacent dysplastic glands in the setting of Barrett's dysplasia. (**b**) Positive synaptophysin immunohistochemistry-neuroendocrine component. (**c**) Positive CDX2 immunohistochemistry-focal

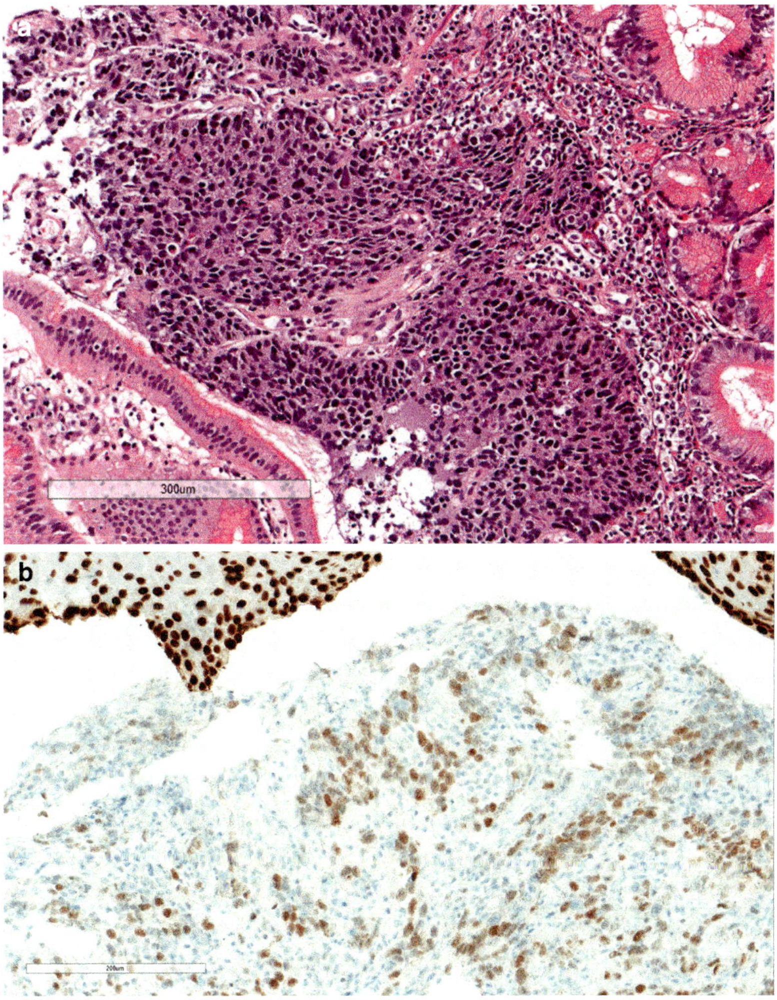

Fig. 3.35 (**a**) Poorly differentiated carcinoma (blue cell pattern) with possible squamous differentiation. (**b**) Moderate to weak P63 positivity but p40 negative (not shown), with strong positivity was overlying squamous mucosa

may be the possibility of a neoplastic squamous lesion. Endoscopic appearance is a vital clue. Although rare, granular cell tumours may show a small risk of malignant potential, and therefore complete removal is recommended in most cases. Complete removal is mostly performed through EMR or Endoscopic Submucosa Dissec tion for larger lesions. Adenocarcinoma with "signet ring cell" differentiation can present in biopsies with single pink and clear cells, but are often accompanied by extracellular mucin (Figure 3.38). "Signet ring" cells seen in mucinous carcinomas can be a degenerate phenomenon in malignant cells ("pseudosignet ring cells"). True signet ring cell adenocarcinomas are rare in the oesophagus compared to signet ring cell adenocarcinomas associated with CDH1 mutations of the stomach.

Spindle Cell Pattern

In an oesophageal biopsy, this pattern warrants excluding spindle cell (sarcomatoid) carcinomas before a diagnosis of a rarer mesenchymal tumour is made. Often a variety of cytokeratins are required for confirmation as cytokeratin expression can be very patchy. Squamous markers such as p63 and p40 are helpful, but again expression can be weak and patchy. The differentiation is important considering implication for treatment and prognosis. P40 is considered as a more specific staining supporting squamous origin than P63. P63 has been shown to be positive in

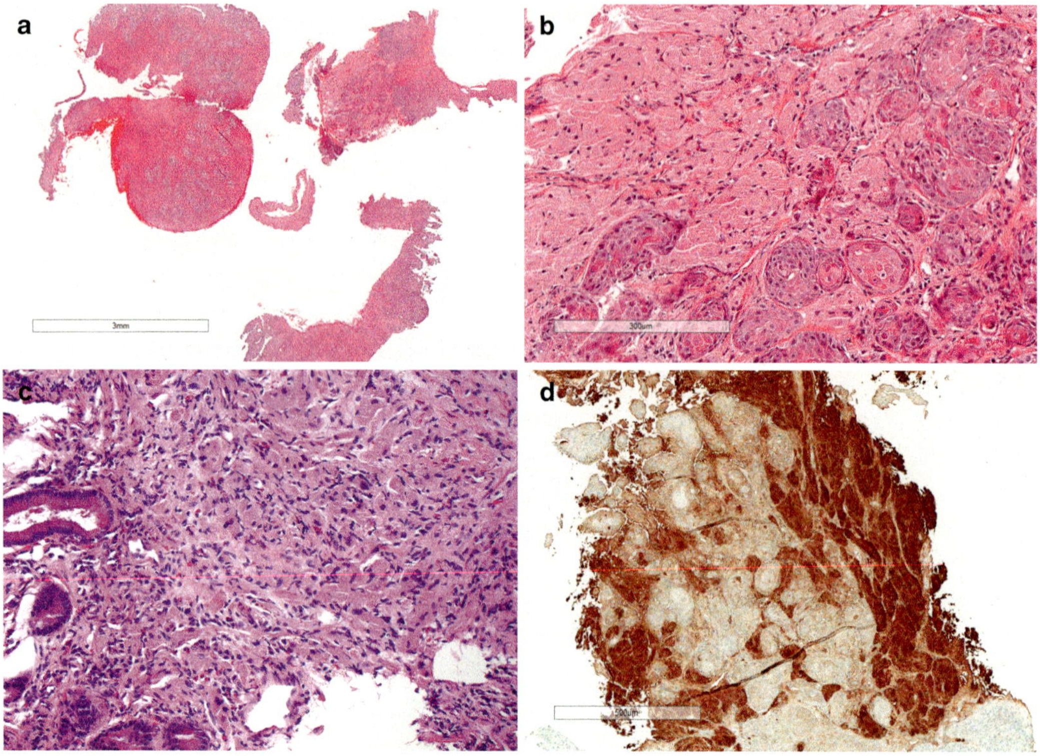

Fig. 3.36 (**a**) Typical low-power appearance of granular cell tumour with hyperproliferative squamous mucosa. (**b**) Pink cell pattern of GCT: epithelioid cells with abundant eosinophilic granular cytoplasm and small uniform nuclei. The overlying epithelium shows pseudoepitheliomatous hyperplasia mimicking "invasive squamous islands". (**c**) Pink cell pattern of GCT: note the more subtle pink tumour cells. (**d**) S100 immunostain: tumour cells are positive compared to the hyperplastic squamous islands that are negative

non-squamous carcinomas including adenocarcinoma, but positivity is focal and weak.

Smooth muscle and neural tumours and gastrointestinal stromal tumours (GIST) are rare tumours that may be presented in oesophageal biopsy. General approach to differentiation is discussed in Chapter 1.

Biomarker Testing for Therapeutic Targets

The major therapeutic biomarker thus far that has a role in BO-associated adenocarcinomas is human epidermal growth factor receptor 2 (HER2) [49–55]. This assertion is based on the results of the landmark ToGA study (trastuzumab for gastric/gastroesophageal junction adenocarcinomas) that showed better survival in HER2 positive cancers treated with trastuzumab-based treatment combinations [49]. In the study cohort, GOJ cancers showed a higher proportion of HER2 amplifications, and most of the GOJ cancers were from Western countries. This is regarded as evidence of response to BO-related adenocarcinomas to trastuzumab. There are independent studies of HER2 status in pure oesophageal adenocarcinomas that have confirmed the occurrence of HER2 amplification [50–54]. Clinical studies on HER2 expression in more proximal oesophageal adenocarcinomas are ongoing [55]. The approach and a guide to HER2 testing in gastric and GOJ cancers are provided in chapter 5.

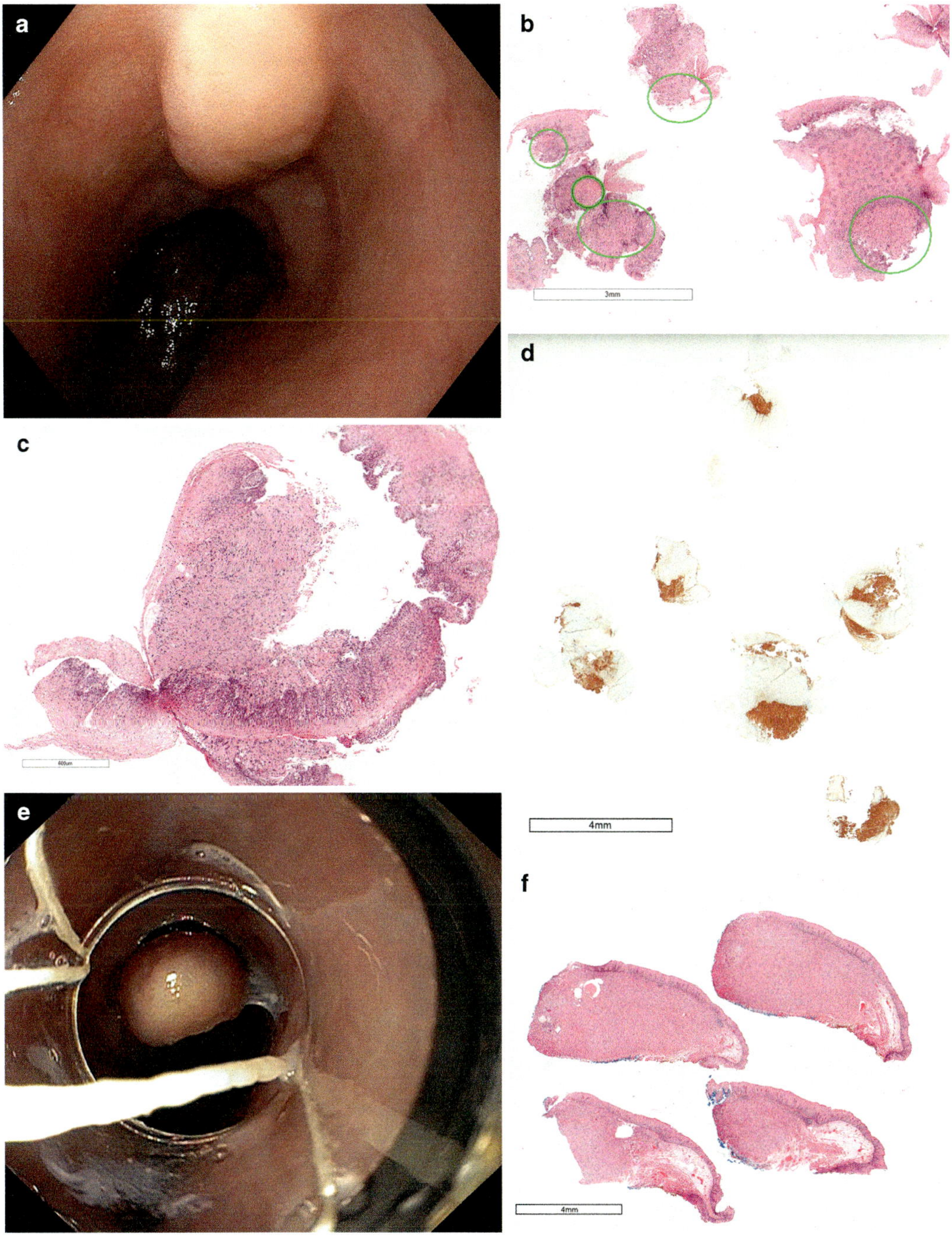

Fig. 3.37 A 44-year-old lady initially referred for evaluation of abdominal bloating. Gastroscopy was performed and revealed a 20-mm ovoid yellowish subepithelial mass (**a**) with tunnel biopsies confirming a GCT (**b**), tumour in all circles and high power of pink cell pattern of GCT); (**c**) S100 positivity in tumour cells (**d**). She was later referred for endoscopic removal, which was performed using an EMR technique with complete removal achieved (**e**) GCT was confirmed on EMR (**f**)

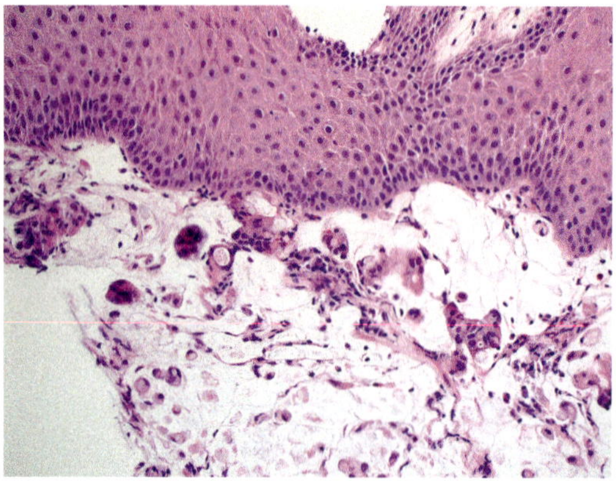

Fig. 3.38 Adenocarcinoma with some "signet ring" cells and extracellular mucin

References

1. Raftopoulos SC, Segarajasingam DS, Burke V, Ee HC, Yusoff IF. A cohort study of missed and new cancers after esophagogastroduodenoscopy. Am J Gastroenterol. 2010;105:1292–7.
2. Anonymous. The Paris endoscopic classification of superficial neoplastic lesions: esophagus, stomach, and colon:November 30 to December 1, 2002. Gastrointest Endosc. 2003;58(6 Suppl):S3–43.
3. Cottreau J, Gruchy S, Kamionek M, Lauwers GY, Arnason T. Prevalence of oesophageal epidermoid metaplasia in 1048 consecutive patients and 58 patients with squamous neoplasms. Histopathology. 2016;68:988–95.
4. Singhi AD, Arnold CA, Crowder CD, Lam-Himlin DM, Voltaggio L, Montgomery EA. Oesophageal leukoplakia or epidermoid metaplasia: a clinicopathological study of 18 patients. Mod Pathol. 2014;27(1):38–43.
5. Dawsey SM, Lewin KJ, Wang GQ, Liu FS, Nieberg RK, Yu Y, et al. Squamous oesophageal histology and subsequent risk of squamous cell carcinoma of the esophagus.A prospective follow-up study from Linxian, China. Cancer. 1994;74:1686–92.
6. Rubio C, Liu F, Zhao H. Histological classification of intraepithelial neoplasias and microinvasive squamous carcinoma of the esophagus. Am J Surg Pathol. 1989;13:685–90.
7. Taylor PR, Abnet CC, Dawsey SM. Squamous dysplasia - the precursor lesion for oesophageal squamouscarcinoma. Cancer Epidemiol Biomarkers Prev. 2013;22(4):540–52.
8. DiMaio MA, Kwok S, Montgomery KD, Lowe AW, Pai RK. Immunohistochemical panel for distinguishing oesophageal adenocarcinoma from squamous cell carcinoma: a combination of p63, cytokeratin 5/6, MUC5AC, and anterior gradient homolog 2 allows optimal subtyping. Hum Pathol. 2012;43(11):1799–807.
9. Wang HH, Zeroogian JM, Spechler SJ, Goyal RK, Antonioli DA. Prevalence and significance of pancreatic acinar metaplasia at the gastroesophageal junction. Am J Surg Pathol. 1996;20(12):1507–10.
10. Fitzgerald RC, di Pietro M, Ragunath K, Ang Y, Kang JY, Watson P, et al. British Society of Gastroenterology guidelines on the diagnosis and management of Barrett's oesophagus. Gut. 2014;63:7–42.
11. Shaheen NJ, Falk GW, Iyer PG, Gerson L. ACG clinical guideline: diagnosis and management of Barrett's esophagus. Am J Gastroenterol. 2015;108:1238–49.
12. Whiteman DC, Appleyard M, Bahin FF, Bobryshev YV, Bourke MJ, Brown I, et al. Australian clinical practice guidelines for the diagnosis and management of Barrett's Esophagus and Early Oesophageal Adenocarcinoma. J Gastroenterol Hepatol. 2015;30:804–20.
13. Bennett C, Vakil N, Bergman J, Harrison R, Odze R, Vieth M, et al. Consensus statements for management of Barrett's dysplasia and early-stage oesophageal adenocarcinoma, based on a delphi process. Gastroenterology. 2012;143(2):336–46.
14. Schlemper RJ, Riddell RH, Kato Y, Borchard F, Cooper HS, Dawsey SM, et al. The Vienna classification of gastrointestinal epithelial neoplasia. Gut. 2000;47:251–5.
15. Coco DP, Goldblum JR, Hornick JL, Lauwers GY, Montgomery E, Srivastava A, et al. Interobserver variability in the diagnosis of crypt dysplasia in Barrett esophagus. Am J Surg Pathol. 2011;35:45–54.
16. Curvers WL, ten Kate FJ, Krishnadath KK, Visser M, Elzer B, Baak LC, et al. Low-grade dysplasia in Barrett's esophagus: overdiagnosed and underestimated. Am J Gastroenterol. 2010;105:1523–30.
17. Skacel M, Petras RE, Rybicki LA, Gramlich TL, Richter JE, Falk GW, et al. p53 expression in low grade dysplasia in Barrett's esophagus: correlation with interobserver agreement and disease progression. Am J Gastroenterol. 2002;97:2508–13.
18. Mahajan D, Bennett AE, Liu X, Bena J, Bronner MP. Grading of gastric foveolar-type dysplasia in Barrett's esophagus. Mod Pathol. 2010;23:1–11.
19. Odze RD. Update on the diagnosis and treatment of barrett esophagus and related neoplastic precursor lesions. Arch Pathol Lab Med. 2008;132:1577–85.
20. Goldblum JR. Current issues in Barrett's esophagus and Barrett's-related dysplasia. Mod Pathol. 2015;28(May 2014):S1–6.
21. Odze RD. Diagnosis and grading of dysplasia in Barrett's oesophagus. J Clin Pathol. 2006;59:1029–38.
22. Odze RD. Barrett esophagus: histology and pathology for the clinician. Nat Rev Gastroenterol Hepatol. 2009;6:478–90.
23. Greenblatt MS, Bennett WP, Hollstein M, Greenblatt MS, Bennett WP, Hollstein M, et al. Mutations in the p53 tumour suppressor gene: clues to cancer

etiology and molecular pathogenesis. Cancer Res. 1994;54:4855–78.
24. McCormick Matthews LH, Noble F, Tod J, Jaynes E, Harris S, Primrose JN, et al. Systematic review and meta-analysis of immunohistochemical prognostic biomarkers in resected oesophageal adenocarcinoma. Br J Cancer. 2015;113:107–18.
25. Brown IS, Whiteman DC, Lauwers GY. Foveolar type dysplasia in Barrett esophagus. Mod Pathol. 2010;23:834–43.
26. Park DY, Srivastava A, Kim GH, Mino-Kenudson M, Deshpande V, Zukerberg LR, et al. Adenomatous and foveolar gastric dysplasia: distinct patterns of mucin expression and background intestinal metaplasia. Am J Surg Pathol. 2008;32(4):524–33.
27. Patil DT, Bennett AE, Mahajan D, Bronner MP. Distinguishing Barrett gastric foveolar dysplasia from reactive cardiac mucosa in gastroesophageal reflux disease. Hum Pathol. 2013;44:1146–53.
28. Khor TS, Alfaro EE, Ooi EMM, Li Y, Srivastava A, Fujita H, et al. Divergent expression of MUC5AC, MUC6, MUC2, CD10, and CDX-2 in dysplasia and intramucosal adenocarcinomas with intestinal and foveolar morphology. Am J Surg Pathol. 2012;36(3):331–42.
29. Lomo LC, Blount PL, Sanchez CA, Li X, Galipeau PC, Cowan DS, et al. Crypt dysplasia with surface maturation. Am J Surg Pathol. 2006;30(4):423–35.
30. Younes M, Lauwers GY, Atilla E, Gulchin E, Verm R, Bridges M, et al. The significance of "'indefinite for dysplasia'" grading in barrett metaplasia. Arch Pathol Lab Med. 2011;135:430–2.
31. Sangle NA, Taylor SL, Emond MJ, Depot M, Overholt BF, Bronner MP. Overdiagnosis of high-grade dysplasia in Barrett's esophagus: a multicenter, international study. Mod Pathol. 2015;28(6):758–65.
32. di Pietro M, Boerwinkel DF, Shariff MK, Liu X, Telakis E, Lao-Sirieix P, et al. The combination of autofluorescence endoscopy and molecular biomarkers is a novel diagnostic tool for dysplasia in Barrett's oesophagus. Gut. 2015;64(1):49–56.
33. Ross-Innes CS, Becq J, Warren A, Cheetham RK, Northen H, O'Donovan M, et al. Whole-genome sequencing provides new insights into the clonal architecture of Barrett's esophagus and oesophageal adenocarcinoma. Nat Genet. 2015;47:1038.
34. Stachler MD, Taylor-Weiner A, Peng S, McKenna A, Agoston AT, Odze RD, et al. Paired exome analysis of Barrett's esophagus and adenocarcinoma. Nat Genet. 2015;47:1047–55.
35. Bhat S, Coleman HG, Yousef F, Johnston BT, McManus DT, Gavin AT, et al. Risk of malignant progression in Barrett's Esophagus patients: results from a large population-based study. J Natl Cancer Inst. 2011;103:1049–57.
36. Prasad GA, Wang KK, Buttar NS, Wongkeesong L, Krishnadath KK, Nichols FC, et al. Long-term survival following endoscopic and surgical treatment of high-grade dysplasia in Barrett's esophagus. Gastroenterology. 2007;132:1226–33.
37. Mojtahed A, Shimoda T. Proper pathologic preparation and assessment of endoscopic mucosal resection and endoscopic submucosal dissection specimens. Tech Gastrointest Endosc. 2011;13:95–9.
38. Kumarasinghe MP, Brown I, Raftopoulos S, Bourke MJ, Charlton A, de Boer WB, et al. Standardised reporting protocol for endoscopic resection for Barrett oesophagus associated neoplasia: expert consensus recommendations. Pathology. 2014;46:473–80.
39. Vieth M, Ell C, Gossner L, May A, Stolte M. Histological analysis of endoscopic resection specimens from 326 patients with Barrett's esophagus and early neoplasia. Endoscopy. 2004;36:776–81.
40. Pennathur A, Farkas A, Krasinskas AM, Ferson PF, Gooding WE, Gibson MK, et al. Esophagectomy for T1 oesophageal cancer: outcomes in 100 patients and implications for endoscopic therapy. Ann Thorac Surg. 2009;87:1048–55.
41. Patil DT, Goldblum JR, Rybicki L, Plesec TP, Mendelin JE, Bennett AE, et al. Prediction of adenocarcinoma in esophagectomy specimens based upon analysis of preresection biopsies of barrett esophagus with at least high-grade dysplasia: a comparison of 2 systems. Am J Surg Pathol. 2012;36:134–41.
42. Downs-Kelly E, Mendelin JE, Bennett AE, Castilla E, Henricks WH, Schoenfield L, et al. Poor interobserver agreement in the distinction of high-grade dysplasia and adenocarcinoma in pretreatment Barrett's esophagus biopsies. Am J Gastroenterol. 2008;103:2333–40.
43. Zhu W, Appelman HD, Greenson JK, Ramsburgh SR, Orringer MB, Chang AC, et al. A histologically defined subset of high-grade dysplasia in Barrett mucosa is predictive of associated carcinoma. Am J Clin Pathol. 2009;132:94–100.
44. Abraham SC, Krasinskas AM, Correa AM, Hofstetter WL, Ajani JA, Swisher SG, et al. Duplication of the muscularis mucosae in Barrett esophagus: an underrecognized feature and its implication for staging of adenocarcinoma. Am J Surg Pathol. 2007;31:1719–25.
45. Lewis JT, Wang KK, Abraham SC. Muscularis mucosae duplication and the musculo-fibrous anomaly in endoscopic mucosal resections for barrett esophagus: implications for staging of adenocarcinoma. Am J Surg Pathol. 2008;32:566–71.
46. Hölscher AH, Vallböhmer D, Bollschweiler E. Early barrett's carcinoma of the esophagus. Ann Thorac Cardiovasc Surg. 2008;14:347–54.
47. Vieth M, Stolte M. Pathology of early upper GI cancers. Best Pract Res Clin Gastroenterol. 2005;19:857–69.
48. Orlowska J, Patchlewski J, Gugulski A, Butruk E. A conservative approach to granular cell tumours of the esophagus: four case reports and literature review. Am J Gastroenterol. 1993;88:311–5.
49. Bang YJ, Van Cutsem E, Feyereislova A, Chung HC, Shen L, Sawaki A, Lordick F, Ohtsu A, Omuro Y, Satoh T, Aprile G, Kulikov E, Hill J, Lehle M, Rüschoff J, Kang YK. Trastuzumab in combination with chemotherapy versus chemotherapy alone for treatment of HER2-positive advanced gastric or

gastro-oesophageal junction cancer (ToGA): a phase 3, openlabel, randomised controlled trial. Lancet. 2010;376:687–97.
50. Flejou J-F, Paraf F, Muzeau F, et al. Expression of c-erbB-2 oncogene product in Barrett's adenocarcinoma: pathological and prognostic correlations. J Clin Pathol. 1994;47:23–6.
51. Nakamura T, Nekarda H, Hoelscher AH, et al. Prognostic value ofDNA ploidy and c-erbB-2 oncoprotein overexpression in adenocarcinoma of Barrett's oesophagus. Cancer. 1994;73:1785–94.
52. Brien TP, Odze RD, Sheehan CE, McKenna BJ, Ross JS. Her-2/neu gene amplification by FISH predicts poor survival in Barrett's esophagus-associated adenocarcinoma. Hum Pathol. 2000;31:35–9.
53. Rossi E, Grisanti S, Villanacci V, et al. HER-2 overexpression/amplification in Barrett's oesophagus predicts early transition from dysplasia to adenocarcinoma: a clinico-pathologic study. J Cell Mol Med. 2009;13:3826–33.
54. Hu Y, Bandla S, Godfrey TE, Tan D, Luketich JD, Pennathur A, Qiu X, Hicks DG, Peters JH, Zhou Z. HER2 amplification, overexpression and score criteria in oesophageal adenocarcinoma. Mod Pathol. 2011;24(7):899–907.
55. Villanacci V, Rossi E, Grisanti S, et al. Targeted therapy with trastuzumab in dysplasia and adenocarcinoma arising in Barrett's esophagus: a translational approach. Minerva Gastroenterol Dietol. 2008;54(4):347–53.

Part III

Stomach

Stomach: Inflammatory Patterns

4

M. Priyanthi Kumarasinghe, Spiro C. Raftopoulos, and Gregory Y. Lauwers

Contents

M. P. Kumarasinghe (✉)
Department of Anatomical Pathology, PathWest Laboratory Medicine, QEII Medical Centre and University of Western Australia, Perth, WA, Australia
e-mail: priyanthi.kumarasinghe@health.wa.gov.au

S. C. Raftopoulos
Interventional Endoscopist and Gastroenterologist, Department of Gastroenterology, Sir Charles Gairdner Hospital, Nedlands, WA, Australia

University of Western Australia, Perth, WA, Australia

G. Y. Lauwers
Gastrointestinal Pathology Service, Department of Pathology, Moffitt Cancer Center, Tampa, FL, USA

M. P. Kumarasinghe, I. Brown (eds.), *Endoscopic Biopsy Interpretation*,
https://doi.org/10.1007/978-3-319-79117-3_4

The most common non- neoplastic process encountered in a gastric biopsy in routine practice is gastritis. Most common causes of "endoscopic gastritis" are *Helicobacter pylori* infection, chemical/medication-induced gastropathy, autoimmune gastritis, and chronic gastritis/gastropathy of undetermined aetiology. However, agreement between endoscopic and histological findings is known to show poor correlation, and thus finding of "gastritis" endoscopically does not necessarily mean inflammation [1, 2].

From a histologic point of view, microscopic inflammation signifies true gastritis, while gastropathy includes mucosal and vasculopathic changes either in combination or alone, with minimal or no inflammation. Aetiology of both may overlap with a primary reactive gastropathy featuring erosion or ulceration and inflammation. Of note, distinction between a true gastritis and gastropathy is not possible on endoscopic appearance alone. Furthermore, overlaps are not uncommon.

A comprehensive clinicopathological or a etiological classification of gastritis is not possible as different entities show morphological overlap. Endoscopic biopsies provide valuable information with regard to the presence of inflammation and acute or chronic nature of the gastritis, but also aetiological clues based on the inflammatory pattern, presence of specific etiological agents (i.e., infections, residual pill substances, toxic material), and in some specific cases the risk of disease progression and cancer risk. Sydney system and Operative Link for Gastritis Assessment (OLGA) system have been proposed to standardise classification and to provide prognostic information concerning cancer risk in cases of chronic atrophic gastritis. However, adoption of any system is not universally accepted, and a more practical approach is required to guide clinical management in routine practice (Box 4.1).

When reviewing histologic samples, it should be emphasised that pathological assessment of a gastric biopsy should not be a mere description of microscopic features but one that guides clinicians to the aetiology and, in some cases, offers information to the next step of management and possibly treatment.

Box 4.1 Guide to Quick and Comprehensive Assessment of "Gastritis"

- **Confirm** inflammation.
  - Define the type (monocytes, eosinophils, neutrophils).
- **Spot** the:
  - Inflammatory pattern (dominant pattern +/− sub-patterns, mixed patterns)
  - Etiological clues
  - Indicators of prognosis and cancer risk, e.g. atrophy, metaplasia

An important first step is to differentiate gastritis from reactive gastropathy. Once gastric inflammation is established, the inflammatory pattern, in many cases, provides a key to possible aetiologies. Consideration should be given to the type and the location of inflammation in the mucosa and topography in terms of diffuse or focal inflammation ("pattern in pattern"). Attention to documentation of a probable causative agent and provision of information regarding atrophy and intestinal metaplasia ought to be expected. It is important to stress that more than one pattern is not uncommon (e.g. chronic, active chronic, and atrophic patterns are frequently intertwined). Also, an easy trap is to overlook a minor secondary pattern that might give important clues to the aetiology (e.g., microthrombi that signifies a vasculopathy in a biopsy of apparent reactive gastropathy or foveolar hyperplasia).

Presence of inflammatory cells in the gastric mucosa is a response to some form of injury but may not necessarily be "pathological" to be responsible for "symptoms". Ideally "normal" gastric mucosa should be devoid of any neutrophils, and mononuclear cells or eosinophils should be extremely scarce if not absent. Unfortunately, this ideal situation is difficult to prove as there are no data based on scientific studies on normal stomachs of asymptomatic people. However, an occasional neutrophil and a few mononuclear cells and rare scattered eosinophils are considered to be non-pathological in a normal healthy individual whereas true mucosal congestion and oedema are regarded as abnormal features in response to injury.

Acute Gastritis Pattern

Acute gastritis pattern is defined by the presence of a neutrophilic infiltrate in the lamina propria. This may be accompanied by intraepithelial neutrophils ("activity"; Fig. 4.1). More severe forms of acute injury are accompanied by erosions and ulceration (Fig. 4.2a–c). Architectural distortion is absent or minimal.

Acute gastritis is a result of acute inflammatory response of the gastric mucosa to injury. Active inflammation is associated with sustained injury to epithelium by inflammatory mediators. Although a rare neutrophil in the lamina propria is not considered pathological, the presence of intraepithelial neutrophils is abnormal. Most injuries to the gastric mucosa have the potential to produce "acute gastritis" pattern in the acute phase that is often not encountered by the gastroenterologist or the pathologist unless the episode is severe as in the case of acute haemorrhagic gastritis (see below). Chronic inflammation is not allowed in pure forms of acute gastritis pattern.

Causes include:

- *Helicobacter pylori* infection (rarely observed as transient phase of infection, at the first encounter of the bacteria and the mucosa).
- Local/topical injury due to medications, chemicals (caustic agents) and alcohol.
- Other infections due to non-*Helicobacter pylori* organisms: CMV and *Herpes*.
- Stress-induced gastritis.
- Zollinger-Ellison syndrome is an uncommon cause.

Helicobacter pylori and other Infections

Most classic descriptions of *Helicobacter pylori* infection are based on the inflammatory pattern that is noted in symptomatic patients. Usually by this stage, the acute phase has passed and the inflammatory response has progressed to chronic stage. Experimental studies have described acute

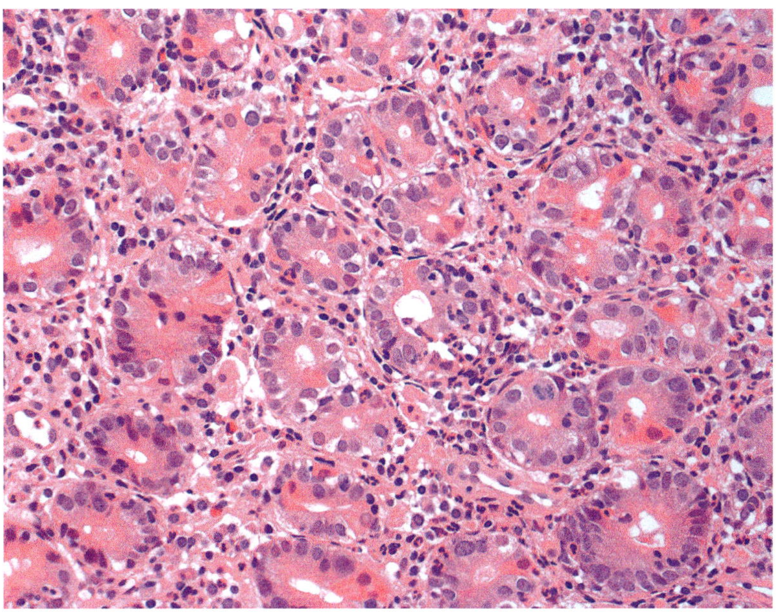

Fig. 4.1 Activity

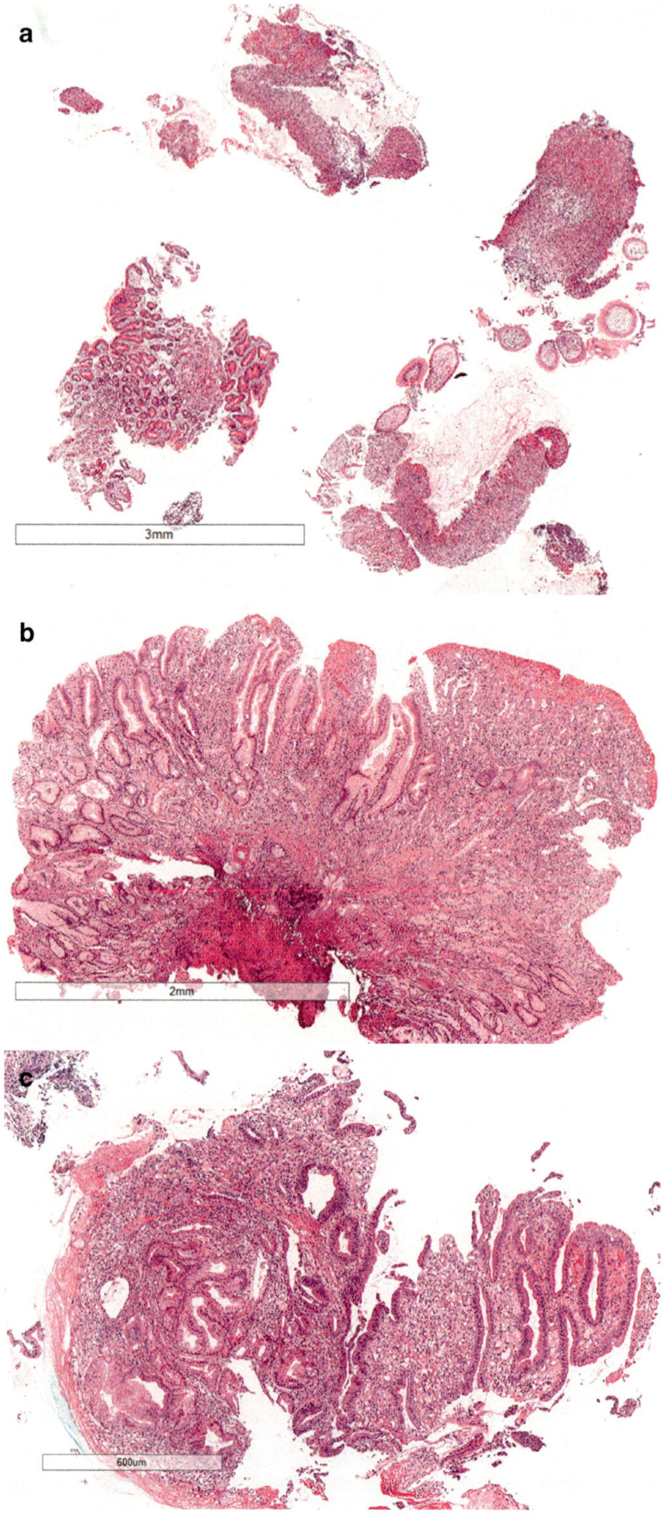

Fig. 4.2 Acute gastritis with ulceration associated with NSAIDs. (**a**) Ulceration; (**b**) granulation tissue underlying ulcerated mucosa; (**c**) reactive changes in adjacent mucosa

inflammation in the form of acute gastritis [3, 4]. However, in routine practice this stage is rarely encountered. Other infections include *Cytomegalovirus* (Fig. 4.3a–e) and *Herpesvirus* infection. Rarely non-*Helicobacter* bacteria such as *Staphylococci* have been responsible for acute gastritis. At times acute injury is multifactorial, as in infections and medication use occurring together.

Local injury due to gastrotoxic agents is known to cause acute gastritis pattern (Fig. 4.4a, b). Such agents are medications including nonsteroidal anti-inflammatory drugs (NSAIDs), iron pills,

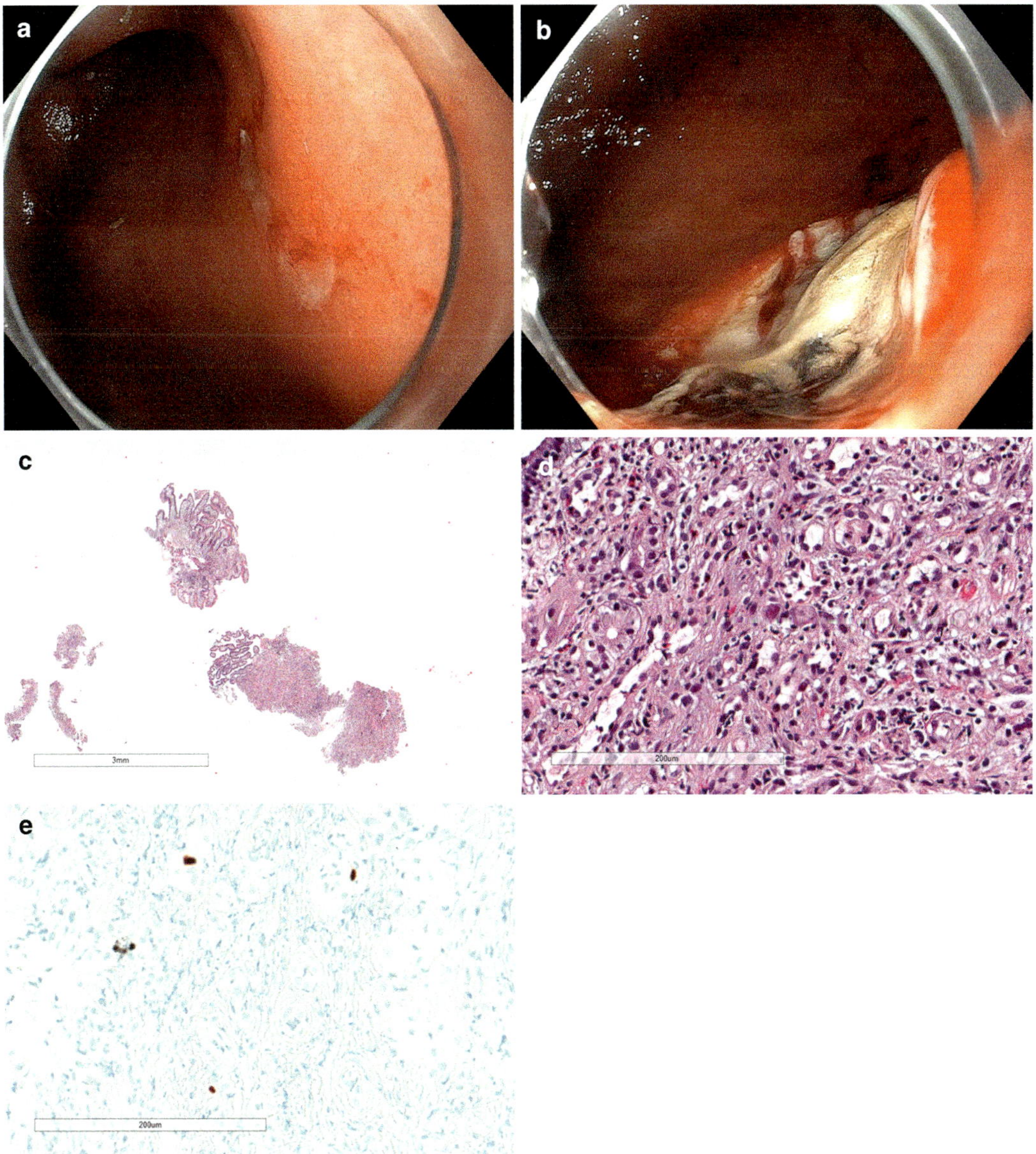

Fig. 4.3 **Case 1** A 45-year-old kidney and pancreatic transplant recipient on multiple immunosuppressive agents presenting for evaluation of gastroparesis-like symptoms. At OGD (oesopago-gastroduodenoscopy) she was noted to have multiple superficial ulcers involving the pyloric channel and antrum (**a**) including a deep ulcer within the posterior wall of the distal gastric body (**b**). Multiple biopsies showed acute gastritis pattern with ulceration (**c**) and very focal cytopathic changes consistent with *cytomegalovirus* (CMV) infection (**d**), a few CMV inclusions confirmed by immunohistochemistry (**e**): Acute gastritis pattern could be multifactorial with CMV infection and others such as medications playing a role together, in the given clinical setting in this patient

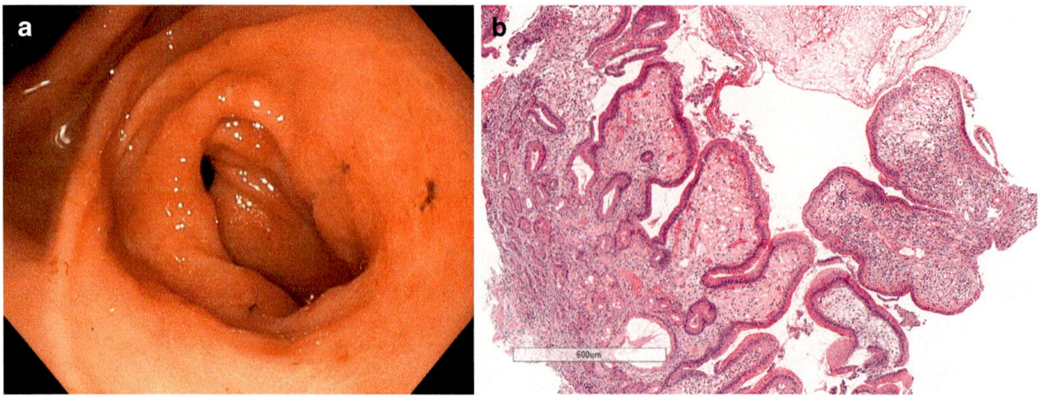

Fig. 4.4 (**Case 2**): An 81-year-old lady on long-term low-dose aspirin without proton pump inhibitor therapy. Presented for OGD to evaluate intermittent epigastric pain. Gastroscopy revealed multiple small antral erosions and surrounding mucosal erythema (**a**). The biopsy shows acute gastritis pattern with erosion (**b**)

bisphosphonates, doxycycline [5], a variety of chemotherapeutic agents, caustic substances, as well as excessive amounts of alcohol. Radiotherapy changes can also cause acute gastritis pattern. Some of above gastrotoxic agents show distinctive patterns in addition to acute injury as a dominant or a secondary pattern and will be discussed under specific distinctive patterns.

Acute gastritis pattern can be associated with haemorrhage ("acute haemorrhagic gastritis"), erosions ("acute erosive gastritis"), or ulceration ("acute ulcerative gastritis") resulting in additional patterns that indicate specific aetiology or severity of the injury.

Acute Gastritis Pattern with Haemorrhage, Erosion, and Ulceration ("Acute Erosive, Ulcerative, and Haemorrhagic Gastritis")

Gastric ulceration in biopsies is represented by fibrinopurulent exudate and inflamed granulation tissue (Fig. 4.2a, b). There may be deep ulceration accompanied by perforation. Adjacent mucosa shows reactive regenerative changes (Fig. 4.2c). Erosions by definition show loss of epithelium but not beyond the muscularis mucosae and indicate less severe injury than frank ulceration.

H. pylori-induced ulcers are common in the antrum, whereas NSAID and related medications commonly produce ulcers in the greater curvature and the fundus. Not infrequently, endoscopy and biopsy are repeated due to non-healing ulcers as a malignancy may be a concern. Gastrotoxic agents and pill substances should be searched for in gastric biopsies with ulceration.

One ought to remember that neoplasia and particularly adenocarcinoma and lymphoma may present with mucosal erosion and ulceration. After considering the clinical and endoscopic picture, adequate levels should be performed, and any suspicion of a neoplasm should prompt the performance of ancillary stains (see chapter 5). On the other hand, reactive changes in the mucosa may mimic epithelial dysplasia (see chapter 5). Ulceration may accompany deposition of various substances (see under "Deposition Pattern").

Stress-Induced Gastritis, Erosions, and Ulcers

Breakdown of the mucosal barrier and a mucosal ischaemic process are thought to be responsible in the pathogenesis of this disorder. Stress-induced acute gastritis and ulceration are seen in a small minority of patients in an intensive care environment (1.5%). Curling ulcers are seen in patients with burns and Cushing ulcers in those with head injuries (Table 4.1)

Table 4.1 Acute gastritis pattern +/− erosion, ulceration, and haemorrhage [3–5]

• Medications: look for pill substances.
• Chemicals, alcohol: clinical history.
• *Helicobacter pylori* infection: rare, transient phase, do special stains and other lab investigations.
• (Other infections) Look for: – CMV: owl's eye intranuclear inclusion bodies and intracytoplasmic inclusions, may be focal (see case 1) – *Herpes*: ground-glass nuclei and eosinophilic intranuclear inclusions surrounded by a halo.
• Rare deposits: amyloid, hyaline in vessels walls (i.e. radiation-induced injury).
• Hidden malignancies: lymphoma, poorly differentiated carcinoma.
• Severe (grades 3–4) GVHD: clinical history.

CMV = *Cytomegalovirus*, *GVHD* = Graft versus host disease.

Chronic Gastritis Pattern

This pattern is characterised by mucosal inflammation composed of chronic inflammatory cells that include lymphocytes, plasma cells, and eosinophils without a noticeable neutrophil component. Lymphoid follicles can be seen. Mucosal architectural distortion is a feature.

Typically, chronic gastritis (CG) pattern is patchy and considered as a nonspecific injury pattern leading to a nonspecific diagnosis of "chronic gastritis" without further qualification. Pathologists feel comfortable in making this "diagnosis" and it is not inaccurate! However, such diagnoses without further qualification are often meaningless to the clinician. Acknowledging that in many instances the aetiology cannot be elicited, the "patterns within pattern" based on topography of inflammation and a "secondary or associated pattern" within the spectrum of chronic gastritis may provide important clues. The most common associated secondary pattern is active inflammation resulting in "active chronic gastritis" pattern (see below). Active inflammation may be subtle and focal or obvious. Many other patterns described below, e.g. lymphocytic, eosinophilic, and granulomatous, may be seen providing important etiological clues. Atrophy, intestinal metaplasia (IM), and pseudopyloric metaplasia (PPM) may be present with important implications for follow-up. Secondary patterns may be focal and subtle and call for judgment to proceed with deep levels and ancillary stains for further analyses.

Two most common aetiologies that result in CG pattern are early stages of autoimmune gastritis (AIG) and late or healed *H. pylori* gastritis (HPG). Appreciating the "pattern in pattern" greatly helps in differentiating AIG form HPG.

CG pattern of classic AIG is antral sparing, and lamina propria reveals an intense mononuclear infiltrate deeply centred on the glands. This feature is in contrast to the superficial inflammation of *H. pylori* gastritis. In particular, superficial plasm cells are uncommon in AIG. Antral predominant plasma cell-rich superficial chronic gastritis should be considered as *H. pylori* related unless proven otherwise, and all efforts should be made to prove current or past infection. Subtle foci of activity will further support a diagnosis. Active inflammation is not a dominant pattern in AIG.

Body/Fundus Predominant Chronic Gastritis Pattern ("Pattern in Pattern") Associated with AIG

This secondary pattern of CG pattern is characterised by a predominant basal, lymphocyte-rich inflammatory infiltrate, often accompanied by atrophy and metaplastic changes (Fig. 4.5a). Distribution and severity of inflammation may vary according to the stage of disease. Early phase shows patchy chronic inflammation with a minor component of neutrophils and eosinophils (Fig. 4.5b). In some cases, eosinophils are prominent. Subtle and patchy loss of oxyntic glands, atrophy, and metaplastic changes, particularly pseudopyloric metaplasia, may also be present. Established stage associated with AIG shows the characteristic pattern of dense and diffuse lymphoplasmacytic infiltrate with marked atrophy, pseudopyloric (PPM) (Fig. 4.5d) and intestinal metaplasia (IM) (Fig. 4.5d), and other metaplastic changes such as pancreatic acinar metaplasia (PAC) (Fig. 4.5e). The antrum may show reactive changes with a variable degree of G-cell hyperplasia in response to hypochlorhydria. Although the antrum is commonly spared of

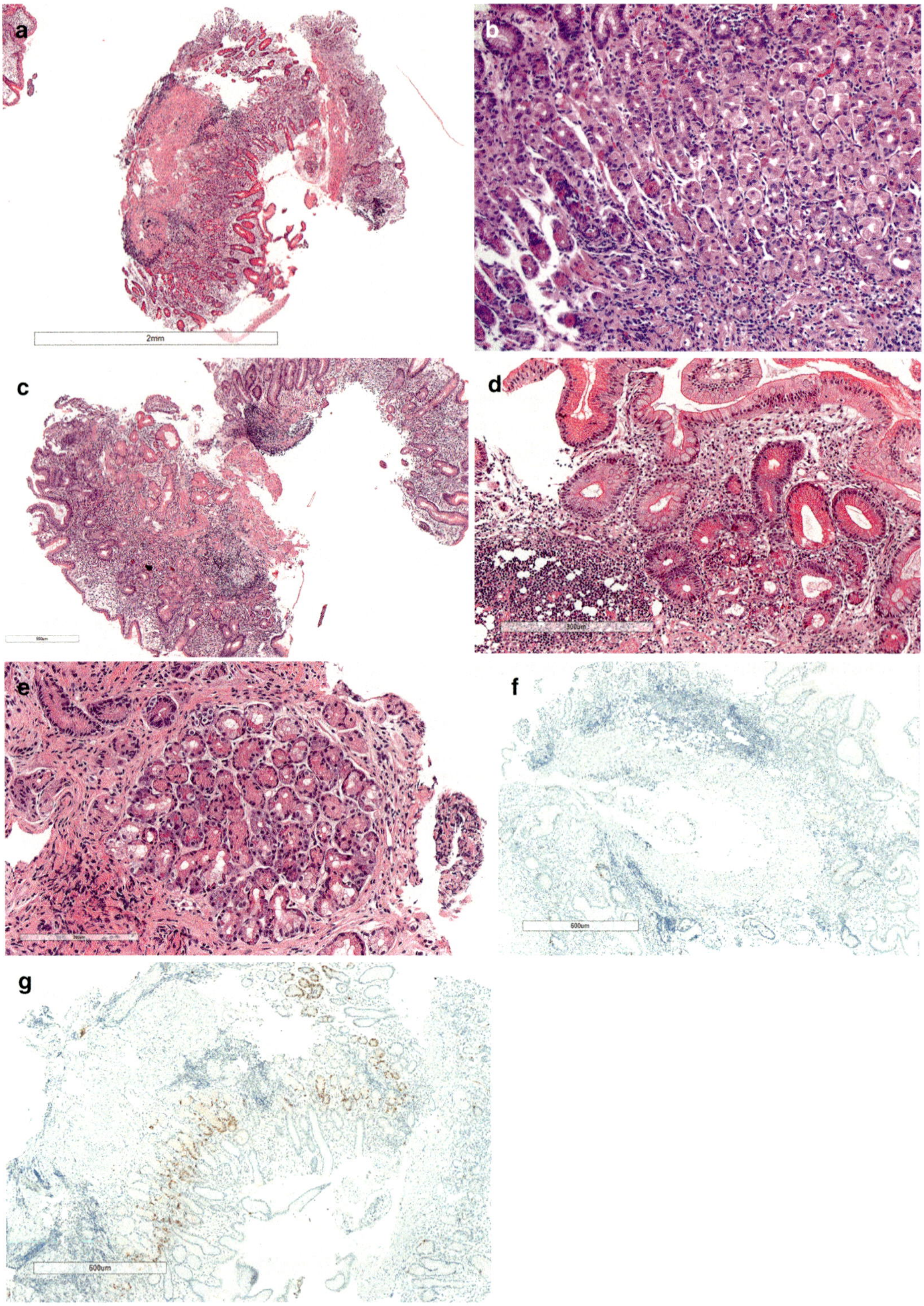

Fig. 4.5 Pattern in pattern characteristic of AIG (a-f). Body predominant chronic gastritis pattern intertwined with atrophic and metaplastic patterns. (**a**) CG pattern often accompanied by atrophy and metaplastic changes. (**b**) Early AIG with patchy chronic inflammation, a few neutrophils, and eosinophils. (**c**) Pseudopyloric metaplasia (PPM). (**d**) Intestinal metaplasia. (**e**) Pancreatic acinar metaplasia (PAC). (**f**) Absence of G cells confirmed by gastrin immunohistochemistry in the gastric body in PPM. (**g**) Atrophic antral gastritis that shows intact G cells to compare

inflammation in AIG, scattered parietal cells in the antrum may be targeted by immune-mediated injury. Therefore, it is not uncommon to find some antral inflammation, that is always milder compared to that of the gastric body [6–8].

Advanced stages of AIG show complete or near complete loss of oxyntic cells accompanied by diffuse pseudo-pyloric metaplasia (Fig. 4.5c); hence, the body mucosa may be mistaken for the antrum. Pancreatic acinar and intestinal metaplasia are also commonly observed. Inflammation may be minimal at this stage. Absence of G cells demonstrated by gastrin immunohistochemistry confirms PPM of body mucosa (Fig. 4.5f) as opposed to atrophic antral gastritis that shows intact G cells (Fig. 4.5g)

Late-stage AIG can be further associated with foveolar hyperplasia, hyperplastic polyps, residual oxyntic nodules resembling polyps (background is atrophic), neuroendocrine cell hyperplasia, low-grade neuroendocrine neoplasm, pyloric gland adenomas, polypoid or flat dysplasia, adenocarcinomas, or gastric lymphomas. An uncommon phenomenon of "pseudohypertrophy" of the remaining parietal cells may be seen [7].

AIG should be considered in the appropriate clinical setting of middle-age females with anaemia. Classic "pattern in pattern" of CG may be the first clue to the diagnosis and coupled with other relevant laboratory investigations can be diagnostic (Fig. 4.6a–c).

Box 4.2 Chronic Gastritis Pattern

- A diagnosis of CG alone is not very useful to the clinician.
- A common mistake is to overlook a subtle secondary pattern/s or "pattern in pattern".
- Body/fundal predominant antral sparing chronic gastritis with a basal lymphoplasmacytic infiltrate: Exclude AIG (clinical information of pernicious anaemia and anti-parietal antibody status should be investigated).
- In advanced stage of AIG, body mucosa may be mistaken for the antrum; gastrin immunohistochemistry is helpful.
- Antral predominant superficial plasmacytic infiltration: Exclude HP gastritis.

Antral Predominant CG Pattern ("Pattern in pattern")

A plasma cell-rich superficial chronic gastritis pattern should be considered as HP related unless otherwise proven (see below). IM and atrophy may be an associated pattern. HP may be demonstrated after vigilant search (Box 4.2).

Active Chronic Gastritis Pattern (ACG pattern)

Active chronic gastritis (ACG) pattern is characterised by a lamina propria infiltrate of plasma cells, lymphocytes, and a few eosinophils and neutrophils. Neutrophils are present both in the lamina propria and within the epithelium (activity). The most common cause of this pattern is *Helicobacter pylori* infection. Neutrophil-induced epithelial inflammation results in "active" inflammation, which is part of an acute inflammatory response. The term "active/activity" refers to neutrophil-induced epithelial injury. Active chronic gastritis pattern can be diffuse or focal and may be superficial or bottom heavy. Similar to CG pattern, "pattern in pattern" within the spectrum of active chronic gastritis may provide important clues to the aetiology, although *H. pylori* infection remains the most common cause of most of these patterns.

The common causes of active chronic gastritis pattern are the following:

- *Helicobacter pylori* infection.
- Medications.
- Autoimmune gastritis.
- Inflammatory bowel disease-related active chronic gastritis.

ACG Pattern: *Helicobacter pylori* Associated (Figs. 4.7 and 4.8a–j)

H. pylori-induced active chronic gastritis is characterised by a dense, band-like infiltrate of

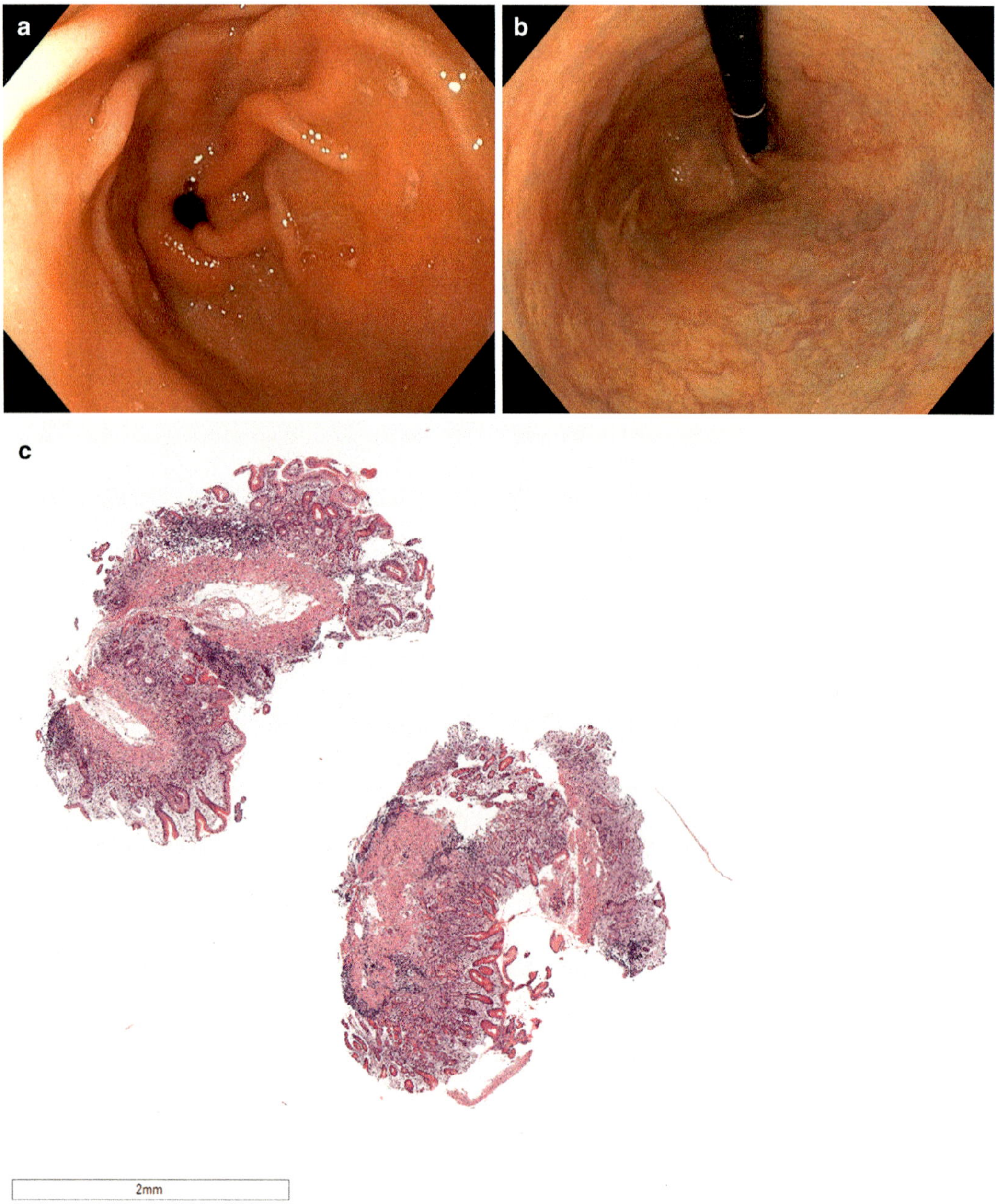

Fig. 4.6 (**Case 3**) An 81-year-old lady referred for evaluation of anaemia and B12 deficiency. Gastroscopy was performed showing normal antral mucosa (**a**); however, the gastric body and funds revealed absence of gastric rugae (**b**) and visible submucosal blood vessels through thin, atrophic, overlying mucosa. Gastric biopsies were consistent with a diagnosis of autoimmune metaplastic atrophic gastritis (**c**) with elevated intrinsic factor antibodies detected on serological testing

lymphocytes, macrophages, and plasma cells in the superficial mucosa with neutrophilic activity resulting in classical "superficial active chronic gastritis pattern" and endoscopic appearance is characteristic (Fig. 4.7). Lymphoid follicles may be encountered, more commonly in the antrum. They are less common in non-HP gastritis. Occasionally neutrophilic pit abscesses

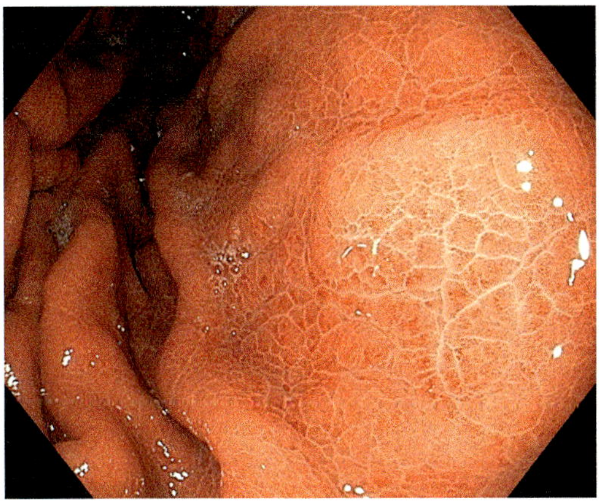

Fig. 4.7 (**Case 4**) A 69-year-old man presenting for gastroscopy to evaluate a history of intermittent epigastric pain. At OGD he was noted to have diffuse mucosal erythema with a "chicken skin" appearance highly suspicious for *H. pylori*-associated gastritis. As he was on a PPI, biopsies were taken from the gastric antrum and corpus, and HP gastritis was confirmed in both

are also noted (Fig. 4.8c). *H. pylori* organisms are often present in these biopsies (Fig. 4.8d). The presence of neutrophils correlates closely with active colonisation of the gastric lumen by *H. pylori* organisms. Although antral predominant superficial active chronic gastritis pattern is the hallmark of HPG, overtime inflammation of the corpus develops, resulting in pangastritis.

Proton pump inhibitors (PPIs) inhibit gastric acid secretions and alleviate symptoms of peptic ulcer disease and facilitate healing. PPIs are frequently used by patients with GORD and those who are on NSAIDs. Low acid secretion results in proximal migration of bacteria that may result in corpus predominant HP gastritis rather than pangastritis. PPIs, in particular omeprazole is also associated with reduction in bacterial load. Therefore, biopsies of such patients may not show demonstrable *H. pylori* organisms, and the diagnosis can be challenging in these cases.

Some cases of *Helicobacter pylori* infection may not respond to conventional therapy and present as cases of "failed therapy". Patients who have had *H. pylori eradicated* may get reinfected even by the same strain through the organism's ability to overcome natural immunity [9]. As such, a related past history does not preclude a diagnosis of HP infection.

It is important to emphasise that non-atrophic antral gastritis, which is the predominant finding in patients with *H. pylori*-associated duodenal peptic ulcer, is not related to an increased cancer risk. It is believed that the HP strain that results in a duodenal ulcer phenotype may produce lower levels of IL-1β, which results in lower risk and is in fact protective against gastric cancer [10].

Other *Helicobacter* Organisms (Fig. 4.8e, i)

Rarely other species of *Helicobacter* organisms can infect humans and are acquired from domestic pets. The organisms are longer and show a tightly coiled morphology. They are not adherent to the surface mucus layer compared to *H. pylori* species. It is believed that there are more than one species that could infect humans; hence, these organisms are referred to as *Helicobacter heilmannii*-like organisms (encompassing others such as *H. felis*, *H. suis*, *H. bizzozeronii*, *H. salomonis*, *H. cynogastricus*, *H. baculiformis*). In addition to domestic pets, cattle, rabbits, swine, and primate are believed to be responsible for direct transmission of the infection [11–13]. Infection with *H. heilmannii*-like organisms classically produces milder inflammation. In our experience, all types of stains including immunohistochemistry are positive in these organisms.

Demonstration of *Helicobacter* organisms [14–21]

In routine haematoxylin and eosin (H&E) stains, organisms appear as thin, curved rod-shaped or seagull-shaped blue rods in association with the classical "superficial active chronic gastritis" pattern. They are typically seen in the mucus-rich layer of the surface foveolar epithelium or superficial gastric pits (Fig. 4.8d). They should be searched for focusing on the mucous layers of

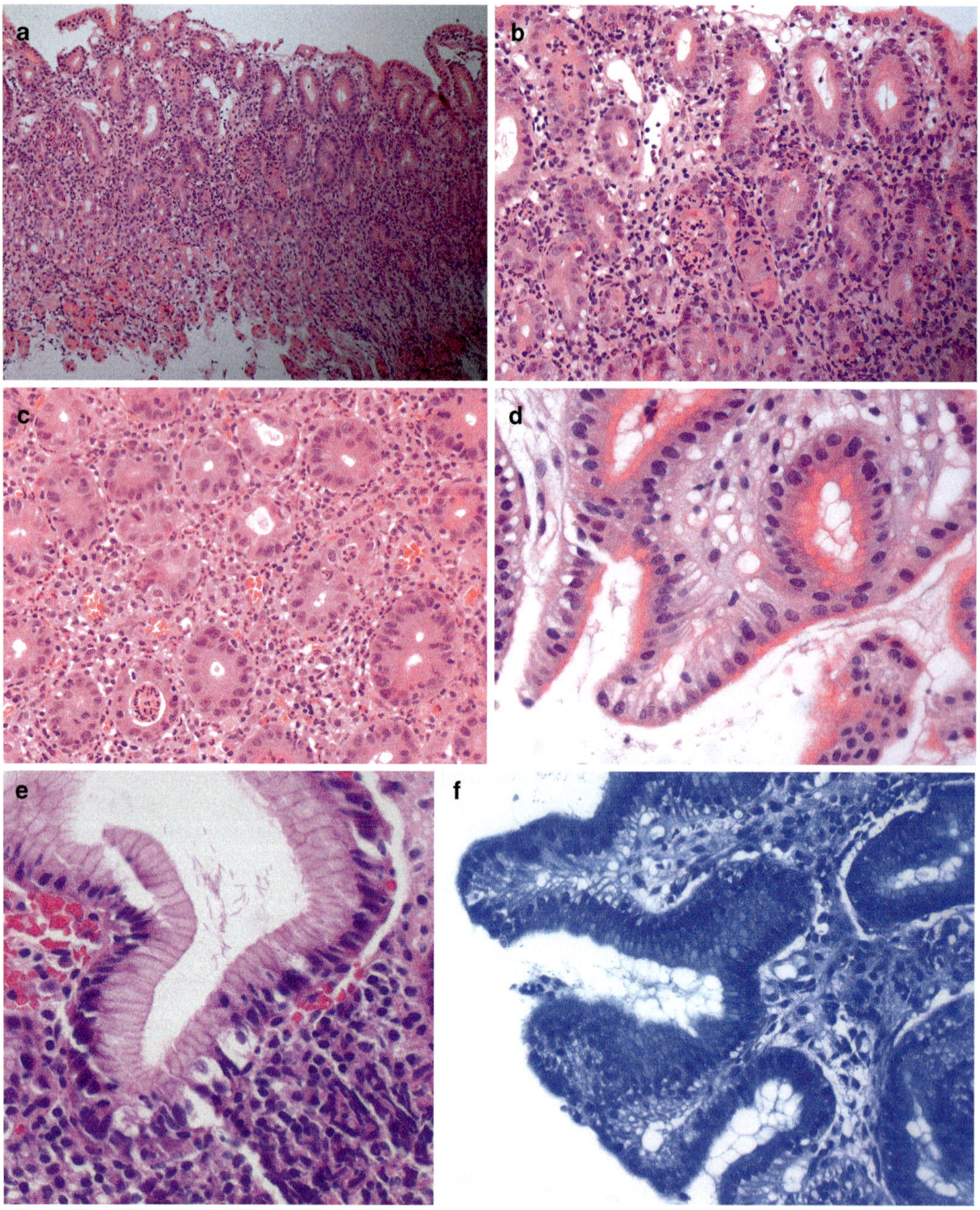

Fig. 4.8 Active chronic gastritis pattern and infective organisms. (**a**, **b**) Superficial active chronic gastritis pattern. (**c**) Neutrophilic pit abscess. (**d**) *Helicobacter pylori* organism (H&E). (**e**) *Helicobacter heilmannii*-like organisms (H&E). (**f**) *Helicobacter pylori* organisms (toluidine blue stain). (**g**) *Helicobacter pylori* organisms (immunohistochemical stain). (**h**) *Helicobacter pylori* organisms in small numbers in deep pits (immunohistochemical stain). (**i**) *Helicobacter heilmannii*-like organisms (immunohistochemical stain). (**j**) Sarcina ventriculi

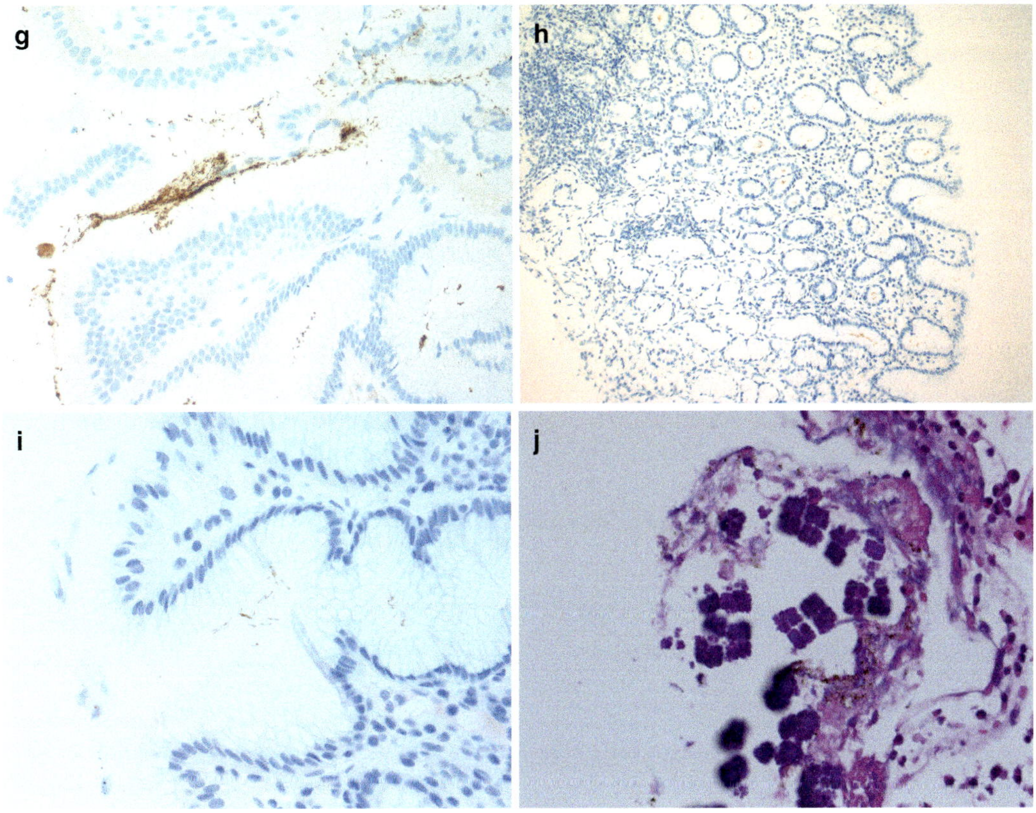

Fig. 4.8 (continued)

acutely inflamed areas away from intestinal metaplasia.

H. pylori are usually absent in foci of intestinal metaplasia, especially complete (type I) intestinal metaplasia, but often present in foci of incomplete (type II) intestinal metaplasia [22].

Caution is needed in patients who are on PPI therapy as antral biopsies may show fewer organisms or none at all [16]. Thus, PCR testing, serology, or evaluation of stool antigen may be considered as an alternative for detection. In order to minimise the percentage of false-negative results, PPI therapy may be discontinued at least 2 weeks before the endoscopic tissue sampling.

Special stains are used to identify the organisms when they are not detected with routine H&E stains. Commonly used non-silver-based stains are Giemsa, toluidine blue (Fig. 4.8f) and Diff-Quik stains. Silver-based stains are Warthin-Starry, Genta, modified Steiner, and El-Zimaity dual stains. Immunohistochemistry (IHC) for *Helicobacter* is highly sensitive and specific (Fig. 4.8g). These are particularly useful when there are fewer organisms as they are readily identifiable with IHC even in small numbers and in deep pits (Fig. 4.8h). The IHC is specific for all *Helicobacter* species differentiating them from other oral and enteric non-HP bacteria. IHC will stain all morphological forms including coccoid forms of bacteria. All above stains including immunohistochemistry will be positive for *H. heilmannii-like organisms* (Fig. 4.8i).

Other infections in the stomach are rare and include non-*Helicobacter* bacterial, fungal, protozoal, nematodal, and viral infections. *Sarcina ventriculi* is a gram-positive anaerobic bacterium that may rarely cause gastric ulcers, emphysematous gastritis, and perforation especially in patients with gastroparesis [23]. These organisms generally do not cause injury in the absence of underlying mucosal defect and are regarded as a bystander. Organisms occur in tetrads or octet packets and found admixed in debris (Fig. 4.8j). They are of the size of a lymphocyte or about 10 μm across. The characteristic appearance is diagnostic in H&E stains. Oral contaminants and normal flora could raise concern for HP occasionally. They do not show specific localisation and are generally seen admixed with debris. These non-HP bacteria do not stain with immunohistochemical stains, and they do not show any specific localisation in the mucosa (Box 4.3).

ACG Pattern: Autoimmune gastritis (AIG)

As described earlier, the dominant inflammatory pattern of AIG is CG pattern commonly accompanied by atrophic and metaplastic patterns and characterised by body/fundus predominant basal inflammation. Active inflammation may be present but is much more rare than HPG. ACG pattern occurs in the early phase of autoimmune gastritis before metaplastic and atrophic changes manifest. Careful scrutiny might show subtle loss of oxyntic glands. History of PPI therapy should be investigated in body/fundus predominant ACG patterns since HPG is a more likely possibility than AIG in which activity is rare.

Box 4.3 Detection of *Helicobacter*-Associated Gastritis

- H&E: Adequate in most cases; focus on the mucus-rich layer of the surface and superficial gastric pits.
- Top-heavy ACG pattern: Associated with HP unless otherwise proven; may recommend non-histological tests for proof (e.g. serology, culture, PCR, and referral to specialist HP laboratory).
- Immunostain: Highly specific for *Helicobacter* species and easy interpretation.
- Histochemical stains: Inferior to IHC.
- Special stains (IHC in particular) indicated: HP negative antral, cardiac, pan and body predominant inflammation (ACG, CG—even mild, with clinical suspicion of HP and LG pattern, GC pattern included) and gastroduodenal ulcers.
- Special stains (IHC in particular) NOT indicated: Normal mucosa, RG pattern with no inflammation +/− confirmed vasculopathy, obvious HP with H&E, uninflamed gastric polyps and adenomas.
- Up-front special stains including IHC: probably not required.
- Patients on PPI therapy: Antral biopsies may be negative while corpus and body may be positive (sometimes deep in the glands). Non-histological test may be considered. Discontinuation of PPI for at least 2 weeks before the endoscopic tissue sampling may be needed.

ACG Pattern: Medications

The spectrum of gastric injury pattern in medication-induced injury may include active chronic gastritis pattern. After excluding HPG and AIG, a positive clinical history coupled with secondary gastrotoxic patterns or presence of culprit material should be actively searched for.

ACG Pattern: Others

Inflammatory bowel disease in particular Crohn's disease (CD) can be associated with ACG pattern without granulomatous inflammation. Granulomatous inflammation is seen in

<1/3 of biopsies of cases of CD. Active chronic inflammation is classically patchy but can fully mimic *H. pylori* gastritis (Box 4.4).

Box 4.4 ACG Pattern

- Classic antral predominant superficial ACG pattern: HPG.
- PPI therapy: Corpus predominant HP gastritis and *H. pylori* organisms may not be demonstrable.
- Some strains of HP may not respond to conventional HP therapy ("failed therapy").
- Patients after eradicating *H. pylori*: May get reinfected by the same strain.
- ACG pattern in AIG: Rarely, some degree of antral involvement in AIG can pose a diagnostic challenge at early stages.
- Gastrin immunostain may be required to differentiate pseudopyloric metaplasia from true antrum if biopsy site is not known.
- Patchy ACG pattern: Exclude inflammatory bowel disease.
- ACG pattern in medications: look for secondary patterns of injury, pill substances and clinical history

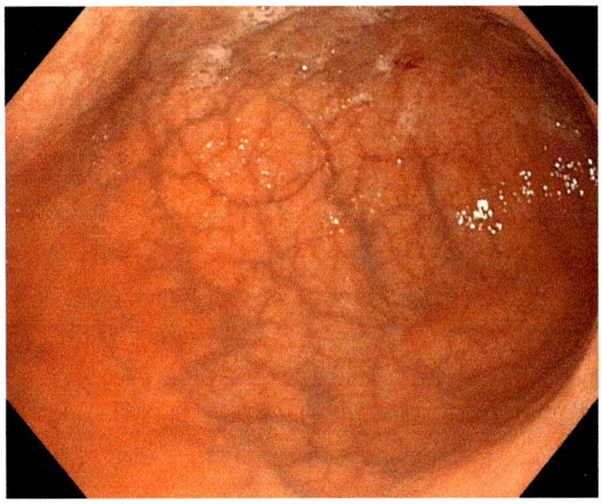

Fig. 4.9 Atrophic antral gastritis (endoscopic appearance)

Atrophic Pattern (Figs. 4.5, 4.6 and 4.9)

Atrophic pattern is characterised by multifocal loss of the original gastric glands with or without metaplasia with or without inflammation. Atrophic pattern as an advanced stage of damage is often accompanied by metaplastic pattern. Therefore, metaplastic and atrophic patterns often coexist as a mixed pattern of atrophic metaplastic gastritis. An overall diagnosis of chronic atrophic gastritis should not be made based on the finding of patchy mucosal atrophy as it may not be of great clinical significance. In such cases, focal atrophy could be documented in the report. A pitfall is mistaking the morphology of transitional zones of the gastric mucosa (antrum and body, and fundus and cardia) that may show a reduction of expected normal components as atrophy. In advanced stages, confluent foci of mucosal atrophy lead to a reduction in mucosal thickness. A diagnosis of atrophic gastritis has important clinical implications indicating altered gastric function and increased risk of cancer [24, 25].

"Pattern in pattern" appearance focused on location gives important etiological clues similar to CG. Chronic atrophic gastritis (CAG) essentially is a progression of CG; therefore, the two most common aetiologies are autoimmune gastritis and *H. pylori* infection. As a result, classically AIG is characterised by oxyntic gland atrophy, while *H. pylori* gastritis shows antropyloric gland atrophy. Antral atrophy is often associated with IM and usually involves the full thickness of the mucosa that may be patchy, and difficult to appreciate in a biopsy.

In atrophy associated with AIG, the metaplastic changes are first seen at the junction of the antrum and oxyntic corporal mucosa. Over time, the foci of metaplasia advance and extend to the mucosa of the corpus. In advanced stages of AIG, atrophy is obvious, accompanied by metaplastic changes but shows less inflammation. The more extensive the atrophic and metaplastic pattern, the greater the cancer risk.

Profound achlorhydria induces increased gastrin secretion by antral G cells as well as Enterochromaffin-like cell (ECL) hyperplasia [8]. ECL cells are seen as small cuboidal clear cells with round nuclei and finely dispersed chromatin with H&E satin. ECL hyperplasia can be seen as linear chains, small nodules, ribbons, and tubules deep in the body/fundic mucosa.

Chronic atrophic gastritis pattern (CAG) can often be diagnosed at gastroscopy by the presence of atrophic-appearing gastric mucosa (Fig 4.9). Advanced stages of atrophic mucosa is recognised by the presence of vessels readily observed in the atrophic mucosa extending throughout the antrum, corpus, or fundus. Distribution of atrophy can assist in determining the aetiology of CAG. Antral predominant CAG is consistent with *H. pylori*-associated chronic atrophic gastritis while antral sparing gastritis is typical of autoimmune gastritis.

CAG is etiologically associated with intestinal-type gastric cancer (GC) and type I neuroendocrine neoplasm (NENs). Later is through a process of hypergastrinaemia with resultant stimulation of enterochromaffin-like cells leading to neuroendocrine hyperplasia and finally development of low-grade NEN.

Box 4.5 Atrophic Pattern

- Transitional zones of the gastric mucosa, i.e. antral and body, and fundus and cardia may be mistaken for atrophy: a pitfall.
- Oxyntic gland atrophy with sparing of antrum: AIG.
- Antro-pyloric predominant atrophy: HPG.
- Atrophy is often accompanied by IM, PPM and PAM, and ECL hyperplasia.

Metaplastic Patterns

Metaplastic pattern is characterised by the replacement of native mucosa with another differentiated cell type. This is an adaptive response to an insult or injury.

In the stomach, intestinal and pancreatic acinar metaplasia of the gastric mucosa and pyloric pseudo-metaplasia of gastric body mucosa are common metaplastic patterns noted.

Intestinal Metaplasia

Intestinal metaplastic (IM) pattern is characterised by the presence of goblet cells with or without absorptive enterocytes. Generally, goblet cells are easily identified by their intracytoplasmic mucin goblet that pushes the nucleus to the base (Fig. 4.10a), and identification does not require special stains. Hyperplastic foveolar epithelial cells with distended gastric mucin and artefactual clearing should not be mistaken for IM (Fig. 4.10b). In routine practice, histochemical and immunohistochemical stains are not required to confirm IM. At endoscopy multiple, white plaques are noted (Fig. 4.10c).

IM pattern can be of two established types [24, 25]. In type I, metaplastic glands phenotypically resemble those of the small intestine, with eosinophilic absorptive enterocytes with a brush border, alternating with mucus-producing goblet cells and Paneth cells. This pattern of complete IM (type I), also known as "small intestinal-type metaplasia" (Fig. 4.10d), when advanced may show villiform architecture. The second pattern of incomplete IM (type II) shows irregular goblet cells interspersed within the gastric epithelium and lacks the brush border, absorptive cells, and Paneth cells and resembles colonic mucosa, alternatively called "colonic metaplasia" (Fig. 4.10e) [23]. Within incomplete IM, presence of sulfomucins within the non-goblet cells (also known as type III or type IIb patterns by some authors) is believed to be associated with an increased risk of progression to gastric cancer [24]. However, the practical application of this division is questionable as a mixture of all types of metaplasia is often seen in individual patients. There appears to be a correlation with the degree of intestinal metaplasia and risk of progression to carcinoma. In routine practice, there is no indication to subtype or comment on the degree of IM, although the information may be requested to guide management in individual, high-risk patients.

Immunohistochemical Markers for Subtyping IM

Complete (type I) metaplasia shows expression of MUC2 in goblet cells (Fig. 4.10f), that is an intestinal mucin, as well as luminal CD10 expression highlighting the presence of enterocytes (Fig. 4.10g) and decreased expression of "gastric" mucins (MUC5AC and MUC6). Instead, incomplete intestinal metaplasia shows "gastric" mucins co-expressed with intestinal mucin MUC2 and lacks CD10 representing an aberrant differentiation. Although more than 20 specific mucin encoding genes associated with secretion of specific mucin proteins have been identified, four are being used routinely in most laboratories (Table 4.2; Fig. 4.10h, i).

Focal intestinal metaplasia may be subtle and missed. Intestinal metaplasia occurs frequently in association with Paneth cells. Paneth cells are easy to recognise due to the intense pink granularity in the cytoplasm at low power. The presence of Paneth cells should prompt a vigilant search for goblet cells in gastric biopsies.

Pseudopyloric Metaplasia (PPM) (Figs. 4.5c and 4.11)

With continuous inflammation and progressive atrophy in the oxyntic mucosa, specialised glands are lost and replaced by mucus cells. The phenomenon is known as "pseudopyloric metapla-

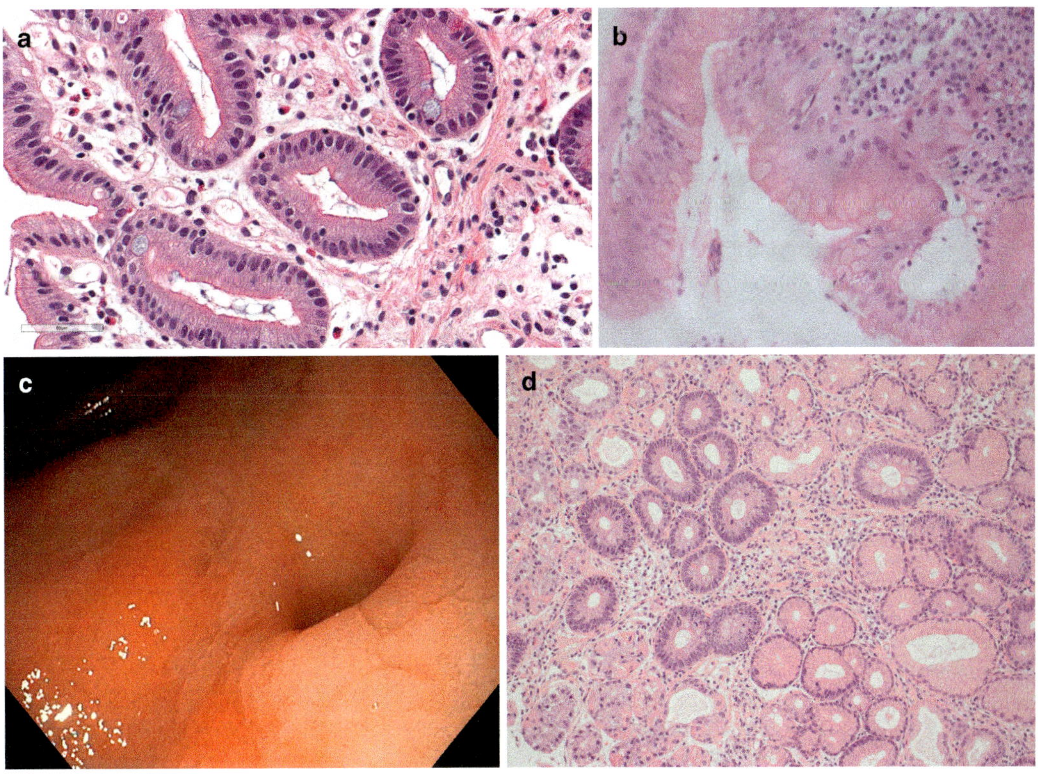

Fig. 4.10 Morphology and immunohistochemical expression in complete and incomplete intestinal metaplasia. Intestinal metaplastic patterns. (**a**) Goblet cells. (**b**) Hyperplastic foveolar epithelial cells with distended gastric mucin and non-goblet cells, a mimic of true goblet cells. (**c**) Endoscopy: multiple white plaques within the antrum and pyloric channel. (**d**) Complete intestinal metaplasia (type 1/small intestinal type). (**e**) Incomplete intestinal metaplasia (type II/colonic type): irregular interspersed goblet cells. (**f**) MUC2 expression in goblet cells. (**g**) CD10 positivity in absorptive cells (brush border) seen in complete intestinal metaplasia (type II). (**h**) MUC5AC: positive in normal foveolar epithelium and negative in the pyloric glands. (**i**) MUC6: positive in normal antropyloric glands and negative in the foveolar compartment (reverse of **h**)

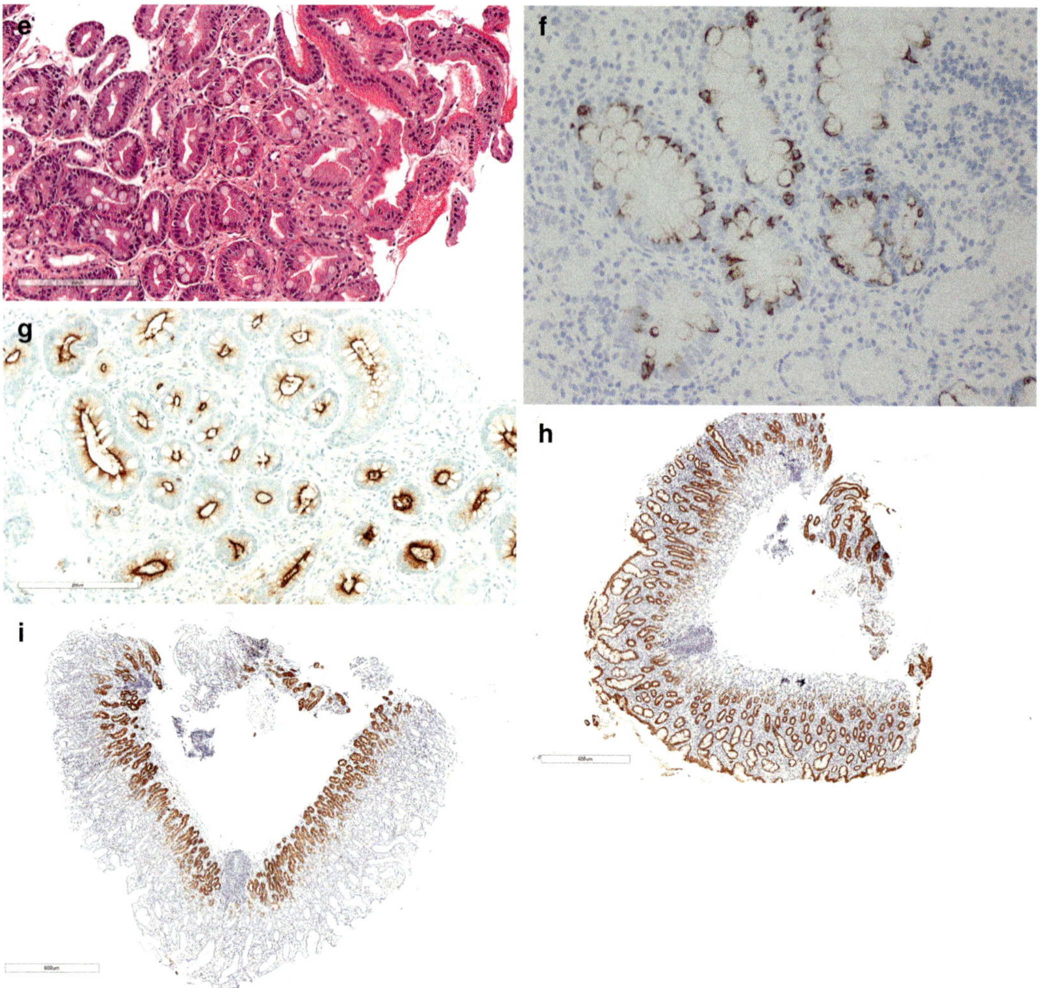

Fig. 4.10 (continued)

Table 4.2 Mucin proteins by immunohistochemistry

Mucin proteins by immunohistochemistry	Cells positive
MUC2	Goblet cells (see Fig. 4.10a)
MUC5AC	Foveolar epithelium (cytoplasmic) (see Fig. 4.10h)
MUC6	Pyloric glands (cytoplasmic) (see Fig. 4.10i)
MUC1	Not expressed in non neoplastic stomach

sia" as the mucosa is not antral. In classic antral sparing AIG, over time "pseudopyloric metaplasia" develops, and oxyntic mucosa may mimic that of antrum (Fig. 4.11). However, gastrin-producing cells (G cells) are not seen in the PPM of the body, and their absence in a biopsy that "looks antral" confirms pseudopyloric metaplasia as opposed to true antral mucosa that contains G cells. Gastrin immunostain is useful for confirmation (Fig. 4.5f, g). PPM also stains for pepsinogen (PG1) that localises to chief and mucus neck cells and transitional cells while absent in antral glands.

Pancreatic Acinar Metaplasia (PAM) (Figs. 4.12 and 4.5e)

Foci of pancreatic acinar metaplasia (PAM) can be seen in association with chronic gastric pattern together with PPM (Fig. 4.12) and IM.

Box 4.6 Atrophic and metaplastic patterns in gastric mucosa

- General rules of antral sparing and body fundus vs. antral predominant atrophy accompanied by metaplasia are important clues to differentiate atrophy due to AIG from HPG.
- ECL hyperplasia and IM, PPM, and PAM are common associations of atrophy.
- Focal IM can be overlooked.
- Subtyping or assessing the extent of IM: not for routine reporting.
- "Antral look" can be deceiving; exclude pseudopyloric metaplasia by endoscopic correlation and attention to inflammatory pattern.
- Gastrin and PG1 IHC are helpful.
- Clinical significance of metaplastic pattern needs to be appreciated and hence documented.

Lymphocytic Gastritis Pattern (Fig. 4.13 a-e)

Lymphocytic gastritis (LG) is defined by intraepithelial lymphocytosis (IEL). The definition requires >25 lymphocytes [26–29] per 100 epithelial cells within the foveolae of gastric mucosa. However, in practice strict counting is often unnecessary as the pattern is striking and rarely missed at low-power screening. The lymphocytes are predominantly regular CD8-positive T lymphocytes. Immunohistochemical stains are not recommended in routine practice.

A number of aetiologies lead to lymphocytic gastritis, the two a most well recognised of which are *Helicobacter pylori* infection and coeliac disease. Other causes of LG pattern include medications (sartans: olmesartan and telmisartan, valsartan and irbesartan, and ticlopidine), immune-mediated disorders (Crohn's disease, CVID), human immunodeficiency virus (HIV), syphilis, EBV infection (Fig. 4.13c, d), lymphoma, hypertrophic gastritis, inflammatory

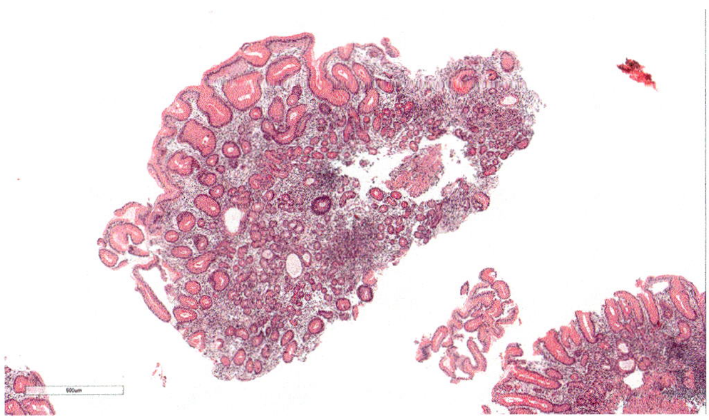

Fig. 4.11 Oxyntic mucosa with pseudopyloric metaplasia mimicking the antrum

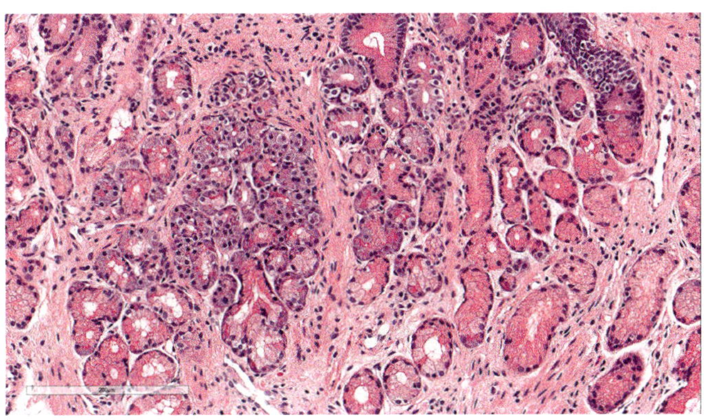

Fig. 4.12 Pancreatic acinar metaplasia (PAM) and pseudopyloric metaplasia (PPM) side by side in a case of AIG

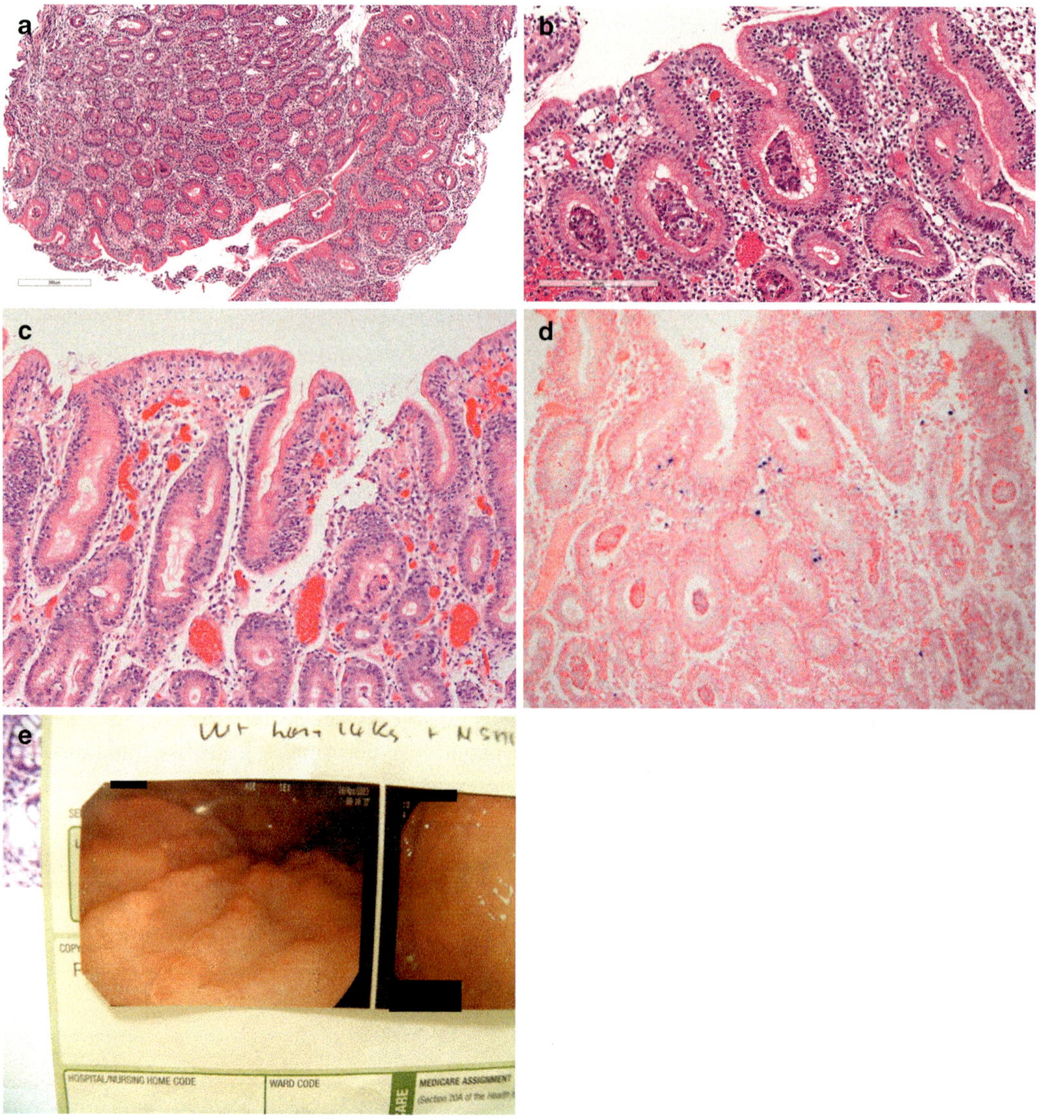

Fig. 4.13 Lymphocytic gastritis pattern. (**a**, **b**) *Helicobacter pylori* associated: organisms are not demonstrated by microscopic examination but proven by serology and culture in this case. (**c**) LG pattern associated with EBV. (**d**) A few scattered EBV positive cells with Epstein-Barr-encoded RNA by ISH (EBER-ISH). (**e**) Endoscopy: a case of varioliform gastritis that shows the LG pattern on biopsies

polyps, and oesophageal carcinoma. In some, the cause is unknown ("idiopathic"). Secondary patterns may indicate important clues.

ACG pattern accompanied by LG pattern is an important clue to HP-related gastritis [26, 27]. HP-related lymphocytic gastritis often does not have demonstrable HP organisms even after employing special stains including IHC. Therefore, lack of demonstrable HP does not exclude HP infection especially when LG pattern is accompanied by ACG pattern. Patients who show mixed ACG and LG pattern in gastric biopsies are known to show evidence of HP infection by serology, culture, and a positive urea breath test. Treatment for HP has resolved inflammation in these cases [27].

Coeliac disease should be strongly considered in LG pattern without activity and no conclusive evidence of HP infection. The duodenum is almost always involved in coeliac disease. In our experience, certain strains of HP are more likely to produce LG pattern than others. Estimated incidence of LG pattern in coeliac disease (CD) varies from 3% to 46%.

LG is usually detected in the corpus and is more common in women, with a median age distribution of 45–49 years. The endoscopic findings are variable and, in many cases, may be normal, but can include thickening of mucosal folds, aphthous erosions, hypertrophic gastropathy, and nodularity commonly denoted as varioliform gastritis [29] (Fig. 4.13e). Patients can have severe symptoms of anorexia, weight loss, epigastric pain, and at times protein-losing enteropathy (Box 4.7) [27–29].

Box 4.7 LG Pattern

- *Helicobacter pylori* infection and coeliac disease.
- LG with ACG pattern—Exclude HP even if organisms are negative; alternative tests may be useful.
- LG pattern is coeliac disease—Duodenum is abnormal.
- Endoscopic features vary from normal to alarmingly nodular (varioliform gastritis).

Eosinophilic Gastritis Pattern (Fig. 4.14)

The normal gastric mucosa ideally should not contain eosinophils, but exact quantification of what is "abnormal" is difficult [30–33]. However, 8–11 eosinophils per HPF, 12/HPF averaged over 5 HPF, and <38 eosinophils per square millimetre have been reported as "normal". Eosinophils can be observed both in the lamina propria and within the epithelium. Important considerations before diagnosing eosinophilic gastritis (EoG) are the infiltrative pattern, the intensity of eosinophilic infiltration, presence of intraepithelial eosinophils (IEE), and associated damage to the mucosa. A description of increased eosinophils or the term eosinophilia is appropriate for the mere presence of eosinophils in the lamina propria. Eosinophils frequently accompany other inflammatory cells. The presence of eosinophils in the epithelium, muscularis mucosa, or submucosa associated with epithelial damage is regarded as eosinophilic gastritis (EoG). It is not clear how vigilantly one should be counting lamina propria eosinophils when other evidence of damage to the mucosa and IEE are lacking [30–33].

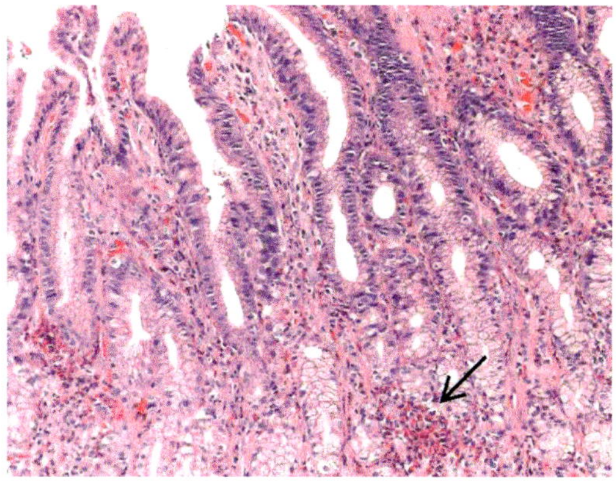

Fig. 4.14 Eosinophilic gastritis pattern (Eosinophils indicated by the arrow)

The stomach may be involved as part of a generalised gastrointestinal process or may be an isolated phenomenon. Although eosinophilic gastritis pattern is often seen in the setting of eosinophilic gastroenteritis, "eosinophilic gastritis pattern" in isolation can be associated with diverse aetiologies such as food allergies (e.g. cow milk, soy protein), certain medications such as NSAIDs, gold, tacrolimus, clozapine), *H. pylori* infection, collagen vascular diseases such as SLE, systemic connective tissue disorders (e.g. scleroderma and polymyositis), vasculitis, Churg-Strauss granulomatosis, hypereosinophilic syndrome, and parasitic infections. Other associated conditions, in particular neoplastic disorders include inflammatory fibroid polyp, Langerhans cell histiocytosis, mastocytosis, lymphoma, and leukaemia. Endoscopic findings are nonspecific and include nodular or polypoid gastric mucosa, erythema, or erosions.

Granulomatous Gastritis Pattern (Figs. 4.15a–c and 4.16a–c)

Granulomatous gastritis (GG) is characterised by aggregates of epithelioid histiocytes admixed with lymphocytes and plasma cell with and without multinucleated giant cells (Fig. 4.15a). Isolated collec-

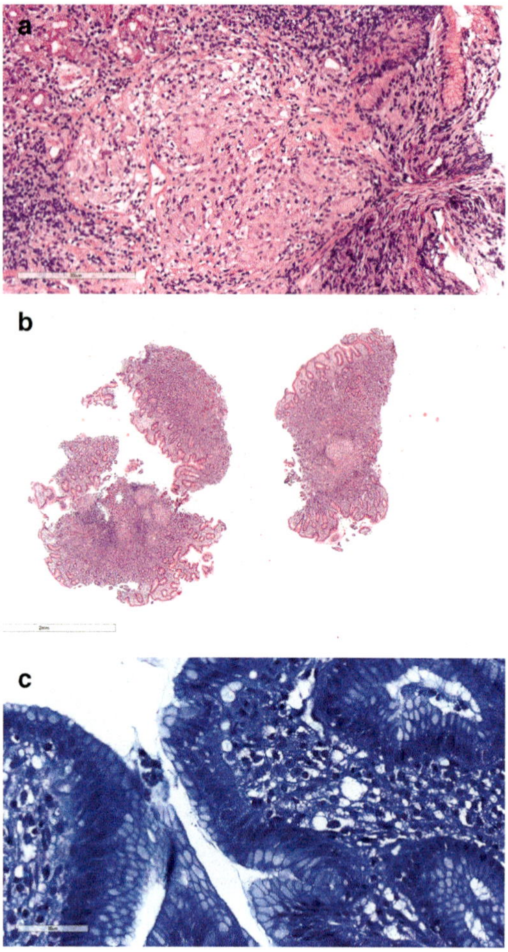

Fig. 4.15 Granulomatous gastritis pattern. (**a**) Well-formed granuloma. (**b**) Chronic granulomatous gastritis in a case with *H. pylori*. (**c**) HP organisms with toluidine blue stain in above case

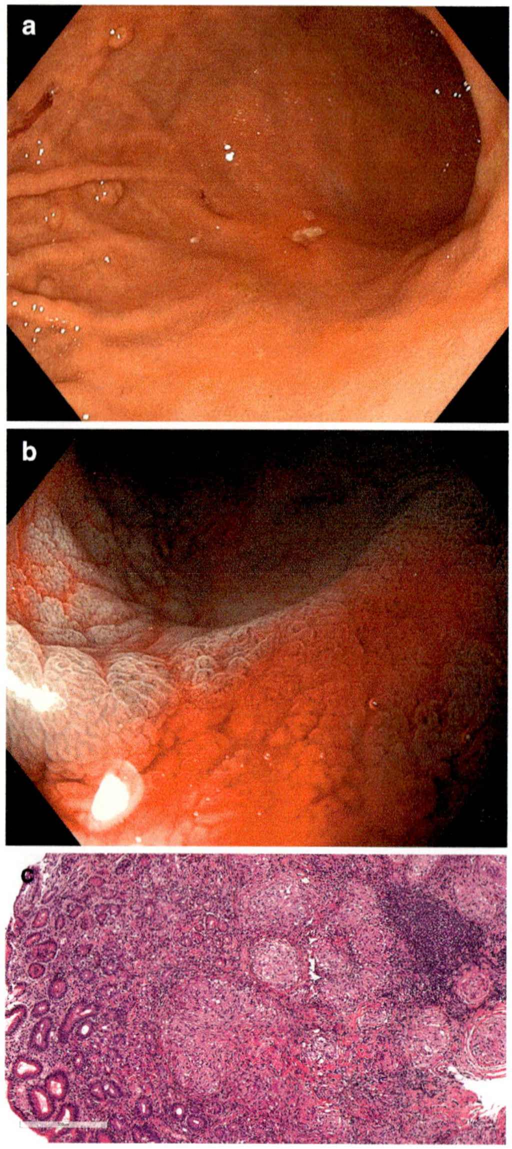

Fig. 4.16 (**Case 5**) A 66-year-old man referred for evaluation of iron deficiency. At OGD he was noted to have mildly erythematous antral mucosa with a low risk antral ulcer seen along the greater curve (**a**). Duodenal examination revealed duodenal mucosal atrophy with mosaic pattern (**b**) with villous blunting noted with NBI zoom magnification (**c**). Anti-tTG antibodies >100 U/ml consistent with a diagnosis of coeliac disease. However, gastric biopsies showed a mixed pattern of granulomatous gastritis and lymphocytic gastritis. In addition to the finding of positive coeliac disease the patient was found to be on angiotensin II inhibitor

tions of histiocytes should not be regarded as granulomatous gastritis, as a confident diagnosis of GG triggers a significant clinical challenge. Gastric granulomas are uncommon, with a reported incidence between 0.08% and 0.35%. When granulomas are numerous, the pattern is obvious. However, more often than not, granulomas may be accompanied by other patterns of inflammation, most common being the chronic gastritis pattern. Specific secondary patterns that may give etiological clues should be investigated.

A large number of diverse aetiologies that include infective and non-infective causes have been associated with a granulomatous response (see chapter 1: granulomatous pattern) [34–39]. Aetiology is believed to vary according to geography and ethnicity. Most cases of granulomatous gastritis in developed countries are believed to be of noninfectious aetiology with the most common causes in adults and children being Crohn disease and sarcoidosis. However, a large series of GG studied in a Western population documented *H. pylori* to be a common association in 92% of their cases [34] (Fig. 4.15b, c). In a Korean study, *H. pylori* were associated with 78% of their cases [35]. Most were single and located in the antrum. Currently it is challenged that *H. pylori* can be regarded as the sole aetiology, and therefore other causes should be searched for when gastric biopsies show GG pattern, even in the presence of HP. Eradication of *H. pylori* should be undertaken when *H. pylori* is found in association with GG.

While the search for an aetiology is one important aspect of handling gastric biopsy with GG pattern, the finding should alert the possibility of underlying immunodeficiency. Morphological and clinical clues of granulomatous inflammation are invaluable (see chapter 1).

Crohn's disease needs to be considered in the paediatric age group with GG. Granulomatous Crohn's disease is often accompanied by involvement of the other sites of the GI tract; therefore, an important step would be to correlate with the finding of luminal biopsies of other sites. Within the stomach, a sub-pattern of FEG may provide a clue to the diagnosis [38]. Sarcoidosis is believed to be common in Western populations before *Helicobacter* was recognised as a potential cause of GG gastritis. The stomach is the most common GI site involved by sarcoidosis. The diagnosis of sarcoid is usually established by identifying associated thoracic or other extraintestinal diseases and by elevated level of angiotensin-converting enzyme. Other bacterial, fungal, and parasitic infections need to be suspected in the setting of immune suppression.

Medications and immunotherapy (interferon) have been known to produce granulomatous inflammation. Drugs associated with GG include cocaine, carbimazole, and interferon.

Foreign body granulomas may be seen with impacted food, suture material, or medications including antacids. Detection of magnesium, aluminium, and silicon has been demonstrated within granulomas by X-ray spectrometry. A granulomatous inflammatory response has also been reported in association with adenocarcinomas and MALT lymphomas.

Rare causes would include Langerhans cell histiocytosis and Whipple's disease. Histiocytic infiltrates are seen in xanthomas, malakoplakia, and Whipple's disease and should not be reported as granulomatous gastritis. Signet ring cells of gastric cancer can be mistaken for histiocytes and can be a near miss. Ancillary stains including those confirming the histiocytic nature would be helpful.

GG pattern occurs without an obvious aetiology in up to 25% of cases. The term idiopathic granulomatous gastritis (IGG) may be used for these after extensive search for a cause both clinically and pathologically. This has been described as a clinicopathologic entity; however, using a descriptive designation of "granulomatous gastritis of uncertain aetiology" likely represents the best practice. Long-term follow-up of these cases is important as some cases of granulomatous inflammation may be the first manifestation of sarcoidosis or Crohn's disease and precede the full spectrum of the disease, sometimes by many years. Therefore, an initial "diagnosis "of IGG should not be regarded as a distinct entity (Box 4.8) [39].

Box 4.8 Association of Aetiological Etiological Agents of GG Pattern, Secondary Patterns and Clues

- With ACG, antrum predominant: look for *H. pylori*
- Non-HP infections
  Mycobacterial: large caseating/necrotising and demonstration of organisms
  Fungal: necrotising and demonstration of organisms
  Syphilis: GG with heavy plasma cells and lymphoid aggregates
  Parasites: EoG pattern is often mixed
- Foreign body granuloma: demonstration of polarisable foreign substances
- Sarcoidosis: isolated, noncaseating with normal surrounding
- Crohn disease: noncaseating with secondary FEG and chronic gastritis pattern
- Medications: secondary FEG and apoptotic pattern
- Associated with malignancy: gastric carcinoma, MALT lymphoma

Collagenous Gastritis Pattern (Fig. 4.17a, b)

Collagenous gastritis (CG) is characterised by deposition of a dense eosinophilic amorphous band under the surface epithelium accompanied by a chronic superficial lymphoplasmacytic infiltrate, scattered eosinophils, and rare neutrophils. Collagenous pattern may be accompanied by secondary patterns of lymphocytic, eosinophilic, or atrophic pattern [40–44]. Intestinal metaplasia is not thought to be a common association. The collagenous band is variably thick (averages from 30 to 70 μm) and composed of types III, IV, and VI collagen. It is often discontinuous, entraps capillaries, and is frequently associated with epithelial detachment. Tenascin immunohistochemistry has shown to be sensitive to detect collagen deposition that is difficult to appreciate otherwise. Masson Trichrome often highlights the collagen band. CG is a rare pattern of uncertain pathogenesis. Diffuse nodularity of the gastric corpus is the characteristic endoscopic finding; however, it is not seen in all cases with some displaying changes ranging from diffuse erythema to normal mucosa. Olmesartan has been reported to produce CG pattern in addition to sprue-like enteropathy.

CG pattern may be accompanied by collagenous or lymphocytic colitis. CG with lymphocytic pattern has been shown to be associated with coeliac disease in some cases. These associations suggest a pan-enteric pathogenic process, although the specific features are unknown. Recent studies have shown female disease predominance. Conditions such as chronic postradiation gastritis and long-standing bile reflux gastritis may rarely mimic collagenous gastritis. Subepithelial collagen deposition may also occur focally in the setting of healed erosion related to local injury (Box 4.9).

Box 4.9 CG Pattern

- Ill-defined pathogenesis.
- Secondary patterns of lymphocytic, eosinophilic, or atrophic pattern are common.
- CG with lymphocytic pattern may be associated with coeliac disease.
- Atrophic pattern may resemble AIG pattern.
- Endoscopic features are variable: Normal to nodularity.
- Overinterpretation of CG pattern: Mimics include chronic postradiation gastritis, longstanding bile reflux gastritis, and setting of healed erosions and ulcers.

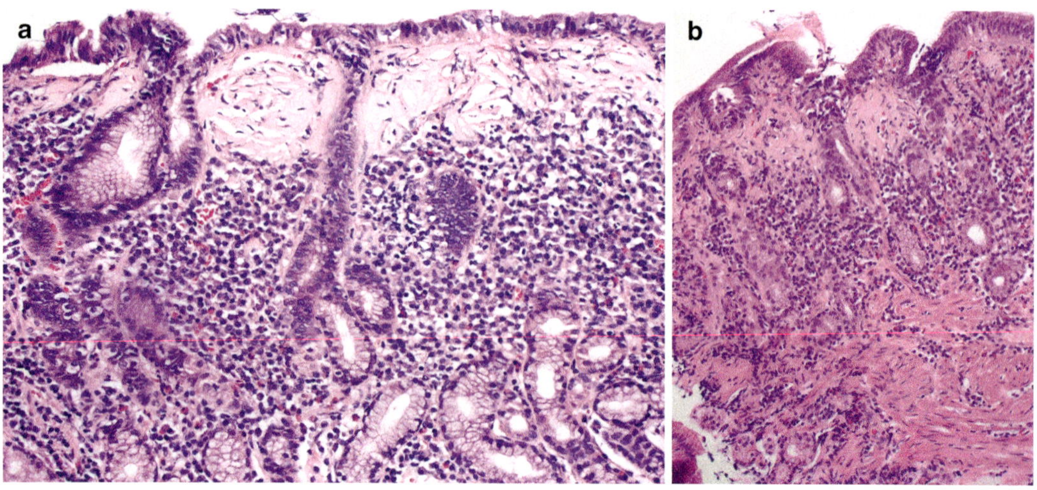

Fig. 4.17 (**a**, **b**) Collagenous gastritis pattern

Apoptotic Pattern (Fig. 4.18)

Apoptotic bodies concentrated in the mucous neck region with various degrees of apoptosis and epithelial injury with or without crypt dilatation and intraluminal granular eosinophilic debris are seen in apoptotic gastropathy ("gastritis") [45–48].

Finding of apoptosis in the gastric biopsies is not common. In the gastric mucosa, one apoptotic body per 100 cells may be regarded as normal; such numbers will rarely be eye-catching. Therefore, if a focus of apoptosis is found in routine evaluation of a gastric biopsy detailed examination is warranted to identify other secondary patterns and clues. The proliferative compartment of the gastric mucosa is in the neck area, and foveolar and surface epithelium is usually unaffected. An important rule is to differentiate apoptotic cell death of neutrophils infiltrating the epithelium from true epithelial apoptosis. The former may be accompanied by other foci of activity. Occasionally, degenerate intraepithelial lymphocytes can cause concern for apoptosis.

Common causes of apoptotic pattern are graft versus host disease (GVHD); infections, in particular CMV and *H. pylori* and HIV; medications, NSAIDs; chemotherapeutic and immunomodulatory agents, e.g. ipilimumab and mycophenolate; and autoimmune enteropathy [45–48]. Confirmative diagnosis often requires a positive clinical history. Immune-mediated diseases including autoimmune enteropathy may show apoptotic pattern in gastric biopsies. Duodenal biopsies may show associated pathology (Box 4.10).

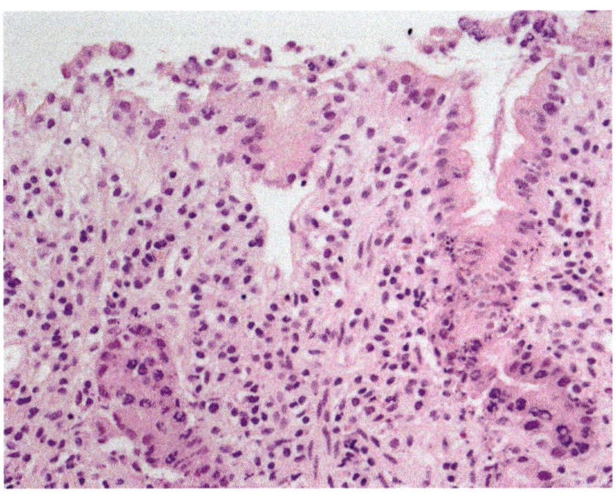

Fig. 4.18 Apoptotic pattern: Apoptotic bodies in the mucous neck region with epithelial injury

In the setting of well-described apoptotic pattern in graft versus host disease (GVHD), the mucous neck region shows the diagnostic features with various degrees of apoptosis and epithelial injury. Crypt dilatation with intraluminal granular eosinophilic debris may also be seen. In severe forms, gland destruction with fibrosis and eventual complete loss of mucosa are seen. Characteristically, the lamina propria shows only a sparse lymphocytic infiltrate.

Infections such as CMV are a well-known cause of epithelial apoptosis throughout the GI tract. Other infections such as those due to *H. pylori* and HIV are also known to cause apoptosis. Medication-induced injury has emerged as an important cause; offending medications include NSAIDs, and chemotherapeutic and immunomodulatory agents such as ipilimumab and mycophenolate. With emergence of cancer immunotherapy, GI pathologists are likely to see this pattern more often than in the past. Immune modulators are being increasingly used in the treatment of metastatic melanomas. If apoptotic pattern is noted, the biopsy should not be reported without the knowledge of medication history. Patient's full clinical history should include medications related to non-GI malignancies, organ transplantation, and herbal therapies.

Box 4.10 Apoptotic Pattern

- Graft versus host disease (GVHD): Classical pattern
- Infections, in particular CMV and *H. pylori* and HIV: Demonstrable organisms and clinical setting
- NSAIDs: Mixed patterns with ACG with erosion, EoG and LG patterns
- Chemotherapeutic and immunomodulatory agents, e.g. ipilimumab, mycophenolate (with "funny-looking" crypts), others
- Autoimmune enteropathy: Common site outside the small intestine
- Radiation: Other radiation-induced changes including vasculopathic pattern
- Overinterpretation: Neutrophilic and lymphocytic apoptosis as epithelial apoptosis

Deposition Pattern (Fig. 4.19a–m)

Endogenous or exogenous pigmented material is not uncommonly encountered in gastric biopsies [49, 50]. A variety of mucosal injury patterns is commonly associated with depositions. Deposits may be striking or subtle at low power and show a variety of colours with H&E.

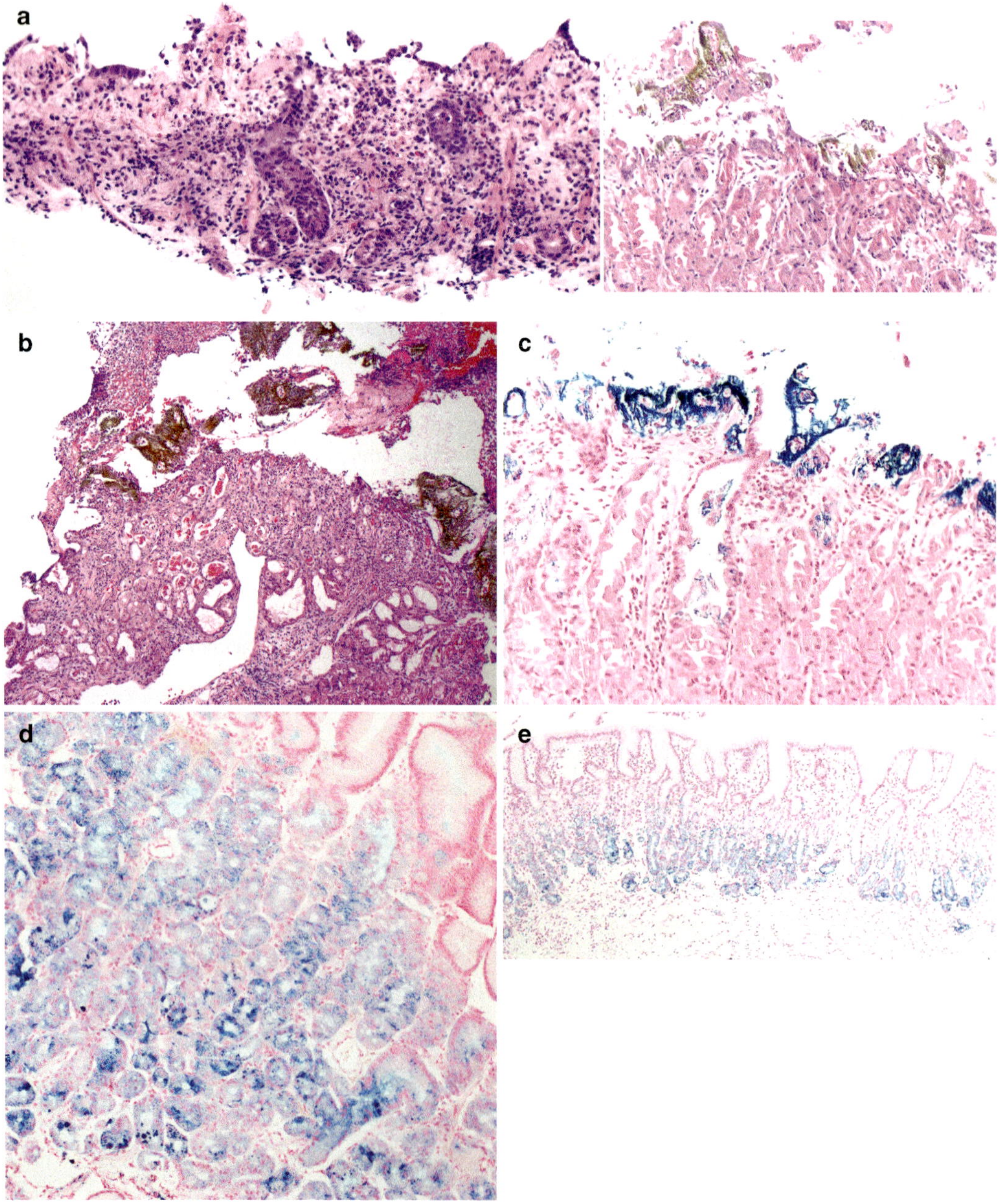

Fig. 4.19 (**a**, **b**) Deposition pattern of iron. (**c**) Iron stains. (**d**, **e**) Gastric glandular siderosis with iron stain. (**f**) Lanthanum carbonate deposition. (**g**) Amyloid deposition. (**h**) Amyloid deposition: globular deposits. (**i**) Amyloid with Congo red stain. (**j**) Amyloid showing apple green birefringence. (**k**) Calcium deposition. (**l**, **m**) SIRT beads and radiation-induced vasculopathy

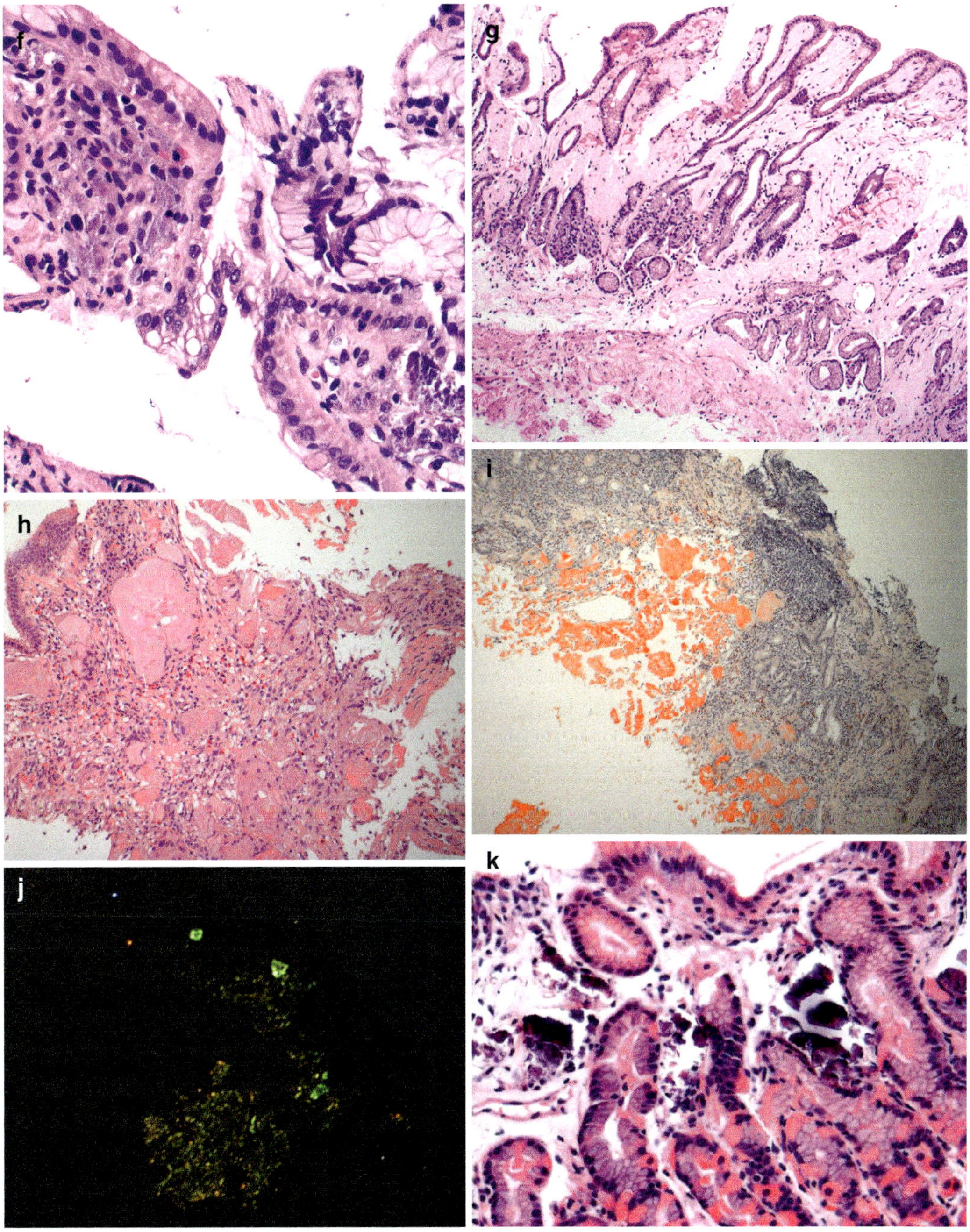

Fig. 4.19 (continued)

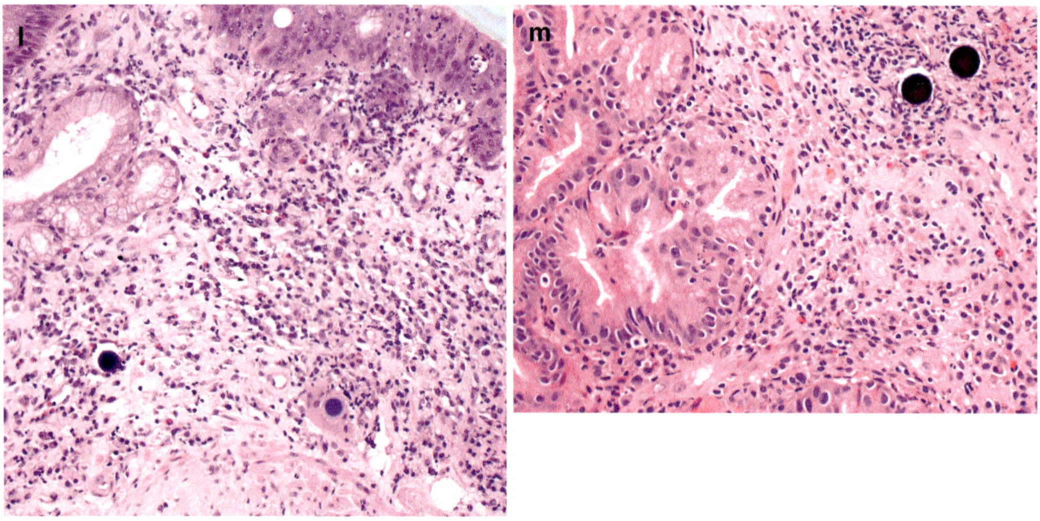

Fig. 4.19 (continued)

Brown-Black Deposits

Iron

Iron deposits in gastric mucosal biopsies may be subtle or striking. The striking deposits appear as extracellular golden brown crystals commonly seen in surface exudate and granulation tissue or encrusted in the superficial mucosa that is often damaged (Fig. 4.19a, b).

They also may be entrapped in the lamina propria, or may be present in stromal cells. The pigments are usually easily visible, but may be highlighted by an iron stain (Fig. 4.19c). Iron deposition pattern with gastric epithelial injury induced by iron is famously known as "iron pill gastritis/gastropathy". The associated reactionary pattern is usually mixed and includes reactive gastropathy, hyperplastic/polypoid pattern and ACG pattern with or without erosions, and infarct-like necrosis. Reactive epithelial changes show worrying atypia that may mimic dysplasia.

Less obvious subtle deposits of iron may be identified in macrophages and stroma and believed to be associated with previous mucosal injury and microhaemorrhages. Iron stains highlight these subtle deposits in the absence of an obvious inflammatory response and epithelial injury.

Iron deposition in "gastric glandular siderosis" (Fig. 4.19d, e) is an uncommon finding that may be associated with systemic iron overload or haemochromatosis. This deposition pattern is subtle and should be differentiated from "iron pill gastritis" and secondary iron deposition. Gastric glandular siderosis shows iron deposition in the epithelial cells deep in the antral and specialised glands unaccompanied by epithelial damage and inflammation.

Pseudomelanosis

These are dark brown-black pigments of unknown aetiology, deposited in macrophages of superficial lamina propria. Metastatic melanoma can be ruled out with lack of any cytological atypia and immunohistochemical stains. Positive staining for macrophage markers (e.g. CD68) and negativity for melanoma markers confirm this rare pattern.

Lanthanum Carbonate (Fig. 4.19f)

Lanthanum carbonate is a phosphate binder for the treatment of hyperphosphatemia in dialysis patients. Fine, granular, brownish deposits are observed in macrophages or multinucleated giant cells.

Pink Deposits

Amyloid

Deposits are extracellular, lightly eosinophilic, homogeneous, and amorphous with haematoxylin and eosin (Fig. 4.19g) and may appear globular (Fig. 4.19h). They are orange with Congo red stain under direct light (Fig. 4.19i) and show bright apple green birefringence under polarised light (Fig. 4.19j). In mucosal biopsies, deposits are seen in the lamina propria, muscularis mucosae, or vessel wall. Submucosal deposits are more common but may not be included in mucosal biopsies. Amyloid needs to be distinguished from other pink deposits such as vascular thrombi, collagen deposits, and radiation changes. Occasionally amyloid deposits may be globular resembling Waldenstrom protein. Systemic amyloidosis can involve the stomach in about 10% of cases. It may occur in isolation too. Amyloid deposition can accompany haemorrhagic gastritis due to vascular damage. In such cases vasculopathic pattern may be the primary pattern with focal deposition of subtle amyloid deposits.

Waldenstrom Protein

Brightly eosinophilic immunoglobulin material within vascular spaces may be rarely confused with globular amyloid deposits. These deposits are characteristically brightly eosinophilic, PASD positive, and Congo red negative. They are also immunoreactive for IgM.

Vascular Thrombi

These are accompanied by other features of vasculopathic pattern (discussed elsewhere), and special stains should resolve the issue in difficult cases (CD16, PASD, Congo red).

Collagen

Collagen deposition is seen in radiation injury (often accompanied by radiation pattern) and collagenous gastritis with the typical subepithelial deposition pattern.

Deep Pink-Purple Deposits

Calcium

Crystalline deep pink or purple deposits indicate calcium. Presence of small, deeply pink to purple (cyanophilic) and partially calcified refractile crystals typically observed beneath the surface epithelium of the antrum signifies "gastric mucosal calcinosis" (Fig. 4.19k). Deposition is mainly in the antrum and may be rimmed by macrophages. Mucosal injury patterns include reactive gastropathy and foveolar hyperplasia accompanied by oedema. This is frequently seen in the setting of renal transplantation or in patients with chronic renal failure on aluminium-based antacids or sucralfate. The crystals can contain aluminium, phosphorus, calcium, and chlorine. Calcium deposition is most commonly associated with metastatic calcification associated with calcium dysregulation. They may be seen with other forms of epithelial damage associated with dystrophic calcification. Clinical setting is important.

Purple Blue Deposits

OsmoPrep Preparations

They have been recently identified as large purplish granules resembling calcium deposits. They are von Koss positive but negative for alizarin red and also for Perl's iron stain. OsmoPrep, a tablet-based colonoscopy preparation, has been identified as the culprit [50].

Kayexalate

Characteristic purple rhomboid plate-like crystals of Kayexalate in sorbitol are deposited within ulcer debris and exudate, or seen adherent to intact mucosa. The mucosa usually shows reactive changes and erosions. Kayexalate in sorbitol is prescribed to manage hyperkalaemia, which can lead to gastric injury in addition to the more common and severe ischaemic colonic necrosis.

Deep Blue Deposits

SIRT Spheres/beads

They are haematoxophilic purple or dark blue rounded structures that are seen often in association with ulceration (see more details under radiation pattern) (Fig. 4.19 l and m). They are strictly not depositions but can be mistaken as such. The striking deep purple spheres are diagnostic once you are aware of the clinical circumstances.

Orange-Red Deposits

Cholestyramine deposits are smooth orange and not associated with mucosal injury. Rarely bile can be seen in gastric mucosal epithelial damage and ulceration associated with bile leaks into the stomach following surgical complications (Fig. 4.20a–d). Colesevelam also appears red-orange-brown (Box 4.11)

Box 4.11 Coloured Deposits

Brown-Black

- Iron—often associated with mucosal injury patterns, iron stain positive
- Lipofuscin—no inflammation
- Melanin
- Carbon
- Lanthanum carbonate

Pink

- Amyloid—light pink, Congo red positive
- Waldenstrom protein—bright pink, Congo red negative, PASD positive, IgM positive
- Collagen: collagenous gastritis—sub-epithelial, pink, Congo red negative
- Hyaline: radiation gastritis—pink, Congo red negative, other radiation changes
- Vascular thrombi—pink, Congo red negative + vasculopathic pattern

CD16+ (marker may highlight microthrombi)

Yellow-Pink

- Sevelamer—with typical fish scale pattern

Blue-Purple

- Calcium—bright purple, Von Kossa positive
- OsmoPrep preparations: Purplish and large granules, Von Kossa positive, Alizarin red and Iron stain negative
- Kayexalate—purple with typical fish scale pattern

Deep Blue

- SIRT/yttrium-80—deep purple, round, unique, radiation pattern

Orange-Red

- Cholestyramine—smooth orange with no mucosa injury
- Bile—bile that leaks into the stomach
- Colesevelam

Grey

Barium—granular refractive

Clear

- Lipid
- Glycogen

Mixed Patterns

This pattern is regarded as a red flag to investigate further for medication-induced injury and also the possibility of having more than one aetiology. Depending on the underlying mechanism of injury inflicted by medications, various combinations can be seen as illustrated by examples discussed here. The greatest clue will be the presence of pill material or other related substances (i.e. "iron pill gastritis") [49–51].

Site-Specific and Special Patterns

Gastropathy Pattern

Two main patterns are based on mucosal and vascular changes. Mucosal changes (reactive gastropathy) are much more common than vascular (vasculopathy) changes.

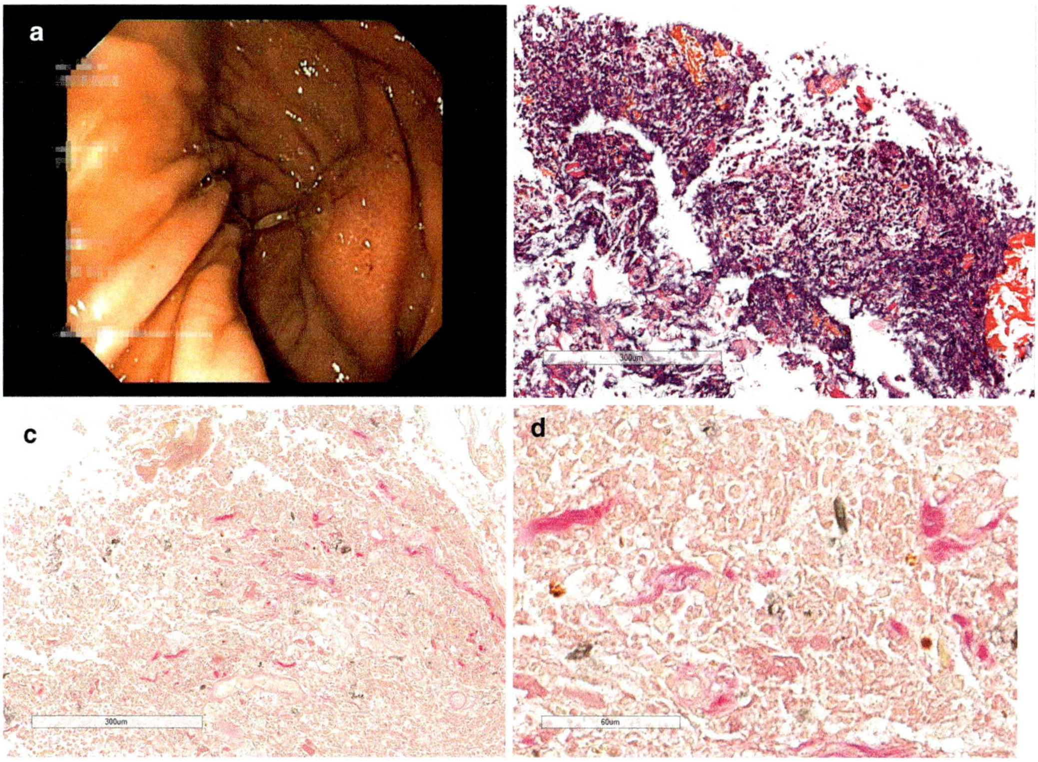

Fig. 4.20 **Case 6**: A 71-year-old man with a complex past surgical history of left haemihepatectomy for intraductal papillary neoplasm of the bile duct. Referral made for gastroscopy to evaluate a single episode of melaena stool. At gastroscopy, he was noted to have a 30 mm subepithelial mass with central ulceration (**a**). Biopsies showed extensively ulcerated specialised gastric mucosa with associated mixed inflammation and yellow/orange material favoured to represent bile (**b**) and confirmed by Fouchet's stain (**c**, **d**). Subsequent CT revealed a chronic biloma related to previous surgery with likely fistulisation of the biloma within the gastric antrum

Reactive Gastropathy Pattern (Fig. 4.21)

This pattern is signified by reduction of foveolar mucin cap resulting in darker foveolar surface, corkscrew-like changes in the gastric pits, superficial mucosal oedema with dilated capillaries, and "tongues" of smooth muscle fibres extending from the muscularis mucosae upward into the lamina propria (muscularisation). A few eosinophils may be present; otherwise inflammation is uncommon. The unique finding of subnuclear vacuolisation of foveolar cells has been seen specifically in operated stomachs [51].

Reactive gastropathy (RG) pattern is the most common pattern of gastric injury seen in routine practice and is considered to represent a nonspecific mucosal response to a variety of gastric irritants. Gastric erythema is a common finding at endoscopy. Common aetiological considerations are bile reflux, medications and alcohol, as well as increased gastric pH and bacterial contamination by faecal-type microflora [51, 52]. Reactive gastropathy (RG) is common in the antrum.

A dominant RG pattern may be accompanied by a secondary pattern including acute injury pattern associated with erosions, ulceration, and diagnostic clues such as gastrotoxic and pill substances as well as vasculopathic, radiation, metaplastic, and granulomatous patterns that may be responsible for the primary pathology. It is easy to overlook the more sinister secondary pattern with the striking RG pattern. Darker foveolar surface with mucin depletion may mimic low-grade dysplasia, particularly foveolar subtype. This appearance can be alarming, and such biopsies are not infrequent consults (see under foveolar hyperplastic pattern and foveolar dysplasia in chapter 5) (Box 4.12).

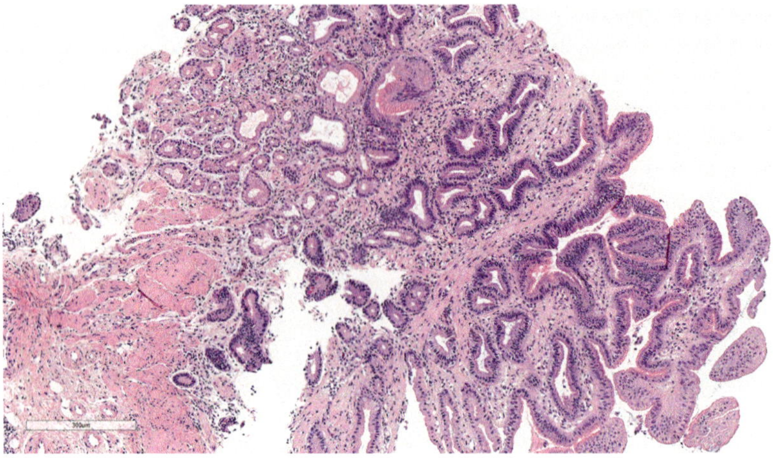

Fig. 4.21 Reactive gastropathy pattern

> **Box 4.12 Reactive Gastropathy Pattern**
>
> - The most common pattern of gastric injury seen in gastric biopsies.
> - May be the dominant pattern of injury undermining specific clues and secondary patterns that may be diagnostic.
> - Severe foveolar reactive changes may mimic foveolar dysplasia.

Mucosal Vasculopathic Pattern

The pattern is characterised by congested and ectatic vessels; either the number of these vessels or their luminal diameter is increased. Background mucosa often shows a reactive gastropathy pattern. Vasculopathic injury may be subtle especially in mild cases, and mucosal gastropathy pattern may be the dominant feature, although the primary injury is centred on mucosal blood vessels. This diagnostic feature may be focal and easily overlooked at screening. Portal hypertensive gastropathy, gastric antral vascular ectasia (GAVE), gastric lymphocytic phlebitis, amyloid deposition, and radiation changes can result in mucosal vasculopathic pattern. Specific features when present, together with clinical and endoscopic information will clinch the etiological diagnosis.

Portal Hypertensive Gastropathy (PHG) (Figs. 4.22 and 4.23)

PHG pattern is characterised by typical vasculopathic changes that show prominent vascular ectasia, irregularity and tortuosity, and variable mural thickening of mucosal and submucosal capillaries and veins. The body and fundus are commonly involved although the entire stomach is affected by the setting of high-pressure high-resistance system often created by advanced hepatic fibrosis.

Changes may be more marked in deeper submucosal vessels; therefore, normal biopsies do not rule out a diagnosis of PHG. On the other hand, presence of capillary dilatation in mucosal biopsies is a nonspecific finding that may be seen in patients with and without portal hypertension, and in isolation is not a reliable diagnostic criterion for PHG. Mucosal gastropathy pattern may be more obvious, and the primary vasculopathy pattern may be missed in low-power magnification (Fig. 4.23). Marked vasculopathic and mucosal changes in the body and fundus as opposed to the antrum should alert the GI pathologist to the possibility of PHG.

Clinical history of cirrhosis as well as noncirrhotic portal hypertension, extrahepatic portal vein obstruction, and Budd-Chiari syndrome are vital for a conclusive diagnosis [53, 54]. The endoscopic appearance of PHG is variable. An oedematous red mucosa with a mosaic pattern also known as "snake skin pattern" is seen in early and mild disease; friable, cherry red mucosal red spots that actively bleed on touch are present in severe disease.

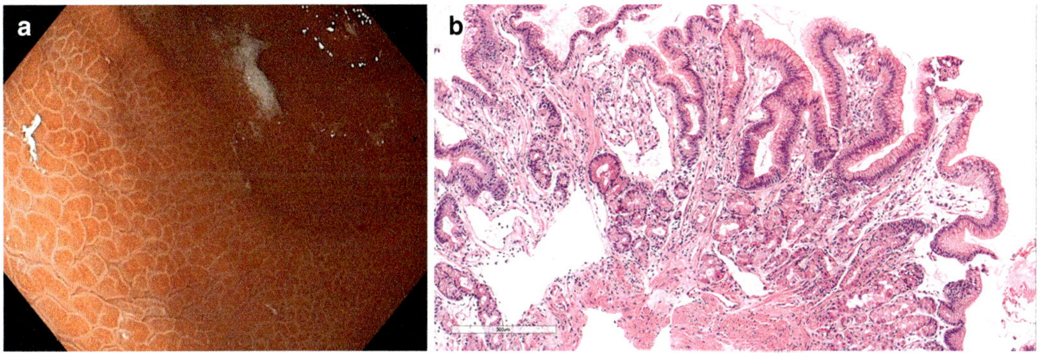

Fig. 4.22 (**Case 7**) A 71-year-old man presenting for gastroscopy to evaluate a recent episode of hematemesis. There was no past history of significant alcohol use. Gastroscopy revealed a fine, white, reticular pattern (**a**) separating areas of pinkish mucosa, giving the gastric mucosa a snakeskin appearance consistent with a likely diagnosis of portal hypertensive gastropathy (PHG). As there was no history of chronic liver disease or risk factors for cirrhosis, biopsies were taken given similar appearances in *H. pylori*-associated gastritis. Histology reported dilated submucosal and mucosal veins and ectatic capillaries consistent with a diagnosis of PHG (**b**). Liver biopsy was performed confirming non-alcoholic steatohepatitis with established early cirrhosis

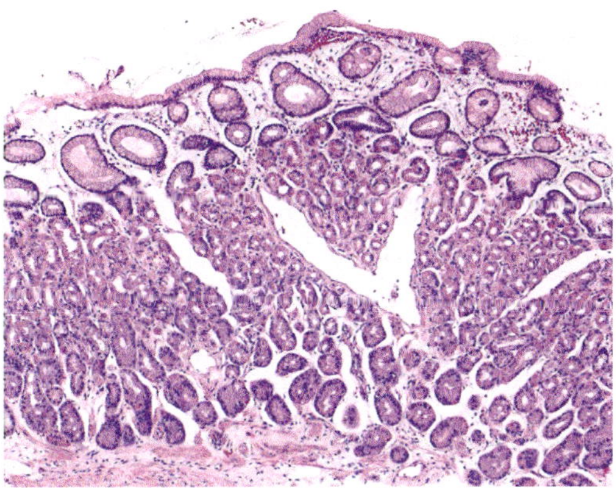

Fig. 4.23 Portal hypertensive gastropathy

Gastric Antral Vascular Ectasia (GAVE) (Fig. 4.24a, b)

GAVE is characterised histologically by abnormalities in the gastric antral mucosal and/or submucosal blood vessels [55–58]. Inflammation is conspicuously absent. Vascular dilatation and intravascular microthrombi (Fig. 4.24b) are present in about 50% of cases. Reparative spindle cell myofibroblastic proliferation in the lamina propria may be seen. Mucosal gastropathy pattern featuring foveolar hyperplasia and regenerative epithelial changes may be the dominant feature. Microthrombi may be highlighted by immunohistochemical stains for platelet marker CD 61.

The antrum is affected most often, but proximal extension into the corpus and cardia has been described. Antral involvement is an important feature that differentiates GAVE from PHG. GAVE is less common than PHG. Distinction between the two types of vasculopathies is important as management is different.

Clinical and endoscopic features of GAVE are characteristic, and such information gives clues to establish a clinicopathological diagnosis. The typical patient is elderly and frequently a woman suffering from autoimmune connective tissue disease with evidence of chronic occult blood loss. Endoscopic appearance is typically described as a "watermelon stomach" (Fig. 4.24a, b) (raised, red mucosal stripes of dilated and tortuous blood vessels involving the antrum and converging on the pylorus) but is present in only about half the cases. About 30% of patients with GAVE may have cirrhosis, and the distinction PHG can be a challenge.

Dieulafoy Lesions

Occasionally gastric biopsy may show ulceration and an unusually larger calibre, tortuous, aneurysmal artery at the base and thought to be a congenital vascular abnormality that may also be seen in the small and large intestine. Specific diagnosis on a mucosal biopsy may be very difficult.

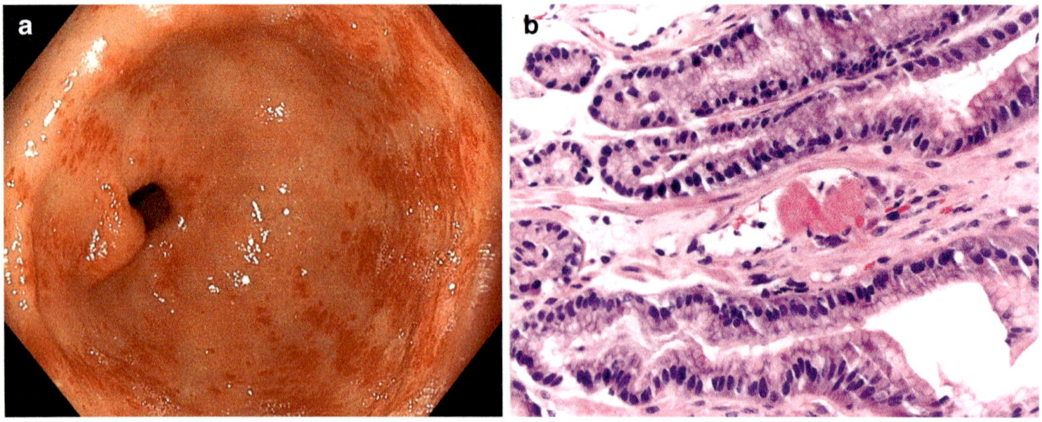

Fig. 4.24 Gastric antral vascular ectasia (GAVE). (a) "Watermelon stomach". (b) Thrombin in dilated vessels

Doxycycline Effect

A distinctive type of eosinophilic fibrinoid degeneration of superficial capillaries with platelet microthrombi with erosions has been described. Concurrent oesophageal mucosa injury has a distinctive pattern that is different to this pattern of injury (see Chapter 2) (Box 4.13) [5, 59].

Box 4.13 Vasculopathic Pattern and Clues

- Common to all vasculopathies: Mucosa capillary dilatation, congestion with mucosal reactive change (reactive gastropathy).
- PHG—May be subtle, mucosal gastropathy may be more obvious, may be prominent in body and fundus but involves the entire stomach.
- GAVE—Vascular ectasia with thrombi mostly in the antrum, occasionally involves the entire stomach.
- RIV—Vascular damage and fibrinoid necrosis in extensive damage. Specific clues, e.g. yttrium beads. Exclude residual malignancy and other associations, e.g. CMV.
- Amyloid—Amyloid deposits.
- Diagnostic vasculopathic pattern may be undermined by the dominant reactive gastropathy pattern.
- Medications: Emerging patterns, e.g. doxycycline.

Radiation-Induced Vasculopathy (RIV) (Fig. 4.25a, b, and Fig. 4.19l and m)

In addition to the common vasculopathic pattern accompanied by mucosal changes, hyalinisation, and damage of vascular wall, lamina propria hyalinisation and atypical stromal ("radiation fibroblasts"), epithelial, and endothelial cells are seen in RIV [60]. Nuclear karyorrhexis and cytoplasmic eosinophilia are noted in the pit epithelium as early alterations. Inflammation is usually insignificant but an eosinophilic infiltrate can be seen.

Glandular necrosis may develop in some cases and, if extensive, is associated with ulceration and haemorrhage. Additional vasculitic changes such as endothelial proliferation and fibrinoid necrosis may be seen. RIV is usually seen in the setting of upper abdominal neoplasia or in bone marrow transplant recipients. At gastroscopy, diffuse erythema, dilated capillaries, and active bleeding can be seen (Fig. 4.25a, b).

It is important to exclude residual malignancy in the biopsy. Conversely, glandular and stromal atypia can mimic malignancy, but the almost unique involvement of pit zone location is a clue. Other associated processes such as infections in particular CMV need to be excluded. Special and immunohistochemical stains may be useful.

Haemotoxyphilic microsphere is a unique finding in a gastric biopsy in patients who have received selective internal radiation therapy (SIRT) for primary and metastatic hepatic malignancies that are unsuitable for resection.

These are resins labelled with yttrium-80 injected via the hepatic artery system to the vascular supply of the tumour with the aim of providing high-dose targeted radiation to the neoplastic cells with least effect to the nonneoplastic parenchyma. Occasionally and often in the setting of aberrant blood supply, the beads may travel in vessels supplying the gastroduodenal region. They can be seen in the biopsy at screening power as round, deep purple, opaque beads lying within arterioles accompanied by changes of the radiation pattern described above. If the clinical setting is uncertain, they have the potential to be mistaken for psammoma bodies, dystrophic calcifications, foreign substances, and even *Schistosoma*. However, the bead that measures around 30–40 μm has a unique appearance and once seen is never missed! Clinical setting confirms the diagnosis (Fig. 4.24a, b).

Polypoid and Hyperplastic pattern

Polypoid hyperplastic pattern is characterised by expansion of foveolar or oxyntic mucosa or combination of both. Expansion of the mucosa is often accompanied by hyperplastic changes of individual cells and architectural changes such as dilatation and tortuosity. Such pattern may represent a genuine hyperplastic polyp, foveolar hyperplasia, oxyntic hyperplasia, or a mucosal prolapse [61]. Hyperplastic pattern in a mucosal biopsy may also represent superficial parts of genuine neoplastic and syndromic polyps, and the diagnosis may be challenging especially when there is discordance between the endoscopic and microscopic features. There are hardly any specific features that distinguish sporadic from syndromic polyps in gastric mucosal biopsies with certainty. However, larger polypoid fragments or polypectomy specimens may show subtle but important clues. Clinical and endoscopic features are of paramount importance to suspect polyposis syndromes. Endoscopic features of gastric mucosal hyperplasia are often dramatic, but mucosal biopsy features can be deflating. Clinical appearance can vary from thickened folds, giant folds, and polyps (Fig. 4.26a–c).

Foveolar Hyperplastic Pattern

This pattern shows superficial elongation of the foveolar region with a minimal inflammatory component in the lamina propria. A few wisps of smooth muscle fibres may be seen. Foveolar hyperplasia is a nonspecific response of the mucosa to injury. Hyperplastic polyps and polypoid foveolar hyperplasia are diagnosed when a polyp has been detected endoscopically (Fig. 4.26a), whereas similar but early changes are noted in non-polypoidal reactive gastropathy pattern. Surface foveolar changes may overlap in different pathological processes, and distinction may be difficult. Focal foveolar hyperplasia and polypoid regenerative mucosa (Fig. 4.26b, c) often occur in chemically induced gastritis in which the mucosa shows reactive gastropathy pattern. Some experts are of the opinion that foveolar hyperplasia is an early change that may progress to a genuine hyperplastic polyp and distinction is a matter of the size. Others are of the opinion that genuine hyperplastic polyps are commonly found in active and atrophic autoimmune gastritis and corpus predominant *Helicobacter pylori* gastritis. In fact, the pathological basis of both foveolar hyperplasia and a hyperplastic polyp may be similar.

Hyperplastic Polyp Pattern

Typically, the pattern is characterised by marked elongation of the pit region with a corkscrew appearance with significant branching and cystic dilatation resulting in architectural disarray (Fig. 4.27). There is mixed acute and chronic inflammation of the lamina propria accompanying early erosion at times. Glandular components are depleted. Hyperplastic polyps are the second most common gastric polyps. Differential diagnoses to consider in the appropriate clinical setting are juvenile polyposis, Peutz-Jeghers syndrome, PTEN syndrome, Cronkhite-Canada syndrome, and Menetrier disease (see neoplastic section).

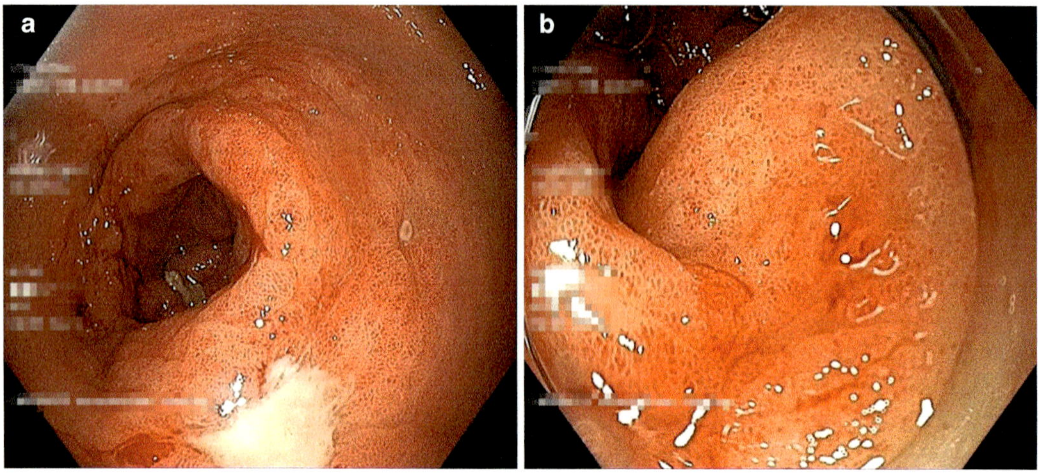

Fig. 4.25 (**a**, **b**) Radiation-induced vasculopathy (RIV) endoscopy

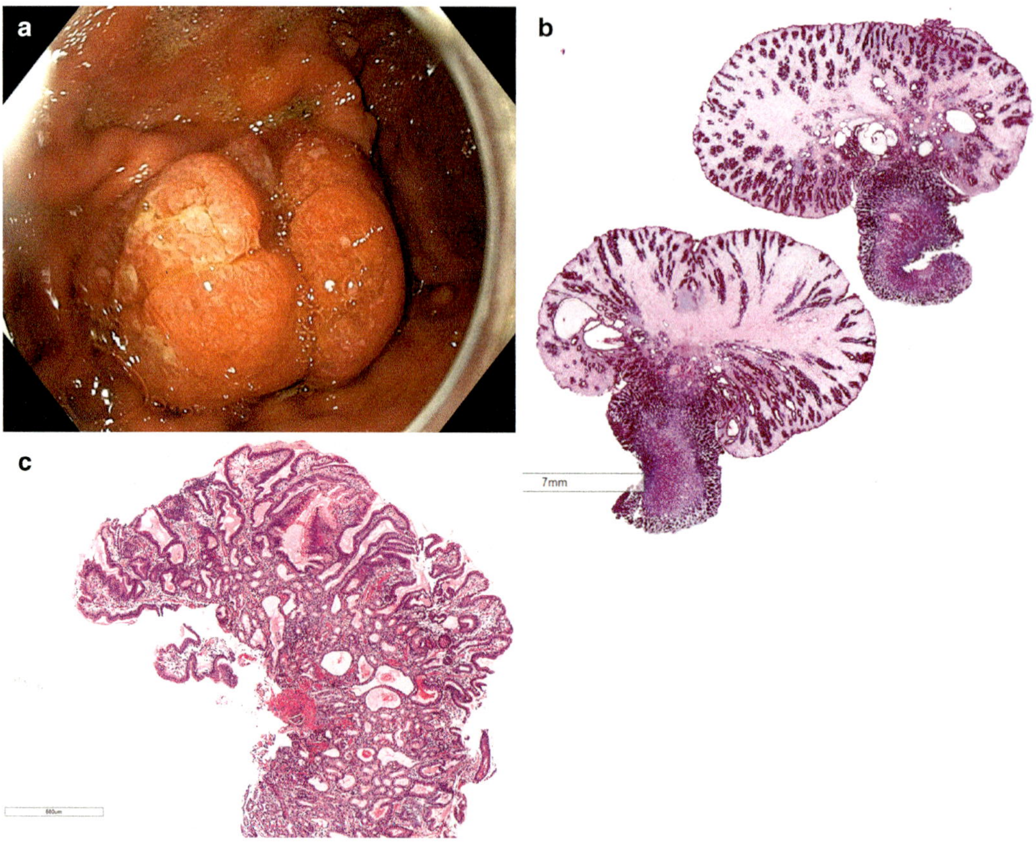

Fig. 4.26 (**a**) Polyp—endoscopy. (**b**) Polypoid foveolar hyperplasia with PASD to show hyperlytic foveolar compartment. (**c**) Foveolar hyperplasia and polypoid regenerative mucosa

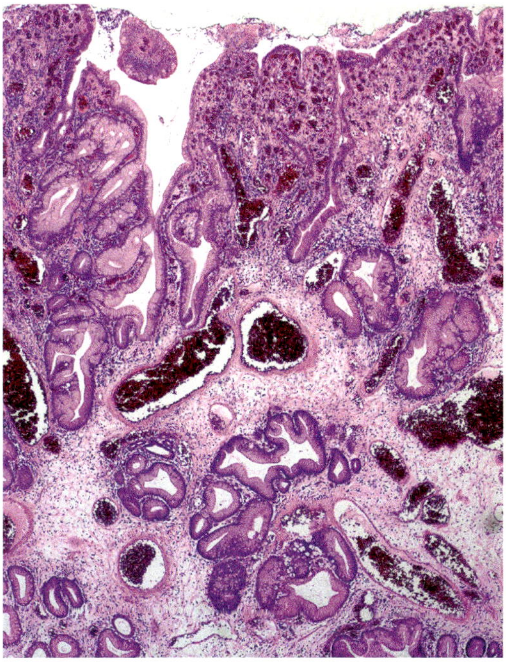

Fig. 4.27 Hyperplastic polyp pattern

Oxyntic (Parietal and Chief cell) Hyperplastic Pattern

Prototype of this pattern is fundic gland polyps (FGPs){Fig. 4.28a} resulting from oxyntic hyperplasia (Fig. 4.28b, c). Chief cell hyperplasia and associated oxyntic adenomas, some featuring chief cell predominance, have been described lately with a weak association related to PPI therapy [62].

Oxyntic hyperplasia may also produce giant folds. Oxyntic hyperplastic pattern is most commonly described with PPI therapy in sporadic setting. In early stages, there is expansion of the oxyntic mucosa with depletion of foveolar compartment and hypertrophic parietal cells that prolapse into the glandular lumen; in established FGPs, there is dilatation of oxyntic glands lined by hypertrophic and flattened parietal cells. FGPs can show dysplasia, and when there are multiple and dysplastic associated syndromes needs to be considered. These include Familial Adenomatous Polyposis (FAP), MUTYH-associated polyposis, sporadic FGP syndrome, Zollinger-Ellison syndrome (sporadic and familial), and Gastric Adenocarcinoma and Proximal Polyposis (GAPPs).

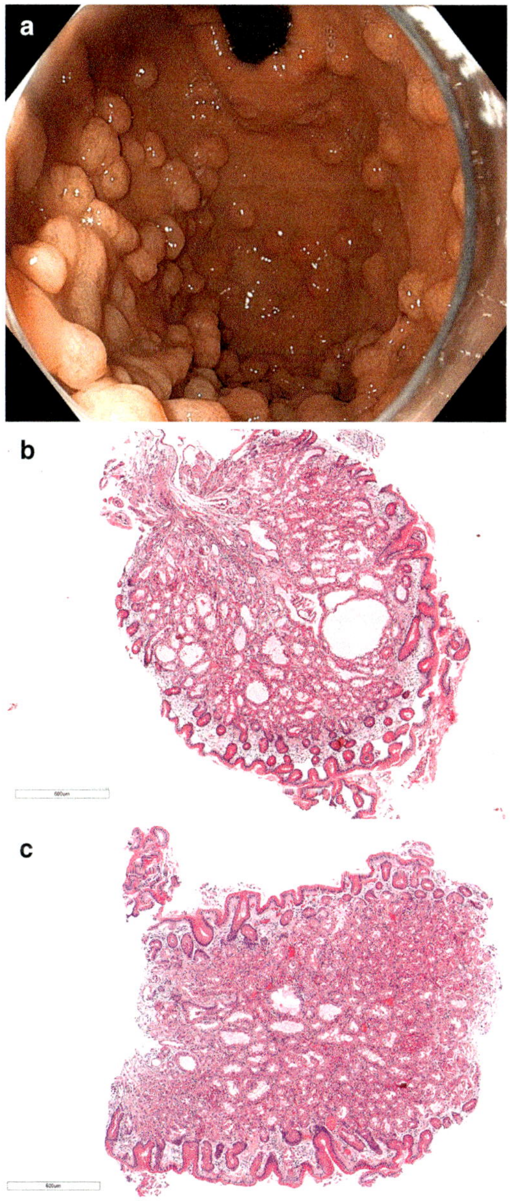

Fig. 4.28 (**a**) Fundic gland polyps—endoscopy. (**b**) Fundic gland polyp—histology. (**c**) Oxyntic cell hyperplastic pattern

Mucosal Prolapsing Pattern (Fig. 4.29)

This pattern is characterised by variable elongation of foveolar regions and cystic dilatation of the pit region and presence of thick-walled blood vessels with organised arborising thick bundles of the muscle. A distinctive feature is also the presence of

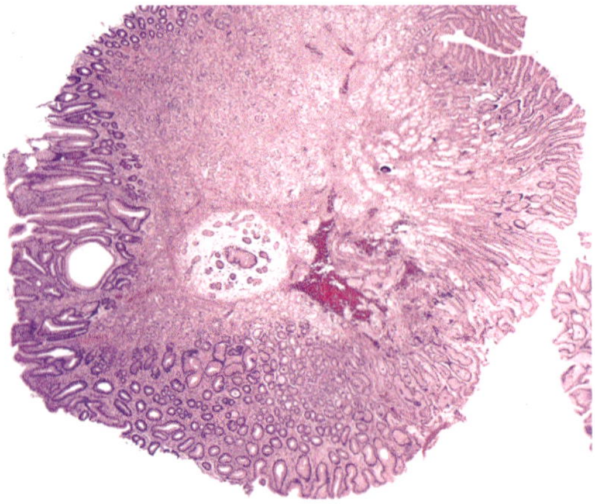

Fig. 4.29 Mucosa prolapsing pattern

large-calibre thick-walled vessels that is unusual for normal gastric mucosa. A distinguishing feature from a hyperplastic polyp is the presence of either pyloric or oxyntic glandular component depending on the location. The diagnostic feature may not be observed in a mucosal biopsy (Box 4.14) [61].

Box 4.14 Polypoid/Hyperplastic Pattern

- Endoscopic features are often dramatic, but microscopic features can be deflating.
- Foveolar hyperplasia—elongated foveolar compartment with minimal inflammation.
- Hyperplastic polyp—Hyperplastic polyp - marked elongation of foveolar regions and dilatation of pits with branching and inflammation +/– erosion with depletion of glandular component.
- Mucosal prolapse—cystic dilatation of the pits, thick-walled blood vessels, organised arborising thick bundles of muscle with the presence of the glandular component.
- Oxyntic hyperplasia—the combination of parietal and chief cell hyperplasia, most commonly seen with PPI therapy.
- Superficial parts of the neoplastic polyp—subtle clues should be observed.
- Consider syndromic polyps—clinical setting is important.

Focally Enhanced Gastritis Pattern (Fig. 4.30a, b)

Focally enhanced gastritis (FEG) is characterised by the presence of focal inflammatory lesions comprising lymphocytes and histiocytes and occasional neutrophils that involve either one or a few adjacent foveolae/glands. The lesion is more commonly noted in the antrum in an otherwise normal mucosa. This pattern basically refers to a form of focally active gastritis that was first thought to be specific to Crohn's disease but was subsequently noted in patients with ulcerative colitis and *H. pylori* infection and in those taking NSAIDs. Focal enhanced gastritis has been shown to be a relatively good positive predictive marker for Crohn's disease in the paediatric population. FEG also has been noted in bone marrow transplant patients and autistic children [39, 63–65].

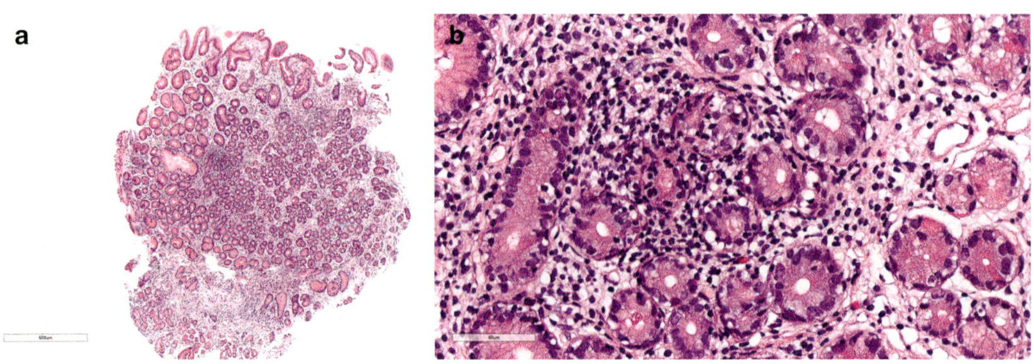

Fig. 4.30 (**a**, **b**) Focally enhanced gastritis pattern

Colchicine Effect

Nuclear pseudostratification and loss of polarity with numerous mitotic figures arrested in metaphase with characteristic "ring" mitoses represent the most common epithelial alteration. Apoptosis can be observed, particularly in the proliferative region of the gastric pits or the gland neck. The appearance may be alarming at screening. Colchicine is commonly prescribed for gout. Mucosal changes are observed only when this alkaloid reaches toxic levels in patients with failing renal or hepatic function. The histologic changes reflect the inhibition of tubulin polymerisation. Taxol (see below) used predominantly in the treatment of breast cancer can initiate similar morphologic changes (see below).

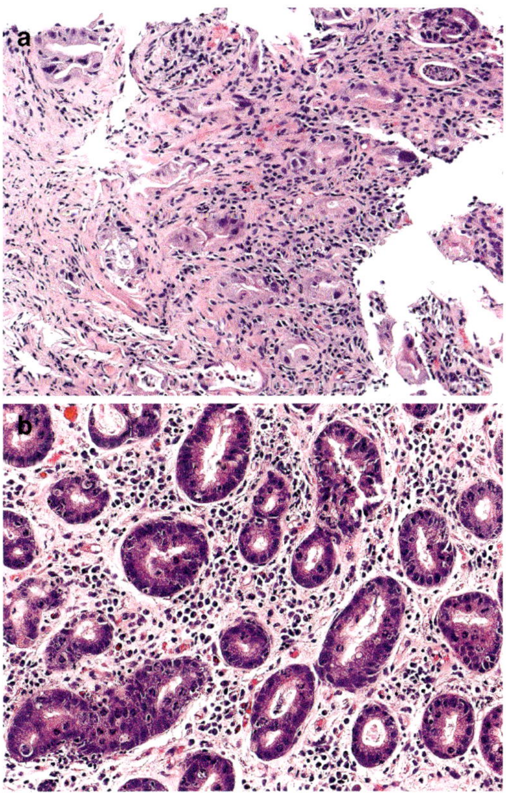

Fig. 4.31 (**a**) A biopsy from a patient who have received radiation therapy for biliary duct cancer. Abortive or cystic distended glands with nuclear atypia are scattered. Considering the involvement of irradiation as well as the degenerative type appearance with a low nuclear density, this is interpreted as radiation injury. (**b**) A gastric biopsy from a patient under chemotherapy including docetaxel. Glands show mild nuclear enlargement and many mitoses, worrisome features for malignancy. Looking carefully, most of the mitoses are ring mitosis, which represents mitosis arrest caused by taxane-based anticancer agent like docetaxel. Therefore, this is considered as chemotherapy effect. Clinical information is critical for an accurate interpretation of this kind of gastric biopsy

Chemoradiation injury (Fig. 4.31)

Chemo radiation injury can elicit various patterns with gastric mucosal damage. The list is fast growing with many new emerging agents in medical oncology. These include mitomycin C, 5-fluoro-2-deoxyuridine, floxuridine, and Taxol, among others. It can be challenging to differentiate an adenocarcinoma from these changes, which may include ulceration and bizarre epithelial atypia accentuated at the base of the glands, as well as increased apoptosis. Prominent eosinophilia, vacuolisation, and pleomorphic nuclei can be seen as well, but mitoses are usually limited. Similar changes can be seen in endothelial cells and fibroblasts.

References

1. Elta GH, Appelman HD, Behler EM, Wilson JA, Nostrant TJ. A study of the correlation between endoscopic and histological diagnoses in gastroduodenitis. J Gastroenterol. 1987;82(8):749.
2. Tytgat GN. The Sydney System: endoscopic division. Endoscopic appearances in gastritis/duodenitis. J Gastroenterol Hepatol. 1991;6(3):223.
3. Marshall BJ, Armstrong JA, DB MG, Glancy RJ. Attempt to fulfil Koch's postulates for pyloric campylobacter. Med J Aust. 1985;142:436–9.
4. Graham DY, Opekun AR, Osato MS, El-Zimaity HMT, Lee CK, Yamaoka Y, Qureshi WA, Cadoz M, Monath TP. Challenge model for Helicobacter pylori infection in human volunteers. Gut. 2004;53:1235–43.
5. Xiao S-Y, Zhao L, Hart J, Semrad CE. Doxycycline-induced gastric and oesophageal mucosal injuries with vascular degeneration. Am J Surg Pathol. 2013;37:259–63.
6. Neumann WL, Coss E, Rugge M, Genta RM. Autoimmune atrophic gastritis--pathogenesis, pathology and management. Nat Rev Gastroenterol Hepatol. 2013;10(9):529–41.
7. Krasinskas AM, Abraham SC, Metz DC, Furth EE. Oxyntic mucosa pseudopolyps: a presentation of atrophic autoimmune gastritis. Am J Surg Pathol. 2003;27(2):236–41.

8. Torbenson M, Abraham SC, Boitnott J, Yardley JH, Wu TT. Autoimmune gastritis: distinct histological and immunohistochemical findings before complete loss of oxyntic glands. Mod Pathol. 2002;15(2):102–9.
9. Stenström B, Windsor HM, Fulurija A, Benghezal M, Kumarasinghe MP, Kimura K, Tay CY, Viiala CH, Ee HC, Lu W, Schoep TD, Webberley KM, Marshall BJ. Helicobacter pylori overcomes natural immunity in repeated infections. Clin Case Rep. 2016;4(11):1026–33.
10. Fox JG, Wang TC. Inflammation, atrophy, and gastric cancer. J Clin Invest. 2007;117(1):60–9.
11. Yakoob J, Abbas Z, Khan R, Naz S, Ahmad Z, Islam M, Awan S, Jafri F, Yakoob JW, et al. Prevalence of non-helicobacter pylori species in patients presenting with dyspepsia. BMC Gastroenterol. 2012;12:3.
12. Heilmann KL, Borchard F. Gastritis due to spiral shaped bacteria other than Helicobacter pylori: clinical, histological, and ultrastructural findings. Gut. 1991;32(2):137–40.
13. Singhal AV, Sepulveda AR. Helicobacter heilmannii gastritis: a case study with review of literature. Am J Surg Pathol. 2005;29(11):1537–9.
14. Batts KP, et al. Appropriate use of special stains for identifying Helicobacter pylori: recommendations from the Rodger C. Haggitt Gastrointestinal Pathology Society. Am J Surg Pathol. 2013;37(11):e12.
15. Genta RM, Sonnenberg A. Helicobacter-negative gastritis: a distinct entity unrelated to Helicobacter pylori infection. Aliment Pharmacol Ther. 2015;41: 218–26.
16. Dickey W, Kenny BD, McConnell JB. Effect of proton pump inhibitors on the detection of Helicobacter pylori in gastric biopsies. Aliment Pharmacol Ther. 1996;10:289–93.
17. Kalantar J, Xia HHX, Wyatt JM, et al. Determination of optimal biopsy sites for detection of H. pylori in patients treated or not treated with antibiotics and antisecretory drugs. Gastroenterology. 1997;112:A165.
18. Ramırez-Lazaro MJ, Lario S, Casalots A, et al. Realtime PCR improves Helicobacter pylori detection in patients with peptic ulcer bleeding. PLoS One. 2011;6:1–7.
19. Fallone CA, Loo VG, Lough J, Barkun AN. Hematoxylin and eosin staining of gastric tissue for the detection of Helicobacter pylori. Helicobacter. 1997;2(1):32–5.
20. Rotimi O, Cairns A, Gray S, Moayyedi P, Dixon MF. Histological identification of Helicobacter pylori: comparison of staining methods. J Clin Pathol. 2000;53(10):756–9.
21. Jonkers D, Stobberingh E, de Bruine A, Arends JW, Stockbrügger R. Evaluation of immunohistochemistry for the detection of Helicobacter pylori in gastric mucosal biopsies. J Infect. 1997;35(2):149–54.
22. Ota H, Katsuyama T, Nakajima S, El-Zimaity H, Kim JG, Graham DY, Genta RM. Intestinal metaplasia with adherent Helicobacter pylori: a hybrid epithelium with both gastric and intestinal features. Hum Pathol. 1998;29(8):846–50.
23. Ratuapli SK, Lam-Himlin DM, Heigh RI. Sarcina ventriculi of the stomach: a case report. World J Gastroenterol. 2013;19(14):2282–5.
24. El-Zimaity HMT, Ramchatesingh J, Ali Saeed M, Graham DY. Gastric intestinal metaplasia: subtypes and natural history. J Clin Pathol. 2001;54:679–83.
25. El-Zimaity HM, et al. Patterns of gastric atrophy in intestinal type gastric carcinoma. Cancer. 2002;94: 1428.
26. Green C, Kumarasinghe MP, Fulurija A, Hooi E, Blanchard J, Nilsson HO, Benghezal M, Marshall B. Helicobacter pylori associated 'lymphocytic gastritis' unravelled. Pathology. 2016;48(Suppl 1):S126.
27. Madisch A, Miehlke S, Neuber F, Morgner A, Kuhlisch E, Rappel S, Lehn N, Bayerdörffer E, Seitz G, Stolte M. Healing of lymphocytic gastritis after Helicobacter pylori eradication therapy--a randomized, double-blind, placebo-controlled multicentre trial. Aliment Pharmacol Ther. 2006;23(4):473–9.
28. Nielsen JA, Roberts CA, Lager DJ, Putcha RV, Jain R, Lewin M. Lymphocytic gastritis is not associated with active helicobacter pylori infection. Helicobacter. 2014;19:349–55.
29. Haot J, Jouret A, Willette M, Gossuin A, Mainguet P. Lymphocytic gastritis - prospective study of its relationship with varioliform gastritis. Gut. 1990;31:282–5.
30. De Brosse CW, Case JW, Putnam PE, et al. Quantity and distribution of eosinophils in the gastrointestinal tract of children. Pediatr Dev Pathol. 2006;9(3):210–8.
31. Lewin T, Melton SD, Genta RM. Eosinophilic gastritis: histopathological characterization and quantification of the normal gastric eosinophil content. Mod Pathol. 2011;24(4):556–63.
32. Lucendo AJ, Arias A. Eosinophilic gastroenteritis: an update. Expert Rev Gastroenterol Hepatol. 2012;6(5):591–601.
33. Rothenberg ME. Eosinophilic gastrointestinal disorders (EGID). J Allergy Clin Immunol. 2004;113(1):11–28. quiz 29.
34. Ectors NL, Dixon MF, Geboes KJ, et al. Granulomatous gastritis: a morphological and diagnostic approach. Histopathology. 1993;23:55–61.
35. Maeng L, Lee A, Choi K, Kang CS, Kim KM. Granulomatous gastritis: a clinicopathologic analysis of 18 biopsy cases. Am J Surg Pathol. 2004;28:941–5.
36. Pai M, Riley LW, Colford JM Jr. Interferon-gamma assays in the immunodiagnosis of tuberculosis: a systematic review. Lancet Infect Dis. 2004;4(12):761–76.
37. Hirokawa M, Shimizu M, Terayama K, Tamai M, Takeda M, Iida M, Manabe T. Bamboo-joint-like appearance of the stomach: a histopathological study. APMIS. 1999;107(10):951–6.
38. Oberhuber G, Püspök A, Oesterreicher C, Novacek G, Zauner C, Burghuber M, Vogelsang H, Pötzi R, Stolte M, Wrba F. Focally enhanced gastritis: a frequent type of gastritis in patients with Crohn's disease. Gastroenterology. 1997;112(3):698–706.

39. Shapiro JL, Goldblum JR, Petras RE. A clinicopathologic study of 42 patients with granulomatous gastritis. Is there really an "idiopathic" granulomatous gastritis? Am J Surg Pathol. 1996;20:462–70.
40. Vesoulis Z, Lozanski G, Ravichandran P, Esber E. Collagenous gastritis: a case report, morphologic evaluation, and review. Mod Pathol. 2000;13:591–6.
41. Lagorce-Pages C, Fabiani B, Bouvier R, et al. Collagenous gastritis: a report of six cases. Am J Surg Pathol. 2001;25:1174–9.
42. Winslow JL, Trainer TD, Colletti RB. Collagenous gastritis: a long-term follow-up with the development of endocrine cell hyperplasia, intestinal metaplasia, and epithelial changes indeterminate for dysplasia. Am J Clin Pathol. 2001;116:753–8.
43. Groisman GM, Meyers S, Harpaz N. Collagenous gastritis associated with lymphocytic colitis. J Clin Gastroenterol. 1996;22:134–7.
44. Arnason T, Brown IS, Goldsmith JD, Anderson W, O'Brien BH, Wilson C, Winter H, Lauwers GY. Collagenous gastritis: a morphologic and immunohistochemical study of 40 patients. Mod Pathol. 2015;28(4):533–44.
45. Masia R, Peyton S, Lauwers GY, Brown I. Gastrointestinal biopsy findings of autoimmune enteropathy: a review of 25 cases. Am J Surg Pathol. 2014;38(10):1319–29.
46. Washington K, Jagasia M. Gastrointestinal biopsy findings of autoimmune enteropathy: a review of 25 cases. Pathology of graft-versus-host disease in the gastrointestinal tract. Hum Pathol. 2009;40(7):909–17.
47. Snover DC. Graft-versus-host disease of the gastrointestinal tract. Am J Surg Pathol. 1990;14(Suppl 1):101–8.
48. Nguyen TDO, Park JY, Scudiere JR, Montgomery E. Mycophenolic acid (cellcept and myofortic) induced injury of the upper GI tract. Am J Surg Pathol. 2009;33(9):1355–63.
49. Abraham SC, Yardley JH, Wu TT. Erosive injury to the upper gastrointestinal tract in patients receiving iron medication: an underrecognized entity. Am J Surg Pathol. 1999;23(10):1241–7.
50. Matsukuma K, Gui D, Olson KA, Tejaswi S, Clayton EF, Thai A. OsmoPrep-associated gastritis: a histopathologic mimic of iron pill gastritis and mucosal calcinosis. Am J Surg Pathol. 2016;40(11):1550–6.
51. Rubio CA, Slezak P. Foveolar cell vacuolization in operated stomachs. Am J Surg Pathol. 1988;12:773–6.
52. Lauwers GY, Furman J, Michael LE, Balis UJ, Kubilis PS. Cytoskeletal and kinetic epithelial differences between NSAID gastropathy and Helicobacter pylori gastritis: an immunohistochemical determination. Histopathology. 2001;39:133–40.
53. Patwardhan VR, Cardenas A. Review article: the management of portal hypertensive gastropathy and gastric antral vascular ectasia in cirrhosis. Aliment Pharmacol Ther. 2014;40(4):354–62.
54. Cubillas R, Rockey DC. Portal hypertensive gastropathy: a review. Liver Int. 2010;30(8):1094–102.
55. Rawlinson WD, Barr GD, Lin BP. Antral vascular ectasia--the "watermelon" stomach. Med J Aust. 1986;144(13):709–11.
56. Stotzer PO, Willén R, Kilander AF. Watermelon stomach: not only an antral disease. Gastrointest Endosc. 2002;55(7):897–900.
57. Suit PF, Petras RE, Bauer TW, Petrini JL Jr. Gastric antral vascular ectasia. A histologic and morphometric study of "the watermelon stomach". Am J Surg Pathol. 1987;11(10):750–7.
58. Yusoff I, Brennan F, Ormonde D, Laurence B. Argon plasma coagulation for treatment of watermelon stomach. Endoscopy. 2002;34(5):407–10.
59. Affolter K, Samowitz W, Boynton K, Kelly ED. Doxycycline induced gastrointestinal injury. Hum Pathol. 2017;66:212.
60. Novak JM, Collins JT, Donowitz M, et al. Effects of radiation on the human gastrointestinal tract. J Clin Gastroenterol. 1979;1:9–39.
61. Gonzalez-Obeso E, Fujita H, Deshpande V, Ogawa F, Lisovsky M, Genevay M, Grzyb K, Brugge W, Lennerz JK, Shimizu M, Srivastava A, Lauwers GY. Gastric hyperplastic polyps: a heterogeneous clinicopathologic group including a distinct subset best categorized as mucosal prolapse polyp. Am J Surg Pathol. 2011;35:670–7.
62. Chan K, Brown IS, Kyle T, Lauwers GY, Kumarasinghe MP. Chief cell-predominant gastric polyps: a series of 12 cases with literature review. Histopathology. 2016;68(6):773–948.
63. Sharif F, McDermott M, Dillon M, Drumm B, Rowland M, Imrie C, Kelleher S, Harty S, Bourke B. Focally enhanced gastritis in children with Crohn's disease and ulcerative colitis. Am J Gastroenterol. 2002;97(6):1415–20.
64. Xin W, Greenson JK. The clinical significance of focally enhanced gastritis. Am J Surg Pathol. 2004;28(10):1347–51.
65. Torrente F, Anthony A, Heuschkel RB, Thomson MA, Ashwood P, Murch SH. Focal-enhanced gastritis in regressive autism with features distinct from Crohn's and Helicobacter pylori gastritis. Am J Gastroenterol. 2004;99(4):598–605.

Stomach: Neoplastic Patterns and Mimics

5

Tetsuo Ushiku, Spiro C. Raftopoulos, Gregory Y. Lauwers, and M. Priyanthi Kumarasinghe

Contents

The most common neoplastic pattern encountered in a gastric biopsy is the "epithelial pattern" as adenocarcinomas are the most common tumours in the stomach. Lymphomas account for 5–10% of gastric malignancies. Mesenchymal tumours account for <1% of gastric tumours. However,

T. Ushiku (✉)
Department of Pathology, The University of Tokyo, Tokyo, Japan
e-mail: usikut-tky@umin.ac.jp

S. C. Raftopoulos
Interventional Endoscopist and Gastroenterologist, Department of Gastroenterology, Sir Charles Gairdner Hospital, Nedlands, WA, Australia

University of Western Australia, Perth, WA, Australia

G. Y. Lauwers
Gastrointestinal Pathology Service, Department of Pathology, Moffitt Cancer Center, Tampa, FL, USA

M. P. Kumarasinghe
Department of Anatomical Pathology, PathWest Laboratory Medicine, QEII Medical Centre and University of Western Australia, Perth, WA, Australia
e-mail: priyanthi.kumarasinghe@health.wa.gov.au

M. P. Kumarasinghe, I. Brown (eds.), *Endoscopic Biopsy Interpretation*,
https://doi.org/10.1007/978-3-319-79117-3_5

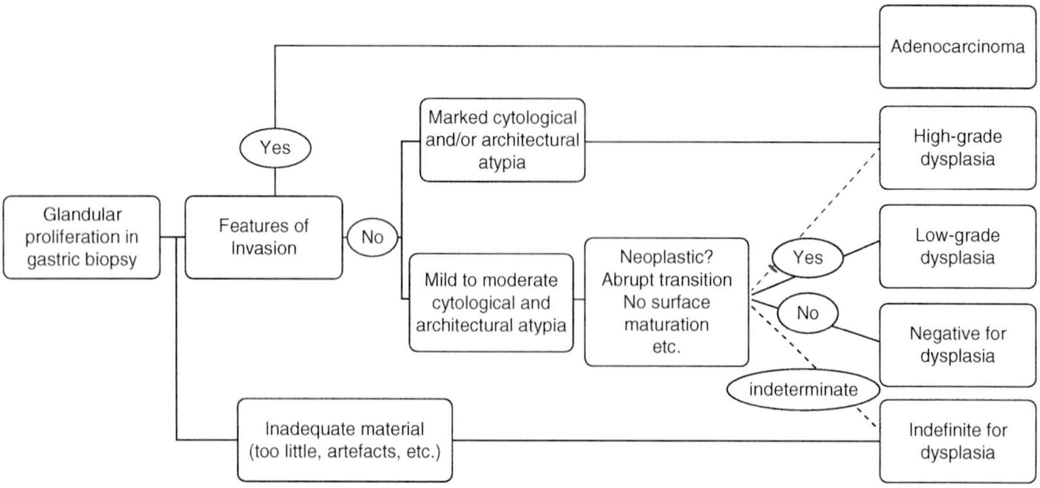

Fig. 5.1 Algorithm for interpretation of the neoplastic pattern

60–70% of gastrointestinal stromal tumours arise in the stomach. Neuroendocrine neoplasm (NENs) account for approximately 1% of gastric tumours.

The patterns related to common neoplasms are further discussed here and uncommon patterns are listed in Chap. 2.

Considering the prevalence of gastric neoplasms, the most common low-power, dominant "neoplastic pattern" on a gastric biopsy is characterised by architectural abnormalities and cytonuclear atypia ("epithelial pattern"). A standard diagnostic algorithm of biopsy interpretation is shown in Fig. 5.1. In parallel additional secondary patterns that may give clues to rare types and variants of primary gastric tumours as well as metastatic tumours should be noted (i.e. diffuse round cells, pink cell, clear cell, spindle cell, biphasic patterns).

If invasion can be definitely identified with the epithelial pattern, a diagnosis of adenocarcinoma will be established. Alternatively, in a biopsy featuring "neoplastic epithelial pattern" with no evidence of invasion, the diagnostic clues that are immediately recognised and then confirmed at higher magnification are abrupt transition, lack of surface maturation and stromal change such as inflammation. When marked cytological or architectural atypia are present, making a diagnosis of high-grade dysplasia/adenoma or even adenocarcinoma is possible. However, at times, marked epithelial atypia may be seen in non-neoplastic conditions such as a regenerative process or epithelial injury induced by chemotherapy and irradiation.

Epithelial Pattern with No Stromal Invasion

When an endoscopic biopsy of the stomach presents the glandular proliferative pattern, the approach is similar to the rest of the GIT to differentiate a non-neoplastic glandular proliferation from neoplasms. Inflammatory and hyperplastic polyps and polypoid mucosal lesions constitute the main non-neoplastic lesions. Most of these are discussed in the preceding sections in this chapter under polypoid and hyperplastic pattern.

Hamartomatous lesions introduced in Chap. 2 may involve the stomach. Polyps of Peutz-Jeghers syndrome and Cronkhite-Canada syndrome may present in endoscopic biopsies. Confirmative diagnosis may be difficult on a gastric biopsy alone. When a glandular proliferation pattern without atypia is noted in an endoscopic biopsy, endoscopic appearance should always be correlated as some syndromes may show important clues. Pancreatic heterotopia presenting as a proliferation of benign acinar structure may be recognised in biopsies.

Epithelial Pattern with Cellular Atypia: No Stromal Invasion (Intraepithelial Neoplasia)

The dysplastic glandular pattern comprises a glandular proliferation characterised by architectural abnormality of glands coupled with cytological atypia with lack of surface maturation and abrupt transition with the adjacent epithelium. Most lesions retain the glandular pattern. These lesions are called "dysplasia" (or "adenoma" if it is a polyp or nodule) or intraepithelial neoplasia (IEN) and divided into low- and high-grade categories throughout the GIT [1, 2].

Abrupt transition, lack of surface maturation and stromal change such as inflammation and absence of desmoplasia are important diagnostic clues that are immediately recognised on low-power examination and then confirmed at higher magnification.

Abrupt Transition

Abrupt transition in a biopsy fragment is a highly valuable finding for a diagnosis of gastric neoplasia. This feature is considered to represent clonal nature of the epithelium. In general, neoplastic glands are morphologically sharply demarcated from non-neoplastic gastric pits or glands, and constitutive cells are often more atypical and monomorphic compared to adjacent non-neoplastic epithelium (Fig. 5.2). This contrasts with reactive changes, which are less uniform, are not sharply

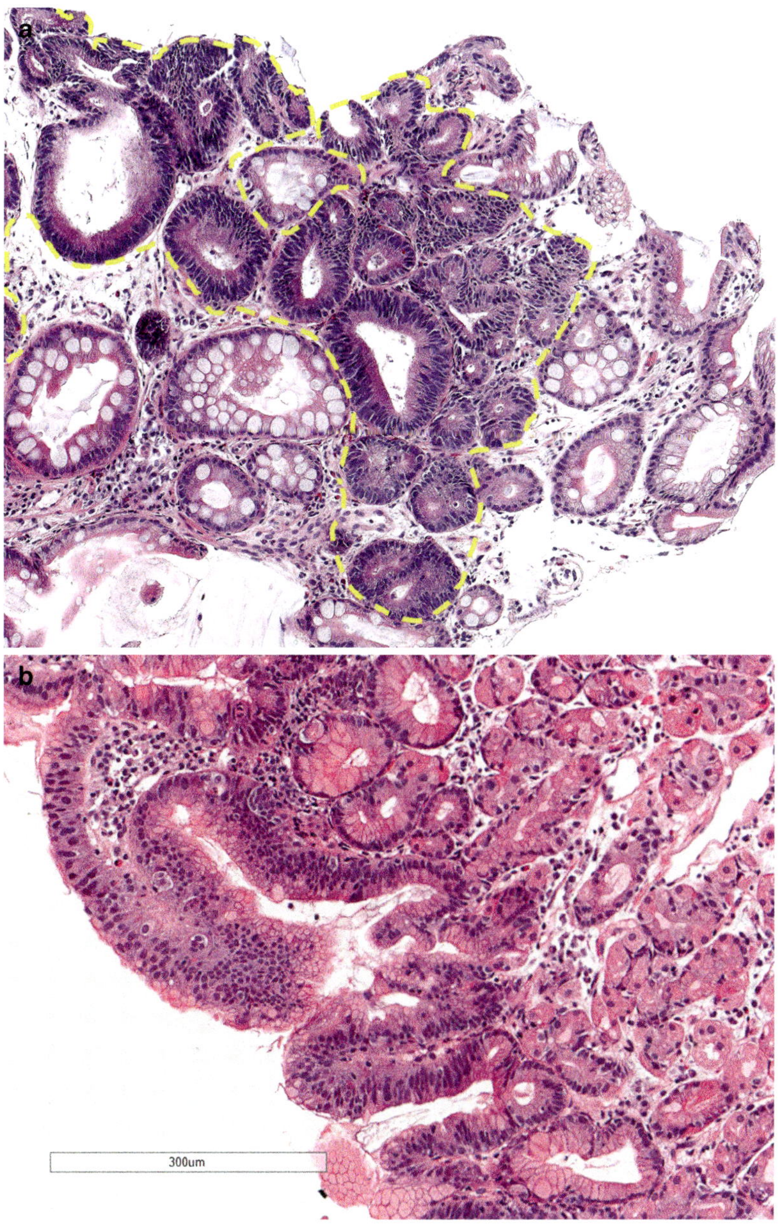

Fig. 5.2 (**a**) Abrupt transition from non-neoplastic metaplastic glands to adenomatous glands. The boundary between the two components is well defined (yellow dotted line). (**b**) Abrupt transition on the surface

demarcated and gradually transit to unremarkable neighbouring mucosa. However, it should be noted that a sharp transition can also be seen between metaplastic and non-metaplastic epithelium.

Surface Maturation

The presence of surface maturation in a biopsy is a feature that would help pathologists exclude a diagnosis of dysplasia, because dysplasia most frequently involves surface epithelium (Fig. 5.3a). In normal or most reactive processes, as the epithelium moves towards the luminal surface, the nuclei become smaller and the cytoplasm becomes larger ("maturation") (Fig. 5.3b). However, lack of surface maturation is not a specific feature to dysplasia, because it can also be caused by inflammation and regeneration (Fig. 5.3c). In addition, several studies reported intestinal metaplasia with basal gland atypia, which showed cytological atypia consistent with dysplasia, without surface involvement ("pit dysplasia") [3]. These observations suggest that early dysplastic change in chronic gastritis may be limited to the basal pit epithelium. Furthermore, some neoplastic polyps are frequently covered with non-neoplastic foveolar epithelium (i.e. oxyntic gland adenoma/polyp) [4].

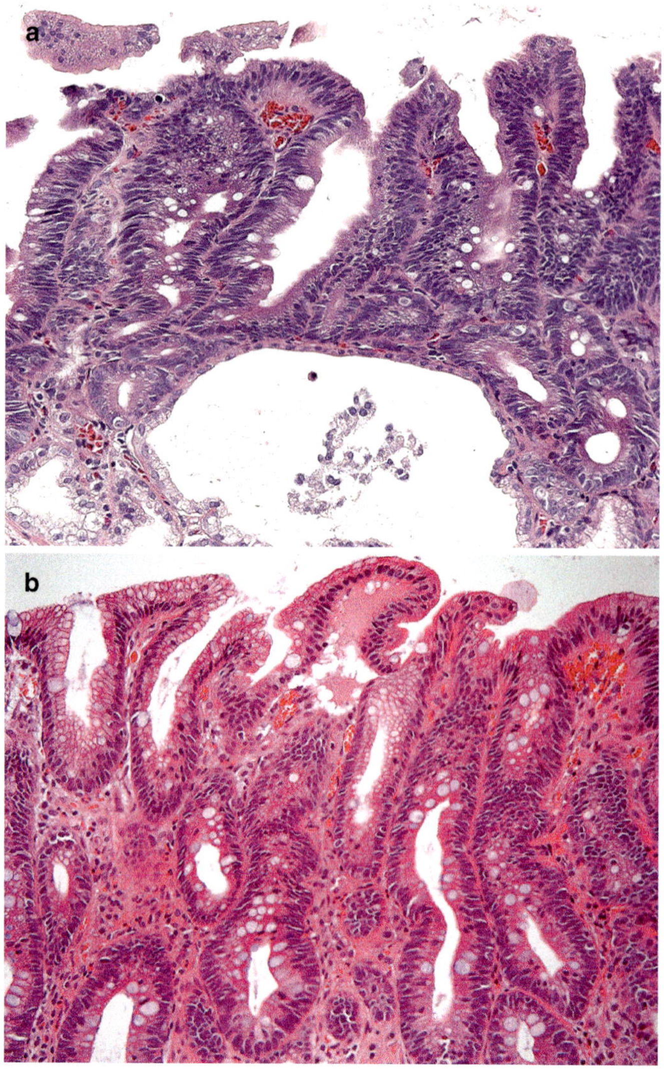

Fig. 5.3 Surface maturation: (**a**) Low-grade dysplasia/adenoma. Neoplastic cells involve the entire gland uniformly without surface maturation. (**b**) Reactive mucosa with intestinal metaplasia featuring surface maturation. Metaplastic glandular epithelium shows nuclear elongation in the bottom part resembling an adenoma but has smaller nuclei with a lower N/C ratio towards the surface. (**c**) Regenerative mucosa without surface maturation. Note that nuclear enlargement and prominent nucleoli can be seen even in the surface epithelium in early phase of regenerative process

Fig. 5.3 (continued)

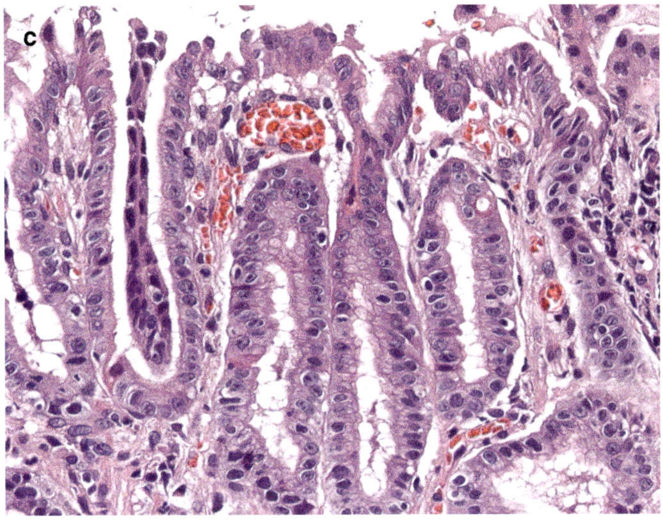

Stromal Changes

Stromal changes, such as increased inflammatory cells, fibrosis, healed granulation tissue or haemorrhage, should also be included into consideration because these may suggest reactive aetiology. However, myxoid transformation can represent early desmoplastic changes

Dysplastic Sub-patterns

On the basis of cellular phenotype, gastric intraepithelial neoplasia can be divided into five categories forming unique patterns (Table 5.1). They are intestinal, foveolar, pyloric, oxyntic (and chief cell) and signet ring patterns. Gastric intraepithelial neoplastic lesions are intestinal-type (type I, adenomatous) dysplasia/adenoma which resemble colonic adenoma (Fig. 5.4a, b; Box 5.1), gastric phenotype including foveolar-type (type II) dysplasia/adenoma (Fig. 5.5a, b; Box 5.2) and pyloric gland adenoma (Figs. 5.6a, b and 5.7) [5, 6]. Intraepithelial neoplasia of pyloric gland type is always polypoid and therefore called pyloric gland "adenoma" (Fig. 5.7), whereas those of intestinal type and foveolar type may be polypoid or flat (or even slightly depressed). Some of these sub-patterns share similarities with those in the setting of Barrett's neoplasia (Chap. 3).

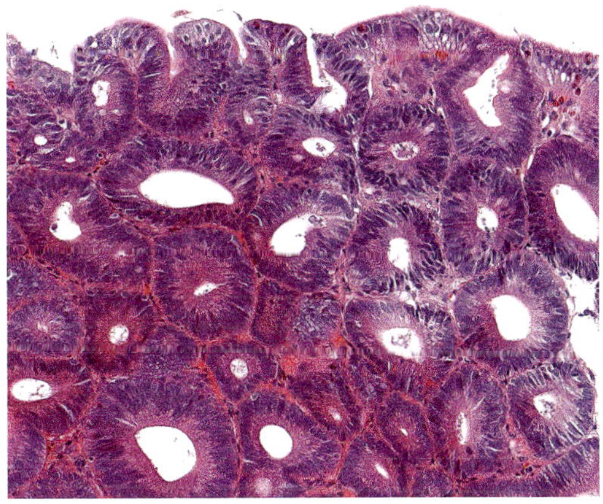

Fig. 5.4 Intestinal-type dysplastic pattern/adenoma (low grade)

Table 5.1 Phenotypic classification of glandular proliferations with no stromal invasion

("Dysplastic pattern")
Intestinal (type I, adenomatous)
Foveolar (type II)
Pyloric gland
Oxyntic (and chief cell)[a]
Signet ring cell carcinoma in situ

[a]It is still under debate whether this is invasive (i.e. adenocarcinoma) or noninvasive (i.e. adenoma)

Box 5.1 Dysplastic Intestinal Pattern (See Fig. 5.4)

- Proliferated of intestinal (colonic)-type glands with typical pencillate hyperchromatic nuclei
- Identical to colonic adenomas
- MUC 2 and CDX2, always positive; MUC5AC, may be weakly and focally positive, accentuated on the surface and superficial glands; MUC6, negative

Box 5.2 Dysplastic Foveolar Pattern (See Fig. 5.5a, b)

- Often villiform and glands featuring a frayed border with apical mucin cap, nuclei are oval or rounded and basal.
- Resembles the foveolar epithelium closely. Resemblance is more in low-grade lesions.
- MUC5AC, always positive; MUC 6 and MUC 2 and CDX2, variable.

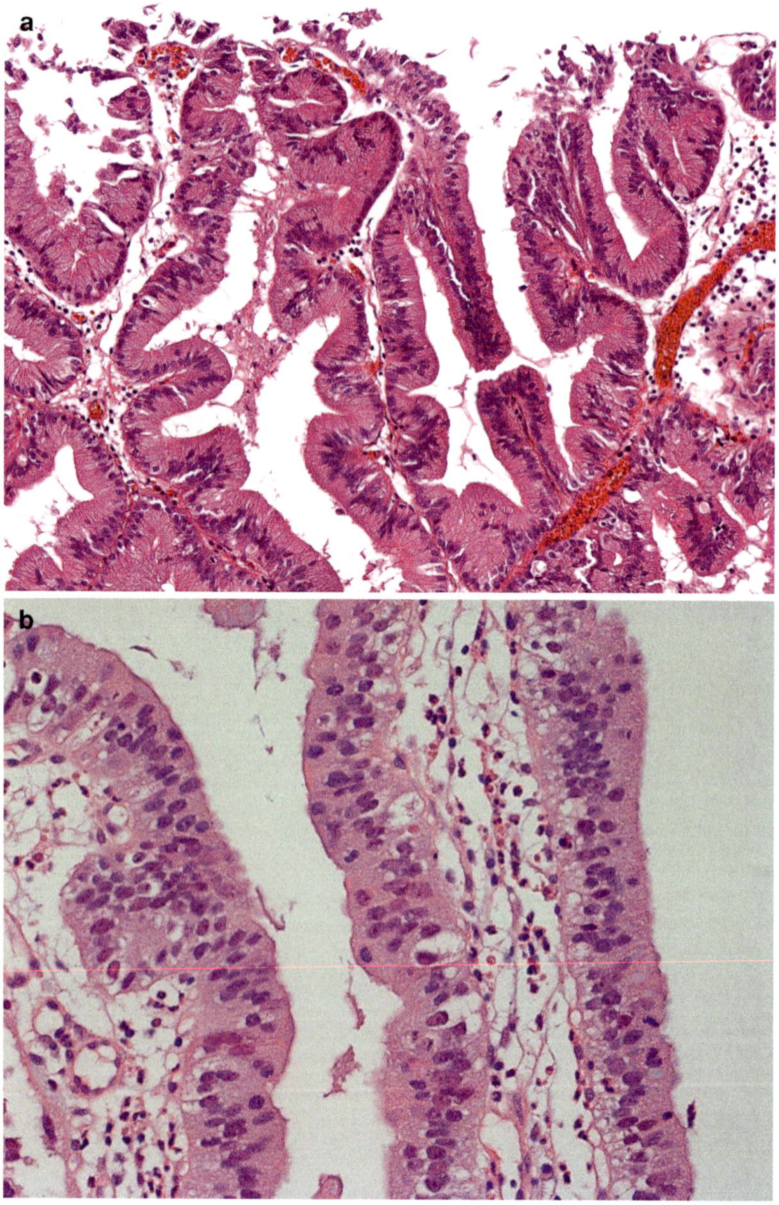

Fig. 5.5 (**a**, **b**) Foveolar-type dysplasia (low grade)

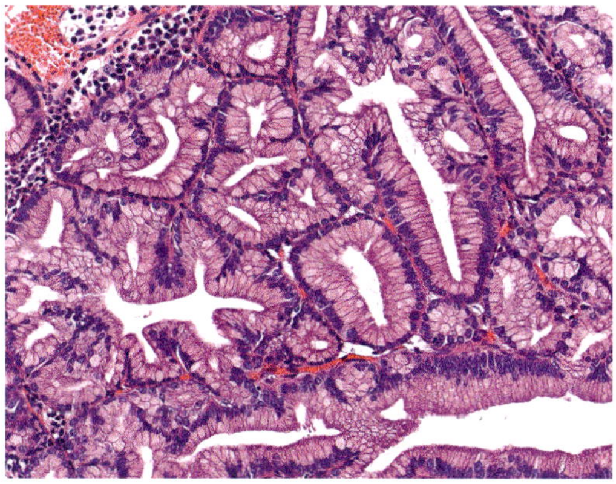

Fig. 5.6 Pyloric gland adenoma (low grade)

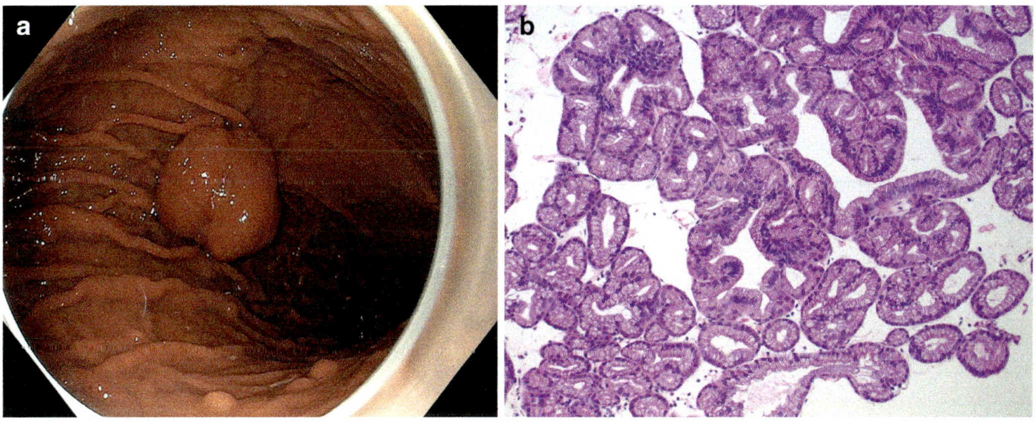

Fig. 5.7 **Case 1:** An 88-year-old lady presenting with constipation, bloating and recurrent iron deficiency anaemia. Abdominal CT was by her primary care practitioner revealing a mid-gastric body mass along the anterior gastric wall. Referral was made for further endoscopic evaluation. A gastroscopy note was made of a benign appearing 40 mm gastric polyp within the mid-gastric body greater curve on a short stalk (Paris Ip) (**a**). The polyp was resected in multiple pieces and retrieved for histopathology. The diagnosis is a pyloric gland adenoma (**b**)

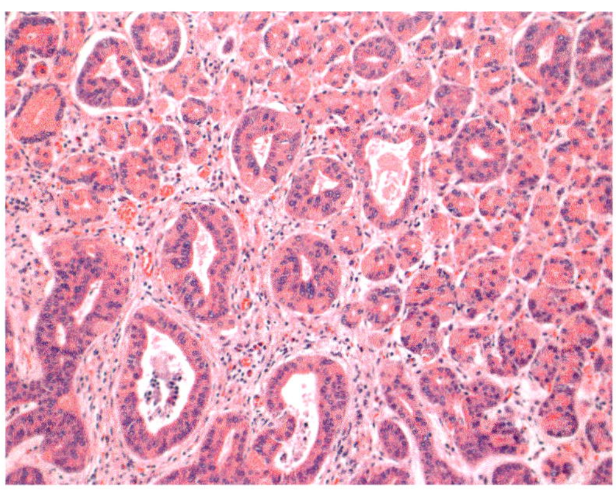

Fig. 5.8 Oxyntic/chief cell predominant pattern/adenoma

Rarer neoplastic lesions of oxyntic mucosa have been recognised recently. Recent studies have recognised novel low-grade neoplastic lesions differentiating to oxyntic glandular epithelium, predominantly of chief cell type (Figs. 5.8 and 5.9; Box 5.3). This entity was first reported as "adenocarcinoma of fundic gland type" on the basis of the significant glandular architectural abnormality and frequent submucosal involvement, but subsequent studies suggested a term "oxyntic gland polyp/ adenoma" and "chief cell predominant adenoma" for this entity because of its benign clinical nature as well as a lack of unequivocal invasion [4, 7, 8]. Another emerging dysplastic lesion associated with expansion of oxyntic compartment has been documented in the newly described genetic syndrome known as GAPPS syndrome (Fig. 5.10a) [9]. Fundic gland-type polyps with hyper-proliferative aberrant pits (HPAPs—Fig. 5.10a) progressing to dysplasia (Fig. 5.10b) and to carcinoma are described. In addition, although very rare, "signet ring cell carcinoma in situ" is considered to be a precursor of signet ring cell carcinoma, and this is usually seen in the setting of hereditary diffuse-type gastric carcinoma.

Box 5.3 Oxyntic (Chief Cell Predominant) Pattern (See Figs. 5.8 and 5.9)

- Closely packed mixture of parietal and chief cells.
- A range of architectural patterns: clustered and or solid glands with or without well-defined lumina, anastomosing cords, dilated glands with or without infoldings, complex glands with multiple layers of cells and cribriform glands.
- MUC6 and MUC5AC, positive; CDX2 and MUC2, negative; pepsinogen-I, positive; H-K-ATPase, variable.
- Rarely extends to submucosa ("invasion")—metastases have not been reported to date.
- Terminology is controversial—reported as adenocarcinoma of fundic gland-type by Japanese authors.

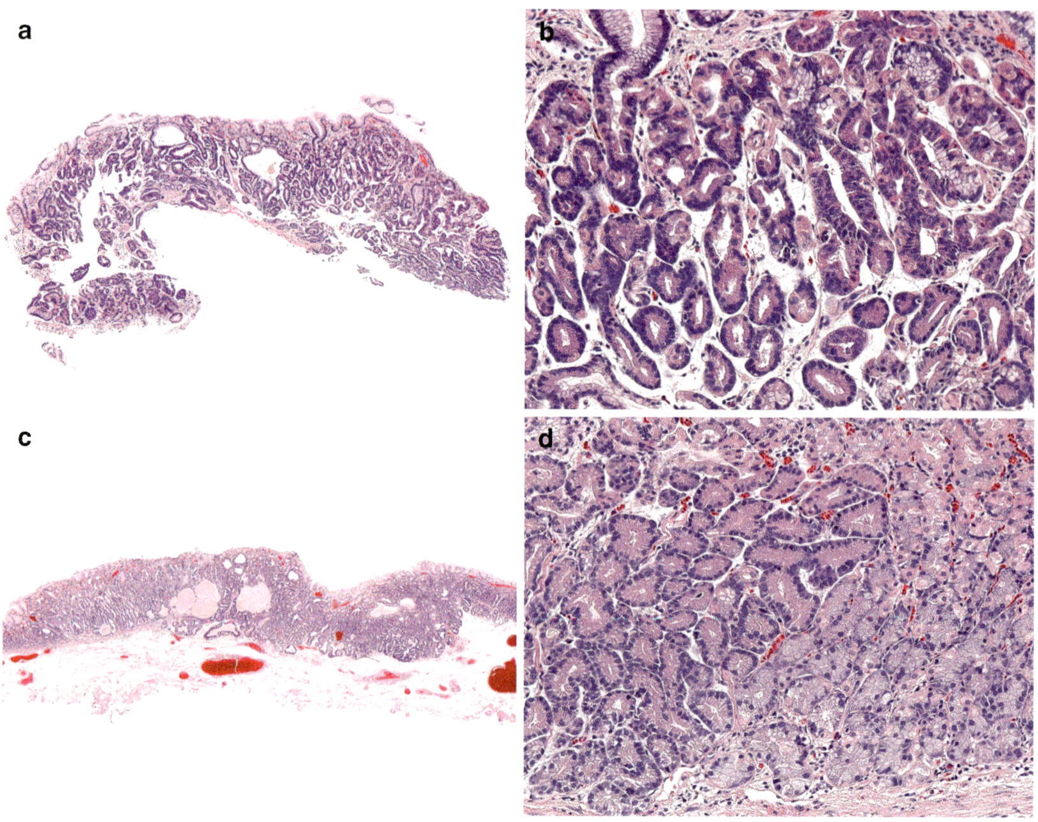

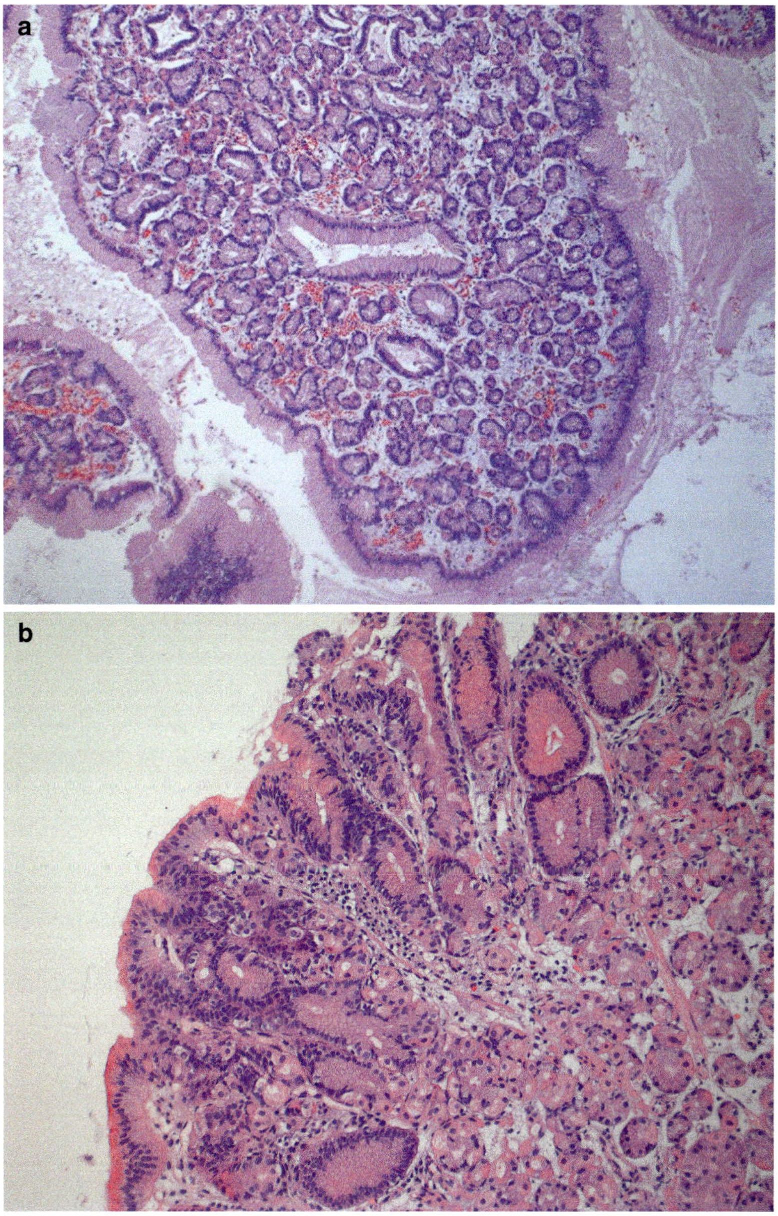

Fig. 5.10 (**a**) Polyps in GAPPS syndrome: "fundic gland-type" polyps with hyper-proliferative aberrant pits (HPAPs). (**b**) Dysplasia on the surface of a GAPPS polyp

Fig. 5.9 **Case 2:** "Oxyntic gland polyp/adenoma" and "chief cell predominant adenoma". (**a**) This biopsy is from a small elevated lesion (about 1 cm) at the gastric body. (**b**) At high-power magnification, the lesion is composed of oxyntic-type glands. Looking at this for the first time, it may be difficult to interpret it as neoplastic. However, there is mild glandular architectural disarray, while cytological atypia is minimal. This is a typical example of adenocarcinoma of fundic gland-type or oxyntic gland polyp/adenoma, which has been recently recognised. (**c**) Endoscopic resection was performed and demonstrated the tumour showed pushing growth into the submucosa, a finding frequently seen in this type of tumour (**d**) Compared to normal oxyntic mucosa (right), neoplastic mucosa (left) shows a higher nuclear density and a mild nuclear enlargement of oxyntic and chief cells

Grading of Dysplasia

Low-grade dysplasia (or low-grade adenoma/IEN) has mild architectural abnormality and cytological atypia, whereas high-grade dysplasia (or high-grade adenoma/IEN) is characterised by marked cytological atypia or architectural complexity. Altered nuclear features are nuclear enlargement, elongation, stratification, loss of polarity, hyperchromasia, prominent nucleoli, increased nuclear-to-cytoplasmic ratio, increased mitoses and atypical mitoses. Architectural abnormalities may include branching, crowding, irregular shapes, villiform or papillary structures. However, if pronounced these changes in addition of budding and cribriforming become diagnostic of intramucosal adenocarcinoma. Of note, phenotypic characteristics of dysplastic sub-patterns get blurred in higher-grade lesions.

The distinction between low grade and high grade in a gastric biopsy is important, because the management will be different. Higher-grade lesions usually need treatment by endoscopic mucosal resection or submucosal endoscopic dissection, while low-grade lesions can be followed by endoscopy and biopsies. Unfortunately, grading is not a perfect marker for the risk of progression to adenocarcinoma due to lack of uniform diagnostic criteria resulting in interobserver disagreement. There is also limited data of natural history of dysplastic lesions. Tumour heterogeneity plays a role too [10, 11].

There are differences between Japan and Western countries in the interpretation of biopsies of intraepithelial neoplasia [12]. Invasion into the lamina propria and architectural complexity (irrespective of invasiveness) are the essential features of intramucosal adenocarcinoma according to Western criteria, but cytonuclear atypia is considered of paramount importance for the diagnosis of adenocarcinoma in Japan. Consequently, intraepithelial neoplasia with high-grade cytonuclear atypia is diagnosed as "adenocarcinoma" in Japan, while similar lesions are diagnosed as "high-grade dysplasia" in most Western countries (Fig. 5.11). However, this disagreement may not be of great importance, because both intramucosal adenocarcinoma and high-grade dysplasia are usually treated with conservative approach through endoscopic resection. In addition, among many Japanese pathologists, a diagnosis of "adenoma" is reserved only for a low-grade pyloric gland adenoma or typical example of low-grade intestinal-type adenoma, which is small (usually 1 cm or less).

When marked cytological or architectural atypia is present, making a diagnosis of high-grade dysplasia/adenoma is not difficult. At times, marked epithelial atypia may be seen in non-neoplastic condition such as regenerative process or epithelial injury by chemotherapy and irradiation. As mentioned earlier, characteristic features of phenotypic sub-patterns as well as immunohistochemical features become less dis-

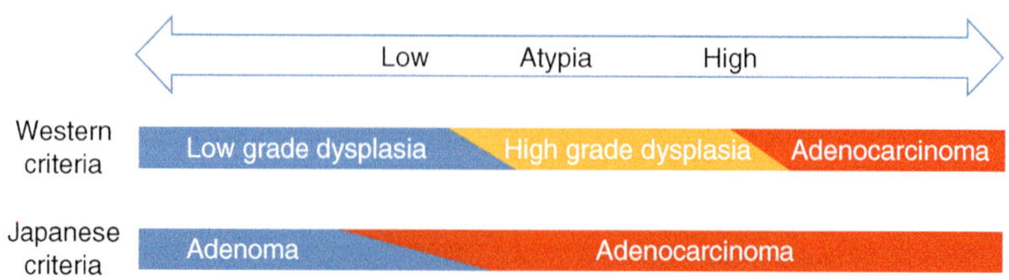

Fig. 5.11 Difference in the diagnostic criteria between the West and Japan

tinctive as the neoplastic processes progress to high-grade and ultimately to invasive carcinoma.

Epithelial Pattern with Mild to Moderate Atypia "Noninvasive Atypical Epithelium"

A major problem in gastric biopsy interpretation includes differentiating neoplastic conditions from reactive or regenerative changes. Abrupt transitions, surface maturation and stromal changes in addition to the degree of architectural and cytological abnormalities are key features to be focused.

On the basis of these core features in combination, distinction between neoplastic and non-neoplastic lesion can be made in most biopsies. A diagnosis of "indefinite for neoplasia/dysplasia" is reserved for biopsies in which a reliable differentiation between neoplastic and non-neoplastic is not possible. Such a diagnosis should not be ignored since some of these changes are either genuine neoplastic lesions or flag bearers of more sinister lesions [13, 14].

Reasons for a diagnosis of "indefinite for neoplasia" are diverse and include technical problems, such as too little amount of atypical epithelium for concern, marked cautery or crushed artefacts, poor orientation, tangential cutting, denuded surface epithelium, etc. In such cases, cutting deeper level sections or obtaining additional biopsies may solve the diagnostic dilemma.

A useful rule in such a situation is to describe the reason for the diagnosis of "indefinite for neoplasia" and the degree of concern. This approach is valuable for clinical management.

Correlation with the endoscopic appearance and review of previous biopsies (if any) and a dialogue with the clinician can reveal important information such as medication history may resolve the uncertainty to a great extent (Fig. 4.31). Other clinical information such as past medication history may facilitate further follow-up and investigations.

Epithelial Pattern (Glandular Proliferations) with Stromal Invasion ("Invasive Pattern")

This pattern signifies invasive carcinoma acknowledging the criteria used by Japanese pathologists described above. This category includes adenocarcinoma, excluding intraepithelial adenocarcinoma in Japanese criteria and in situ signet ring cell carcinoma.

In addition to cytoarchitectural disturbances described above, features of stromal invasion are present represented by single-cell/small cluster infiltration, angulated/abortive glands, sheetlike growth, never-ending/anastomosing gland pattern, highly complex cribriform arrangement of glands and stromal desmoplasia. Again, there are similarities to adenocarcinomas in Barrett's setting (Chap. 3) (Box 5.4).

Box 5.4 Invasive Patterns in Gastric Adenocarcinoma

Recognition of the wide morphologic spectrum (sub-patterns) within the established histological types is important not to miss early GAC in a biopsy.

- Tubular, papillary, mucinous, poorly cohesive, and mixed (five main WHO histologic types)
- Sub-patterns/types
  - "Very well-differentiated adenocarcinoma" pattern (WHO tubular)
  - Micropapillary
  - Mixed neuroendocrine carcinomas (MANEC/MiNEN)
  - AFP-positive adenocarcinoma
  - EBV-positive adenocarcinoma

Although many schemes have been proposed for gastric cancer classification, two major classification schemes internationally used in pathology practice are WHO classification and Laurén classification (Table 5.2) [13, 15]. The WHO classification system recognises five main histological types, namely, tubular adenocarcinoma, papillary adenocarcinoma, mucinous adenocarcinoma, poorly cohesive carcinoma (including signet ring cell carcinoma and other variants) and mixed carcinoma. A molecular classification of GAC with four molecular subtypes has been proposed recently. They are EBV-positive, microsatellite-unstable (MSI), genomically stable tumours and tumours with chromosomal instability (CIN)

However, gastric adenocarcinoma is characterised by a wide morphologic spectrum with respect to cellular differentiation, architecture and growth pattern and shows heterogeneity (Fig. 5.12). Thus, it is important to recognise these sub-patterns within the spectrum of the invasive pattern in an endoscopic biopsy to accurately diagnose early gastric carcinoma.

Table 5.2 Classification of gastric adenocarcinoma

Laurén classification	Intestinal
	Diffuse
	Mixed
	Indeterminate
WHO classification	Tubular
	Papillary
	Mucinous
	Poorly cohesive
	Mixed
	Other rare variants

WHO World Health Organization

Tubular Pattern

Tubular adenocarcinoma is composed of irregularly distended, fused or branching tubules of various sizes, often with intraluminal mucin or debris (Fig. 5.13). Acinar structures or cribriform pattern may also be present. Tumour with solid pattern is considered as a poorly differentiated form of this type. Of note, rare cases of tubular adenocarcinoma have minimal architectural

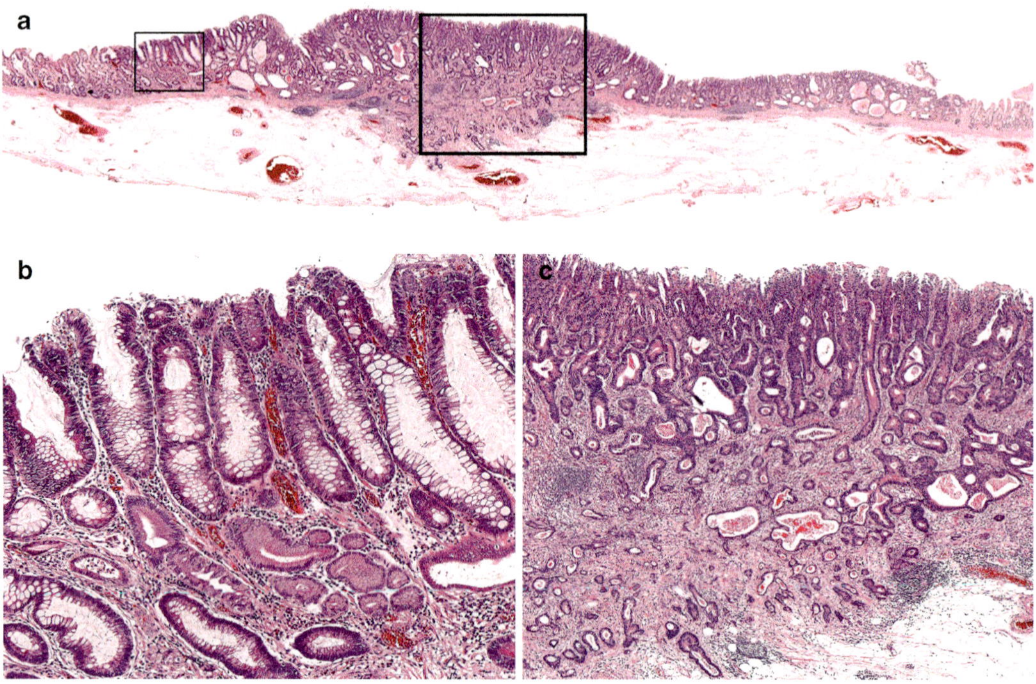

Fig. 5.12 **Case 3:** Heterogeneity of gastric carcinoma. (**a**) Endoscopic resection was performed for an elevated lesion of the stomach. (**b**) Peripheral area of the lesion is composed of low-grade intestinal-type dysplasia (smaller square of A). (**c**) At the centre (larger square of A), submucosal invasive adenocarcinoma is noted. It is important to know that gastric neoplasm often shows heterogeneity within a lesion like this case and to take multiple biopsies if the endoscopic appearance is heterogeneous

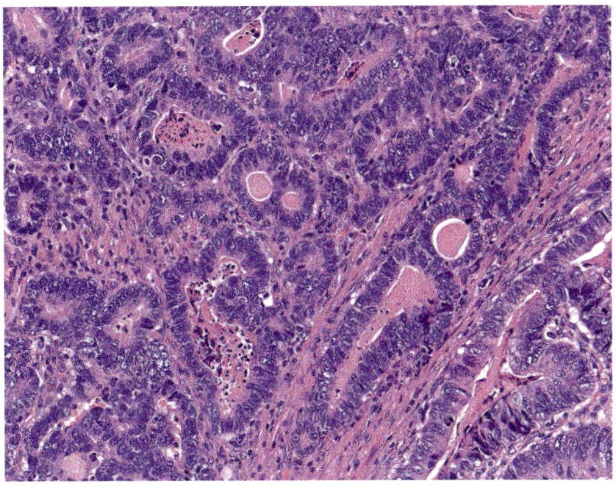

Fig. 5.13 Tubular adenocarcinoma

abnormality as well as subtle cytological atypia, for which a term "very well-differentiated adenocarcinoma" may be used.

Papillary Pattern

Papillary adenocarcinoma is characterised by epithelial fingerlike projections with central fibrovascular cores (Fig. 5.14a). Some tumours show tubulopapillary architectures. Micropapillary pattern can be present in a rare tumour (Fig. 5.14b) [16].

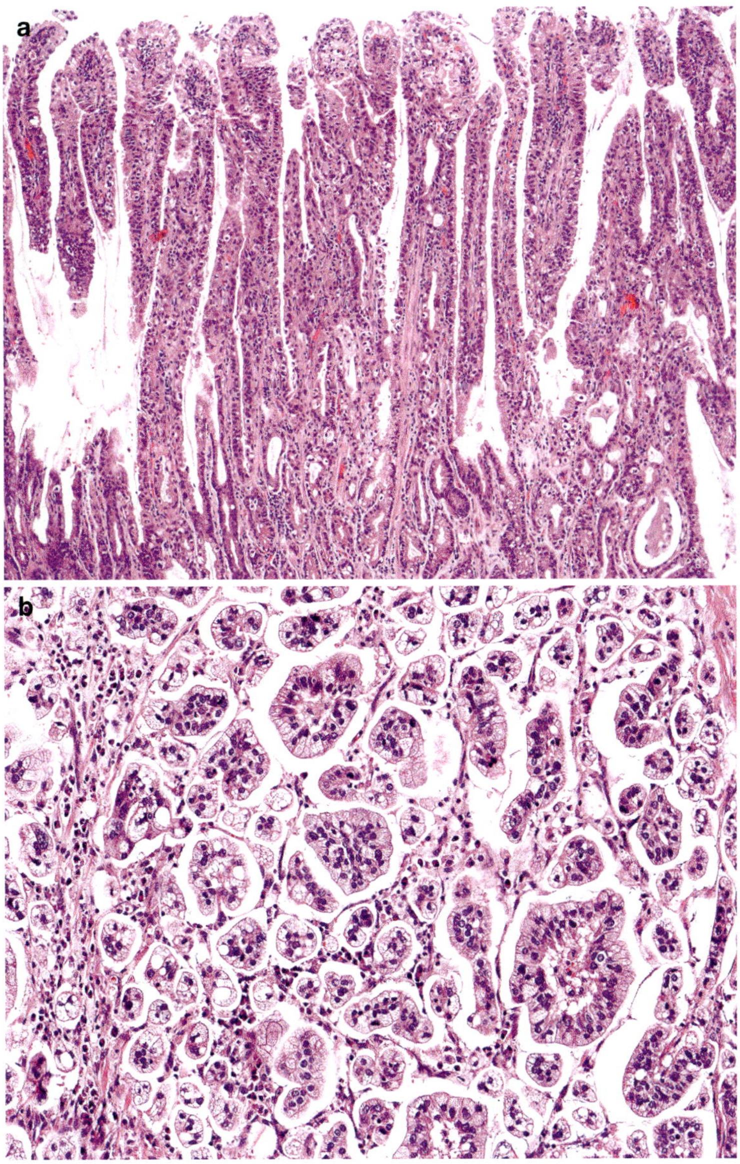

Fig. 5.14 (**a**) Papillary adenocarcinoma. (**b**) Adenocarcinoma showing micropapillary pattern

Mucinous Pattern

Mucinous adenocarcinoma is characterised by extracellular mucinous pools, which constitute at least 50% of tumour volume. The tumour cells form glandular structures, irregular cell clusters or scattered signet ring cells floating in the mucin pools (Fig. 5.15).

Poorly Cohesive Pattern

Poorly cohesive carcinoma includes signet ring cell carcinoma and other variants and is often composed of a mixture of both of them. Signet ring cell is characterised by abundant mucin-filled cytoplasm and eccentrically placed nucleus (Fig. 5.16a). Poorly cohesive non-signet ring carcinoma cells are those that morpho-

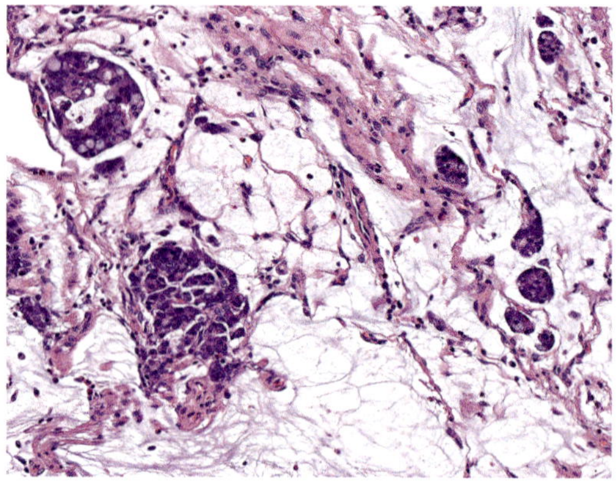

Fig. 5.15 Mucinous adenocarcinoma

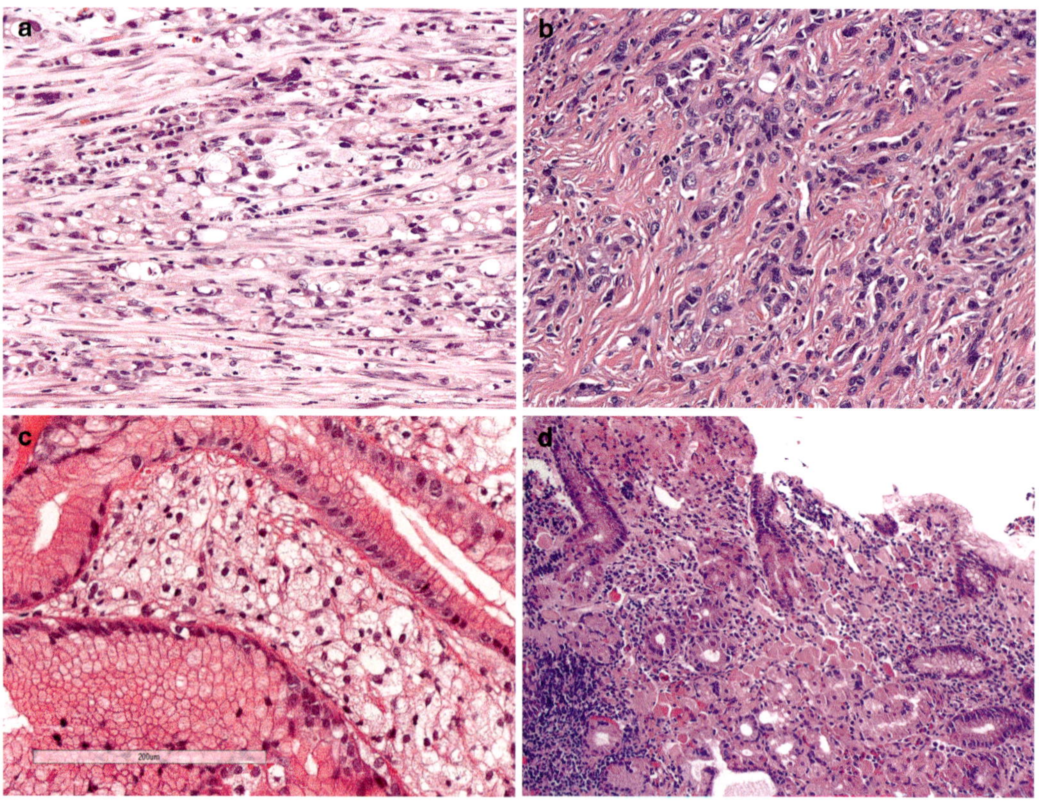

Fig. 5.16 Poorly cohesive carcinoma. (**a**) Signet ring cell carcinoma. (**b**) Non-signet ring cell-type poorly cohesive carcinoma. (**c**) Xanthoma cells—mimic of signet ring cells. (**d**) Russel body gastritis—mimic of signet ring cells. (**e**) Capillary filled with plasma—mimic of signet ring cells

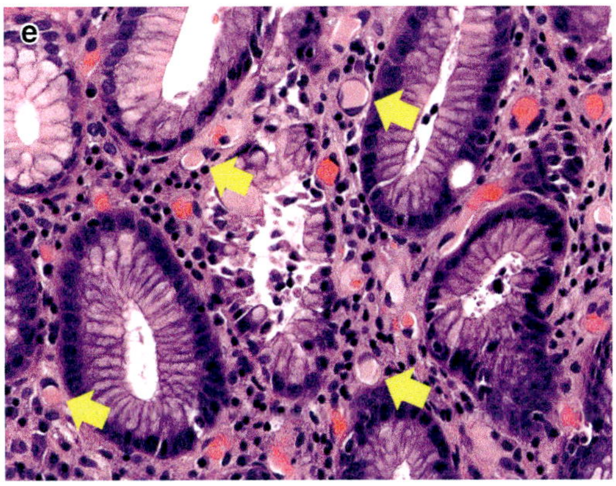

Fig. 5.16 (continued)

logically resemble histiocytes, lymphocytes, plasma cells and even spindle fibroblast-like cells. Those tumour cells can form irregular micro-trabeculae or lacelike abortive glands. This type of tumour is often accompanied by marked stromal desmoplasia in the submucosal or deeper invasive area, whereas intramucosal component consists of dense aggregation of signet ring cells with minimal stromal change (Fig. 5.16b). Histiocytes, xanthoma cells (Fig. 5.16c), plasma cells with abundant brightly eosinophilic cytoplasm of plasma cells in Russell body gastritis (Fig. 5.16d) and small dilated vessels filled with eosinophilic plasma constituents (Fig. 5.16e) may mimic signet ring cells in small biopsies raising concern.

Mixed Pattern

In the Laurén classification, tumours are classified into intestinal and diffuse types. Intestinal type essentially corresponds to tubular and papillary adenocarcinoma in WHO scheme, whereas diffuse type falls into the poorly cohesive carcinoma category. Tumours containing both of intestinal and diffuse components are termed mixed type. Undifferentiated tumours are classified as indeterminate.

"Invasive Epithelial Pattern": Others

Other patterns include EBV-positive adenocarcinoma, AFP-producing carcinoma, rarer sub-patterns of well-differentiated adenocarcinoma and those with the neuroendocrine sub-pattern.

AFP-producing carcinoma is characterised by the AFP expression by neoplastic cells, which is usually demonstrated by positive AFP immunostaining or increased serum AFP level. Histologically, AFP-producing carcinoma has two major histological types: adenocarcinoma with enteroblastic differentiation, a tubular or papillary adenocarcinoma composed of columnar neoplastic cells with glycogen rich clear cytoplasm resembling foetal gut epithelium at early gestation (Fig. 5.17a), and hepatoid adenocarcinoma, which consists of polygonal eosinophilic neoplastic cells similar to hepatocellular carcinoma (Fig. 5.17b). Yolk sac tumour-like carcinoma can be less frequently noted in a component of AFP-producing carcinoma. It may be important to recognise this entity because it is associated with highly aggressive phenotype with frequent liver metastasis and serum AFP levels can be used as a sensitive tumour marker.

EBV-positive adenocarcinoma is a carcinoma with EBV positivity in almost all neoplastic cells. This tumour has distinct clinicopathological and molecular features, which reflect peculiar viral carcinogenesis [17, 18]. The presence of EBV in tumour cells is confirmed by in situ hybridisation targeting an EBV-encoded small RNA (*EBER-ISH*), whereas immunohistochemistry of LMP1 or EBNA2 is always negative in this tumour. EBV-positive adenocarcinoma typically shows a pushing tumour border and is usually composed of moderately to poorly differentiated tubular

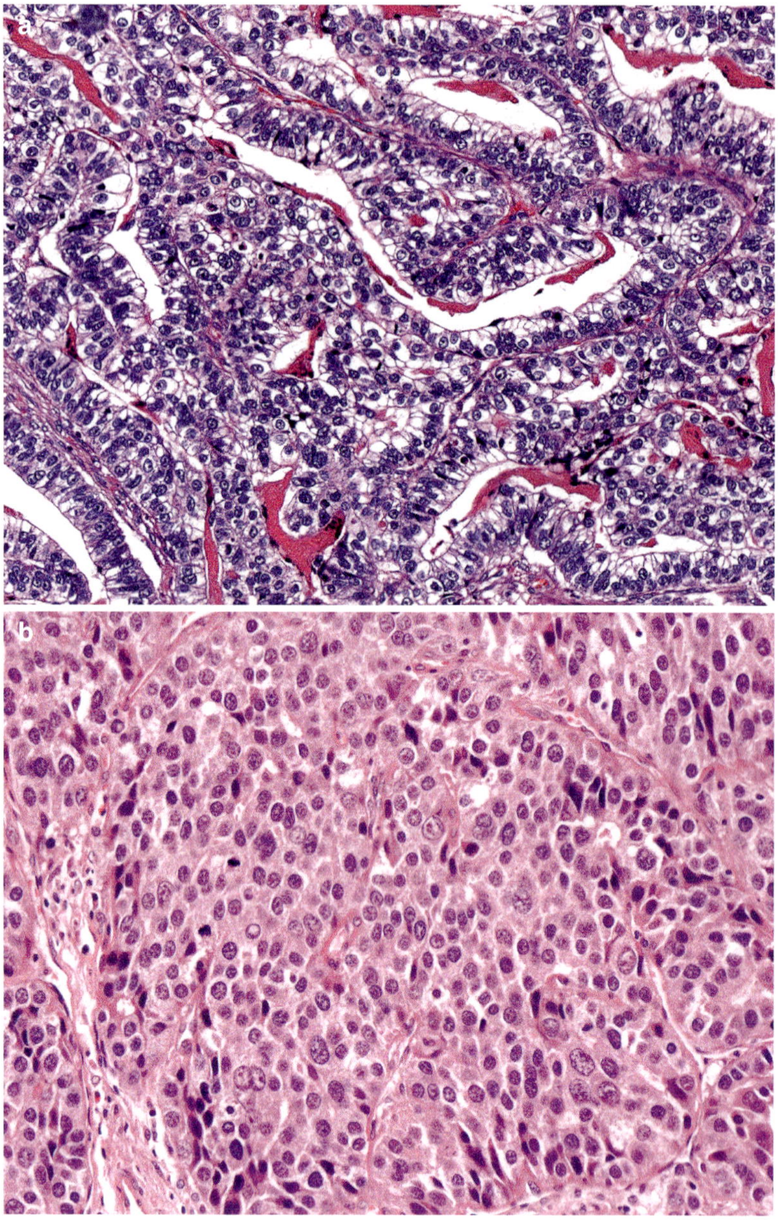

Fig. 5.17 AFP-producing adenocarcinoma. (**a**) Adenocarcinoma with enteroblastic differentiation. (**b**) Hepatoid adenocarcinoma

adenocarcinoma accompanied by lymphoid stroma (Fig. 5.18). Cases with prominent lymphoid infiltrates are called "gastric carcinoma with lymphoid stroma" (also reported as "lymphoepithelioma-like carcinoma"). More than 80% of gastric carcinomas with lymphoid stroma are EBV positive. Clinical features of EBV-positive gastric cancer include male predominance, a proximal location, low rate of nodal metastasis in early cancer and a relatively favourable prognosis.

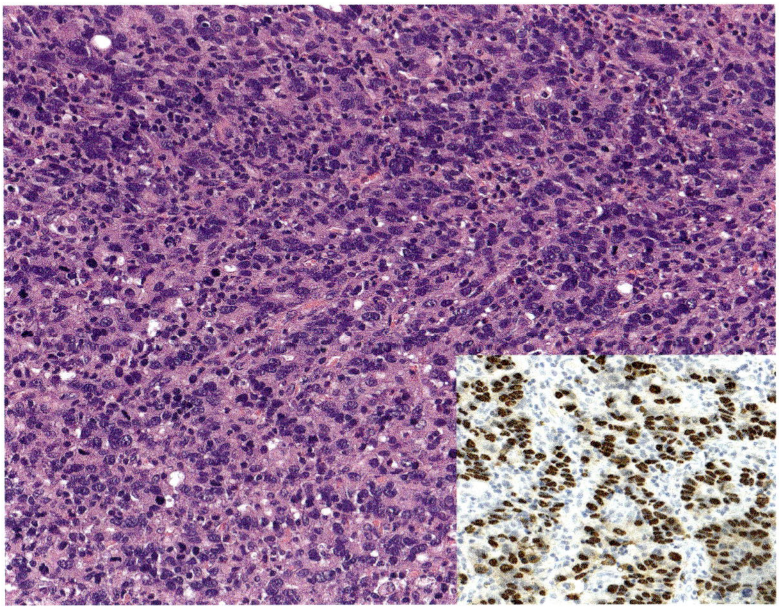

Fig. 5.18 EBV-associated adenocarcinoma. Abundant lymphocytes infiltrate in poorly differentiated adenocarcinoma. EBV infection is demonstrated by EBER-ISH (inset)

Cases with very rare histological types, such as adenosquamous/squamous cell carcinoma, yolk-sac tumour-like carcinoma, choriocarcinoma, carcinosarcoma, malignant undifferentiated/rhabdoid carcinoma, mucoepidermoid carcinoma, parietal cell carcinoma, pancreatic-type acinar/mixed acinar and endocrine carcinoma, and gastroblastoma have been reported.

Rare Differentiated Patterns of GAC

In general, because most gastric carcinomas have significant architectural abnormality and cytological atypia as well as invasive features, a diagnosis of adenocarcinoma is straightforward in adequate biopsies. Exceptionally, rare gastric adenocarcinomas show minimal cytological and/or architectural abnormalities even though they are clearly invasive (Figs. 5.19a, b and 5.20). Biopsy diagnosis for such a lesion is often difficult and can be misinterpreted. In addition, metastatic carcinoma needs to be considered in the differential diagnoses.

Gastric adenocarcinoma with low-grade atypia include a several subtypes, including very well-differentiated adenocarcinoma of intestinal type which resembles intestinal metaplasia and that of gastric type mimicking foveolar epithelium (Fig. 5.19a, b) [19]. These lesions are rare and exhibit minimal cytological atypia, and therefore recognising architectural abnormalities is important for a diagnosis. Characteristic architectural features of gastric adenocarcinoma with low-grade atypia include pit and glandular anastomosis, spiky glands, distended glands, discohesive cells, abortive glands and budding. A subset of this tumour may transform into poorly cohesive carcinoma and behave aggressively (Fig. 5.19c).

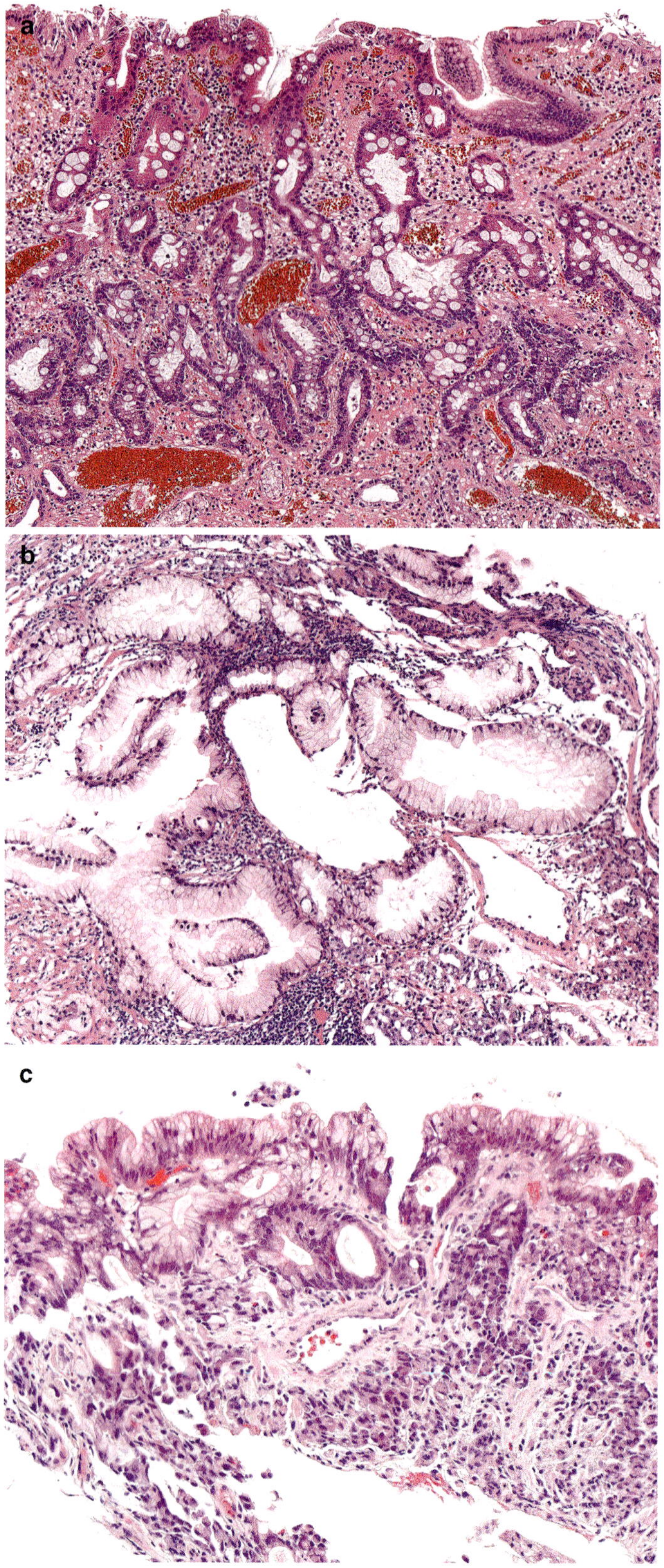

Fig. 5.19 Very well-differentiated adenocarcinoma. (**a**) Very well-differentiated adenocarcinoma of intestinal type closely mimicking intestinal metaplasia. Cellular atypia is minimal, but neoplastic glands show characteristic "hand-in-hand"-type anastomoses. (**b**) Very well-differentiated adenocarcinoma of gastric type resembling hyperplastic foveolar epithelium. (**c**) Very well-differentiated adenocarcinoma of gastric type with transformation into signet ring cell carcinoma

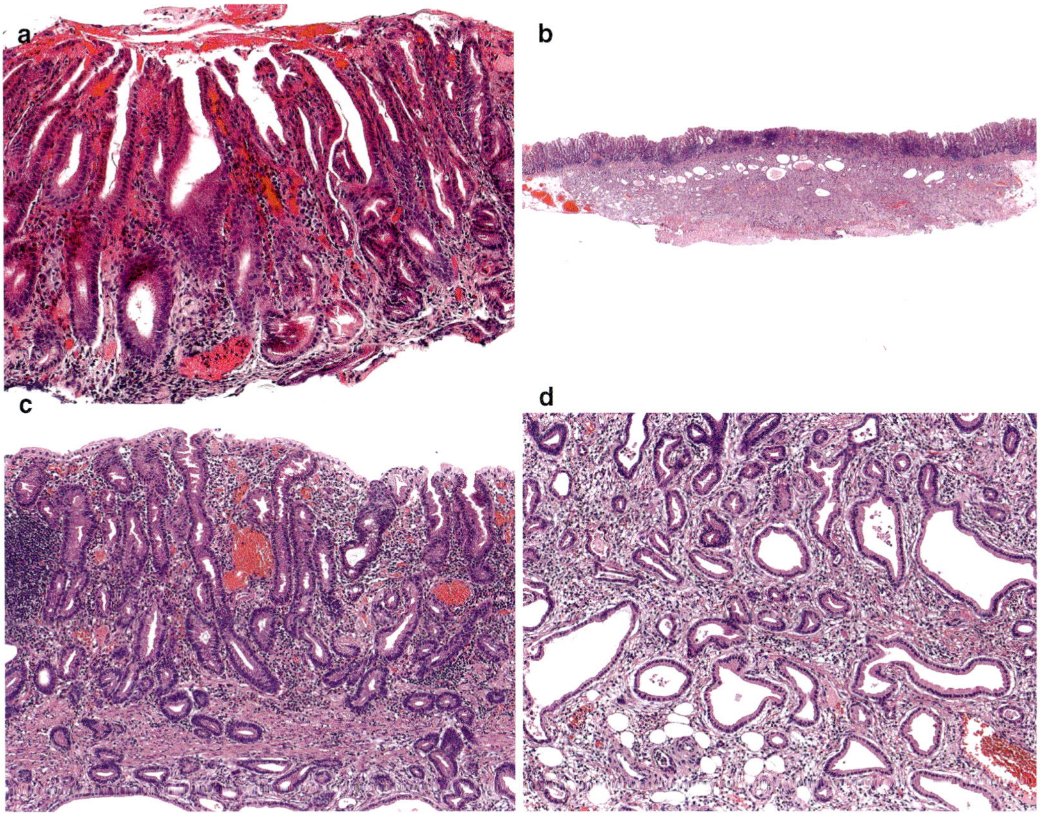

Fig. 5.20 **Case 4:** Very well-differentiated adenocarcinoma. (**a**) This biopsy is from a slightly elevated lesion measuring 2 cm in size. This looks like a reactive gastropathy with mild architectural disarray. It may be very difficult to make a diagnosis of cancer for this biopsy. (**b**) This lesion is actually an advanced cancer invading into the muscularis propria composed of very well-differentiated adenocarcinoma of intestinal type. (**c**) Neoplastic glands show mild distortion and mild nuclear enlargement. (**d**) The deeply invasive area also consists of glandular proliferation with minimal cytological atypia

Neuroendocrine Pattern

The characteristic pattern consists of relatively uniform round cells with variable amounts of eosinophilic cytoplasm and central nuclei with granular, speckled ("salt and pepper") chromatin (Figs. 5.21 and 5.22a, b). Nucleoli are inconspicuous. Well-differentiated neuroendocrine neoplasms (NENs) or neuroendocrine carcinomas (NECs) uncommonly may present with the "epithelial pattern" especially those exhibiting pseudo glandular formations. Additional subpatterns of insular (nested), trabecular and solid patterns are often noted. As neuroendocrine neoplasm often show the epithelial pattern in endoscopic biopsies, they can be mistaken for GAC. The cells may appear blue or pink and also show other cellular patterns in an endoscopic biopsy (see Table 5.4). In general, the neuroendocrine nature is appreciated on H&E sections and confirmed by neuroendocrine markers.

Neuroendocrine carcinoma (NECs), in particular poorly differentiated tumours, may show the epithelial pattern but with more cytological variability, nuclear hyperchromasia, frequent mitoses and prominent nucleoli together with necrosis and may be of small-cell (Fig. 5.22c) or large-cell type (Fig. 5.22d). Cytological features of small-cell type include a small size, a round-to-fusiform shape, scant cytoplasm, finely granular nuclear chromatin, absent or inconspicuous nucleoli and a high mitotic ratio (>20 mitoses per 10 HPF).

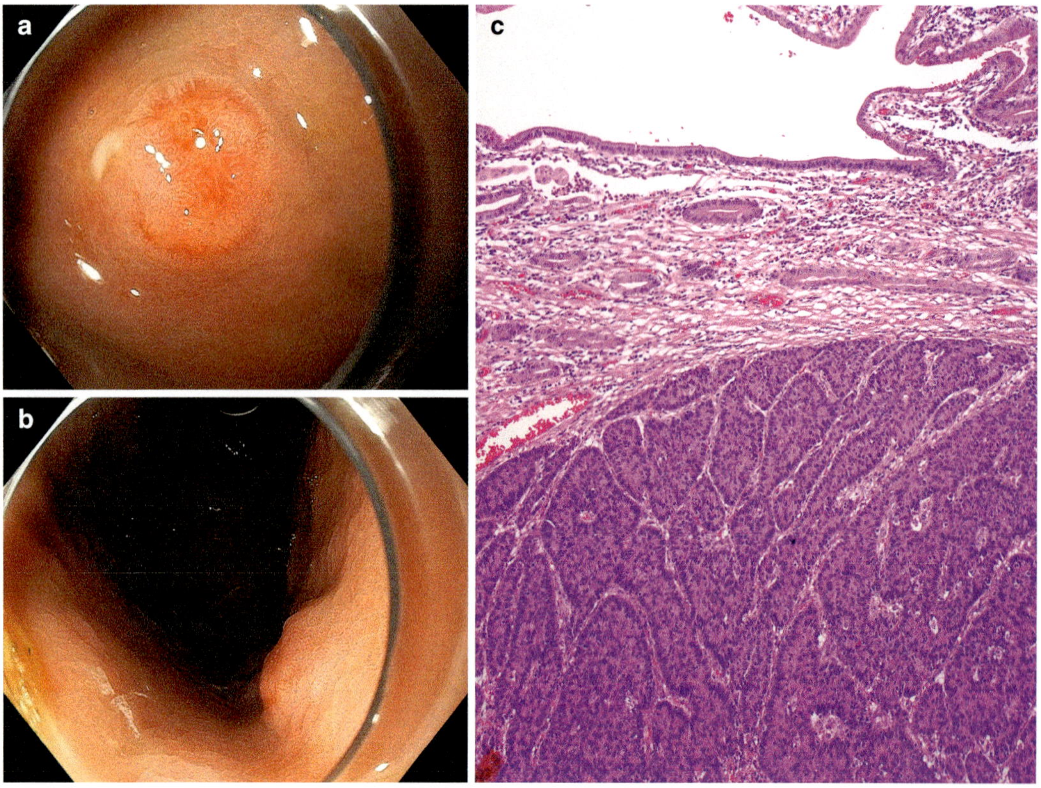

Fig. 5.21 **Case 5:** Well-differentiated (WHO Grade 1) neuroendocrine neoplasm in the setting of AIG (Type 1). A 72-year-old man referred for evaluation of macrocytic anaemia with B12 deficiency. Gastroscopy revealed atrophic appearing corpus gastric mucosa with antral sparing suggesting likely autoimmune atrophic gastritis. In addition to this, there was a 9 mm nodule noted on the mid-gastric body greater curve (**a**, **b** featuring retroflexion view). The nodule was resected and sent for histopathology. Diagnosis was a well-differentiated (Grade 1) neuroendocrine neoplasm (**c**)

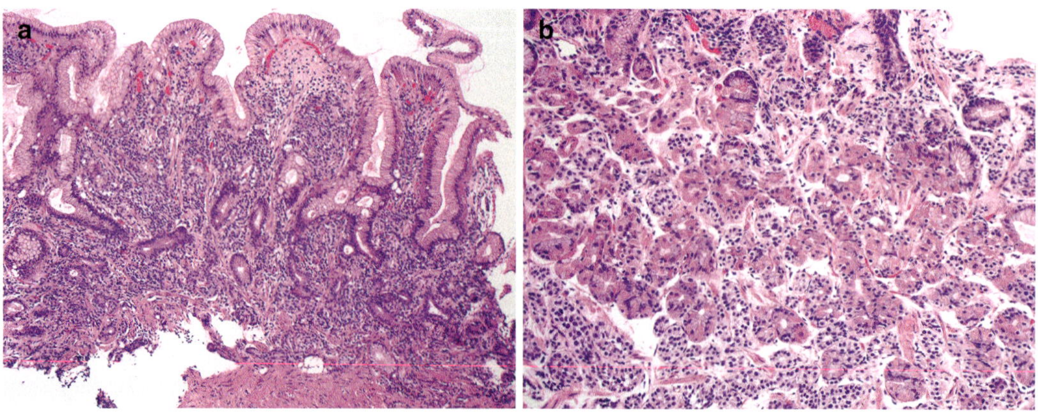

Fig. 5.22 (**a**) Neuroendocrine neoplasm—associated with AIG. (**b**) Neuroendocrine neoplasm—sporadic. (**c**) Neuroendocrine carcinoma—small-cell type. (**d**) Neuroendocrine carcinoma—large-cell type

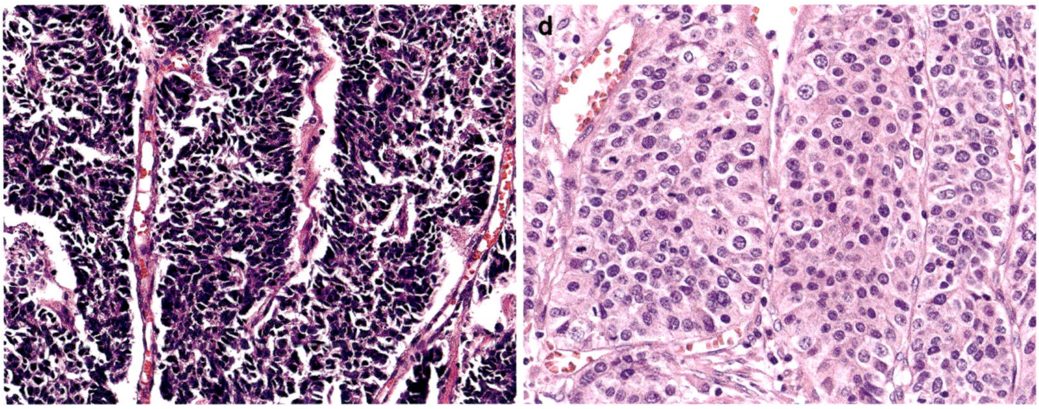

Fig. 5.22 (continued)

Table 5.3 Differential diagnoses and diagnostic markers of tumours with spindle cell pattern

Cell of origin	Diagnosis	Markers
Interstitial cells of Cajal	GIST	c-Kit, DOG1, CD34
Smooth muscle	Leiomyoma, leiomyosarcoma	Smooth muscle actin, caldesmon, Desmin
Neural	Schwannoma, neurofibroma, perineurioma, granular cell tumour, MPNST Gangliocytic paraganglioma, ganglioneuroma/ganglioneuromatosis	S100, EMA (perineural), synaptophysin (ganglion cell)
Fibroblastic/ myofibroblastic	Inflammatory fibroid polyp	CD34, smooth muscle actin, fascin
	Solitary fibrous tumour	CD34, STAT6
	Inflammatory myofibroblastic tumour	ALK, smooth muscle actin
	Fibromatosis (desmoid tumour)	Beta-catenin (nuclear staining)
	Plexiform fibromyxoma	Smooth muscle actin
Vascular	Angiosarcoma	CD31, CD34
	Kaposi sarcoma	HHV8, CD31, CD34
	Glomus tumour	Smooth muscle actin
Adipose	Dedifferentiated liposarcoma	MDM2, CDK4, p16, *MDM2* amplification
Epithelial	Sarcomatoid carcinoma	Cytokeratin
Unknown	Synovial sarcoma	EMA, cytokeratin, *SS18-SSX1/2* fusion
	Clear cell sarcoma	S100, *EWSR1-ATF1/CREB1* fusion
Metastasis	Sarcoma, melanoma, sarcomatoid carcinoma	

GIST gastrointestinal stromal tumours

Large-cell type shows more vesicular nuclei with more prominent nucleoli as well as larger cell size and lower nuclear-cytoplasmic ratios than small-cell type. The cells are usually positive for neuroendocrine markers but may be patchy.

A tumour with both neuroendocrine carcinoma and adenocarcinoma components (with each component exceeding 30%) is referred to as a "mixed adenoneuroendocrine carcinoma", MANEC, now called MiNEN in the new WHO 2017 endocrine tumour classification.

Confirmation of Neuroendocrine Nature

The most useful confirmative immunostains include chromogranin, synaptophysin and CD56 although routine immunohistochemical stains may not be necessary to identify the neuroendocrine pattern but are used for confirmation in particular in NECs and mixed neoplasms. Immunostains for neuropeptide hormones are not routinely performed.

Grading of NENs

Once a diagnosis of a neuroendocrine neoplasm or neuroendocrine carcinoma is confirmed, mitotic count and proliferation index (PI) determined nuclear staining by Ki-67 immunohistochemistry are performed. Manual counting (2000 cells per ENETS), "eyeballed" estimate and digital image analysis are methods used for assessment of proliferation index. Readers are advised to refer to texts that would detail recommendations and discuss controversies of grading criteria of NENs. In spite of heterogeneity reported in NENs and NECs, grading of NENs/NECs should be performed on endoscopic biopsies. This is important for therapeutic decisions in patients with inoperable and/or high-grade NENs and NECs in which the only diagnostic material available may be endoscopic biopsies. NECs by definition are high grade and proliferation index is often irrelevant.

An endoscopic biopsy report of a confirmed neuroendocrine neoplasm/carcinoma should include any relevant associated pathology such as autoimmune gastritis considering the clinical setting in view of their tendency for recurrences yet good prognosis. A common pitfall is crushed neuroendocrine cells in small biopsies that could be easily missed especially those found in random endoscopic biopsies. A comment on the margin status may be required for those tumours that present as small polyps and subject to polypectomy.

Gastric NENs are of three types with important prognostic and clinical differences. Type I tumours arise in the setting of autoimmune gastritis (70–80%). Type II tumours are associated with MEN1-Zollinger-Ellison syndrome and account for 5–10% of NENs. Type III tumours are sporadic, are nearly always solitary and are generally aggressive (Fig. 5.22b). Type 1 tumours (Fig. 5.22a) show indolent behaviour, whereas the biology of type II tumours is intermediate.

In the stomach if the tumour is confined to the mucosa measuring more than 500 μm (0.5 mm) or invades the submucosa, the lesion is considered NEN. The WHO defined these nodules that are < 0.5mm (500μm) as micro carcinoids. The lesions measuring 150–500 μm are termed neuroendocrine dysplasia. Those <150 μm are classified as hyperplasia. However, the size may be an arbitrary criterion and inadequate to determine the clinical significance.

Long-standing hypergastrinaemia is consistently associated with endocrine cell (enterochromaffin-like cells) hyperplasia. Corpus predominant chronic AIG is the most common cause. Less commonly AIG may supervene over chronic *Helicobacter pylori* gastritis. In a minority of cases, corpus predominant *Helicobacter pylori* gastritis may be responsible. Less commonly unrelated causes may be responsible for ECL oncogenesis (i.e. MEN syndrome) [20–27].

Non-epithelial Pattern

This category includes many neoplastic entities common to the entire GI tract, and a general introduction is given in Chap. 2. On the basis of morphologic pattern, non-epithelial patterns in a gastric mucosa biopsy are with diffuse round cell (or epithelioid-like) pattern (Table 5.4), spindle cell pattern (Table 5.3) and an admixture, biphasic pattern (Table 5.5). Epithelial tumours when differentiated may assume a diffuse architectural pattern with sparse or no glandular differentiation. When rounded epithelioid growth patterns are noted, non-glandular epithelial neoplasms, in particular squamous cell and neuroendocrine neoplasm, as well as lymphoma, melanoma and epithelioid mesenchymal tumours should be considered. Dominant cytoplasmic tinctorial quality (blue cell, pink cell or clear cell) on the H&E stain can give a clue to the diagnosis. Tumours that develop specifically in the stomach include plexiform fibromyxoma and gastroblastoma, a diagnosis unlikely to be made in a gastric biopsy.

Table 5.4 Differential diagnoses and diagnostic markers of tumours with diffuse round cell (or epithelioid-like) pattern

	Diagnosis	Markers
Blue cells	Lymphoma	LCA (CD45)
(Small round cell tumours)	Plasma cell tumours	CD138, light chain
	Leukaemia	MPO, CD34
	Less differentiated gastric adenocarcinoma	AE1/AE3
	Neuroendocrine neoplasm	Chromogranin A, synaptophysin, CD56
	Mastocytosis	CD117, CD25
	Sarcoma, e.g. Ewing's/PNET	CD99 (membranous), *EWSR1-FLI-1/ERG* fusion
	Melanoma	S100, HMB45, MelanA/MART-1
	Metastasis, e.g. breast lobular carcinoma	ER, PgR, GCDFP-15
Pink cells	GIST	CD117, DOG1, CD34
	Histiocytic tumours	CD68
	Glomus tumour	SMA
	Granular cell tumour	S-100, SOX10
	Langerhans cell histiocytosis	CD1a
	Epithelioid smooth muscle tumour	SMA, desmin, H-caldesmon
	Melanoma	S100, HMB45, MelanA/MART-1
	Metastasis, e.g. hepatocellular carcinoma	Glypican-3, Hep Par-1, AFP, arginase
Clear cells	GIST	CD117, DOG1, CD34
	Histiocytic lesions (xanthoma)	CD68
	Lymphoma	LCA
	Carcinoma	AE1/AE3
	Neuroendocrine neoplasm, clear cell type	Chromogranin A, synaptophysin, CD56
	Mastocytosis	CD117, CD25
	Langerhans cell histiocytosis	S-100, CD1a
	Clear cell sarcoma	S100, HMB45, MelanA/MART-1, *EWSR1-CREB1* fusion
	PEComa	HMB45, MelanA/MART-1
	Epithelioid smooth muscle tumour	SMA, desmin, H-caldesmon
	Metastasis, e.g. clear cell renal cell carcinoma	CD10, vimentin, RCC, PAX8

GIST gastrointestinal stromal tumours

Table 5.5 Differential diagnoses and diagnostic markers of tumour with biphasic pattern—glandular and stromal proliferation

Diagnosis	Markers
Carcinosarcoma	AE1/AE3, EMA
Synovial sarcoma	AE1/AE3, EMA, TLE1, *SS18-SSX1/2* fusion
Endometriosis	ER, PgR
Mesothelioma	calretinin, WT-1, D2-40
Teratoma	
Gastroblastoma	GLI1 (IHC) and MALAT1-GLI1

Diffuse Round Cell Pattern

The most common neoplasm that presents with "diffuse round small blue cell pattern" in a gastric biopsy is MALT lymphoma characterised by a monotonous infiltrate of monocytoid B cells that expand and replace the normal structures of the lamina propria (Fig. 5.23a). Infiltration of the gastric glands by neoplastic lymphoid cells in the form of lymphoepithelial lesions is a characteristic feature. Presence of larger blue cells should raise the possibility of transformation to diffuse large

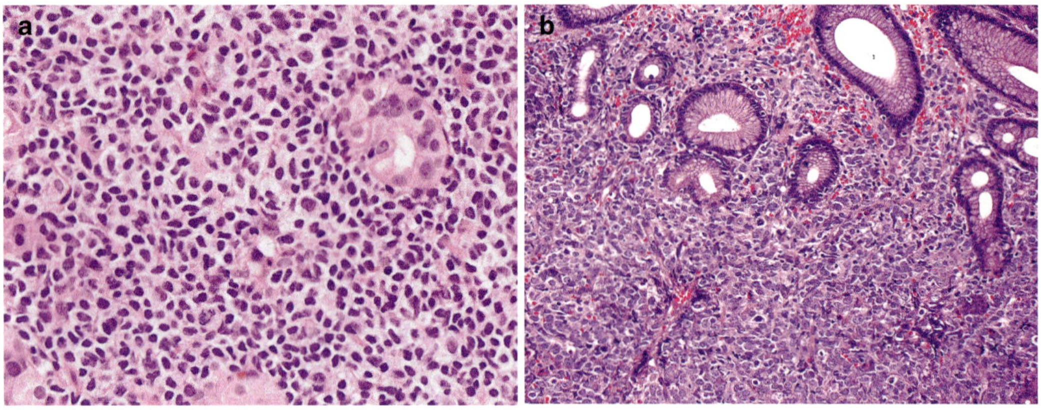

Fig. 5.23 (**a**) MALT lymphoma. (**b**) Diffuse large B-cell lymphoma

B-cell lymphoma. Genuine diffuse large B-cell lymphomas (DLBCL) show large blue cell pattern (Fig. 5.23b) and are more likely to present with macroscopic lesions compared MALT lymphomas that often present in mucosal biopsies. Florid *H. pylori gastritis* with a diffuse lymphoplasmacytic infiltrate can be alarming. In fact, distinction may be very difficult. B-cell clonality studies by advanced polymerase chain reaction technology (using Wotherspoon criteria) may be helpful in the distinction. Other neoplasms that may present as small round blue pattern are listed in Table 5.4.

The stomach is one of the most common sites of gastrointestinal MALT lymphomas. Approximately 50% of MALT lymphomas occur in the GI tract, and about 85% of these occur in the stomach. Around 50% of gastric lymphomas are MALT lymphomas. *Helicobacter pylori* is the major cause of gastric MALT lymphoma and is present in 75–90% of cases. Eradication of *H. pylori* with antibiotics results in complete histological remission in about 70% cases. Histological response can be scored on endoscopic biopsies according to GELA recommendations.

Eradication of *H. pylori* with antibiotics induces complete histological remission in about 70% of gastric MALT lymphoma (GML) cases, and time to achieve remission may last up to 24 months [28–30].

Blue Cell Pattern

Blue cell pattern in a gastric biopsy can mimic a lymphoma. Lymphomatoid gastropathy (or NK-cell enteropathy) is a rare NK-cell proliferation in the gastrointestinal mucosa [31, 32]. This is essentially a benign lesion and usually self-limited disease, but unfortunately overdiagnoses and overtreatment frequently occur because of its close resemblance to malignant lymphoma. Endoscopically, lymphomatoid gastropathy shows slightly elevated haemorrhagic appearance and is always small (around 1 cm) and localised or has multiple lesions. Mucosal biopsy shows expansion of the lamina propria by confluent infiltrates of medium to large-sized atypical lymphoid cells with abundant clear or slightly eosinophilic cytoplasm (Fig. 5.24a, b). Mitoses or apoptosis are not prominent. Characteristically, eosinophilic granules are often observed in the cytoplasm (Fig. 5.24b). In immunohistochemistry, lymphomatoid gastropathy shows NK-cell phenotype, i.e. cytoplasmic CD3+, CD7+, CD56+, and cytotoxic molecules +. T-cell markers (surface CD3, CD4, CD5, TCRαβ), B-cell markers (CD20) and EBV infection (EBER-ISH) are negative. Ki-67 positive ratio is about 10–30%.

Spindle Cell Pattern

Spindle cell pattern in a gastric biopsy is characteristic of gastrointestinal stromal tumour (GIST) although rare epithelial tumour cells may be spindle-shaped, such as poorly differentiated carcinoma and sarcomatoid carcinoma (or sarcomatous component of carcinosarcoma). The vast majority of mesenchymal tumours

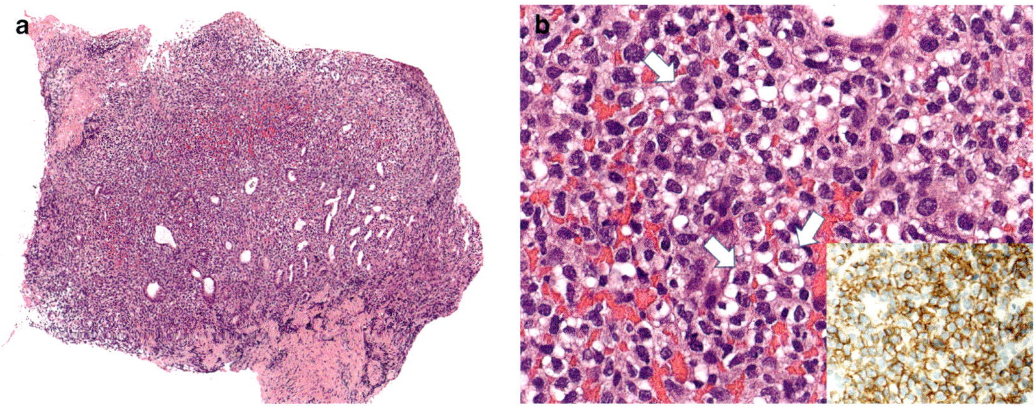

Fig. 5.24 Lymphomatoid gastropathy. (**a**) A biopsy shows diffuse cellular infiltration in the lamina propria with haemorrhage and erosion. (**b**) Medium-sized atypical lymphoid cells with abundant clear or slightly eosinophilic cytoplasm diffusely infiltrate the lamina propria. Some of them have eosinophilic granules in their cytoplasm (arrow). These atypical lymphoid cells are positive for CD56 immunostaining (inset)

within the GI tract are GIST, and in this section the major emphasis is on this neoplasm. GISTs must be distinguished from other spindle cell proliferations in the GI tract (Table 5.3) (Fig. 5.25a, b).

Many have overlapping histologic features, and their accurate diagnosis can be challenging in the setting of limited endoscopic biopsy material. Because most of these lesions develop as a submucosal mass, mucosal biopsy often fails to obtain tissues sufficient for a diagnosis, although several approaches such as boring biopsy (tunnel biopsy) and endoscopic ultrasound/fine-needle aspiration (EUS-FNA) biopsy are currently used. In this setting, a panel of immunohistochemistry (and molecular testing) is often needed to make a definitive diagnosis (Table 5.3). The histomorphology of GIST has a wide spectrum, but most GISTs show spindle cell tumours, and a minority (20–25%) has epithelioid, mixed spindle and epithelioid or rarely pleomorphic histology. Spindle cell GISTs are composed of uniform elongated cells arranged in intersecting fascicles. Perinuclear vacuoles are frequently present in gastric GISTs (Fig. 5.25a). Nuclear palisading, resembling Antoni A areas of a schwannoma, is occasionally encountered. The stroma may show myxoid change (Fig. 5.25c, d), hyalinisation or calcification. Nearly one half of small intestinal GISTs contain oval or elongated eosinophilic aggregates of extracellular collagen fibres, so-called skeinoid fibres. Epithelioid GISTs are characterised by rounded cells arranged in nests or sheets, with variably eosinophilic to clear cytoplasm and vesicular nuclei (Fig. 5.25e). Pleomorphic morphology is unusual in GISTs but can be seen especially in a rare example of dedifferentiated GIST, in which a transition from a conventional KIT-positive spindle cell pattern to an anaplastic or pleomorphic morphology with frequent loss of KIT immunoreactivity is noted [33]. Tumour size and mitotic activity are key parameters in assessing the biologic potential and should be reported when enough tissue samples are biopsied [34]. In immunohistochemistry, the key feature of GIST is positivity for the Kit (CD117; Fig. 5.25f); it is expressed in more than 95% of GISTs. DOG1 antibody is an equally sensitive and specific marker for GISTs (Fig. 5.25g). CD34 is also commonly expressed in about 70% of GISTs but less specific than Kit and DOG1. A minority of GISTs are variably positive for smooth muscle actin (20–30%), S100 (5%) and keratin (CK18) or Desmin (1–2%). Since a subset of malignant melanomas express KIT, melanoma should be excluded by performing a panel of melanocytic markers in a case with significant atypia and mitotic activity. SDH-deficient GISTs, which especially include paediatric GISTs and those associated with Carney triad or Carney-Stratakis syndromes, are identified by immunohistochemical loss of SDHB.

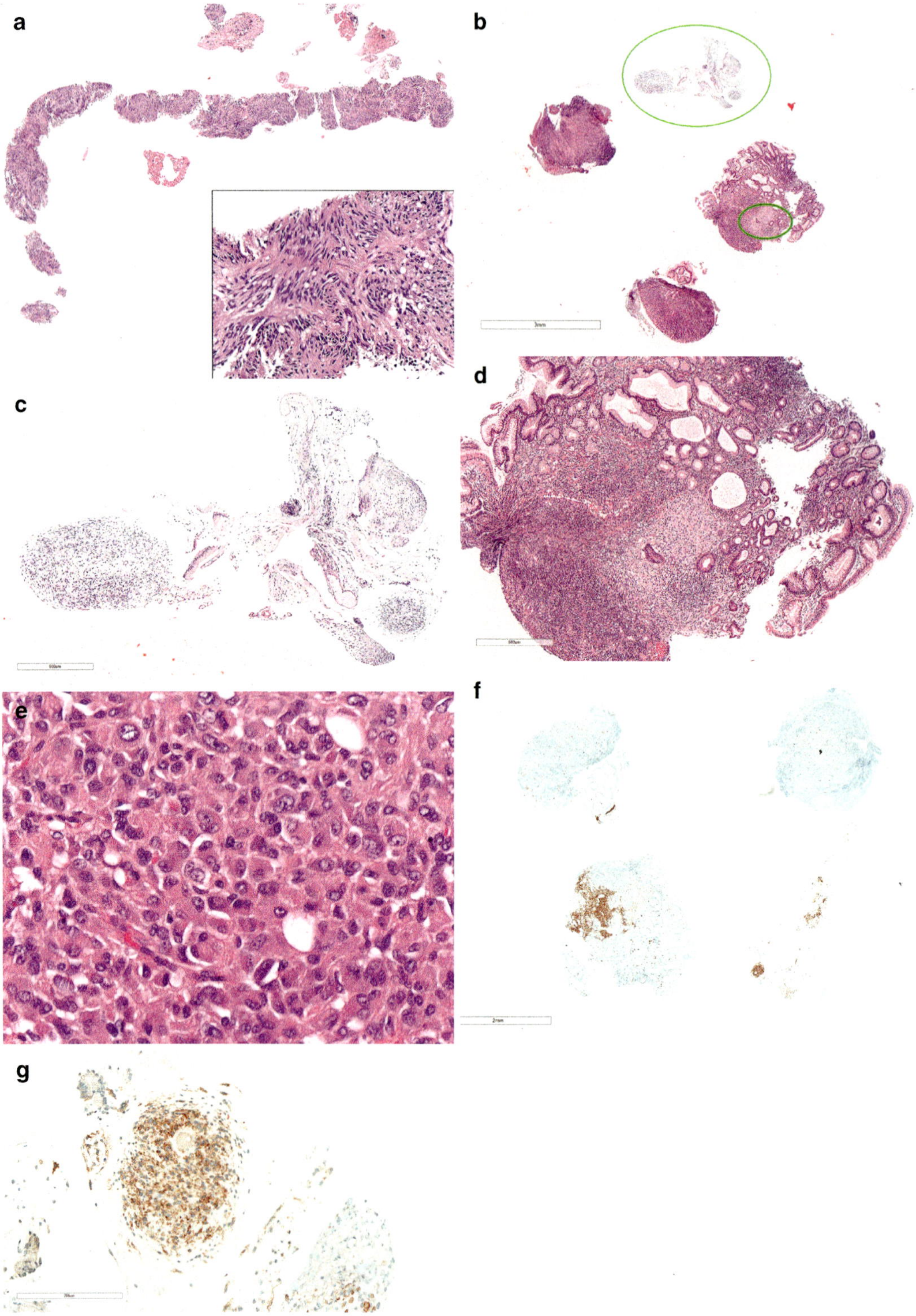

Fig. 5.25 Gastrointestinal stromal tumour (GIST). (**a**) Tissue sample of this gastric submucosal tumour was taken by endoscopic ultrasound-guided fine-needle aspiration. Tumour is a spindle cell GIST composed of uniform spindle cells with perinuclear vacuoles and nuclear palisading. (**b**) Endoscopic biopsy of a GIST. (**c**, **d**). Spidle and myxoid areas (highlighted in **b** in high power) (**e**) Epithelioid GIST composed of epithelioid cells with moderate nuclear pleomorphism. (**f**) CD117 and (**g**) DOG-1 stain with immunohistochemistry in case shown in (**b**)

Table 5.6 Immunohistochemical markers useful for differentiating gastric primary from metastasis

Primary sites	Markers
Lung adenocarcinoma	TTF-1, napsin A
Breast cancer	Oestrogen receptor, progesterone receptor, GCDFP-15, mammaglobin, GATA-3
Squamous cell carcinoma	p40, p63, CK5/6
Malignant melanoma	S100, HMB45, MelanA/MART1

Metastatic Patterns

The characteristic metastatic pattern is submucosal tumour-like appearance, lack of intraepithelial neoplastic component (i.e. precursor lesion of dysplasia/adenoma), distribution predominantly involving deep mucosal or submucosal layer rather than mucosal surface and invasion between non-neoplastic glands, although none of them are specific to metastatic diseases.

A diagnosis of metastatic carcinoma is usually established by confirming the morphologic similarity between the gastric biopsy and the primary tumour. Even if the histology of primary tumour is not available for review, the diagnosis is often possible based on the characteristic morphology and immunophenotype specific to tumours of each primary site. When the presence of extragastric lesion or past medical history of cancer is not recognised clinically, the diagnosis can be challenging. Common primary sites developing gastric metastases include lung cancer, breast cancer, oesophageal cancer and malignant melanoma. Table 5.6 summarises markers of these tumours that are useful for differential diagnosis. Other primary tumours from the kidney, pancreas, testis, cervix, colon, liver, etc. have been reported as well. Notably, stomach metastasis from the breast lobular carcinoma may mimic primary poorly cohesive carcinoma histologically and endoscopically, because it may show morphology of signet ring cell carcinoma and extensive infiltration involving stomach wall similar to scirrhous-type gastric cancer (Fig. 5.26).

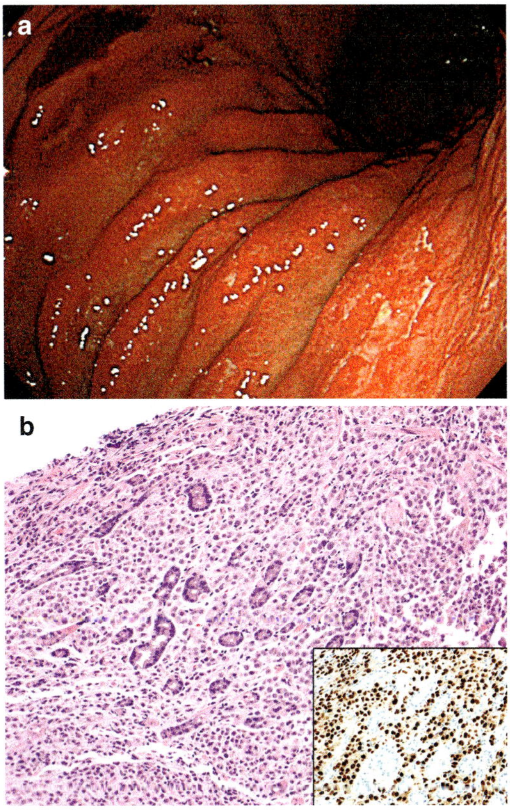

Fig. 5.26 Metastatic lobular carcinoma of the breast. (**a**) This patient has a past medical history of breast cancer 5 years ago. Upper endoscopic examination shows diffuse mucosal erythema and thickened folds, worrisome feature for scirrhous carcinoma. (**b**) Mucosal biopsy shows diffuse infiltration of discohesive neoplastic cells, consistent with primary diffuse-type gastric cancer. Immunohistochemistry of oestrogen receptor was performed to rule out metastatic breast cancer and revealed the neoplastic cells were diffusely positive. This is a typical example of metastatic lobular carcinoma of the breast. It is important to know that metastatic lobular carcinoma often mimics poorly cohesive carcinoma endoscopically and histologically

HER2 (Human Epidermal Growth Factor Receptor 2) and Gastric Carcinomas

Recent advances in targeted therapy have identified HER2 as an important target for anticancer therapy of gastric and gastroesophageal junctional adenocarcinomas. The ToGA study showed clinically and statistically significant benefit in response rates, median progression-free survival and overall survival with the addition of the anti-HER2 biological agent, trastuzumab, to standard chemotherapeutic regimens in advanced and metastatic G/GOJ carcinoma [35, 36]. Amplification of the human epidermal growth factor receptor 2 (HER2) gene resulting in overexpression of the protein products has been identified in 10–20% of G/GOJ carcinomas. The reported frequency of HER2 overexpression ranges from 8.2% to 53.4% in gastric carcinoma. Therefore, HER2 testing in G/GOJ carcinomas should be routinely performed to identify those who will benefit from trastuzumab-based therapy.

When a G/GOJ carcinoma is diagnosed in an endoscopic biopsy, there are a few important factors to consider with regard to routine HER2 testing.

Selection of the Correct Patient for Targeted Therapy

HER2 positivity determines the eligibility for HER2 targeted therapy. HER2 status can be determined by estimation of protein expression by immunohistochemistry (IHC) or assessment of HER2 amplification by in situ hybridisation (ISH). Accurate testing is dependent on several pre-analytical and analytical factors including sample selection, laboratory techniques and accurate interpretation of HER2 test results.

Material Suitable for Testing?

As most patients with G/GOJ carcinoma present with advanced disease, endoscopic biopsy may be the only material available for diagnosis and biomarker testing. Samples that could be tested are endoscopic biopsies, resection specimens and metastatic tumours including cytology samples. Formalin-fixed paraffin-embedded tissue is ideal for HER2 testing by any method. Cold ischaemic time and duration of fixation are important pre-analytical issues that may influence test results. Archival material may be used for testing; however, freshly cut sections should be used for testing.

Testing Methods Employed

Gene amplification is tested by in situ hybridisation (ISH) and protein expression by IHC methods. ISH can be performed by bright-field (chromogen (CISH) or silver (SISH)) and dark-field {fluorescence (FISH)} techniques. Bright-field method is preferred for HER2 testing.

Who Should Be Interpreting and Reporting Results?

Interpretation of both IHC and ISH requires specific expertise on the subject. Centralised testing has shown to give more reliable testing. Ideally gastrointestinal pathologists who have been specially trained to deal with pre-analytical, analytical and post-analytical issues should be dealing with HER2 interpretation and reporting. It is of paramount importance that invasive carcinoma cells are assessed separating them from preinvasive lesions and indeed reactive epithelial and stromal cells. Diagnostic problems of invasive carcinoma, in particular signet ring cell and poorly cohesive carcinomas, and problems of differentiating dysplasia, reactive changes and invasion are discussed above. HER2 assessment is essentially a manual exercise that needs to be coupled with in-depth understanding of diagnostic issues of endoscopic biopsies and knowledge of technical issues. The optimum number of tumour fragments for accurate result is 5 or more due to heterogeneity of HER2 expression in G/GOJ carcinomas.

Standardised reporting with documentation of specimen adequacy, methods employed, interpretation and final test result are mandatory items.

Testing Algorithm

Hoffman et al. validated IHC scoring for HER2 protein expression before the landmark ToGA trial. Scoring criteria and adequacy criteria for biopsies (and resections) were recommended (Fig. 5.27). The main differences from assessing HER2/neu in breast cancer are that gastric cancers

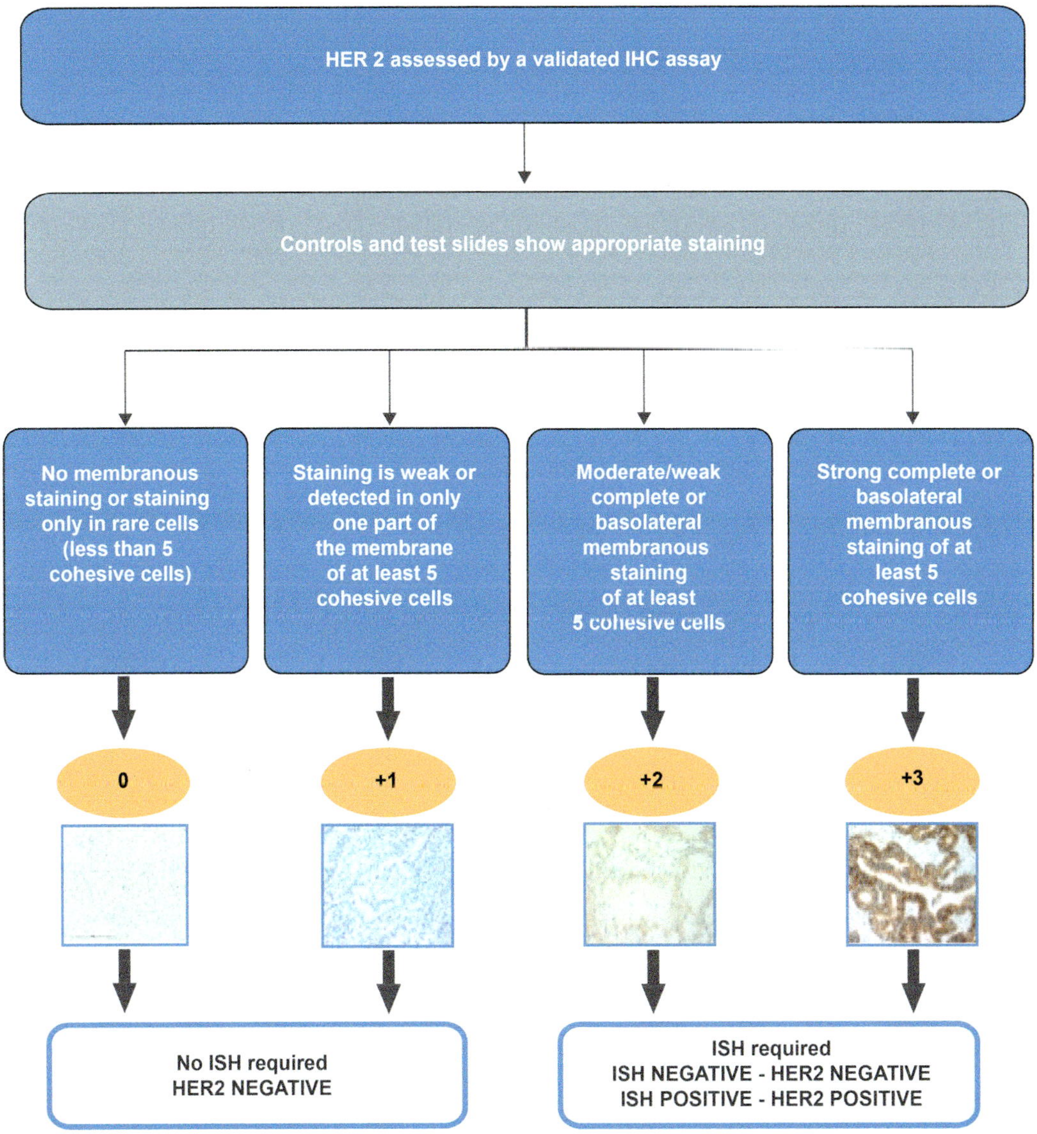

Fig. 5.27 HER2 testing algorithm

often do not show complete membranous staining (i.e. staining is often basolateral) and that only five cells in a biopsy specimen are required to show immunoreactivity to be considered for a positive. Heterogeneity of the overexpression/amplification of HER2 in gastric cancer is more prevalent up to 40% in GC. The recent ASCO/CAP guidelines recommend ISH confirmation for IHC 2+ cases only. The cut-offs for HER2 ISH positivity have been defined as ratio >2 or CN >6 even in the presence of a ratio. Others recommend ISH confirmation for IHC3+ cases to avoid false-positive results [37–44].

References

1. Rugge M, Correa P, Dixon MF, et al. Gastric dysplasia: the Padova international classification. Am J Surg Pathol. 2000;24:167–76.
2. Raftopoulos SC, Kumarasinghe P, de Boer B, Iacobelli J, Kontorinis N, Fermoyle S, Olynyk J, Forrest C, Ee HC, Yusoff IF. Gastric intraepithelial neoplasia in a

Western population. Eur J Gastroenterol Hepatol. 2012;24:48–54.
3. Shin N, Jo HJ, Kim WK, et al. Gastric pit dysplasia in adjacent gastric mucosa in 414 gastric cancers: prevalence and characteristics. Am J Surg Pathol. 2011;35:1021–9.
4. Ueyama H, Yao T, Nakashima Y, et al. Gastric adenocarcinoma of fundic gland type (chief cell predominant type): proposal for a new entity of gastric adenocarcinoma. Am J Surg Pathol. 2010;34:609–19.
5. Park DY, Srivastava A, Kim GH, et al. Adenomatous and foveolar gastric dysplasia: distinct patterns of mucin expression and background intestinal metaplasia. Am J Surg Pathol. 2008;32:524–33.
6. Vieth M, Kushima R, Borchard F, et al. Pyloric gland adenoma: a clinico-pathological analysis of 90 cases. Virchows Arch. 2003;442:317–21.
7. Singhi AD, Lazenby AJ, Montgomery EA. Gastric adenocarcinoma with chief cell differentiation: a proposal for reclassification as oxyntic gland polyp/adenoma. Am J Surg Pathol. 2012;36:1030–5.
8. Chan K, Brown IS, Kyle T, Lauwers GY, Kumarasinghe MP. Chief cell-predominant gastric polyps: a series of 12 cases with literature review. Histopathology. 2016;68(6):825–33.
9. Priyanthi Kumarasinghe W, Bastiaan de Boer M, Hooi E. Neoplasia in gastric adenocarcinoma and proximal polyposis syndrome (GAPPS): gastric rather than intestinal phenotype. Pathology. 2016;48(Suppl 1):S1–S164.
10. Cho SJ, Choi IJ, Kim CG, et al. Risk of high-grade dysplasia or carcinoma in gastric biopsy-proven low-grade dysplasia: an analysis using the Vienna classification. Endoscopy. 2011;43:465–71.
11. Yamada H, Ikegami M, Shimoda T, et al. Long-term follow-up study of gastric adenoma/dysplasia. Endoscopy. 2004;36:390–6.
12. Lauwers GY, Shimizu M, Correa P, et al. Evaluation of gastric biopsies for neoplasia: differences between Japanese and Western pathologists. Am J Surg Pathol. 1999;23:511–8.
13. WHO. WHO classification of tumours of the digestive system. Lyon: IARC; 2010.
14. Shepherd NA, Warren BF, Williams GT, Greenson JK, Lauwers GY, editors. Morson and Dawson's gastrointestinal pathology. 5th ed. New York, NY: John Wiley and Sons; 2013.
15. Lauren P. The two histological main types of gastric carcinoma: diffuse and so-called intestinal-type carcinoma. An attempt at a histo-clinical classification. Acta Pathol Microbiol Scand. 1965;64:31–49.
16. Ushiku T, Matsusaka K, Iwasaki Y, et al. Gastric carcinoma with invasive micropapillary pattern and its association with lymph node metastasis. Histopathology. 2011;59:1081–9.
17. Shinozaki-Ushiku A, Kunita A, Fukayama M. Update on Epstein-Barr virus and gastric cancer (review). Int J Oncol. 2015;46:1421–34.
18. Min BH, Tae CH, Ahn SM, et al. Epstein-Barr virus infection serves as an independent predictor of survival in patients with lymphoepithelioma-like gastric carcinoma. Gastric Cancer. 2016;19:852–9.
19. Ushiku T, Arnason T, Ban S, et al. Very well-differentiated gastric carcinoma of intestinal type: analysis of diagnostic criteria. Mod Pathol. 2013;26:1620–31.
20. Modlin IM, Lye KD, Kidd M. A 5-decade analysis of 13,715 carcinoid tumours. Cancer. 2003;97(4):934–59.
21. Modlin IM, Shapiro MD, Kidd M. An analysis of rare carcinoid tumours: clarifying these clinical conundrums. World J Surg. 2005;29:92–101.
22. Rindi G, Petrone G, Inzani F. The 2010 WHO classification of digestive neuroendocrine neoplasms: four years after its introduction. Endocr Pathol. 2014;25:186–92.
23. Tang LH, Gonen M, Hadvat C, Modlin IM, Klimstra DS. Objective quantification of the Ki67 proliferative index in neuroendocrine tumours of the gastroenteropancreatic system: a comparison of digital image analysis with manual methods. Am J Surg Pathol. 2012;36:1761–70.
24. Yang Z, Tang LT, Klimstra DS. Effect of tumour heterogeneity on the assessment of Ki67 labeling index in well-differentiated neuroendocrine tumours metastatic to the liver: implications for prognostic stratification. Am J Surg Pathol. 2011;35:853–60.
25. Abraham SC, Carney JA, Ooi A, et al. Achlorhydria, parietal cell hyperplasia, and multiple gastric carcinoids. A new disorder. Am J Surg Pathol. 2005;29:969–75.
26. Borch K, Ahren B, Ahlman H, Falkmer S, Granerus G, Grimelius L. Gastric carcinoids: biologic behaviour and prognosis after differentiated treatment in relation to type. Ann Surg. 2005;242:64–73.
27. Ishida M, Sekine S, Fukagawa T, et al. Neuroendocrine carcinoma of the stomach: morphologic and immunohistochemical characteristics and prognosis. Am J Surg Pathol. 2013;37:949–59.
28. Ruskone-Fourmestraux A, Fischbach W, Aleman BMP, et al. EGILs consensus report: gastric extranodal marginal zone B-cell lymphoma of MALT. Gut. 2011;60:747–58.
29. Nakamura S, Sugiyama T, Matsumoto T, et al. Long-term clinical outcome of gastric MALT lymphoma after eradication of Helicobacter pylori: a multicentre cohort follow-up study of 420 patients in Japan. Gut. 2012;61:507–13.
30. Copie-Bergman C, Wotherspoon AC, Capella C, Motta T, Pedrinis E, Piler SA, Berton F, Concon A, Zucca E, Ponzoni M, Ferreri AJM. Gela histological scoring system for post-treatment biopsies of patients with gastric MALT lymphoma is feasible and reliable in routine practice. Br J Haematol. 2012;160:47–52.
31. Mansoor A, Pittaluga S, Beck PL, et al. NK-cell enteropathy: a benign NK-cell lymphoproliferative disease mimicking intestinal lymphoma: clinicopathologic features and follow-up in a unique case series. Blood. 2011;117:1447–52.
32. Takeuchi K, Yokoyama M, Ishizawa S, et al. Lymphomatoid gastropathy: a distinct clinicopathologic

entity of self-limited pseudomalignant NK-cell proliferation. Blood. 2010;116:5631–7.
33. Antonescu CR, Romeo S, Zhang L, et al. Dedifferentiation in gastrointestinal stromal tumour to an anaplastic KIT-negative phenotype: a diagnostic pitfall: morphologic and molecular characterization of 8 cases occurring either de novo or after imatinib therapy. Am J Surg Pathol. 2013;37:385–92.
34. Miettinen M, Lasota J. Gastrointestinal stromal tumours: pathology and prognosis at different sites. Semin Diagn Pathol. 2006;23:70–8.
35. Bang YJ, Van Cutsem E, Feyereislova A, Chung HC, Shen L, Sawaki A, Lordick F, Ohtsu A, Omuro Y, Satoh T, Aprile G, Kulikov E, Hill J, Lehle M, Rüschoff J, Kang YK. Trastuzumab in combination with chemotherapy versus chemotherapy alone for treatment of HER2-positive advanced gastric or gastro-oesophageal junction cancer (ToGA): a phase 3, openlabel, randomised controlled trial. Lancet. 2010;376:687–97.
36. Jørgensen JT. Targeted HER2 treatment in advanced gastric cancer. Oncology. 2010;78:26–33. https://doi.org/10.1159/000288295. PMID: 20185938.
37. Kim KC, Koh YW, Chang HM, Kim TH, Yook JH, Kim BS, Jang SJ, Park YS. Evaluation of HER2 protein expression in gastric carcinomas: comparative analysis of 1,414 cases of whole-tissue sections and 595 cases of tissue microarrays. Ann Surg Oncol. 2011;18:2833–40. https://doi.org/10.1245/s10434-011-1695-2. PMID: 21468783.
38. Wong DD, Kumarasinghe MP, Platten MA, de Boer WB. Concordance of HER2 expression in paired primary and metastatic sites of gastric and gastro-oesophageal junction cancers. Pathology. 2015;47:641–6.
39. Fox SB, Kumarasinghe MP, Armes JE, et al. Gastric HER2 Testing Study (GaTHER): an evaluation of gastric/gastroesophageal junction cancer testing accuracy in Australia. Am J Surg Pathol. 2012;36:577–82.
40. Hofmann M, Stoss O, Shi D, Büttner R, van de Vijver M, Kim W, Ochiai A, Rüschoff J, Henkel T. Assessment of a HER2 scoring system for gastric cancer: results from a validation study. Histopathology. 2008;52:797–805.
41. Wang T, Hsieh ET, Henry P, Hanna W, Streutker CJ, Grin A. Matched biopsy and resection specimens of gastric and gastroesophageal adenocarcinoma show high concordance in HER2 status. Hum Pathol. 2014;45:970–5.
42. Bartley AN, Washington MK, Colasacco C, et al. HER2 testing and clinical decision making in gastroesophageal adenocarcinoma: guideline from the College of American Pathologists, American Society for Clinical Pathology, and the American Society of Clinical Oncology. J Clin Oncol. 2017;35:446–64.
43. Lee S, de Boer WB, Fermoyle S, Platten M, Kumarasinghe MP. Human epidermal growth factor receptor 2 testing in gastric carcinoma: issues related to heterogeneity in biopsies and resections. Histopathology. 2011;59:832–40.
44. Priyanthi Kumarasinghe M, Morey A, Bilous M, Farshid G, Francis G, Lampe G, McCue G, Von Neumann-Cosel V, Fox SB. HER2 testing in advanced gastric and gastro-oesophageal cancer: analysis of an Australia-wide testing program. Pathology. 2017;49:575–81.

Part IV

Small Intestine

Proximal Small Intestine: Inflammatory Patterns

6

Ian Brown

Contents

I. Brown
Envoi Pathology, Kelvin Grove, QLD, Australia
e-mail: ianbrown@envoi.com.au

Acute Inflammation (and/or Erosion)

Peptic Duodenitis

Peptic duodenitis results from increased gastric acid exposure of the proximal duodenum. Typically only the duodenal cap region is affected. Predisposing factors include gastric *Helicobacter* infection, [1–3] excessive gastric acid production from a gastrin-producing tumour (Zollinger-Ellison syndrome) and chronic renal disease. Environmental influences that potentiate the injurious effect of gastric acid include medications, e.g. NSAIDs, cigarettes and alcohol.

Histologically there is variable degree of villous blunting, gastric antral metaplasia and acute inflammation in the lamina propria (Fig. 6.1) [1–3]. Erosion and ulceration may develop. Chronic inflammation increases over time. Secondary features include reactive cytological changes in the inflamed and regenerating epithelium which may be mistaken for dysplasia, *Helicobacter* colonisation of the metaplastic gastric epithelium and Brunner's gland hyperplasia producing nodularity of the mucosa.

The differential diagnoses are:

1. NSAID enteropathy which has a relevant clinical history and usually a conspicuous eosinophil infiltrate with lamina propria hyalinisation.

M. P. Kumarasinghe, I. Brown (eds.), *Endoscopic Biopsy Interpretation*,
https://doi.org/10.1007/978-3-319-79117-3_6

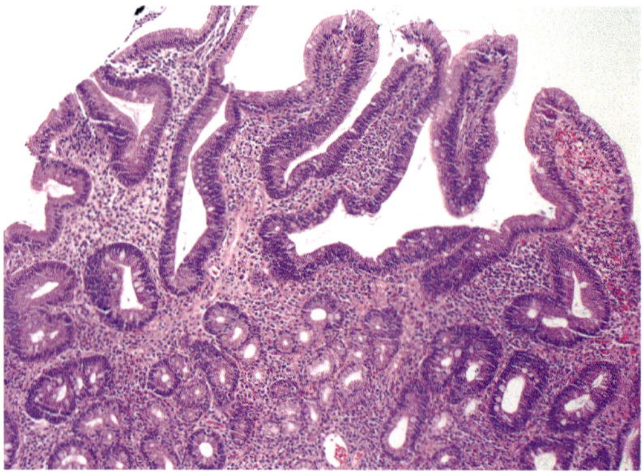

Fig. 6.1 Peptic duodenitis - surface antral metaplasia and lamina propria chronic inflammation

2. Peptic duodenitis-like pattern of coeliac disease. Associated intraepithelial lymphocytosis and the finding of villous blunting and inflammation beyond the duodenal bulb are found in coeliac disease [4].
3. Duodenal involvement by Crohn's disease is more variable in intensity. Ulceration is often present and granulomas may be found [1–4].

NSAID Enteropathy

NSAIDs cause injury of the small intestine mediated by microvascular changes. In addition to acute inflammation and erosion, there may be diaphragm-like strictures [5–7].

Histologically, villous blunting, sometimes leading to a flat mucosa, is usual. Inflammation is usually mild, but conspicuous eosinophils may be seen. Erosion and gastric metaplasia of antral or pseudopyloric gland type occur with chronic injury. Sometimes prominent lipid-induced cytoplasmic vacuolation of the surface epithelium associated with epithelial serration occurs (see Fig. 6.2). Hyalinisation of the lamina propria may also be appreciated in some cases.

Other Causes

The peptic duodenitis pattern of coeliac disease, sartan-induced enteropathy and Crohn's disease are other common causes of acute inflammation and ulceration discussed below.

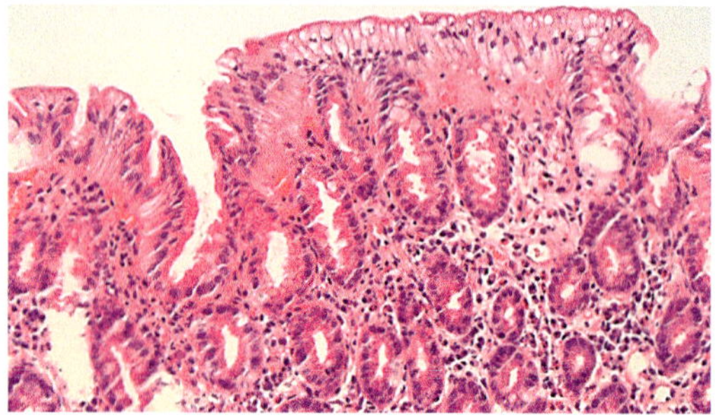

Fig. 6.2 NSAID enteropathy - villous flattening, cytoplasmic vacuolation and eosinophil infiltration

Active Chronic Inflammation

Crohn's Disease

Crohn's disease affects the duodenum in up to one third of the occasions that ileocolonic involvement is encountered [7]. Mucosal biopsies display patchy variable intensity active chronic inflammation with architectural disturbance and pseudopyloric gland metaplasia. Ulceration is frequent, and granuloma formation is seen in about one quarter of biopsies. patchy mild intraepithelial lymphocytosis may be seen (Box 6.1) [8, 9].

The differential diagnosis is:

Box 6.1 Diagnostic Clues: Acute Inflammation ± Chronic Inflammation and Erosion

Peptic duodenitis—Antral metaplasia, Brunner's gland hyperplasia

NSAID injury—Hyalinisation of the lamina propria, eosinophils

Autoimmune enteropathy—Prominent crypt apoptosis, other autoimmune conditions

Coeliac disease—Prominent intraepithelial lymphocytosis

Crohn's disease—Patchy inflammation, ulceration and granuloma formation

Sartan enteropathy—Prominent eosinophils, intraepithelial lymphocytosis, sometimes subepithelial collagen

1. Medication injury—NSAID injury is devoid of granulomata and generally has less chronic inflammation. Eosinophils may be frequent.

Sartan enteropathy usually is not associated with ulceration and granulomata. The inflammation is more diffuse with prominent eosinophils. Subepithelial collagen deposition may be seen. Intraepithelial lymphocytosis is generally more than seen with Crohn's disease.
2. Severe peptic duodenitis.
3. A diffuse pattern of active chronic duodenal inflammation may rarely follow colectomy for severe ulcerative pancolitis.
4. Autoimmune enteropathy—the presence of crypt apoptosis, absence of ulceration and granuloma formation and history of other autoimmune conditions point to autoimmune enteropathy.

Intraepithelial Lymphocytosis

This pattern is characterised by increased intraepithelial T lymphocytes above the normal range. The upper limit of normal for the duodenum is 25 IEL/100EC with 25–29 IEL/100EC regarded as a borderline abnormality and ≥30 IEL/100EC definitely abnormal [10–12]. A total count of ≥30 IELs in a span of 20 enterocytes at the tip of 5 randomly chosen villi is the best way to document subtle abnormality [10]. Intraepithelial lymphocytosis produces epithelial cell injury, and depending on the extent of this, there will be associated villous blunting. It is useful to consider this pattern in terms of situations with no or minimal associated villous blunting and conditions associated with villous blunting or flat mucosa.

Intraepithelial Lymphocytosis with Normal Villous Architecture (Lymphocytic Duodenitis, Lymphocytic Duodenosis) (Box 6.2)

This pattern is encountered in 1.3–6% of proximal small intestinal biopsies. Multiple conditions potentially cause this inflammatory pattern (see Box 6.2) [10–21]. Coeliac disease is responsible in between 9% and 30% of cases and typically displays villous tip predominance of the IEL infiltrate with reduction in IEL density from villous tip to base ("decrescendo sign") (see Fig. 6.3). Although not a specific feature, if absent, coeliac disease is unlikely. Unfortunately, no specific morphological features allow separation of most of the causes of this pattern, and the histopathology report should reflect this. An example report is shown below:

> The duodenal mucosa has normal villous architecture and a preserved villous:crypt ratio. There is an increase of intraepithelial lymphocytes in the surface villous epithelium.

Box 6.2 Intraepithelial Lymphocytosis with Normal Villous Architecture (Lymphocytic Duodenitis): Causes/Associations [10–21]

Common:

- Gluten sensitivity—including dermatitis herpetiformis, first-degree relatives of coeliac patients, and coeliac patients on GFD
- Infection—viral enteritis, *Helicobacter pylori* infection, *Giardia*, cryptosporidia, tropical sprue, and HIV
- Drugs—NSAIDs, and sartan family medications
- Autoimmune disease—rheumatoid arthritis, systemic lupus erythematosus, Hashimoto thyroiditis, Graves' disease, psoriasis, ankylosing spondylitis, type 1 diabetes, and scleroderma
- Idiopathic (many meet clinical criteria for irritable bowel syndrome)

Uncommon:

- Non-gluten food hypersensitivity—cereals, cow's milk, soy products, fish, rice, and chicken
- Autoimmune enteropathy
- Immunodeficiency disorders—IgA deficiency and common variable immunodeficiency
- Inflammatory bowel disease
- Lymphocytic and collagenous colitis
- Morbid obesity
- Bacterial overgrowth
- Secondary to local GIT inflammation

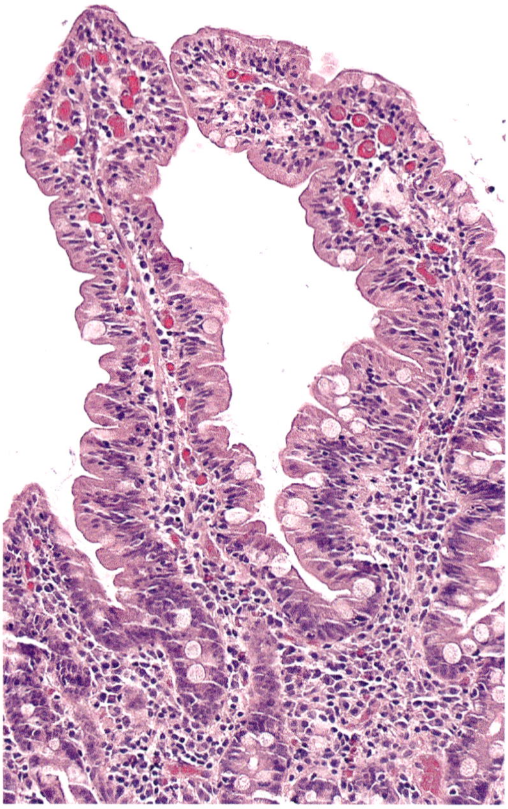

Fig. 6.3 Duodenal intraepithelial lymphocytosis with normal villous architecture—high power view

Comment: This pattern of intraepithelial lymphocytosis with normal villous architecture is not specific. Approximately 10–30% of cases represent an early form of coeliac disease. Other causes include recent viral infection, concurrent autoimmune disease and NSAID effect.

Intraepithelial Lymphocytosis with Villous Blunting (Box 6.3)

The cause and associations of this inflammatory pattern are listed in Box 6.3. Coeliac disease is the most common association and it needs to be considered in all the cases where this pattern is identified. The diagnosis of coeliac disease requires:

1. A suggestive clinical history, although asymptomatic and atypical presentations are common. The following clinical features are an indication to investigate for celiac disease:
   - Persistent unexplained abdominal or gastrointestinal symptoms
   - Faltering growth
   - Prolonged fatigue
   - Unexpected weight loss
   - Severe or persistent mouth ulcers
   - Unexplained iron, vitamin B12, or folate deficiency
   - Type 1 diabetes, at diagnosis
   - Autoimmune thyroid disease, at diagnosis
   - Irritable bowel syndrome (in adults)
   - First-degree relatives of people with coeliac disease.
2. Positive coeliac serology (tissue transglutaminase and/or deamidated gliadin peptide). Note that not all coeliac disease cases have positive coeliac serology.
3. Proximal small-intestinal inflammation with intraepithelial lymphocytosis.
4. A histological improvement in the small-bowel inflammation on commencing a gluten-free diet.
5. Carriage of the HLADQ2 or 8 haplotypes in essentially all coeliac disease patients but also about one-third of the population of Western countries.

Points 3 and 4 are the most important in establishing a diagnosis of coeliac disease. The absence of points 2, 3, 4, and/or 5 is against a diagnosis of coeliac disease.

Box 6.3 Intraepithelial Lymphocytosis with Villous Blunting/Flat Mucosa: Causes/Associations

Coeliac Disease (Majority of Cases)

Non-gluten food hypersensitivity (e.g. cereals, cow's milk, soy products, fish, rice and chicken)

Infection, e.g. viral/bacterial enteritis, tropical sprue and HIV enteropathy

Bacterial overgrowth

Autoimmune enteropathy

Immunodeficiency disorders, e.g. IgA deficiency and CVID

Drugs (e.g. NSAIDs, sartan family, methotrexate, immunomodulatory medications, idelalisib)

Inflammatory bowel disease

Collagenous sprue

Idiopathic

Coeliac Disease

Coeliac disease is a malabsorption disorder resulting from small intestinal epithelial injury induced by an immunological response to ingested gliadin-rich gluten protein. Gliadins contain proline and glutamine amino acids with abundant sulfhydryl groups that are deamidated by tissue transglutaminase. Deamidated gliadin binds to HLA-specific receptors on antigen-presenting cells inducing both cell-mediated and humoral immune response. This immune response generated the anti tissue transglutaminase and anti diamidated gliadin antibodies that are the serological markers of coeliac disease. The endoscopic pattern is characterised by mucosal ridges (see Fig. 6.4). The earliest histological change is increased intraepithelial CD3/CD8 positive T lymphocytes (≥30/HPF) [22, 23] which are associated with enterocyte apoptosis [22–24]. Plasma cells and lymphocytes infiltrate the lamina propria (see Fig. 6.5). In some cases, eosinophils may be conspicuous, and occasionally, neutrophils are found in the lamina propria, surface or crypt epithelium. Injured enterocytes may fail to adequately package and process absorbed lipid leading to cytoplasmic vacuolation ("lipid hang-up sign") (Fig. 6.6) [25]. This should not be interpreted as representing collagenous sprue. As the villi shorten, goblet cells become less readily identified, particularly at the surface. Gastric metaplasia may be observed in up to two thirds of biopsies but is never as prominent as seen in peptic duodenitis [23].

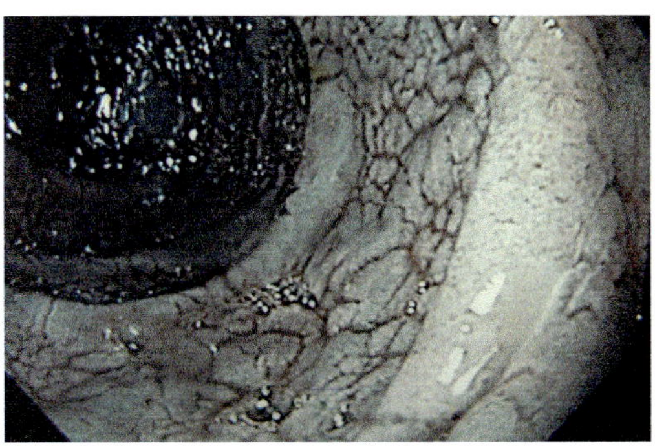

Fig. 6.4 The endoscopic pattern of coeliac disease is characterised by mucosal ridges

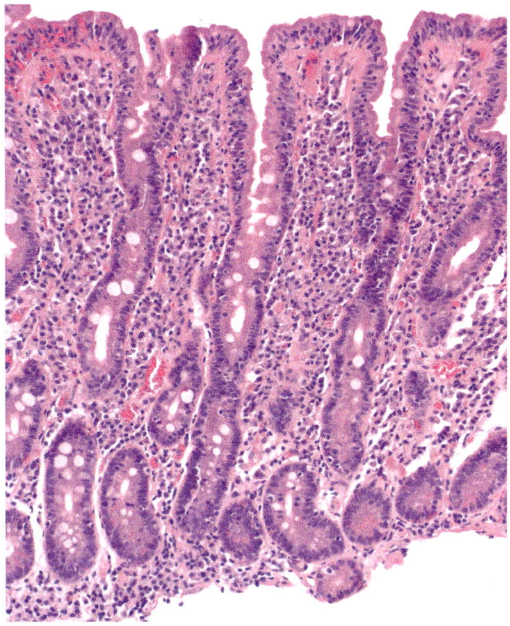

Fig. 6.5 Coeliac disease (×200) - crypt elongation and villous blunting. Intraepithelial lymphocytosis and prominent plasma cell rich lamina propria inflammation

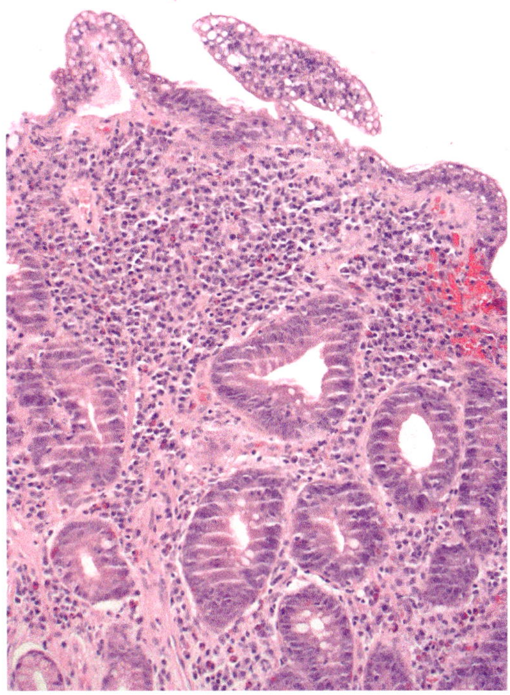

Fig. 6.6 Coeliac disease - lipid retention in surface epithelium. Slight thickening of the subepithelial collagen

Table 6.1 Modified Marsh classification scheme

	0	1	2	3a	3b	3c
IEL	<30	≥30	≥30	≥30	≥30	≥30
Crypts	Normal	Normal	Hypertrophic	Hypertrophic	Hypertrophic	Hypertrophic
Villi	Normal	Normal	Normal	Atrophy +	Atrophy ++	Absent

Table 6.2 Villanacci-Corazza classification scheme

Type A	Infiltrative, non-atrophic; incorporating types 1 and 2
Type B1	Atrophic with shortened but still detectable villi; incorporating types 3a and b
Type B2	Complete atrophy without detectable villi; corresponding to type 3c

The extent of villous and crypt architectural abnormality has been used for two morphological classification schemes—Marsh classification (Table 6.1) and Corazza and Villanacci classification (Table 6.2) [26]. Variability in the degree of injury between biopsy fragments and even within individual biopsy fragments occurs in up to 50% of coeliac disease biopsies (Box 6.4) [27, 28].

Box 6.4 Histological Features of Coeliac Disease

- Intraepithelial lymphocytosis ≥30/100 epithelial cells
- Villous blunting (variable)
- Lamina propria inflammation—plasma cell rich

Positive Serology (tissue transglutaminase ± deamidated gliadin peptide), HLADQ status (must carry HLADQ2 or 8) and demonstration of a histological response to gluten-free diet remain the mainstays in separating coeliac disease from its histological mimics [22–29].

Refractory Coeliac Disease

This is coeliac disease that either does not show improvement despite 6–12 months of a strict gluten-free diet or requires further intervention because of severe or deteriorating clinical symptoms [30]. Histologically, there is persisting enteropathy with minimal or no improvement in villous architecture, intraepithelial lymphocytosis or lamina propria inflammation. There may be subepithelial collagen deposition (collagenous sprue), a basal pattern of lymphocyte infiltration, crypt atrophy [31] and a reduction in Paneth cell numbers [32]. Refractory coeliac disease (RCD) is divided on the basis of IEL immunophenotype into type 1, normal immunophenotype, and type 2, aberrant IEL immunophenotype. Type 2 is at risk for development of overt enteropathy-type T cell lymphoma (ETTL). Distinction relies on immunohistochemical and/or flow cytometric profiling of the intraepithelial T cells by CD3 and CD8. Polymerase chain reaction (PCR) T cell receptor (TCR) clonality studies may also be performed but lack discriminatory value [33–36].

In *type 1 RCD*, the IEL phenotype is identical to usual coeliac disease with expression of surface CD3, CD7, CD8, CD103 and TCRβ on flow cytometry. Immunohistochemical expression of CD8 is identified in the majority of the CD3-positive IEL. TCR gene rearrangement should be polyclonal, although, a dominant clone can occasionally produce a false monoclonal result.

Type 2 RCD (see Figs. 6.7, 6.8, and 6.9) is characterised by loss of multiple surface T cell markers including CD3, CD7 and CD8 on flow cytometry. CD103 and cytoplasmic CD3 (due to preservation of the immunoreactive epsilon component) are demonstrable by immunohistochemistry. Loss of surface markers CD3, CD7 and CD8 in >20% of IEL by flow cytometric analysis and immunohistochemical loss of CD8 in >50% of IEL are indicative of RCD2. Monoclonal TCR is consistently identified but

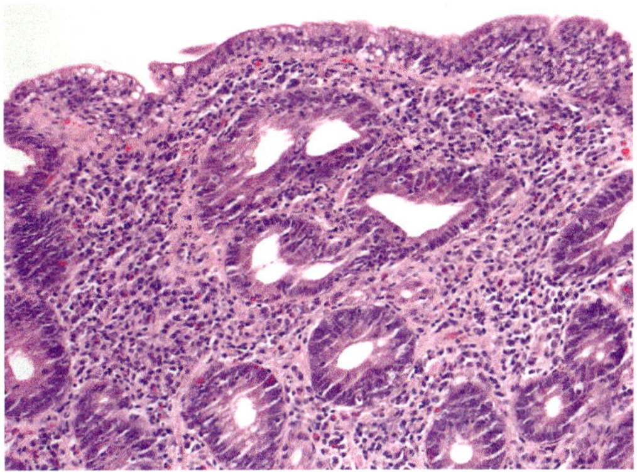

Fig. 6.7 RCD2 H&E

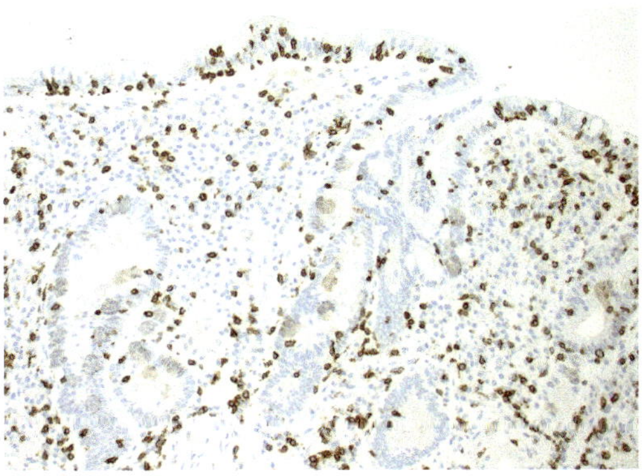

Fig. 6.8 RCD2 CD3 stain highlighting intraepithelial T lymphocytes

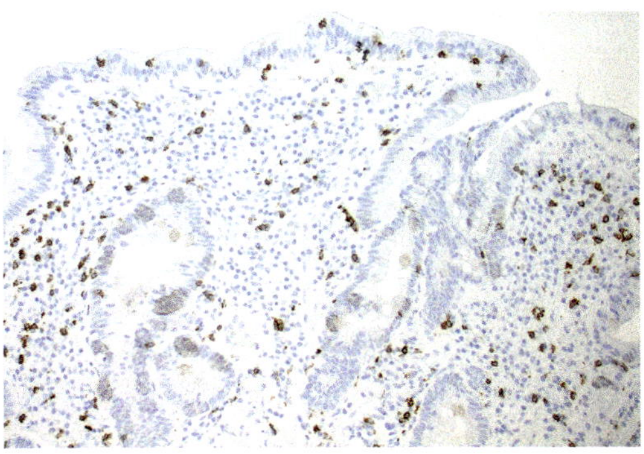

Fig. 6.9 RCD2 CD8 stain - reduced expression in intraepithelial T lymphocytes

is of less help because of the occasional finding of a clonal T cell population in RCD1 (Table 6.3).

Two other important causes for apparently refractory coeliac disease are:

1. Patients are not taking a strict gluten-free diet.
2. A coeliac disease-like enteropathy exists. This includes sartan enteropathy, collagenous sprue, autoimmune enteropathy, tropical sprue and immunodeficiency disorders, e.g. CVID, and Crohn's disease.

Sartan Enteropathy

Sartan family of angiotensin II receptor inhibitors are used primarily in treatment of hypertension and are therefore used mainly by an older population. They are now well recognised to induce gastrointestinal inflammation particularly involving the small intestine. Olmesartan induced injury is most common, because of particular pharmacokinetics of this medication, and therefore is best characterised. Patients have typically been using this medication for at least 1 year prior to onset of symptoms. The clinical onset of symptoms is often quite dramatic with severe diarrhoea and weight loss. Histological features include villous blunting, mild intraepithelial lymphocytosis and prominent lamina propria inflammation which is often rich in eosinophils and often has neutrophils (see Fig. 6.10). Occasional findings include subepithelial collagen deposition and crypt apoptosis. Cessation of the medication usually leads to rapid clinical improvement and disappearance of histological changes within several weeks [37].

Table 6.3 Differentiation of RCD1 and RCD2

	TCR rearrangement	CD3/CD8 immunohistochemistry	Flow cytometry
Coeliac disease	Polyclonal	Preserved CD8 expression	No loss of surface T cell markers
RCD1	Polyclonal (usually)	Preserved CD8 expression	No loss of surface T cell markers
RCD 2	Monoclonal	CD8 lost in >50% of CD3 positive IEL	Loss of surface CD3, CD7 and CD8 in >20% of IEL

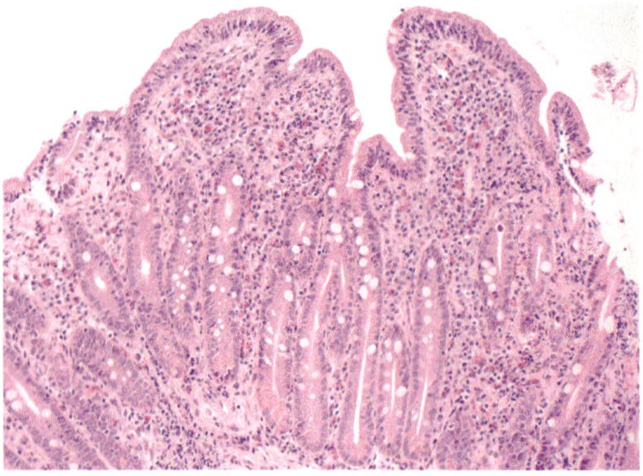

Fig. 6.10 Sartan enteropathy - villous blunting and lamina propria inflammation rich in eosinophils

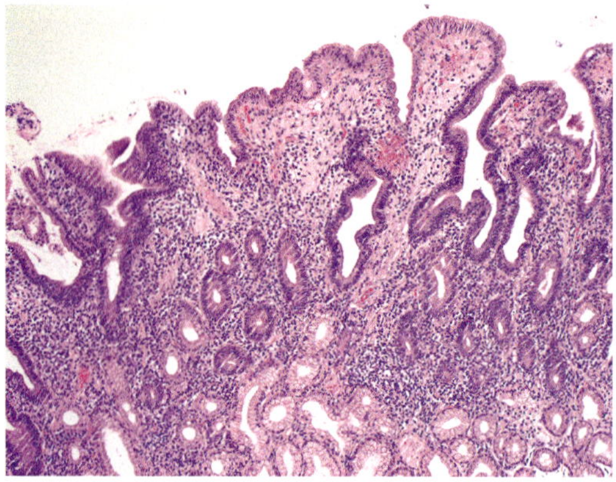

Fig. 6.11 Autoimmune enteropathy - villous blunting and lamina propria inflammation

Autoimmune Enteropathy

Autoimmune enteropathy represents mucosal injury induced by autoantibodies to mucosal epithelial cells, principally to the enterocytes, but sometimes Paneth cells and goblet cells. Most cases present in childhood; however, adult cases are increasingly recognised, and represent an acquired autoimmunity (e.g. thymoma associated, immunomodulatory medication, CVID). [38, 39].

The precipitant for autoantibody development is unknown in many cases. The disorder is a heterogeneous condition resulting from a variety of mechanisms of immune dysregulation leading to loss of self-tolerance and development of autoantibodies. An example of this is seen in IPEX syndrome, an X-linked recessive disorder that is characterised by immune dysregulation, polyendocrinopathy and enteropathy in the affected infant males [40, 41]. Mutations in the FOXP3 gene result in reduced CD25+, CD4+ regulatory T cells allowing development of autoantibodies targeting self-antigens such as gut enterocytes.

Four main patterns of morphological abnormality are recognised:

- Active chronic duodenitis (ACD): villous blunting, expansion of the lamina propria by mixed but predominantly mononuclear inflammation and neutrophilic cryptitis (with or without crypt abscesses), with or without increased apoptosis in crypt epithelium. Crypt architectural disturbance is often present and pseudopyloric gland metaplasia may be seen.
- Coeliac disease-like (CD-like): villous blunting and an increase in intraepithelial lymphocytes in surface epithelium (>= 30 IELs/100 enterocytes). Crypt epithelial apoptosis is present but typically inconspicuous. In contrast to coeliac disease, the $\gamma\sigma$ TCR density is not increased.
- Graft-versus-host disease-like (GvHD-like): increased apoptosis in crypt epithelium with or without crypt dropout, with minimal inflammation.
- Mixed/no predominant pattern: admixture of $\geq$2 patterns or insufficient features to qualify for any the above 3 patterns (see Fig. 6.11).

Circulating autoantibodies against enterocytes, goblet cells and/or Paneth cells are often detected, but are not specific to AIE as they can develop in other chronic inflammatory gut disorders, such as inflammatory bowel disease. Indirect immunofluorescence can confirm the diagnosis, but is rarely needed.

In contrast to coeliac disease, the presence of basal crypt apoptosis or the absence/reduced density of one cell type are important pointers to AIE. Coeliac serology (elevated TTG) is typically negative. HLADQ2/8 haplotype will help exclude coeliac disease if absent.

Food Protein-Induced Enterocolitis Syndrome (FPIES)/Food Protein-Induced Enteropathy

Food protein-induced enterocolitis syndrome is the name for a non-IgE, cell-mediated hypersensitivity of some patients, usually presenting in childhood, to ingested proteins and polypeptide components of cow's milk, soy protein, oats, peanuts, egg, fish, rice or chicken [42–45].

Histologically this manifests as variable severity villous blunting and an increase in intraepithelial lymphocytes [43–45]. Lymphonodular hyperplasia of the duodenal bulb is typically seen and there is an eosinophil infiltrate which may be numerous enough to produce eosinophilic enteritis [42]. Neutrophils are frequently identified in the lamina propria and sometimes the crypt epithelium. Return to normal mucosal morphology and rapid improvement in symptoms follow withdrawal of the offending antigen is usual and helps confirm the diagnosis.

Tropical Sprue

Tropical sprue (enteropathy) is an acquired chronic inflammatory disorder of the intestinal mucosa affecting residents and visitors to tropical regions (30° North or South of the equator, in particular India, much of South East Asia, Puerto Rica, parts of the Caribbean, northern South America and West Africa are high-prevalence locations) [45–49]. The aetiology is proposed to be an enteric acquisition of enterotoxigenic coliforms that induces the inflammatory process injuring the epithelium; hence, the disease is sometimes referred to as "post-infective tropical malabsorption". Particular HLA haplotypes may confer higher risk [48].

The histological features throughout the small intestine closely resemble coeliac disease with villous blunting, inflammation of the lamina propria and intraepithelial lymphocytosis [50–52]. The IEL infiltrate may be marked and involves both crypts and surface epithelium. Villous blunting is typically mild to moderate with progression to flat mucosa being infrequent [52]. The changes involve the entire small intestine, and in contradistinction to coeliac disease, the ileum is often more severely affected than the duodenum (see Figs. 6.12 and 6.13) [50–52]. Eosinophils are prominent in many cases, which can serve as a diagnostic clue [52].

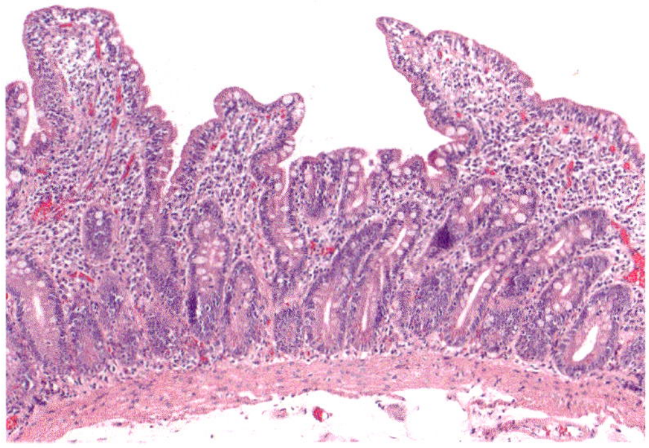

Fig. 6.12 Tropical sprue duodenum (×100) - mild villous blunting

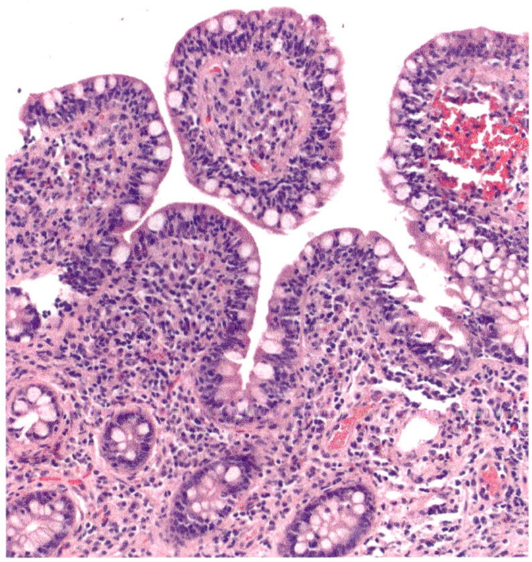

Fig. 6.13 Tropical sprue ileum (×200) - note the prominent intraepithelial lymphocytosis

Separation from coeliac disease is based on a clinical history of travel to a tropical region, negative coeliac serology and failure to respond to a gluten-free diet. Prominent ileal inflammation and uniformity of the IEL density from crypt to villous tip are additional features favouring tropical sprue [52]. Other diagnostic considerations include bacterial overgrowth, which probably shares a similar pathogenesis to tropical sprue; however, the clinical setting allows distinction. Neutrophils in the surface epithelium favour bacterial overgrowth, as they are rarely seen in tropical sprue. Infective enteritis is a further diagnostic consideration. It is usually short lived and is associated with more prominent acute inflammation.

Small Intestinal Bacterial Overgrowth

This condition results from colonisation of the small intestine by aerobic gram-negative bacteria or anaerobic bacteria derived from the colon or less commonly the oropharynx. This process may cause malabsorption or diarrhoea. It is diagnosed when >10 [53] colony-forming units (cfu)/ml of bacteria are identified in small intestinal aspirates[1]. Numerous predisposing conditions are associated with SIBO, including blind loop, surgical adhesions, surgical fistulae scleroderma, chronic renal failure, resections involving the ileocaecal valve, chronic pancreatitis, reduced gastric acid secretion and intestinal dysmotility [53].

The mucosa may appear histologically normal or can show villous blunting accompanied by crypt hyperplasia and mucosal inflammatory changes which typically have a patchy distribution [54–56]. An increase in intraepithelial lymphocytes [55] and a mild neutrophil infiltrate in the lamina propria and in the surface epithelium may be found. The latter is a helpful clue for SIBO [54]. Lymphoid follicles may be found. Seldom does the villous blunting become severe. A clinical setting predisposing to bacterial overgrowth and the absence of abnormal coeliac serology or coeliac disease appropriate HLADQ type can help distinguish this from coeliac disease. Tropical sprue is excluded by the clinical scenario.

Common Variable Immunodeficiency (CVID)

Common variable immunodeficiency (CVID) is the term for a heterogeneous group of disorders of defective B cell maturation producing hypogammaglobulinaemia. Between 20% and 60% of patients have gastrointestinal manifestations. Most cases are sporadic. Up to 20% exhibit an autosomal dominant inheritance. Mutations of TACI [transmembrane activator and calcium modulator and cyclophilin ligand (CAML) interactor] impeding immunoglobulin formation and/or plasma cell maturation are found in 5–10% [57].

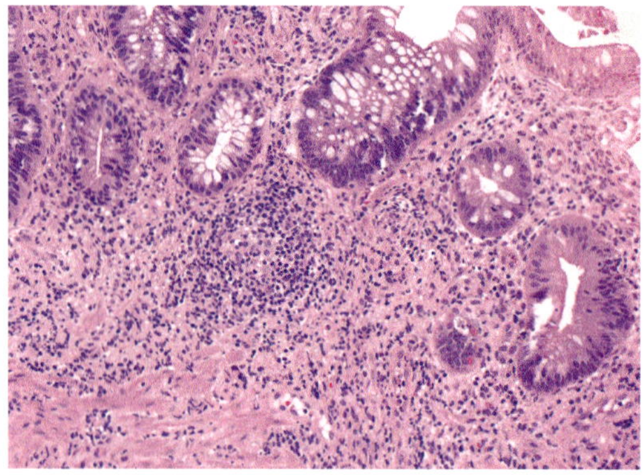

Fig. 6.14 CVID - lamina propria inflammation, intraepithelial lymphocytes and crypt apoptosis. Note the absence of plasma cells

In duodenal biopsies, there is an increase in lymphocytes in the lamina propria with lymphoid nodules composed of T cells. In keeping with the B cell defect, plasma cells are absent or reduced but can be hard to appreciate because lymphocytes may acquire plasmacytoid features. Villous blunting or flat mucosa with intraepithelial lymphocytosis is a common pattern [58–60]. Apoptosis in the crypt epithelium is usually present and may mimic graft-versus-host disease (see Fig. 6.14) [60]. Giardia and other parasitic infections may be found as a result of the immune defect. A histiocyte infiltrate resembling Whipple's disease is sometimes seen, and true granulomata may develop. The differential diagnosis includes:

1. Coeliac disease—Lymphoid nodules, crypt apoptosis and the relative or absolute absence of plasma cells in the lamina propria are the major features suggestive of CVID when a biopsy displays villous blunting and inflammation.

2. GVHD—A clinical history of haematopoietic cell transplant or other transplant will suggest GVHD.
3. Crohn's disease—The granulomatous variant of CVID is often initially misdiagnosed as Crohn's disease. The clinical setting is usually important in distinction. Crypt apoptosis and reduced plasma cell infiltration are histological clues.
4. Whipple's disease—Important for the rare cases with a prominent histiocytic infiltrate. PAS-positive bacilli will be found in the cytoplasm of the histiocytes in Whipple's disease.
5. Other immune dysregulation disorders. i) Autoimmune enteropathy—The relative absence of plasma cells and presence of lymphoid follicles are features suggestive of CVID. ii) X-linked agammaglobulinaemia—Only males are affected and the process has an older age of presentation. iii) Selective IgA deficiency is discussed below.

Selective IgA Deficiency

Immunoglobulin A (IgA) deficiency is the most common primary immunodeficiency. Diagnosis requires demonstration of decreased serum level of IgA in the presence of normal levels of other immunoglobulin isotypes. It is 10–15 times more likely in coeliac disease patients than in general population.

Histological features are similar to CVID with nodular lymphoid hyperplasia, sprue-like and/or GVHD-like patterns and occasional infection by giardia [61]. IgA-secreting plasma cells are absent, but IgM-producing plasma cells are not affected, so the total plasma cell number may not always be appreciably reduced. As coeliac disease is common in IgA deficiency, separation from purely IgA deficiency-related changes is often problematic and may require IgG-based serology, HLADQ haplotype testing and/or a trial of gluten-free diet (Box 6.5).

Box 6.5 Intraepithelial Lymphocytosis and Villous Atrophy: Diagnostic Clues

Coeliac diseases—Positive coeliac serology (increased TTG), carriage of HLADQ2 or HLADQ8 and demonstration of a histological response to gluten-free diet remain the mainstays in separating coeliac disease from its histological mimics.

Tropical sprue—Ileal involvement of similar or greater degree than the duodenum. Conspicuous eosinophils.

Viral infection—Short-lived symptoms with return to normal histology on a normal diet. History of infectious contact.

Autoimmune enteropathy—Young patients. Often a pan-gastrointestinal tract process. History of other autoimmune diseases. Often a poor response to immunosuppressive therapy.

Immunodeficiency related—Reactive lymphoid follicles, reduced or absent plasma cells and crypt apoptosis.

Bacterial overgrowth—History of a predisposing condition.

Sartan enteropathy—Older patients. often incomplete atrophy. Eosinophils and neutrophils are present. There may be inflammation outside of the small intestine.

HIV Enteropathy (See Below)

Subepithelial Collagen

Collagenous Sprue

Collagenous sprue is a heterogeneous disorder characterised by deposition of collagen to a thickness >10 μm in the subepithelial zone of the proximal small intestine [62, 63]. Up to 50% of cases occur in the setting of coeliac disease [62]. Medications such as olmesartan and NSAIDs account for some cases. Common variable immunodeficiency may also be an association. Autoimmune diseases are often present in affected patients.

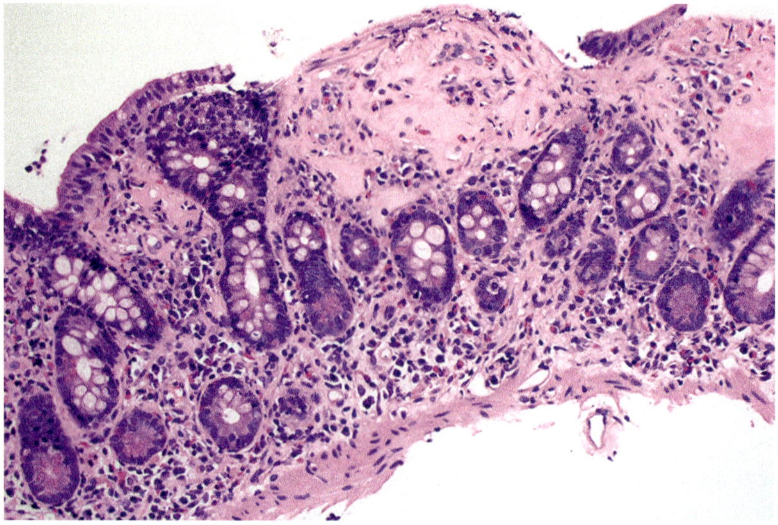

Fig. 6.15 Collagenous sprue H&E demonstrating marked thickening of the subepithelial collagen

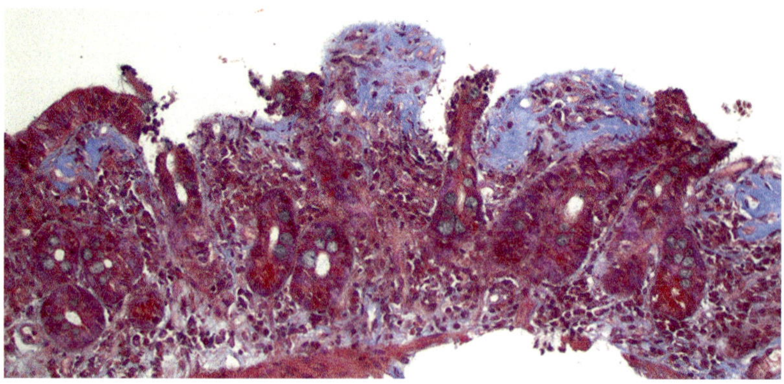

Fig. 6.16 Collagenous sprue trichrome stain confirming collagen thickening

Histologically, the collagen deposition has an irregular lower border with capillary entrapment and dilatation (see Fig. 6.15). The collagen nature can be confirmed by trichrome stain (see Fig. 6.16). There is usually some degree of villous blunting, and an increased chronic inflammatory cells and eosinophils are usually seen in the lamina propria. Intraepithelial lymphocytosis is often present, particularly in the coeliac disease-related cases.

In the small subset of cases associated with refractory coeliac disease, an abnormal intraepithelial lymphocyte population with loss of immunohistochemical reaction for CD8 in the majority of intraepithelial T cells is a good indicator of a neoplastic T cell population (RCD type 2). Clonal T cell receptor gene rearrangement and abnormal findings on flow cytometry further confirm this.

Minimal thickening of the subepithelial collagen layer not exceeding 5 μm, sometimes accompanied by epithelial denudation, is encountered in 36–60% of otherwise typical coeliac disease [63]. Subepithelial collagen deposition may also occur focally in the setting of healed erosion related to local injury. Both circumstances can be separated from true collagenous sprue by the requirement of a diffuse collagen thickening of >10 μm (Box 6.6).

Box 6.6 Causes of Collagenous Sprue

- Coeliac disease—especially refractory type
- Sartan medication
- NSAIDs
- Autoimmune conditions
- Idiopathic

Eosinophil Infiltration

Eosinophilic Duodenitis

Eosinophilic duodenitis remains poorly studied. The normal mean small intestinal eosinophil count is <10/HPF with peak eosinophil counts in paediatric duodenum being 26/HPF. An infiltrate >30/HPF is regarded as abnormal. This is accompanied by villous blunting of variable degree, eosinophil infiltration of epithelium, eosinophilic crypt abscess formation and infiltration of muscularis mucosae (see Fig. 6.17) [64, 65]. Mucosal oedema may be prominent in some case. The duodenum may be involved as part of generalised gastrointestinal process or may be isolated. Parasitic infection, food allergy, certain drugs (e.g. NSAIDs), gold, tacrolimus, clozapine and connective tissue disease (e.g. SLE, vasculitis particularly Churg-Strauss granulomatosis and hypereosinophilic syndrome) are the most common causes; however in most cases, a cause is not established. Exclusion of associated neoplastic disorders such as inflammatory fibroid polyp, Langerhans cell histiocytosis, mastocytosis, lymphoma and leukaemia should be undertaken in all cases.

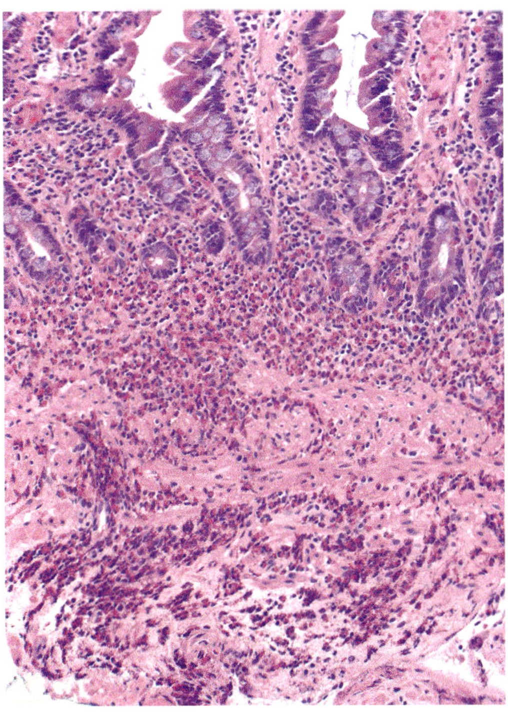

Fig. 6.17 Eosinophilic duodenitis. Note dense eosinophil infiltrate extending through muscularis mucosae

Table 6.4 Causes of histiocytic/granulomatous infiltrates

Histiocytes	• Xanthoma • Malakoplakia • Infections, e.g. Whipple's, MAIC • Lipid storage disorders • Muciphages, lanthanum
Granulomata	• Foreign body granuloma • Sarcoidosis • Crohn's disease • Pneumatosis • CVID • Chronic granulomatous disease • Infections, e.g. *Mycobacterium tuberculosis*

Histiocytic/Granulomatous Infiltrates

These are considered together and the causes are summarised in Table 6.4.

Ischaemic Injury

Ischaemic injury is rarely encountered in the duodenum because of the good collateral blood supply and retroperitoneal location, which protects this site from torsion. An ischaemic pattern may be encountered in some NSAID injury (large doses) or in the setting of vasculitis. In these situations there will be crypt atrophy and hyalinisation of the lamina propria with minimal inflammation.

Apoptosis

Prominent epithelial apoptosis may be encountered in the duodenum in conditions outlined in Box 6.7. It is important to exclude apoptotic cell death of neutrophils infiltrating the epithelium.

Box 6.7 Conditions Associated with Prominent Epithelial Apoptosis in Duodenum

- Medication including chemotherapy and immunomodulatory agents, e.g. ipilimumab, idelalisib, olmesartan and mycophenolate
- Immune mediated—GVHD, CVID, thymoma associated and autoimmune enteropathy
- Infection—HIV and other viruses

Graft-Versus-Host Disease (GVHD)

Graft-versus-host disease occurs in transplant graft recipients either in bone marrow transplantation or in solid organ transplantation, when immunocompetent donor cells induce an immunological reaction against alloantigens of the native cells of the host.

Crypt apoptosis with various degrees of epithelial cell loss is the key finding [66, 67]. With bone marrow transplantation, the background lamina propria is depleted of inflammatory cells. If the mucosa becomes eroded, a neutrophil infiltrate may be seen. Lymphocytes may infiltrate the epithelial near areas of active apoptosis. The severity of changes is graded according to the Lerner system:

Grade	Pathology
Grade 1	Isolated apoptotic epithelial cells, without crypt loss
Grade 2	Loss of isolated crypts, without loss of contiguous crypts
Grade 3	Loss of two or more contiguous crypts
Grade 4	Extensive crypt loss with mucosal denudation

The clinical scenario is usually readily apparent with the main diagnostic issue being exclusion of a medication effect, in particular mycophenolate, as the cause. Prominent eosinophil infiltration is typical of mycophenolate injury and is not found in GVHD.

Toxic Injury Pattern

This is most commonly seen when there is abrupt severe injury to the epithelium leading to obvious epithelial radiation injury that rarely affects the duodenum outside the setting of SIRT spheres.

Radiation Injury Due to SIRT Spheres

SIRT spheres are resin beads labelled with yttrium—80 injected via the hepatic artery system to the vascular supply of an intrahepatic tumour. Occasionally, and often in the setting of aberrant blood supply, the beads may find their way in vessels supplying the gastroduodenal region. In the duodenum, these induce radiation-related epithelial injury. Acute mucosal changes range from oedema to frank mucosal ulceration or necrosis (see Fig. 6.18). Villous blunting and a mild increase in chronic inflammatory cells can be seen. Acute inflammation, crypt apoptosis and crypt loss occur with more severe injury. Atypical appearing stellate cells ("radiation" fibroblasts) may be seen in the granulation tissue of an ulcer. Identification of the haematoxophilic purple or dark blue beads within arterioles in the region of injury and the appropriate clinical history confirms the diagnosis [68].

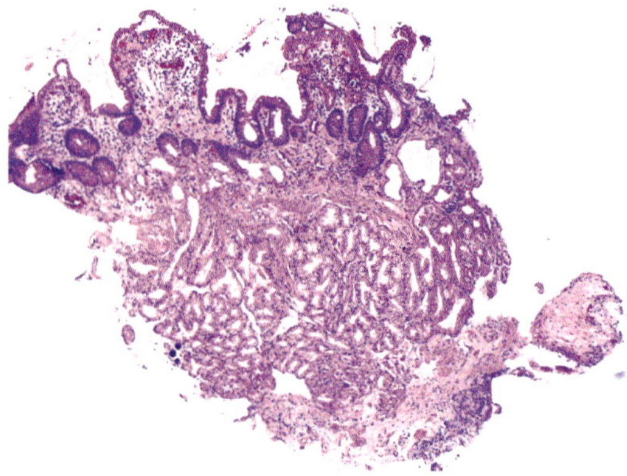

Fig. 6.18 Acute mucosal changes range from oedema to frank mucosal ulceration. SIRT spheres are present in vessels at the base of the mucosa

Mixed Injury Pattern

The most common causes include medications (sartan family, new biological agents e.g. idelalisib) and Crohn's disease.

Depositions

Brown Pigment Depositions

Endogenous or exogenous pigmented material is occasionally encountered in the duodenum. This can be classified into the following causes:

1. Iron [69–71]—Deposition may be related to hereditary haemochromatosis, the result of multiple blood transfusions or administration of oral or parenteral iron. In haemochromatosis the iron deposition can be within the lamina propria and within the epithelium of the both mucosa and Brunner's glands. A similar distribution is encountered with secondary

causes of iron overload. Oral iron tablets may be associated with mucosal erosion, and brown crystalline iron is often seen in the surface exudate.

2. Pseudomelanosis [72, 73]—This is a deposition of brown pigment, usually within the villous stroma. The pigment contains variable amounts of iron, ceroid, sulphur and melanin. A Perls' stain will highlight the iron (Figs. 6.19 and 6.20).
3. True melanosis—May be associated with metastatic melanoma in the local area.
4. "Brown bowel" syndrome [74, 75]—Develops due to deficiency of vitamin E, which is essential for stabilising mitochondrial membranes. Vitamin E deficiency may be primary or secondary fat malabsorption. A smooth muscle "mitochondrial myopathy" results in lipofuscin deposition within the cytoplasm of cells of the muscularis mucosa, muscularis propria and vascular media or within histiocytes throughout the gastrointestinal tract. Lipofuscin pigment granules are cytoplasmic and up to 3 μm in size. Cell atrophy develops with extensive deposition.
5. Lanthanum—A rare Earth used as a phosphate binder that can be taken up and accumulate in lamina propria histiocytes as a light brown to grey material. (see Fig. 6.21).

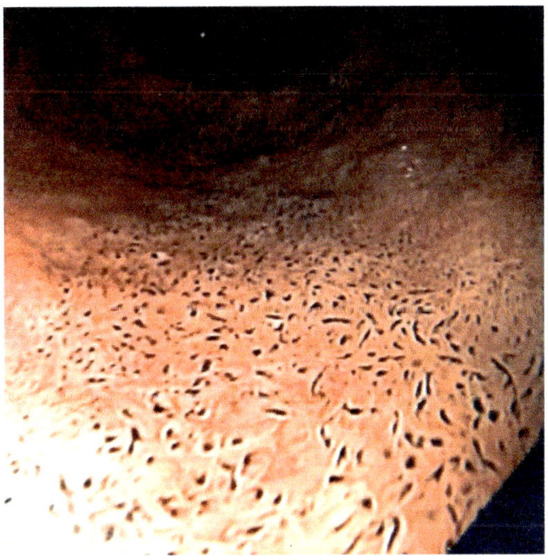

Fig. 6.19 Pseudomelanosis duodeni on endoscopy

Perls' stain highlights the iron in both pseudomelanosis and haemosiderin. Absence of Perls' staining and reaction for Fontana-Masson stain help confirm lipofuscin. Electron microscopy and/or chemical microanalysis may be required in some cases.

Pink Stromal Material Deposition

See Table 6.5.

Waldenstrom Macroglobulinaemia

Waldenstrom macroglobulinaemia is a clinicopathologic disorder characterised by tissue deposition of IgM paraprotein produced by the neoplastic cells of a lymphoplasmacytic lymphoma. The IgM paraprotein is brightly eosinophilic, homogenous

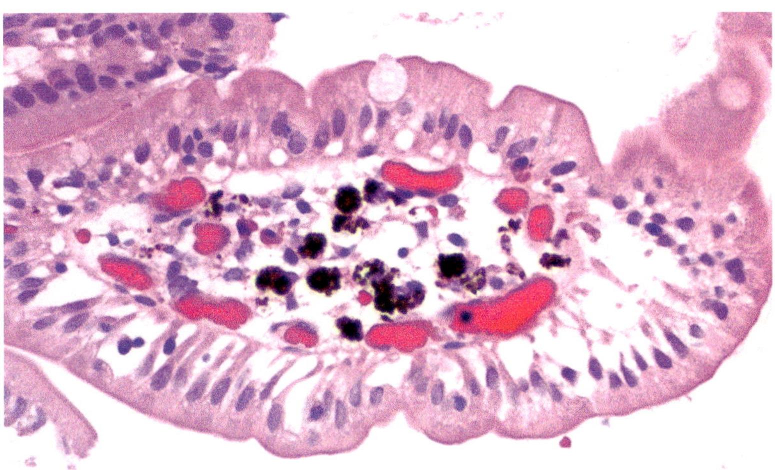

Fig. 6.20 Pseudomelanosis duodeni high-power view of villous tip

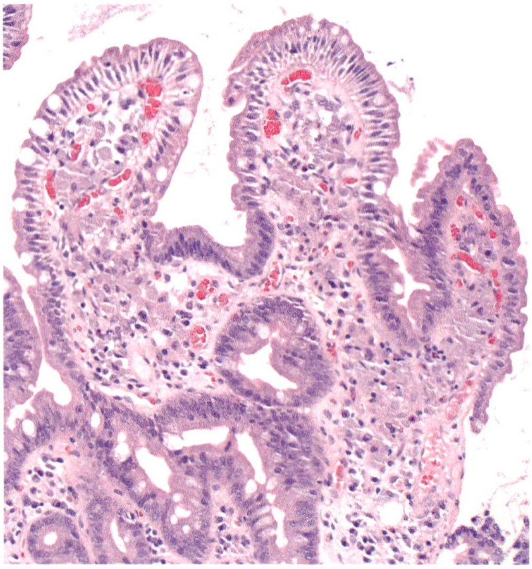

Fig. 6.21 Lanthanum deposition (×100)

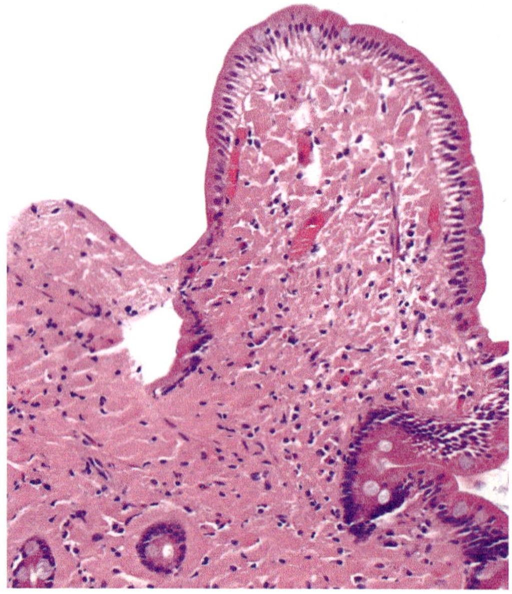

Fig. 6.22 Waldenstrom macroglobulinaemia showing expansion of villous lamina propria by deposits of eosinophilic paraprotein

Table 6.5 Pink stromal material deposition

Material	Special stain
Paraprotein deposition (including light-chain deposition)	PAS
Amyloid	Congo red
Hyaline collagen	Trichrome
Fibroelastosis	Elastin stain (VVG, orcein)

and strongly PAS-positive material. Initially deposition is within the villous lymphatics and between the epithelial cells. Later it fills the lamina propria [76, 77] and is associated with villous blunting and lymphangiectasia (see Fig. 6.22) [78]. Foamy histiocytes are often found within the dilated lymphatics and may be numerous enough to suggest Whipple's disease. Absence of organism products on the PAS stain excludes the later. The associated lymphoma may be seen in the lamina propria. Secondary infection, in particular by giardia, may occur as a result of loss of normal immunoglobulin function. The IgM paraprotein needs to be distinguished from amyloid by a more eosinophilic staining, strong reaction for PAS and absence of Congo red staining.

Amyloidosis

Amyloid is the generic term for various proteins with distinctive structural arrangement (β-pleated sheet) and staining properties (green birefringence with Congo red). Amyloid protein is relatively resistant to degradation and hence accumulates over time in tissues. Three main clinical categories are recognised—AA, AL and hereditary. Classification is also based on the type of amyloid protein as listed in Table 6.6 [77–82].

Amyloidosis is characterised by homogeneous, amorphous and light eosinophilic staining extracellular deposits in haematoxylin and eosin-stained sections (Fig. 6.23). Initially deposition is in the wall of submucosal vessels and around nerves and within the muscularis mucosae. This progresses to a diffuse deposition replacing much of the normal mucosa. Sometimes a globular pattern of deposition is encountered. The initial deposition in familial amyloid polyneuropathy is concentrated around nerve plexus. Secondary changes due to vascular involvement may be seen and include ischaemic ulceration and haemorrhage due to vessel wall weakness.

Confirmation is by way of Congo red staining producing intense red staining (see Fig. 6.24) with apple green birefringence on polarisation. Immunohistochemistry for amyloid P component is confirmatory although staining is finely granular and weak and less easy to interpret.

Table 6.6 Major types of amyloid affecting the small intestine [78–82]

Type of amyloid	Precursor protein	Clinical setting
AA	Serum amyloid A protein	Chronic inflammatory conditions Familial Mediterranean fever
AL	Monoclonal immunoglobulin light chain	Plasma cell neoplasia; B cell lymphoma
ATTR	Transthyretin	Familial amyloidotic polyneuropathy
Alys	Lysozyme	Autosomal dominant systemic amyloidosis with prominent visceral deposition
AApoA1	Apolipoprotein A1	Autosomal dominant systemic amyloidosis with prominent visceral deposition
Aβ_2M	β_2-microglobulin	Renal dialysis associated

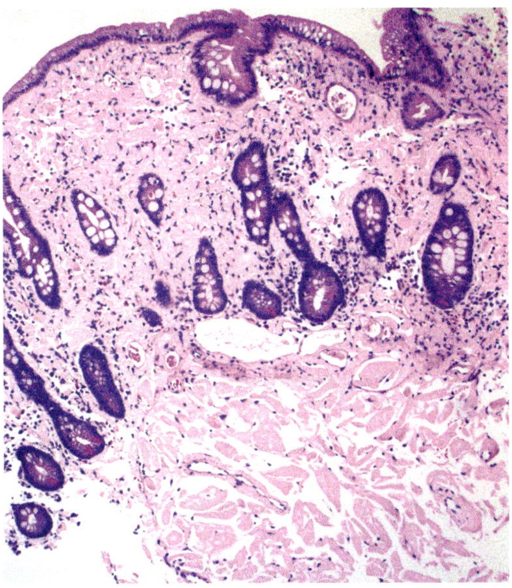

Fig. 6.23 Amyloid deposition in duodenum H&E

Electron microscopy reveals randomly oriented fibrils measuring 7–10 nm in diameter.

Typing

This requires a multidisciplinary approach and including clinical evaluation, immunohistochemical studies and variously biochemical tests, genetic studies and functional imaging. Unfortunately, immunohistochemical studies have low specificity and sensitivity, mostly because of the alterations to the precursor protein in the amyloidogenic process.

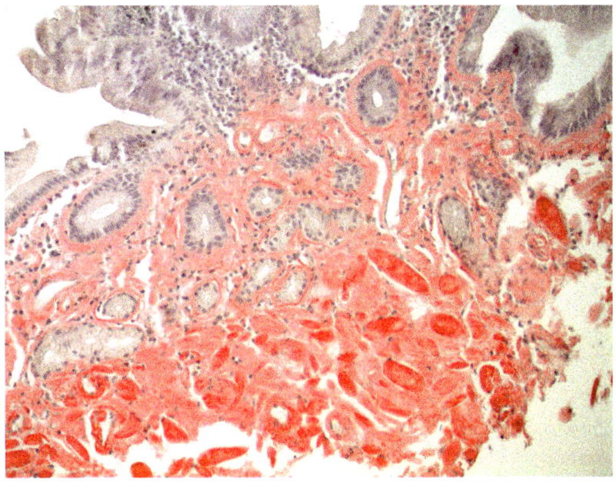

Fig. 6.24 Amyloid in duodenum Congo red stain

Amyloid needs to be separated from hyaline fibrosis, such as occurs in ischaemic injury, and from light-chain paraprotein deposition. Hyaline collagen will be reactive with collagen stains and negative for Congo red or amyloid P stains. Paraproteins are PAS positive and react with light-chain immunohistochemical stains.

Other Deposition Disorders

Light-Chain Deposition Disease

This represents deposition of light chains resulting from a monoclonal B cell lymphoproliferative disorder.

Lipid Storage Disorders

These are usually restricted to paediatric patients with inherited inborn errors of fat metabolism.

Collagen and Elastin Depositions

Collagen and fibroelastotic material accumulate within the lamina propria for a variety of reasons. Most commonly this is related to injury or chronic trauma. Ischaemic injury in particular leads to development of a hyaline pattern of collagen, which may mimic amyloid.

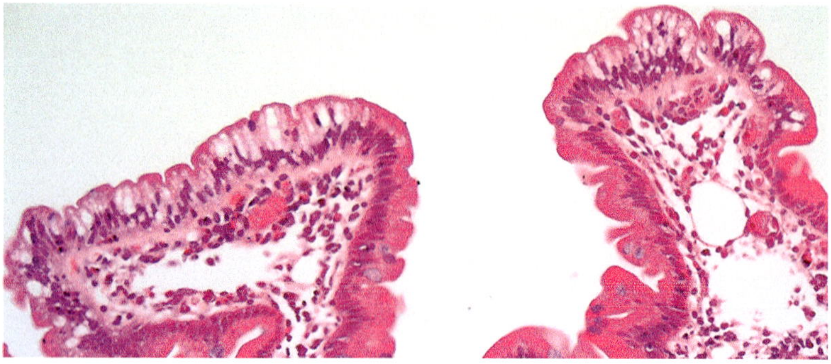

Fig. 6.25 Abetalipoproteinaemia - lipid accumulation in surface enterocytes

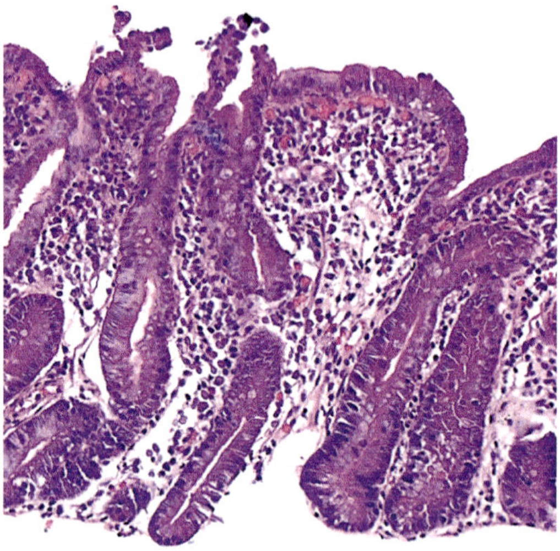

Fig. 6.26 Tufting enteropathy

Special Patterns

These are a diverse range of conditions with characteristic histopathological features that do not fit within the reaction patterns discussed above. These conditions present in early childhood or the neonatal period with severe malabsorption (Figs. 6.25 and 6.26) (Table 6.7) [83–96].

Infections

Giardia

Giardia lamblia infection is acquired via a faecal-oral route or by exposure to contaminated water. Infection is more commonly encountered in children and immunocompromised patients and following travel to underdeveloped countries. Secondary bacterial overgrowth may contribute to the pathological findings.

In most cases the mucosa is normal, and *Giardia* are appreciated in the intervillous space as "kite-shaped" or "sickle-shaped" structures, depending on whether they appear end on or side on in the tissue sections (see Fig. 6.27). Viewed en face, the trophozoites contain two ovoid nuclei. Mucosal inflammation is mild when present and usually contains increased eosinophils. Villous blunting (mild), crypt hyperplasia and intraepithelial lymphocytosis can occur. Sparse or absent plasma cells may indicate a predisposing primary immunodeficiency disease, e.g. CVID or IgA immunodeficiency.

Normal small intestine with epithelial cell sloughing can mimic giardia. Care needs to be taken in assessment of the cellular morphology [96].

Coccidian Protozoan Infections

Cryptosporidia parvum is the most commonly encountered coccidian infection. It is acquired by faecal-oral route or via ingestion of contaminated water. Infection is more common in immunocompromised patients. Organisms are appreciable as 2–5 μm round basophilic "beadlike" structures on the luminal surface (both villous and gland) of the epithelial cells (see Fig. 6.28). The organisms can be highlighted on Giemsa or gram stains and are located both within the apical cytoplasm of the epithelial cells and free within the lumen. A mixed inflammatory cell infiltrate and variable villous blunting are usually seen. Other coccidian infections include *Cyclospora* which are larger organisms located in the cytoplasm but lacking the apical predisposition of cryptosporidia. *Isospora* is characterised by peri-

Table 6.7 Conditions with characteristic histopathological features that do not fit within the reaction patterns discussed in this chapter

Condition	Gene defect	Histology	Special stains
Abetalipoproteinaemia	Autosomal recessive; mutations in the gene encoding for microsomal triglyceride transfer protein	Duodenal biopsies exhibit marked foamy vacuolation of the cytoplasm of enterocytes of the upper two thirds of the villi resulting from retention of absorbed lipid that is not able to be transported to the blood stream. Villous architecture remains normal and there is no inflammation (see Fig. 6.25)	Lipid stains can be performed on fresh tissue
Microvillous inclusion disease	Autosomal recessive; mutation impairs the GTD component of the apo-MyoVa-GTD (class V myosin) structure that is important in apical membrane recycling	Diffuse villous blunting with little or no crypt hyperplasia (so-called crypt hypoplastic atrophy) and normal or even decreased mucosal inflammatory cell infiltrate. Enterocytes have a "bubbly" cytoplasmic appearance which may resemble gastric metaplasia	PAS positive supranuclear cytoplasmic inclusion; cytoplasmic rather than cell membrane immunostaining for CD10; electron microscopy demonstrates vesicles lined by microvilli that are structurally unremarkable
Intestinal epithelial dysplasia (tufting enteropathy)	Autosomal recessive; EpCAM gene mutation; basement membrane disturbance with abnormal cell-matrix and cell-cell matrix interaction	Enterocyte cell tufts representing cells detached from the basement membrane. Tufts exhibit apical rounding producing a teardrop shape. Villous blunting, crypt hyperplasia and normal or increased inflammatory cells in the lamina propria. No intraepithelial lymphocytosis (see Fig. 6.26)	Absence of staining for the mutated gene product EpCAM/MOC31 antibody
Acrodermatitis enteropathica	Autosomal recessive; mutations in the SLC39 gene (at 8q24.3); deficiency of a zinc-specific transporter protein	Normal or show variable villous blunting with crypt hyperplasia and inflammation in the lamina propria[2,3]. Intraepithelial lymphocytes are not increased	Electron microscopy shows distinctive lysosomal inclusions in Paneth cells

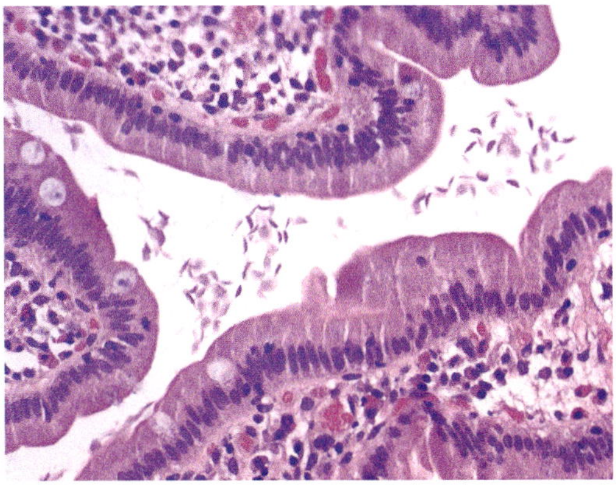

Fig. 6.27 Giardia in the intervillous space. Note the variable shapes of the organisms depending whether they are sectioned en face or side

or subnuclear inclusions which may be banana shaped or rounded with prominent nucleus depending on the stage in the parasite life cycle. Giemsa or silver-based stains can better highlight the organisms. Development of villous blunting with compensatory crypt hyperplasia and associated mixed inflammatory cell infiltrate is present, sometimes with prominent eosinophilia. *Microsporidia* are a similar appearing intracytoplasmic organism previously considered to be a coccidian parasite but now realised to be a fungal relative.

Microsporidia are most commonly encountered in immunosuppressed patients. They are much smaller intracytoplasmic organisms without the apical cytoplasmic location of cryptosporidia. Biopsies often show no abnormality. Minor villous change is sometimes encountered. The

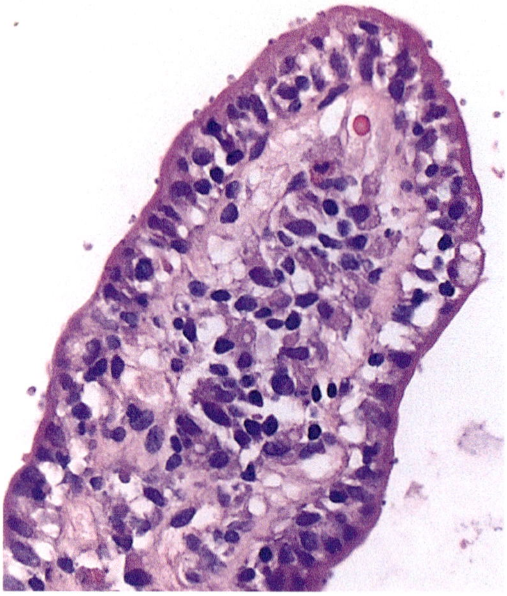

Fig. 6.28 Cryptosporidium on the epithelial surface

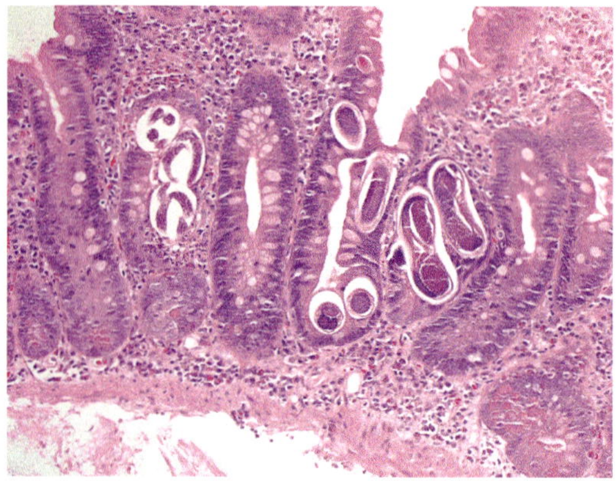

Fig. 6.29 Strongyloides

organisms are identified in supranuclear vacuoles and consist of spore and plasmodial forms. Silver stains best highlight the organisms.

Strongyloides

Infection by the nematode parasite *Strongyloides stercoralis* is endemic in tropical regions and immigrants from these areas. Immunocompromised patients are at particular risk for multisystem disease. In immunocompetent patients there is a marked lamina propria eosinophil infiltrate often accompanied by neutrophils. Adult worms, larvae and eggs may be found in the crypts (see Fig. 6.29). In immunocompromised patients or in the setting of mild disease, there may be minimal inflammation. Serology/stool microscopy is performed for definitive diagnosis. Strongyloides is capable of autoinfection.

Mycobacterial Infection: *Mycobacterium avium*-Intracellulare Complex (MAIC) and *Mycobacterium tuberculosis*

Infection by typical and atypical forms of acid fact mycobacterial infection. MAIC is most commonly acquired in the setting of immunocompromise. *M. tuberculosis* almost always occurs with active pulmonary disease and is more commonly encountered in the ileum and colon.

MAI-associated intestinal disease presents with an infiltrate of histiocytes in the intestinal lamina propria. Villi are distended and secondarily blunted, but inflammation is uncommon. Poorly formed granulomata may be seen. Acid fast stains and a PAS stain will highlight numerous organisms within the cytoplasm of the histiocytes (lesser numbers if immunocompetent).

M. tuberculosis is characterised by well-formed granulomata sometimes with caseous necrosis, a mixed inflammatory cell infiltrate and mucosal ulceration. Architectural distortion, fibrosis and dystrophic calcification are seen in older lesions. PCR of paraffin embedded tissue material can be used to identify the organisms.

The differential diagnosis of MAIC includes Whipple's disease, fungal infection and other histiocyte-rich disorders. For *M. tuberculosis the main differential diagnosis is* Crohn's disease and *Yersinia* infection.

Whipple's Disease

Whipple's disease is an uncommonly encountered infection by the bacterium *Tropheryma whipplei*. It is a multiorgan disease. Small intestine involvement may produce malabsorption.

The key microscopic feature is infiltration of the lamina propria by histiocytes with foamy cytoplasm. Granuloma formation may

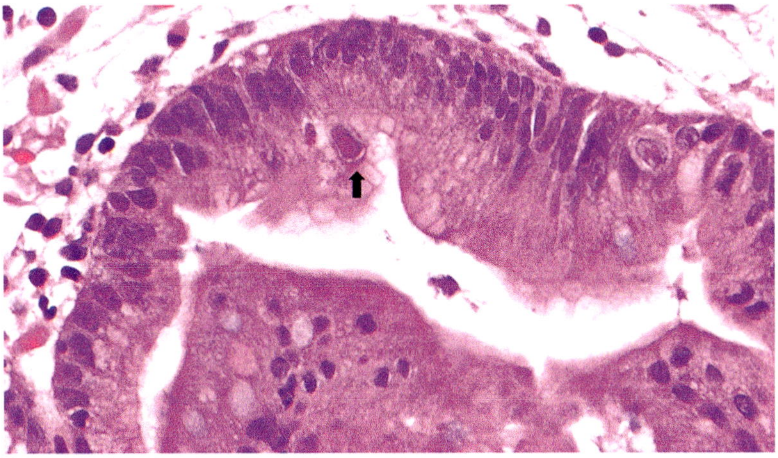

Fig. 6.30 Adenovirus typical inclusion

occasionally be seen. A variable neutrophil infiltrate may be seen. The villi are often blunted, and there may be prominent cytoplasmic vacuolation of enterocytes. Organisms within the histiocytes are strongly PAS positive. A PCR specific for *T. whipplei* is available and can be performed on paraffin shavings from the tissue block. The main differential diagnostic considerations are MAIC; fungal infection, in particular cryptococcus and histoplasmosis; prominent muciphages; and Waldenstrom macroglobulinaemia.

Adenovirus

Adenovirus is a systemic viral infection that only occasionally involves the gastrointestinal tract often in the setting of immunosuppression. Two types of intranuclear changes appreciated on light microscopy are (1) eosinophilic nuclear inclusion bodies and (2) "smudge cells", in which the nucleus is slightly enlarged, homogeneous and basophilic (see Fig. 6.30).

CMV

Is a systemic viral infection of the *Herpesviridae*. Primary gastrointestinal disease is rarely seen. Gastrointestinal involvement is usually the result of reactivation of latent disease due to immunosuppression. Distinctive viral inclusions are found, typically in the endothelial, epithelial or stromal cells. Inflammation or ulceration may develop. CMV can be confirmed by immunohistochemistry.

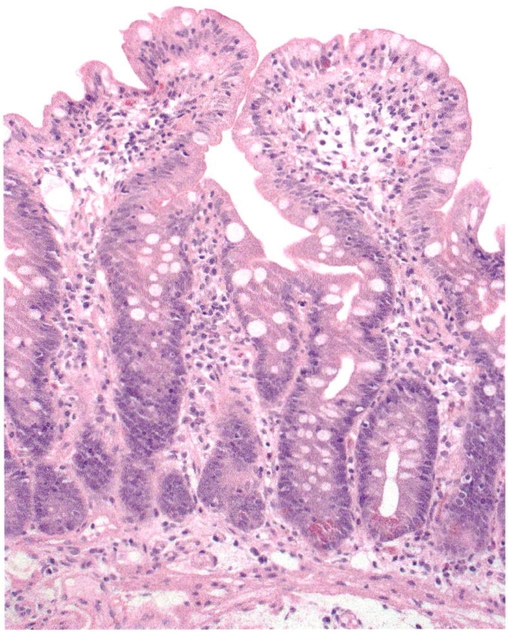

Fig. 6.31 HIV enteropathy - note the intraepithelial lymphocytosis in this example

HIV

HIV targets and depletes CD4-positive T cells. This is particularly prominent in the intestine, so mucosal biopsies exhibit a lamina propria depleted of lymphocytes, and normal lymphoid follicle may show fibrosis. Some cases show an enteropathy that resembled coeliac disease with intraepithelial lymphocytosis and lamina propria inflammation (see Fig. 6.31). In the setting of highly active antiretroviral therapy, commensal infections are uncommon.

References

1. Caselli M, Gaudio M, Chiamenti CM, Trevisani L, Sartori S, Saragoni L, Boldrini P, Dentale A, Ruina M, Alvisi V. Histologic findings and Helicobacter pylori in duodenal biopsies. J Clin Gastroenterol. 1998;26(1):74–80.
2. Wyatt JI, Rathbone BJ, Sobala GM, Shallcross T, Heatley RV, Axon AT, Dixon MF. Gastric epithelium in the duodenum: its association with Helicobacter pylori and inflammation. J Clin Pathol. 1990;43(12):981–6.
3. Khulusi S, Badve S, Patel P, Lloyd R, Marrero JM, Finlayson C, Mendall MA, Northfield TC. Pathogenesis of gastric metaplasia of the human duodenum: role of Helicobacter pylori, gastric acid, and ulceration. Gastroenterology. 1996;110(2):452–8.
4. Moran CJ, Kolman OK, Russell GJ, Brown IS, Mino-Kenudson M. Neutrophilic infiltration in gluten-sensitive enteropathy is neither uncommon nor insignificant: assessment of duodenal biopsies from 267 pediatric and adult patients. Am J Surg Pathol. 2012;36(9):1339–45.
5. De Petris G, López JI. Histopathology of diaphragm disease of the small intestine. Am J Clin Pathol. 2008;130:518–25.
6. Isaacs PE, Sladen GE, Filipe I. Mefenamic acid Enteropathy. J Clin Pathol. 1987;40(10):1221–7.
7. Brown IS, Miller GC, Bettington ML, Rosty C. Histopathological findings of extra-ileal manifestations at initial diagnosis of Crohn's disease-related ileitis. Virchows Arch. 2017;470:597.
8. Satsangi J, Silverberg MS, Vermeire S, Colombel JF. The Montreal classification of inflammatory bowel disease: controversies, consensus, and implications. Gut. 2006;55(6):749–53.
9. Paerregaard A. What Does the IBD Patient Hide in the Upper Gastrointestinal Tract? Inflamm Bowel Dis. 2009;15(7):1101–4.
10. Biagi F, Luinetti O, Campanella J, et al. Intraepithelial lymphocytes in the villous tip: do they indicate potential celiac disease? J Clin Pathol. 2004;57:835.
11. Verress B, Franzen L, Bodin L, Borch K. Duodenal intraepithelial lymphocyte-count revisited. Scand J Gastroenterol. 2004;4:138.
12. Hayat M, Cairns A, Dixon MF, O'Mahony S. Quantitation of intraepithelial lymphocytes in human duodenum: what is normal? J Clin Pathol. 2002;55:393.
13. Brown I, Mino-Kenudson M, Deshpande V, Lauwers GY. Intraepithelial lymphocytosis in architecturally preserved proximal small intestinal mucosa - an increasing diagnostic problem with a wide differential diagnosis. Arch Pathol Lab Med. 2006;130(7):1020–5.
14. Kakar S, Mehra V, et al. Significance of intraepithelial lymphocytosis in small bowel biopsy samples with normal mucosal architecture. Am J Gastroenterol. 2003;98(9):2027–33.
15. Mahadeva S, Wyatt JI, et al. Is a raised intraepithelial lymphocyte count with normal duodenal villous architecture clinically relevant? J Clin Pathol. 2002;55:424–8.
16. Goldstein NS, Underhill J. Morphologic features suggestive of gluten sensitivity in architecturally normal duodenal biopsy specimens. Am J Clin Pathol. 2001;116:63–71.
17. Robert ME. Gluten sensitive enteropathy and other causes of small intestinal lymphocytosis. Semin Diagn Pathol. 2005;22(4):284–94.
18. Chang F, Mahadeva U, Deere H. Pathological and clinical significance of increased intraepithelial lymphocytes (IELs) in small bowel mucosa. APMIS. 2005;113:385.
19. Rosinach M, et al. Lymphocytic duodenosis: aetiology and long-term response to specific treatment. Dig Liver Dis. 2012;44(8):643–8.
20. Aziz I, Evans KE, Hopper AD, et al. A prospective study into the aetiology of lymphocytic duodenosis. Aliment Pharmacol Ther. 2010;32:1392–7.
21. Shmidt E, Smyrk TC, Faubion WA, Oxentenko AS. Duodenal intraepithelial lymphocytosis with normal villous architecture in pediatric patients: Mayo Clinic experience, 2000-2009. J Pediatr Gastroenterol Nutr. 2013;56(1):51–5.
22. Mino-Kenudson M, Brown I, Lauwers GY. Histopathological diagnosis of gluten-sensitive enteropathy. Curr Diagn Pathol. 2005;11(4):274–83.
23. Brown I, Smith J, Rosty C. Gastrointestinal pathology in celiac disease: a case series of 150 consecutive newly diagnosed patients. Am J Clin Pathol. 2012;138(1):42–9.
24. Antonioli D. Celiac disease: a progress report. Mod Pathol. 2003;16(4):342–6.
25. Owens SR, Greenson JK. The pathology of malabsorption: current concepts. Histopathology. 2007;50(1):64–82.
26. Oberhuber G, Granditsch G, Vogelsang H. The histopathology of celiac disease: time for a standardized report scheme for pathologists. Eur J Gastroenterol Hepatol. 1999;11:1185.
27. Corazza GR, Villanacci V. Celiac disease. J Clin Pathol. 2005;58:573.
28. Weir DC, Glickman JN, Roiff T, et al. Variability of histopathological changes in childhood celiac disease. Am J Gastroenterol. 2010;105(1):207–12.
29. Ravelli A, Bolognini S, Gambarotti M, Villanacci V. Variability of histologic lesions in relation to biopsy site in gluten-sensitive enteropathy. Am J Gastroenterol. 2005;100:177.
30. Daum S, Cellier C, Mulder CJ. Refractory celiac disease. Best Pract Res Clin Gastroenterol. 2005;19:413.
31. Robert ME, Ament ME, Weinstein WM. The histologic spectrum and clinical outcome of refractory and unclassified sprue. Am J Surg Pathol. 2000;24:676.
32. Di Sabatino A, Miceli E, Dhaliwal W, et al. Distribution, proliferation, and function of Paneth cells in uncomplicated and complicated adult celiac disease. Am J Clin Pathol. 2008;130:34.

33. Ho-Yen C, Chang F, van der Walt J, Mitchell T, Ciclitira P. Recent advances in refractory celiac disease: a review. Histopathology. 2009;54:783.
34. Al-Toma A, Verbeek WH, Mulder CJ. Update on the management of refractory celiac disease. J Gastrointestin Liver Dis. 2007;16:57.
35. Patey-Mariaud De Serre N, Cellier C, et al. Distinction between celiac disease and refractory sprue: a simple immunohistochemical method. Histopathology. 2000;37:70.
36. Rubio-Tapia A, Murray JA. Classification and management of refractory celiac disease. Gut. 2010;59(4):547–57.
37. Choi EY, McKenna BJ. Olmesartan-associated enteropathy: a review of clinical and histologic findings. Arch Pathol Lab Med. 2015;139(10):1242–7.
38. Akram S, Murray JA, Pardi DS, et al. Adult autoimmune enteropathy: Mayo Clinic Rochester experience. Clin Gastroenterol Hepatol. 2007;5:1282.
39. Montalto M, D'Onofrio F, Santoro L, et al. Autoimmune enteropathy in children and adults. Scand J Gastroenterol. 2009;44:1029.
40. Patey-Mariaud de Serre N, Canioni D, Ganousse S, et al. Digestive histopathological presentation of IPEX syndrome. Mod Pathol. 2009;22:95.
41. Masia R, Peyton S, Lauwers GY, Brown I. Gastrointestinal biopsy findings of autoimmune enteropathy: a review of 25 cases. Am J Surg Pathol. 2014;38(10):1319–29.
42. Kesuaai I, Kuitonen P, Savilahti E, Sippenen P. Mast cells and eosinophils in the jejunal mucosa of patients with intestinal cows' milk allergy and celiac disease of childhood. J Pediatr Gastroenterol Nutr. 1984;3:368.
43. Kokkonen J, Holm K, Karttunen TJ, Mäki M. Children with untreated food allergy express a relative increment in the density of duodenal gammadelta+ T cells. Scand J Gastroenterol. 2000;35:1137.
44. Ament ME, Rubin CE. Soy protein—another cause of the flat intestinal lesion. Gastroenterology. 1972;62:227.
45. Vitoria JC, Camerero C, Sojo A, Ruiz A, Roderiguez-Soriano J. Enteropathy related to fish, rice, and chicken. Arch Dis Child. 1982;57:44.
46. Batheja MJ, Leighton J, Azueta A, Heigh R. The Face of Tropical Sprue in 2010. Case Rep Gastroenterol. 2010;4(2):168–72.
47. Walker MM. What is tropical sprue? J Gastroenterol Hepatol. 2003;18:887.
48. Haghighi P, Wolf PL. Tropical sprue and subclinical enteropathy: a vision for the nineties. Crit Rev Clin Lab Sci. 1997;34:313.
49. Nath SK. Tropical sprue. Curr Gastroenterol Rep. 2005;7(5):343–9.
50. Swanson VL, Thomassen RW. Pathology of the jejunal mucosa in tropical sprue. Am J Pathol. 1965;46:511–51.
51. Wheby MS, Swanson VL, Bayless TM. Comparison of ileal and jejunal biopsies in tropical sprue. Am J Clin Nutr. 1971;24:117–23.
52. Brown IS, Bettington A, Bettington M, Rosty C. Tropical Sprue – revisiting an under recognised condition. Am J Surg Pathol. 2014;38(5):666–72.
53. Rana SV, Bhardwaj SB. Small intestinal bacterial overgrowth. Scand J Gastroenterol. 2008;43:1030–7.
54. Lappinga PJ, Abraham SC, Murray JA, Vetter EA, Patel R, Wu TT. Small intestinal bacterial overgrowth: histopathologic features and clinical correlates in an underrecognized entity. Arch Pathol Lab Med. 2010;134:264–70.
55. Haboubi NY, Lee GS, Montgomery RD. Duodenal mucosal morphometry of elderly patients with small intestinal bacterial overgrowth: response to antibiotic treatment. Age Ageing. 1991;20:29.
56. Riordan SM, McIver CJ, Wakefield D, et al. Small intestinal mucosal immunity and morphometry in luminal overgrowth of indigenous gut flora. Am J Gastroenterol. 2001;96:494.
57. Castigli E, Wilson SA, Garibyan L, et al. TACI is mutant in common variable immunodeficiency and IgA deficiency. Nat Genet. 2005;37:829–34.
58. Malamut G, Verkarre V, Suarez F, Viallard JF, Lascaux AS, Cosnes J, Bouhnik Y, Lambotte O, Béchade D, Ziol M, Lavergne A, Hermine O, Cerf Bensussan N, Cellier C. The enteropathy associated with common variable immunodeficiency: the delineated frontiers with celiac disease. Am J Gastroenterol. 2010;105(10):2262–75.
59. Daniels JA, Lederman HM, Maitra A, Montgomery EA. Gastrointestinal tract pathology in patients with common variable immunodeficiency (CVID): a clinicopathologic study and review. Am J Surg Pathol. 2007;31(12):1800–12.
60. Washington K, Stenzel TT, Buckley RH, Gottfried MR. Gastrointestinal pathology in patients with common variable immunodeficiency and X-linked agammaglobulinemia. Am J Surg Pathol. 1996;20(10):1240–52.
61. Joo M, Shim SH, Chang SH, Kim H, Chi JG, Kim NH. Nodular lymphoid hyperplasia and histologic changes mimicking celiac disease, collagenous sprue, and lymphocytic colitis in a patient with selective IgA deficiency. Pathol Res Pract. 2009;205(12):876–80.
62. Maguire AA, Greenson JK, Lauwers GY, et al. Collagenous sprue: a clinicopathologic study of 12 cases. Am J Surg Pathol. 2009;33:1440.
63. Freeman HJ. Update on collagenous sprue. World J Gastroenterol. 2010;16(3):296–8.
64. DeBrosse CW, Case JW, Putnam PE, et al. Quantity and distribution of eosinophils in the gastrointestinal tract of children. Pediatr Dev Pathol. 2006;9(3):210–8.
65. Lucendo AJ, Arias A. Eosinophilic gastroenteritis: an update. Expert Rev Gastroenterol Hepatol. 2012;6(5):591–601.
66. Washington K, Jagasia M. Pathology of graft-versus-host disease in the gastrointestinal tract. Hum Pathol. 2009;40(7):909–17.
67. Snover DC. Graft-versus-host disease of the gastrointestinal tract. Am J Surg Pathol. 1990;14(Suppl 1):101–8.

68. Ogawa F, Mino-Kenudson M, Shimizu M, Ligato S, Lauwers GY. Gastroduodenitis associated with yttrium 90-microsphere selective internal radiation: an iatrogenic complication in need of recognition. Arch Pathol Lab Med. 2008;132(11):1734–8.
69. Conte D, Velio P, Brunelli L, et al. Stainable iron in gastric and duodenal mucosa of primary hemochromatosis patients and alcoholics. Am J Gastroenterol. 1987;82:237–40.
70. Abraham SC, Yardley JH, Wu TT. Erosive injury to the upper gastrointestinal tract in patients receiving iron medication. Am J Surg Pathol. 1999;23:1241–7.
71. Kaye P, Abdulla K, Wood J, James P, Foley S, Ragunath K, Atherton J. Iron-induced mucosal pathology of the upper gastrointestinal tract: a common finding in patients on oral iron therapy. Histopathology. 2008;53(3):311–7.
72. West B. Pseudomelanosis duodeni. J Clin Gastroenterol. 1988;10(2):127–9.
73. Rex DK, Jersild RA Jr. Further characterization of the pigment in pseudomelanosis duodeni in three patients. Gastroenterology. 1988;95(1):177–82.
74. Foster CS. The brown bowel syndrome: a possible smooth muscle mitochondrial myopathy. Histopathology. 1979;3:1.
75. Horn T, Svendsen LB, Nielsen R. Brown-bowel syndrome. Review of the literature and presentation of cases. Scand J Gastroenterol. 1990;25:66.
76. Brandt LJ, Davidoff A, Bernstein LH, et al. Small-intestine involvement in Waldenstrom's macroglobulinemia. Case report and review of the literature. Dig Dis Sci. 1981;26:174.
77. Gad A, Willén R, Carlén B, Gyland F, Wickander M. Duodenal involvement in Waldenström's macroglobulinemia. J Clin Gastroenterol. 1995;20(2):174–6.
78. Harris M, Burton IE, Scarffe JH. Macroglobulinaemia and intestinal lymphangiectasia: a rare association. J Clin Pathol. 1983;36(1):30–6.
79. Sattianayagam PT, Hawkins PN, Gillmore JD. Systemic amyloidosis and the gastrointestinal Tract. Nat Rev Gastroenterol Hepatol. 2009;6:608–17.
80. Ebert EC, Nagar M. Gastrointestinal manifestations of amyloidosis. Am J Gastroenterol. 2008;103(3):776–87.
81. Hemmer PR, Topazian MD, Gertz MA, Abraham SC. Globular amyloid deposits isolated to the small bowel: a rare association with AL amyloidosis. Am J Surg Pathol. 2007;31:141–5.
82. Gould M, Zarrin-Khameh N, Sellin J. Small Bowel Amyloidosis. Curr Gastroenterol Rep. 2013;350(1-6):15.
83. Cutz E, Rhoads JM, Drumm B, et al. Micro inclusion disease: an inherited defect of brush border assembly and differentiation. N Engl J Med. 1989;320:646.
84. Groisman G, Ben-Izhak O, Schwersenz A, et al. The value of polyclonal carcinoembryonic antigen immunostaining in the diagnosis of micro inclusion disease. Hum Pathol. 1993;24:1232.
85. Groisman GM, Amar M, Livne E. CD10: a valuable tool for the light microscopic diagnosis of microvillous inclusion disease (familial microvillous atrophy). Am J Surg Pathol. 2002;26:902.
86. Al-Daraji WI, Zelger B, Zelger B, Hussein MR. Microvillous inclusion disease: a clinicopathologic study of 17 cases from the UK. Ultrastruct Pathol. 2010;34(6):327–32.
87. Bell SW, Kerner JA Jr, Sibley RK. Microvillous inclusion disease. The importance of electron microscopy for diagnosis. Am J Surg Pathol. 1991;15:1157.
88. Cutz E, Sherman PM, Davidson GP. Enteropathies associated with protracted diarrhea of infancy: clinicopathological features, cellular and molecular mechanisms. Pediatr Pathol Lab Med. 1997;17:335.
89. Sivagnanam M, Mueller JL, Lee H, et al. Identification of EpCAM as the gene for congenital tufting enteropathy. Gastroenterology. 2008;135(2):429–37.
90. Goulet OJ, Brousse N, Canioni D, et al. Syndrome of intractable diarrhoea with persistent villous atrophy in early childhood: a clinicopathological survey of 47 cases. J Pediatr Gastroenterol Nutr. 1998;26:151.
91. Ranganathan S, Schmitt LA, Sindhi R. Tufting enteropathy revisited: the utility of MOC31 (EpCAM) immunohistochemistry in diagnosis. Am J Surg Pathol. 2014;38(2):265–72.
92. Schmitt S, Küry S, Giraud M, et al. An update on mutations of the SLC39A4 gene in acrodermatitis enteropathica. Hum Mutat. 2009;30:926.
93. Kuitunen P, Kosnai I, Savilahti E. Morphometric study of the jejunal mucosa in various childhood enteropathies with special reference to intraepithelial lymphocytes. J Pediatr Gastroenterol Nutr. 1982;1:525.
94. Bohane TD, Cutz E, Hamilton JR, Gall DG. Acrodermatitis enteropathica, zinc, and the Paneth cell. A case report with family studies. Gastroenterology. 1977;73:587.
95. Kobayashi Y, Suzuki H, Konno T, et al. Ultrastructural alterations of Paneth cells in infants associated with gastrointestinal symptoms. Tohoku J Exp Med. 1983;139:225.
96. Oberhuber G, Kastner N, Stolte M. Giardiasis: a histologic analysis of 567 cases. Scand J Gastroenterol. 1997;32:48–51.

Proximal Small Intestine: Neoplastic Patterns and Mimics

7

Ian Brown

Contents

I. Brown
Envoi Pathology, Kelvin Grove, QLD, Australia
e-mail: ianbrown@envoi.com.au

M. P. Kumarasinghe, I. Brown (eds.), *Endoscopic Biopsy Interpretation*,
https://doi.org/10.1007/978-3-319-79117-3_7

Normal Tissue at the Wrong Site (Heterotopias)

Gastric Heterotopia

Gastric heterotopia is most commonly encountered in the duodenal bulb (Fig. 7.1). No aetiology has been established, although an embryological remnant is most likely [1]. The use of proton pump inhibitor medication induces hyperplasia of otherwise incidental rests, probably accounting for the increased prevalence of this finding which is now seen in up to 5% of all duodenal bulb biopsies.

Histologically there are well organised, demarcated gastric body-type glands within the intestinal mucosa (Fig. 7.2) [1–3]. The extent varies from a few glands to extensive replacement of native mucosa. Occasionally Helicobacter can be found. Secondary changes may include:

1. Stromal inflammation

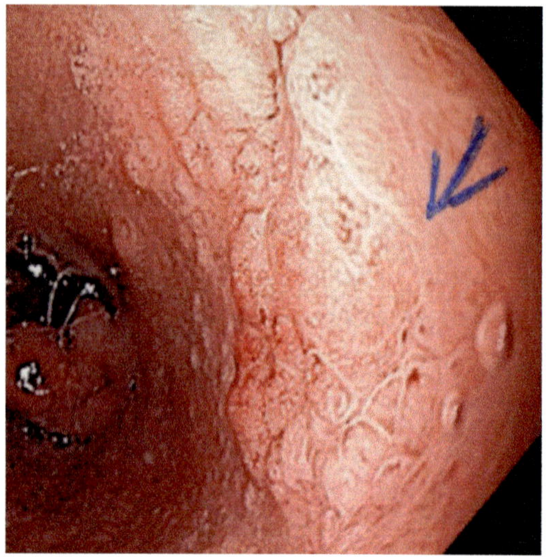

Fig. 7.1 Gastric heterotopia duodenum—endoscopic view

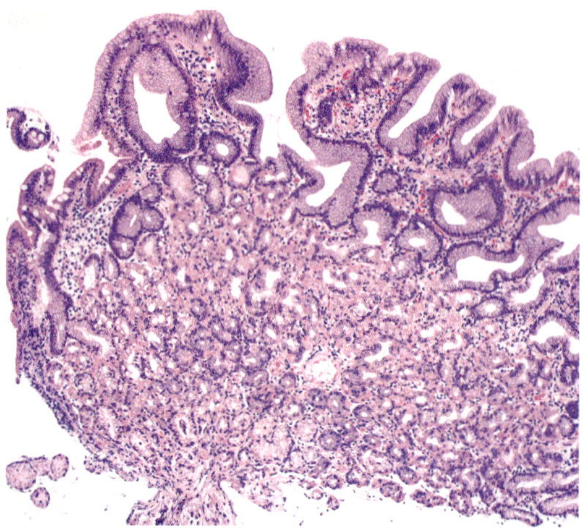

Fig. 7.2 Gastric heterotopia in D1- note the overlying foveolar hyperplasia

2. Helicobacter infection
3. Ulceration (usually with Helicobacter infection)
4. Cystic dilatation resembling cystic fundic gland polyp (particularly in patients taking proton pump inhibitor medication)
5. Foveolar hyperplasia sometimes producing a gastric hyperplastic-type polyp

There is no risk for dysplasia or malignancy. Diagnostic considerations include (1) gastric

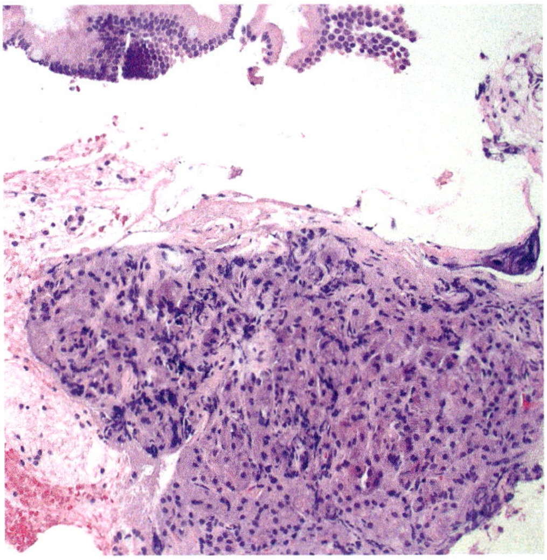

Fig. 7.3 Pancreatic heterotopia with acini

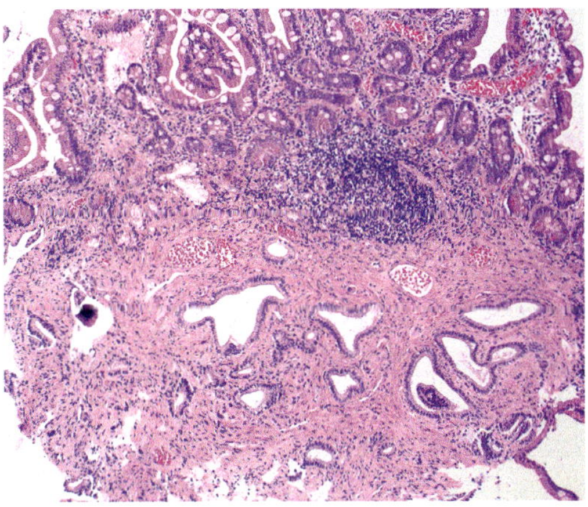

Fig. 7.4 Adenomyoma pattern of pancreatic heterotopia - duct elements within a smooth muscle proliferation

metaplasia, which comprises the antral-type epithelium involving the superficial mucosa of the duodenal bulb region in the setting of duodenitis, and (2) pyloric gland adenoma, which consists of pyloric-type rather than body-type glands.

Pancreatic Heterotopia (Syn. Ectopic Pancreas, Pancreatic Rest)

Pancreatic heterotopia comprises various admixtures of non-neoplastic pancreatic ducts, pancreatic acini and islets of Langerhans. Based on these components, a three-tier classification has been developed [4, 5]:

Class I—all three elements present

Class II—acini and ducts but no islets (Fig. 7.3)

Class III—ducts with rare (or no) acini

A fourth class comprising only endocrine elements also occurs but is exceedingly rare.

The duct structures in Class III lesions may be associated with smooth muscle proliferation and the term "adenomyoma" is alternatively used for this situation (Fig. 7.4).

Pancreatic heterotopia usually resides in the submucosa/base of mucosa and endoscopic biopsies may not include diagnostic tissue.

Cyst formation and development of PanIN in the ductal epithelium can occur.

The differential diagnosis includes (1) ampullary adenomyoma, which is histologically similar to class III pancreatic heterotopias, so knowledge of the site of biopsy is important. In general, ampullary adenomyoma is associated with more smooth muscle proliferation than usual pancreatic heterotopia. The presence of peribiliary glands indicates an ampullary location. (2) Pancreatic metaplasia is very rare in the small intestine and consists of small lobulated collection of pancreatic acinar glands confined to the mucosa; and (3) accessory pancreatic duct is found in the region of the ampulla and has a distinctive duct structure.

Lesions Characterised by Stromal Inflammation and Stromal Expansion (Box 7.1)

Box 7.1 Lesions Characterised by Stromal Inflammation and Stromal Expansion

Mucosal prolapse

Inflammatory fibroid polyp

Hamartomas—juvenile polyposis, Canada-Cronkhite syndrome

Inflammatory pseudopolyp

Pseudopolyp (Benign Mucosal Polyp, Inflammatory Pseudopolyp)

Local trauma or inflammation is most common. Inflammation may be related to Crohn's disease [6] or to medications, e.g. NSAID. Local mucosal ischaemia is a rare cause in the small intestine. It is discussed in more depth in the ileum section.

Mucosal Prolapse-Type Polyps

Mucosal prolapse polyps are a stromal and epithelial expansion induced by traction on the mucosa during peristalsis. Smooth muscle proliferation into the mucosa from a thickened muscularis mucosae is a characteristic feature. Prolapse-type polyps may be related to a submucosal lesion; anatomical abnormality, e.g. sharp angulation in the duodenum; or a mucosal tumour.

The characteristic histological features are crypt elongation and stromal expansion by fibrosis and smooth muscle proliferation from the muscularis mucosae. Inflammation and erosion can occur. Since mucosal prolapse changes may be accompanied by a mucosal-based neoplasm or overlie a submucosal lesion, so careful attention should be paid to these possibilities.

Sometimes the mucosa is normal, and the polyps are due to the expansion of the submucosa, a process akin to that described in the colon as colonic muco-submucosal elongated polyp [6]. The main differential diagnosis is with hamartomatous lesions discussed below. The clinical setting is of most help in separating these two lesions.

Overgrowth of Normal Elements (Hamartomas)

Hamartomas are benign tumour comprising a disorganised collection of tissue elements native to the site of occurrence. They may occur sporadically or as part of several tumour syndromes (discussed below). Solitary hamartomatous polyps of the small intestine are most frequently Peutz-Jeghers type, Brunner's gland type or neuromuscular and vascular type.

The microscopic features of Peutz-Jeghers-type polyp and Brunner's gland hamartoma are discussed below. Neuromuscular- and vascular-type hamartoma comprises an admixture of neural elements, both nerve bundles and ganglion cells, with smooth muscle proliferation. This is mostly within the submucosa and is associated with stricture rather than a discrete polyp. Ectatic vessels may also been seen, particularly at the edge of the areas of frequent mucosal ulceration. There is a clinical and histological overlap with nonsteroidal anti-inflammatory drug-related small bowel diaphragm disease [7]. The absence of a history of NSAID use helps exclude the latter. A well-developed smooth muscle proliferation in the lamina propria and the absence of granulomata are the most helpful features in excluding Crohn's disease (Figs. 7.5 and 7.6) [8].

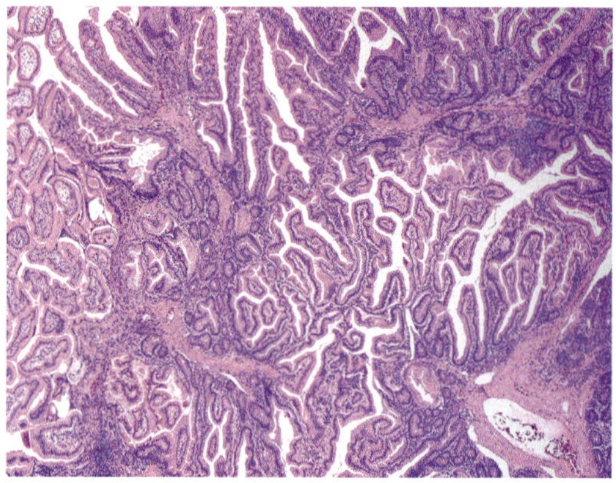

Fig. 7.5 Peutz-Jeghers polyp - arborising smooth muscle core and a proliferation of normal glandular elements

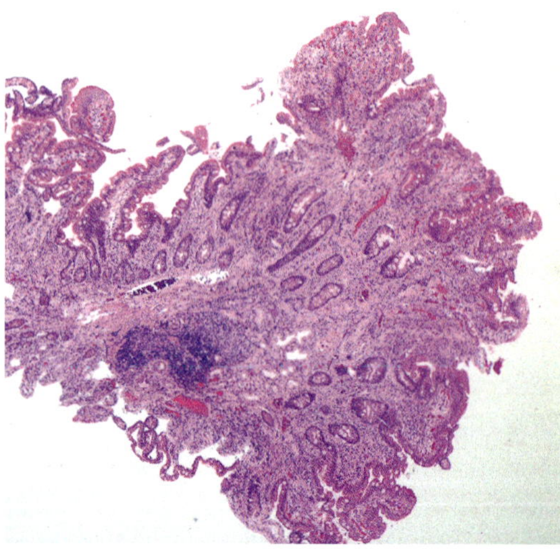

Fig. 7.6 Hamartomatous polyp in duodenum in a patient with Cowden syndrome. Note gland elongation and stromal expansion

Inflammatory Fibroid Polyp

(See page 251)

Cystic Lesions (Box 7.2)

Box 7.2 Cystic Lesions
Brunner's gland cyst
Pneumatosis
Cystic vascular lesions—lymphangiectasia, venous bleb
Post inflammatory

Brunner's Gland Cyst

Brunner's gland cyst is a benign cystic dilatation of a main duct draining the Brunner's glands of the duodenum. It is present in the submucosa but is usually amenable to partial endoscopic sampling (Fig. 7.7). The lesion is underrecognised and is a common cause for a proximal duodenal nodule. It is lined by a single layer of tall columnar mucinous epithelium with clear cytoplasm and basal nuclei. A pseudomicropapillary folded architecture is often present, at least focally (Fig. 7.8) [9]. There is no cytologic atypia, mitotic activity or dysplasia. The adjacent Brunner's gland appears normal. The cyst likely develops as a result of local duct obstruction.

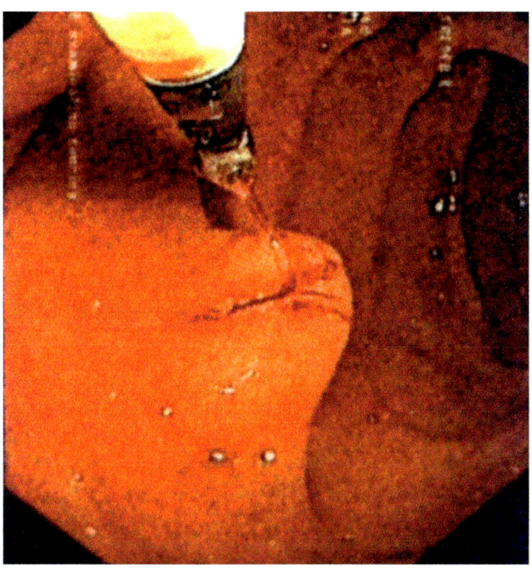

Fig. 7.7 Brunner's gland cyst endoscopic resection picture

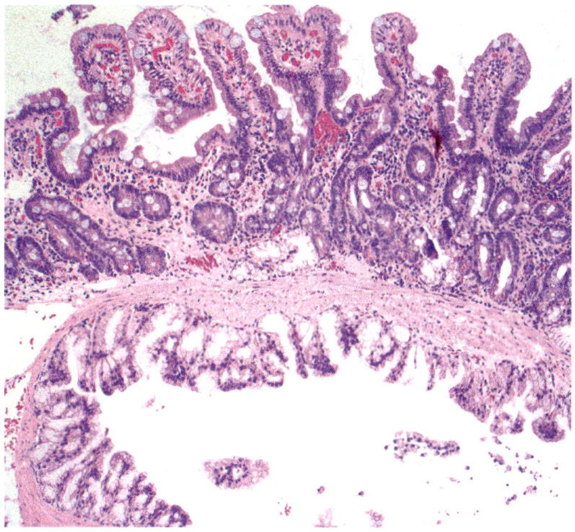

Fig. 7.8 Brunner's gland cyst

Other Cystic Lesions

- Pneumatosis (see page xx)
- Cystic vascular lesions—lymphangiectasia, venous bleb (see page xx)
- Post inflammatory

Glandular Proliferations with No Stromal Invasion

Epithelial Dysplasia

Flat epithelial dysplasia is very uncommon in the duodenum. When present histological features are identical to those described in the large intestine.

Adenoma

Brunner's Gland Adenoma (Syn. Brunneroma, Brunner's Gland Hamartoma)

This is a benign mass of unknown aetiology forming as a result of proliferation of Brunner's glands of the proximal duodenum. It may represent a hamartoma rather than a true neoplasm.

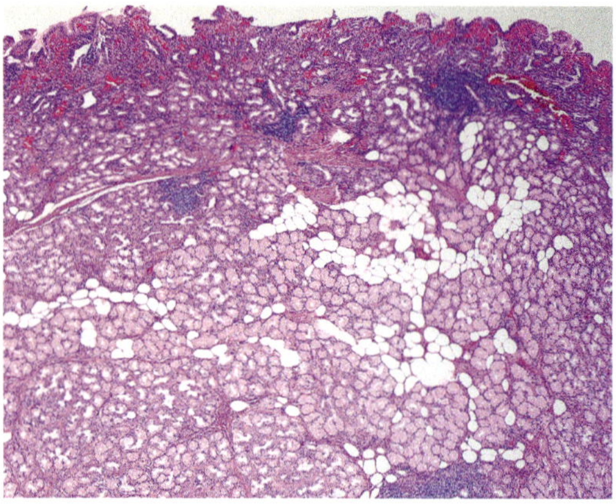

Fig. 7.9 Brunner's gland hamartoma - Brunners gland proliferation, lymphoid follicles and adipose tissue

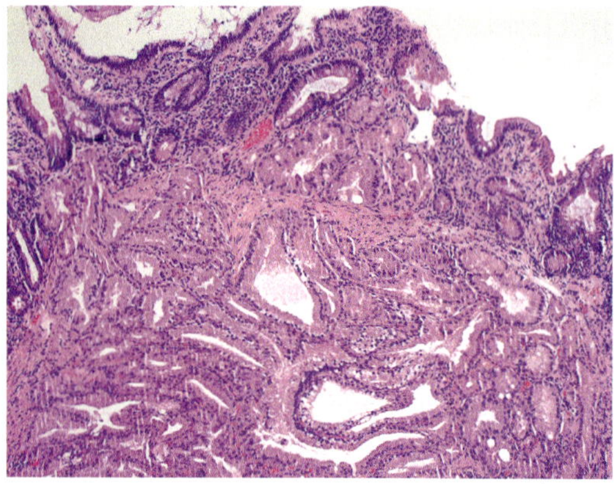

Fig. 7.10 Pyloric gland adenoma - glandular proliferation. The lining cells have clear to light eosinophilic cytoplasm

There is a lobulated proliferation of Brunner's glands within the submucosa and basal mucosa of the duodenum and rarely the proximal jejunum [10, 11]. The lining cells are uniform, cuboidal with pale cytoplasm containing neutral mucin. The gland architecture is regular, although cystic dilatation may occur. There may be admixed smooth muscle proliferation, adipose tissue (Fig. 7.9), lymphoid tissue and/or heterotopic pancreatic acini and ducts. Reactive epithelial changes are often present in the overlying mucosa, particularly in large lesions with surface erosion.

The main differential diagnosis is Brunner's gland hyperplasia resulting from peptic duodenitis. The finding of mucosal inflammation and the less organised architecture are the key distinguishing features. Pyloric gland adenoma is also a consideration; however, the lining cells typically exhibit atypia with prominent nucleoli. Cytoplasmic eosinophilia is usually appreciable in some cells in pyloric gland adenoma but is not found in Brunner's gland adenoma.

Pyloric Gland (Gastric gland-type) Adenoma

Pyloric gland adenoma is a neoplastic proliferation of cells with differentiation towards the gastric pyloric gland cells. Most cases are sporadic, although recent studies suggest an increased prevalence in both Lynch syndrome and familial adenomatous polyposis. Mutations in GNAS and KRAS are frequently found. In the absence of dysplasia, pyloric gland adenoma is characterised by a proliferation of regular, tubular glands lined by cuboidal cells that have clear to eosinophilic cytoplasm and a round nucleus with generally small nucleolus (Fig. 7.10) [12–14]. Development of dysplasia is characterised by architectural irregularity, increase in cell size, increase in nuclear size and increased prominence of nucleoli. Development of invasive carcinoma may be deceptive. A back-to-back gland pattern or infiltration by single tumour cells indicates malignancy.

Pyloric gland adenoma displays cytoplasmic expression of MUC6. Expression of MUC5ac may be found in cells near the luminal aspect of the tumour. Some examples have more extensive MUC5ac expression and the pattern is more of a gastric foveolar type adenoma. The general term of "gastric type adenoma" may be more appropriate for these cases. Differential diagnosis includes gastric heterotopias, which comprise the specialised gastric mucosa distinct from the neutral mucin-producing cells of pyloric gland adenoma. Brunner's gland hyperplasia/adenoma has less cytoarchitectural abnormality than pyloric gland adenoma. Well-differentiated adenocarcinoma may be difficult to separate and require additional tumour material to be examined. Persistent growth or large tumour size is a concerning feature for adenocarcinoma.

Intestinal-Type Adenoma

Intestinal-type adenomas are neoplastic, noninvasive proliferation of dysplastic intestinal lining

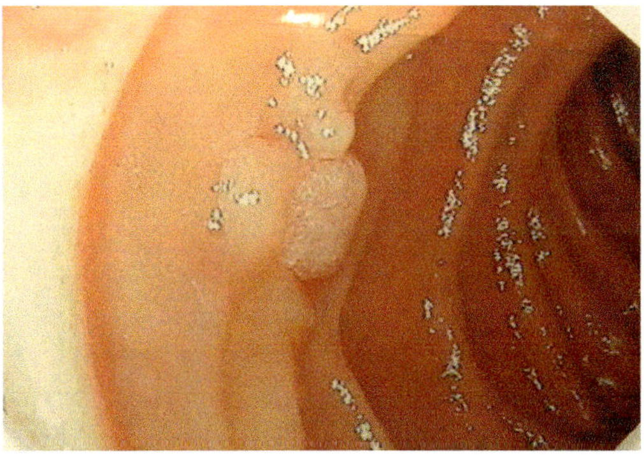

Fig. 7.11 Duodenal adenoma—endoscopic view

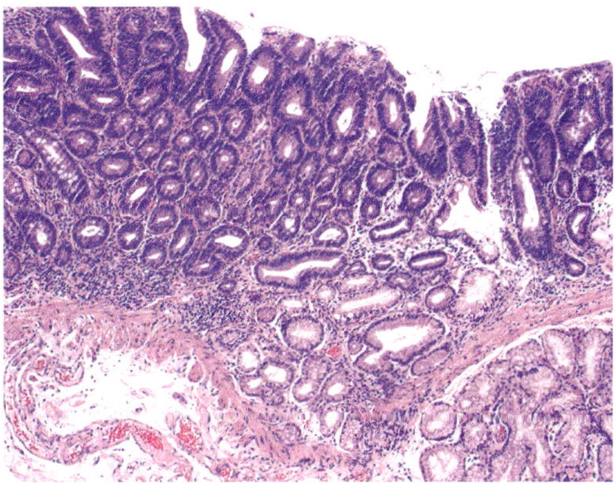

Fig. 7.12 Tubular adenoma of duodenum - morphology identical to the large intestinal counterpart

cells closely akin to their large intestinal counterparts. Most are sporadic; however, some arise in a syndromic setting such as familial adenomatous polyposis syndrome, Lynch syndrome and MutYH associated polyposis.

As with their more common large intestinal counterparts, they may have tubular (Figs. 7.11 and 7.12), tubulovillous or villous architecture, and accompanying dysplasia may be low grade or high grade. Serrated architecture, with a pattern resembling traditional serrated adenoma, may be seen in all or part of the lesion (discussed below; see Fig. 7.12). Gastric surface metaplasia is present in 40% of cases, and a distinctive clear cell change in the cytoplasm of the adenoma cells is present in some cases. Adenomas arising in Lynch syndrome, are likely to be larger, demonstrate tubulovillous architecture and exhibit high grade dysplasia. These generally show a loss of nuclear

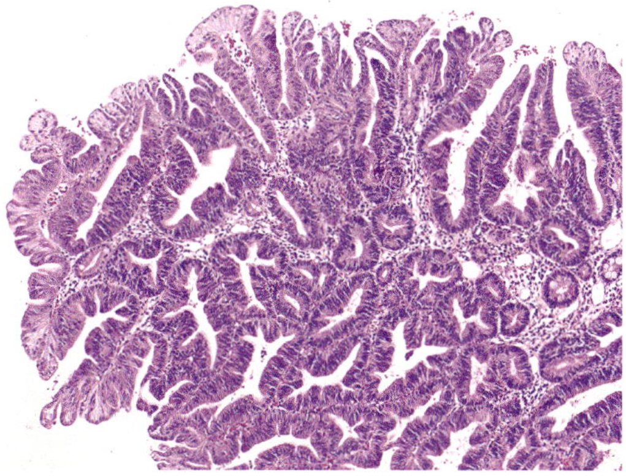

Fig. 7.13 Intestinal adenoma of duodenum with serrated architecture

immunohistochemical reaction for one or more of the mismatch repair proteins, MLH-1, MSH-2, MSH-6 and PMS-2.

Care should be taken to exclude reactive change, seen most commonly at the edge of an ulcer or with acute inflammation. An abrupt change from normal mucosa to the dysplastic epithelium of intestinal adenoma is a helpful feature in this distinction. Intestinal-type adenocarcinoma may arise from an adenoma and the distinction on a small biopsy rests on the finding of complex glandular architecture and stromal desmoplasia or infiltrating single cells. In the ampullary region, pancreatic or biliary tree neoplasia may mimic intestinal-type adenoma particularly on small biopsy.

Serrated Polyps

Serrated lesions of the small intestine remain poorly characterised compared to their colonic relatives (Fig. 7.13). A lesion resembling colonic hyperplastic polyp has been described but is rare [15, 16]. Lesions resembling traditional serrated adenoma of colon, either in pure form or as part of an otherwise conventional intestinal-type adenoma, are reported [17]. Mucosal regeneration after injury, e.g. NSAID induced, may acquire a serrated pattern. Usually there are associated stromal changes of fibrosis and inflammation.

Lesions resembling colonic hyperplastic polyps are innocuous and do not require further

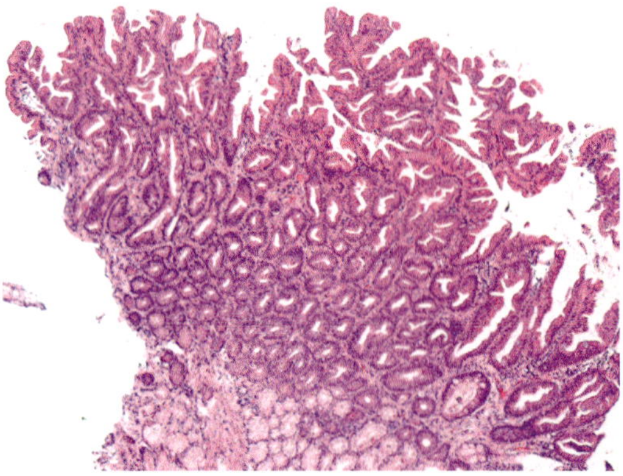

Fig. 7.14 Hyperplastic polyp of duodenum

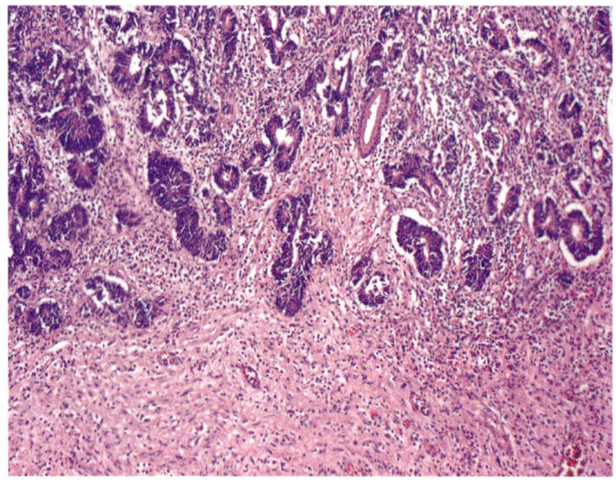

Fig. 7.15 Adenocarcinoma of intestinal type arising in neurofibromatosis with background neurofibroma

treatments (Fig. 7.14). Traditional serrated adenoma-like lesions most likely have a risk for development of malignancy similar to conventional adenomas. Hence, they should be treated and followed up accordingly.

Glandular Proliferations with Stromal Invasion

Blue Cell Pattern

Adenocarcinoma

Usual types of adenocarcinoma are described in Chap. 1. Unusual subtypes include sarcomatoid, choriocarcinoma and hepatoid variants.

Adenocarcinoma: Intestinal Type

This is a malignant neoplasm arising from the glandular epithelium of the small intestine. It is morphologically similar to its colonic counterpart (Fig. 7.15). There is an increased risk in the following conditions:

1. Common:
   - Polyposis syndromes—Familial adenomatous polyposis (FAP), Lynch syndrome (hereditary nonpolyposis colon cancer syndrome, HNPCC), juvenile polyposis syndrome, Peutz-Jeghers syndrome and neurofibromatosis type 1
   - Crohn's disease
2. Uncommon:
   - Celiac disease
   - Congenital abnormalities—Meckel diverticulum, heterotopic pancreas, duplication cysts
   - Chronic inflammation—Ileostomy, ileal pouch radiotherapy

Differential diagnosis of adenocarcinoma in the duodenum:

- Adenocarcinoma of intestinal type (most common).
- Adenocarcinoma of pancreaticobiliary type (see below).
- Adenocarcinoma of pyloric gland type (see below).
- Adenoma with high-grade dysplasia—The absence of clear evidence of lamina propria invasion indicates the lesion is still an adenoma.
- Peutz-Jeghers polyp with pseudoinvasion—Distinction lies in the recognition of the underlying polyp and the absence of cytological dysplasia.
- Adenomyoma of ampulla and heterotopic pancreas devoid of acinar structures. No cytologic atypia is seen.
- Endometriosis—The presence of endometrial stroma and the uniform benign cytology of the endometrial glands allow distinction. A panel of CK7, CK20, CDX-2 and PAX-8 can be applied to difficult cases.

Pink Cell Pattern

Adenocarcinoma of Pancreaticobiliary Type

It presents as a mass arising at the ampulla or periampullary region. In contrast to intestinal-type adenocarcinoma, the component cells are cuboidal and the glands smaller and without the "dirty necrosis" seen in intestinal type adenocarcinoma (Fig. 7.16). As the prognosis of intestinal-type adenocarcinoma is more favourable than pancreaticobiliary-type adenocarcinoma, it is important to make this distinction. A panel of immunohistochemical stains has been shown to be useful (Table 7.1) [18].

Adenocarcinoma of Pyloric Gland (Gastric gland-type) Type

It typically arises from a pre-existing pyloric gland adenoma. Invasion may be difficult to establish on biopsy. Suspicious features are a complex cribriform or small gland pattern. The tumour cells are cuboidal and have clear or lightly eosinophilic cytoplasm in contrast to the pencillate, brightly eosinophilic cells of intestinal-type adenocarcinoma. Immunohistochemical stains aid differentiation of pyloric gland adenocarcinoma (MUC2−, MUC6+, CDX-2−, CK20−) from intestinal adenocarcinoma (MUC2+, MUC6−, CDX-2+, CK20+).

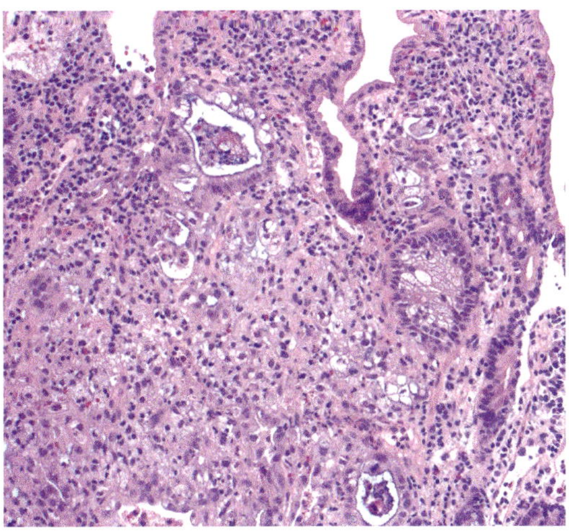

Fig. 7.16 Pancreatic adenocarcinoma in ampulla

Clear Cell Pattern

It is uncommon but may be seen in signet ring cell carcinoma, pyloric gland adenocarcinoma, clear cell sarcoma, metastatic clear cell renal cell carcinoma and clear cell patterns of biliary and pancreatic adenocarcinoma. Rarely neuroendocrine neoplasm may assume a clear cell pattern.

Neuroendocrine Neoplasm

Neuroendocrine neoplasm of the small intestine may be derived from neuroendocrine cells originating in the foregut (duodenum) or midgut (jejunum, ileum). A variety of terms are used for tumours in the small intestine that have in common the feature of neuroendocrine differentiation. For example, tumours are often designated based on their active hormone production or lack there of—gastrinoma, somatostatinoma and non-functional neuroendocrine neoplasm ("carcinoids") (Figs. 7.17 and 7.18). General features are listed in Table 7.2 [19, 20].

Neuroendocrine neoplasm in the proximal small intestine show morphological features of neuroendocrine differentiation as described in Chap. 1. There is a spectrum of cell size and of cytoplasmic characteristic with pink cyto-

Table 7.1 Immunohistochemical stains

	Immunohistochemical stain				
Adenocarcinoma type	MUC 1	MUC 2	CDX 2	CK7	CK20
Intestinal	−	+	+	±	+
Pancreaticobiliary	+	−	−	+	±

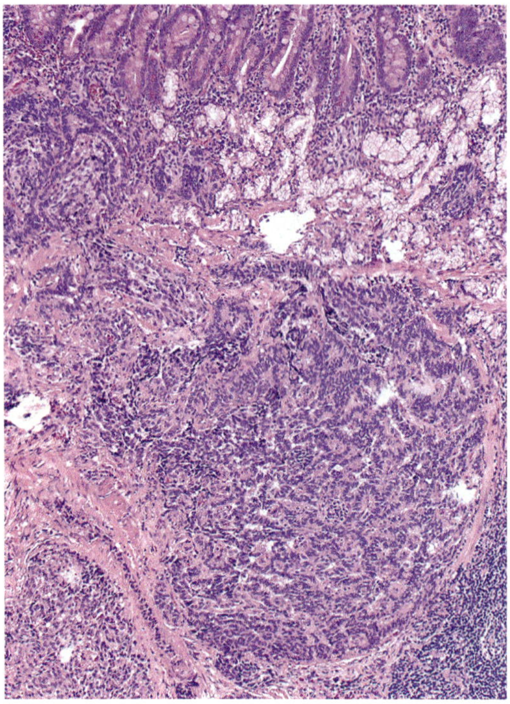

Fig. 7.17 "Carcinoid" tumour duodenum

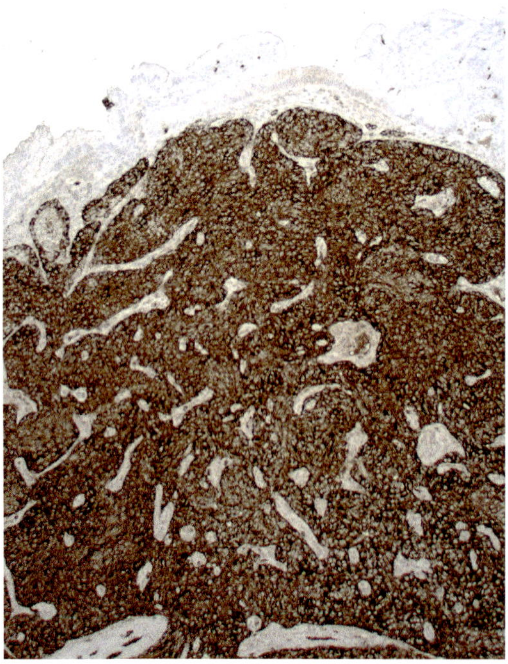

Fig. 7.18 "Carcinoid" tumour duodenum - chromogranin stain with positive reaction

Table 7.2 Neuroendocrine neoplasm of the proximal small intestine: summary features

• 20% of all GIT NENs
• 1–3% all primary duodenal neoplasms • M:F = 2:1 • Mean age sixth decade • Syndromic—MEN1, —6%; NF1, rare • 90% nonfunctional • 10%—functional (mostly gastrinoma producing Zollinger-Ellison syndrome. This is associated with MEN1 in 50%) • Multiple—10% • Periampullary/ampullary location in 20% • 75% are <2 cm (mucosa/submucosa) • Regional lymph node metastases in 50% (early) • Liver metastases in 10% • Prognosis 5-year survival I. Localised—80–95% II. Regional LN—65–75% III. Distant metastases—5–10%

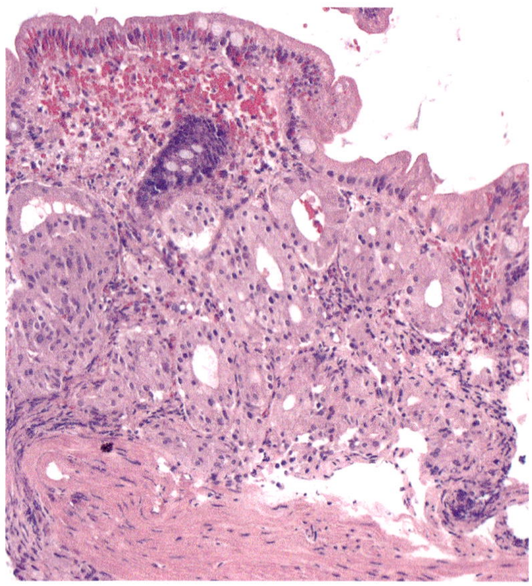

Fig. 7.19 Somatostatinoma - pseudoglandular architecture

plasm being most common but clear cell and the light base of the change are also seen. Pseudoglandular architecture and psammomatous-type dystrophic calcification may occur with somatostatinoma (Fig. 7.19), and amyloid deposition may be encountered in any functional tumour.

In addition to usual immunohistochemical markers of neuroendocrine differentiation, there may be specific hormone production in tumour cells (which does not necessarily correlate with release into the blood or with the production of a specific clinical syndrome), e.g. insulin, gastrin, glucagon and somatostatin. However, demonstration of this is not necessary for histological classification. Because of the variable appearance, duodenal neuroendocrine neoplasm may elicit a wide differential diagnosis. This includes melanoma, GIST, neuroectodermal tumour, lymphoma, paraganglioma (and gangliocytic paraganglioma) and clear cell sarcoma. A panel of immunohistochemical stains that includes neuroendocrine markers, keratin, CD117, S-100 and LCA will usually allow distinction.

Pseudoinvasion

Pseudoinvasion may be seen in intestinal-type adenoma and also in Peutz-Jeghers polyps. The absence of stromal desmoplasia is an important finding in favour of pseudoinvasion. In Peutz-Jeghers polyps, the lining epithelium will be bland and these will be associated prominent smooth muscle proliferation.

Mixed Epithelial and Stromal Pattern

See Box 7.3.

Box 7.3 Mixed Epithelial and Stromal Pattern
Gangliocytic paraganglioma
Synovial sarcoma
Metastases
Endometriosis

Gangliocytic Paraganglioma

Gangliocytic paraganglioma is a distinctive neuroendocrine neoplasm usually developing in the ampullary region of the duodenum and characterised by differentiation towards neuroendocrine cell, Schwann cell and ganglion cell lineages (Figs. 7.20, 7.21, 7.22, 7.23, and 7.24).

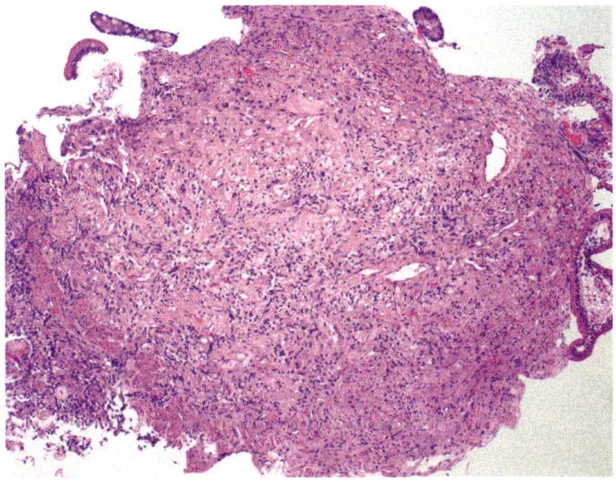

Fig. 7.20 Gangliocytic paraganglioma - note the admixture of elements

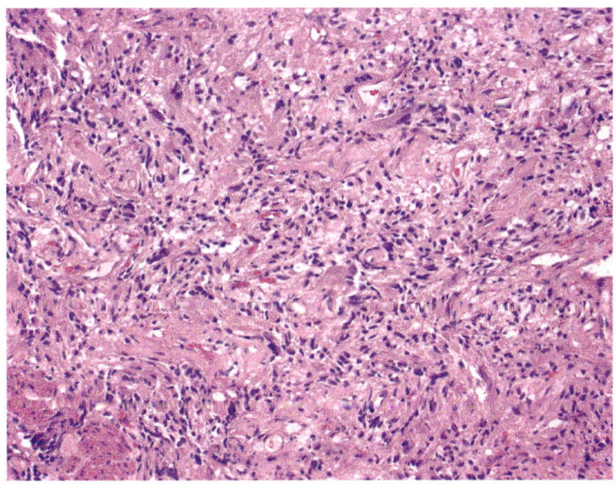

Fig. 7.21 Gangliocytic paraganglioma - neuroendocrine and schwann cell elements

Histologically, the components are an admixture of:

1. Spindle-shaped Schwann cells forming background supporting stroma (S-100 positive).
2. Ganglion cells—either clustered or dispersed within the Schwann cell stroma—S-100 and synaptophysin positive.
3. Well-differentiated neuroendocrine cells in nested, trabecular or papillary arrangements—immunoreactive for keratin and neu-

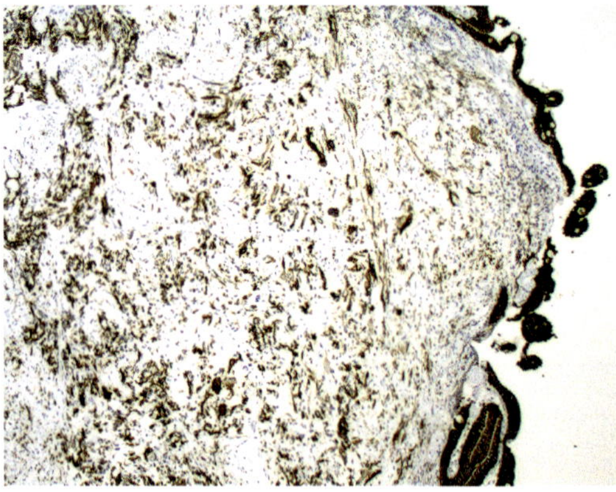

Fig. 7.22 Gangliocytic paraganglioma Keratin stain

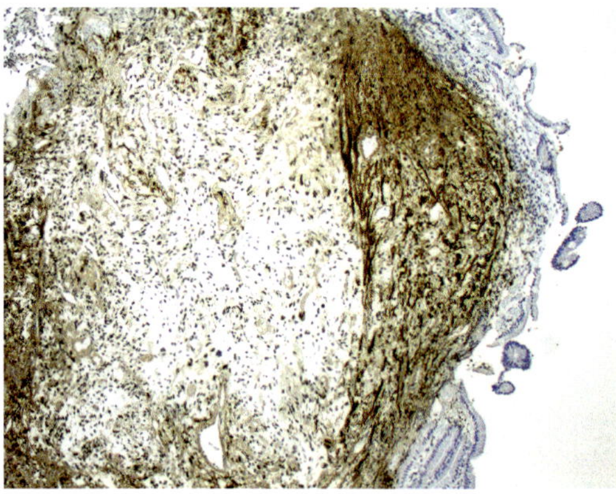

Fig. 7.23 Gangliocytic paraganglioma S-100 stain

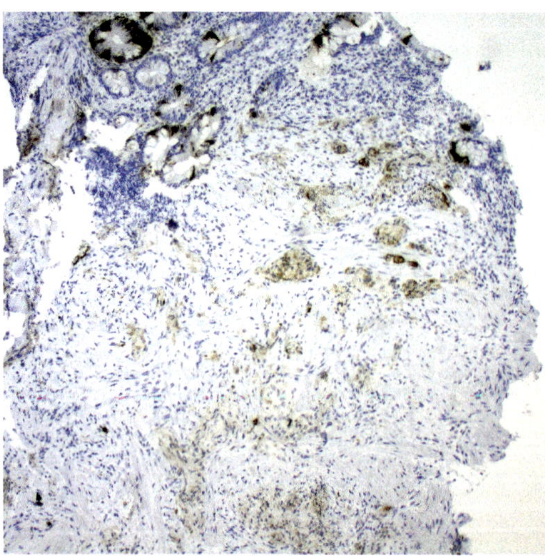

Fig. 7.24 Gangliocytic paraganglioma chromogranin stain

roendocrine stains (e.g. synaptophysin, chromogranin, CD56).

Spindle or epithelial elements might also dominate the appearance, and deeper levels can be useful in identifying other cell types. The differential diagnosis includes:

1. Spindle cell elements—nerve sheath tumour and GIST. GIST can be separated on the basis of immunohistochemical positivity for CD117 and/or DOG-1 stains.
2. Epithelial elements—neuroendocrine neoplasm, as discussed above, are devoid of other elements. Paraganglioma does not contain ganglion cells and exhibits a sustentacular pattern of S-100 reactive cells around the tumour cell nests. Adenocarcinoma should not be reactive for S-100 or neuroendocrine markers such as chromogranin and synaptophysin.
3. Ganglion cells—ganglioneuroma. The presence of neuroendocrine elements is important to this distinction.

Although rare reports of regional lymph node metastases exist [21], there have been no tumour-related deaths and the neoplasm is regarded as indolent.

Diffuse Round Cell Pattern

The causes of this pattern are described below in the following tables.

Blue Cell Pattern

See Table 7.3.

Pink Cell Pattern

See Table 7.4.

Clear Cell Pattern

See Table 7.5.

Table 7.3 Blue cell pattern

Diagnosis	Immunohistochemical profile
Lymphoma	LCA, CD3 or CD20
Plasma cell tumours	CD138
Leukaemia	MPO, CD43
Carcinoma—adenocarcinoma	AE1/AE3
Neuroendocrine neoplasm	AE1/AE3, neuroendocrine markers
Mastocytosis	CD117, CD25
Sarcoma—Ewing's/PNET	CD99
Metastasis	Variable pattern

PNET = primitive neuroectodermal tumour

Table 7.4 Pink cell pattern

Diagnosis	Immunohistochemical profile
GIST	CD117, DOG1
Histiocytic tumours	CD68
Glomus tumour	SMA
Granular cell tumour	S-100, SOX10
Langerhans cell histiocytosis	S-100, CD1a
Epithelioid smooth muscle tumour	SMA, desmin, H-caldesmon
Carcinoma—squamous	P63, High molecular weight CK
Metastasis	Variable pattern

GIST = gastrointestinal stromal tumour

Table 7.5 Clear cell pattern

Diagnosis	Immunohistochemical profile
GIST	CD117, DOG1
Carcinoma—any	AE1/AE3
Histiocytic lesions (xanthoma)	CD68
Lymphoma	LCA
Mastocytosis	CD117, CD25
Langerhans cell histiocytosis	S-100, CD1a
Clear cell sarcoma	S-100, HMB45
PEComa	HMB45
Epithelioid smooth muscle tumour	SMA, desmin, H-caldesmon
Metastasis—clear cell renal cell carcinoma	CD10

GIST = gastrointestinal stromal tumour

Table 7.6 Primary small intestine non-Hodgkin's lymphoma [22]

Tumour type	Frequency compared to all GIT lymphoma sites
Diffuse large B-cell lymphoma	38%
Follicular lymphoma	23%
Enteropathy-associated T-cell lymphoma	10%
Post-transplant lymphoproliferative disorder	10%
Burkitt's lymphoma	8%
MALT	5%

MALT = mucosa-associated lymphoid tissue

Table 7.7 Small and large cell patterns of lymphomas

Small cell pattern	Large cell pattern
Follicular lymphoma MALT lymphoma Chronic lymphocytic leukaemia IPSID	Diffuse large B-cell lymphoma Hodgkin's lymphoma Plasmablastic lymphoma Burkitt's lymphoma T-cell lymphoma
Usually B cell	B or T cell

MALT = mucosa-associated lymphoid tissue; IPSID = immunoproliferative small intestine disease

Lymphoma

The small intestine is a common site for gastrointestinal tract lymphoma. Follicular lymphoma and diffuse large B-cell lymphoma are most frequent (Table 7.6) [22].

It is useful for the initial workup to divide lymphomas of the small intestine in terms of predominant cell size. The differential diagnosis and required immunohistochemical panel can then be applied more effectively (Table 7.7).

In this chapter, Lymphomas that may be encountered in endoscopic biopsy material from the proximal small intestine are described below.

B-Cell Non-Hodgkin's Lymphoma

Follicular B-Cell Lymphoma of the Gastrointestinal Tract

It is a distinctive subset of B-cell follicular lymphoma with generally indolent behaviour, developing as a primary lesion in the gastrointestinal

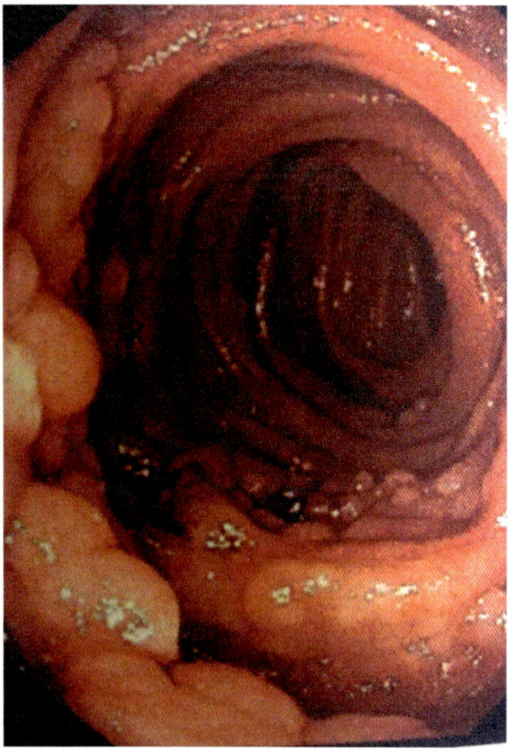

Fig. 7.25 Endoscopic picture of follicular lymphoma in duodenum

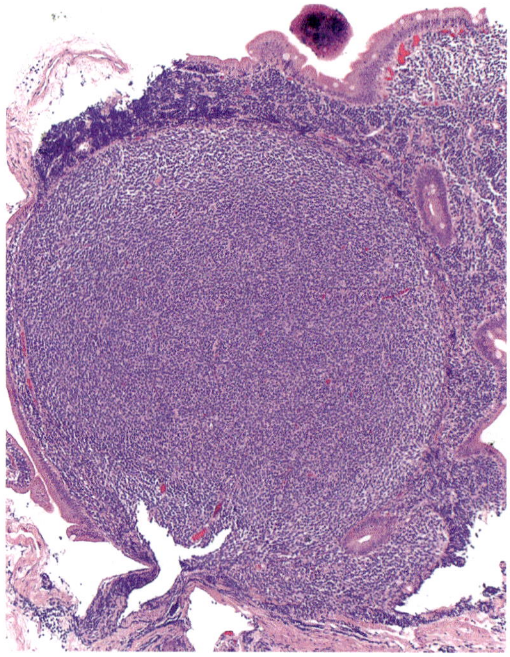

Fig. 7.26 Follicular lymphoma

tract, in particular the second part of duodenum (Fig. 7.25). Follicular architecture is characteristic. The tumour cells are small with irregular nuclear outline resembling centrocytes (Figs. 7.26). Variable numbers of blastic cells resembling centroblasts may be seen; however, tingible body macrophages are conspicuously absent. Centrocyte-like cells may extend in a diffuse fashion into the adjacent lamina propria.

Duodenal follicular lymphoma exhibits the following:

1. Immunophenotype: CD10 (+) (Fig. 7.27), B-cell lymphoma 2 (BCL-2) (+) (Fig. 7.28), BCL-6 (+) and loose CD21 (+) follicular dendritic cell network (often located at the periphery of the follicle). CD10 (+) cells extending in a sheet-like pattern into the lamina propria are particularly suggestive of this lymphoma. It has recently been suggested that the cell of origin may be a memory B cell, although previously follicular lymphoma in the gastrointestinal tract was likened to mucosa-associated lymphoid tissue (MALT) lymphoma. The combination of (1) expression of α-4-β-7 integrin, which is a mucosal homing receptor, (2) VH gene deviation and (3) IgA production suggests that tumour cells are derived from mucosal B cells.

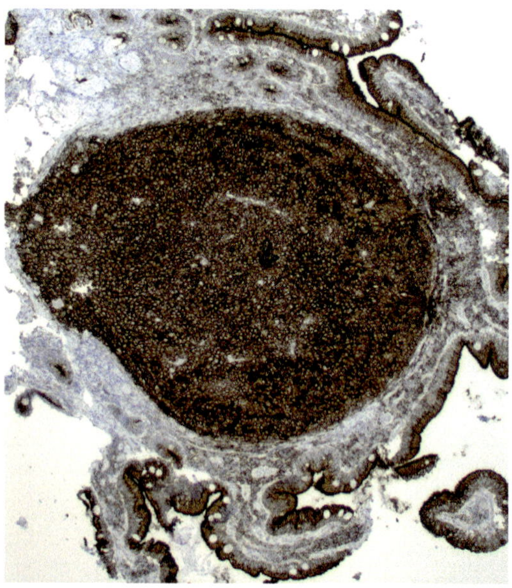

Fig. 7.27 Follicular lymphoma CD10

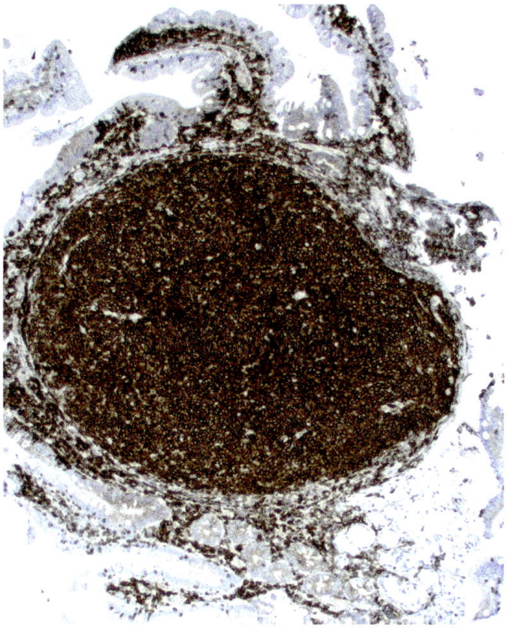

Fig. 7.28 Follicular lymphoma bcl2

2. Flow cytometry: See table (Chapter 1).
3. Molecular: Clonal restriction for Ig heavy and light chain genes. Bcl-2 rearrangement.

Follicular lymphoma should be distinguished from [23, 24]:

1. Reactive lymphoid hyperplasia—features of reactive lymphoid hyperplasia include the presence of tingible body macrophages; absence of Bcl-2 and CD10 confined to germinal centres only
2. MALT lymphoma. Follicular lymphoma differs by having CD10 positive B cells extending into the lamina propria; and no lymphoepithelial lesions

Extranodal Marginal Zone Mucosa-Associated Lymphoid Tissue (MALT) Lymphoma

May present as a primary lesion in the small intestine as a single mass or rarely as a lymphomatoid polyposis. Diagnostic features are discussed in the gastric tumour chapter. IPSID is a distinct subset presenting in the small intestine and is discussed below.

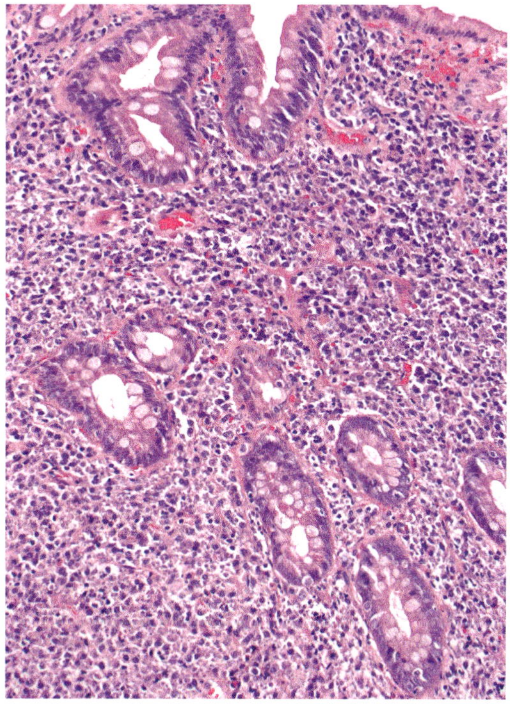

Fig. 7.29 IPSID - note plasmacytoid cell rich infiltrate

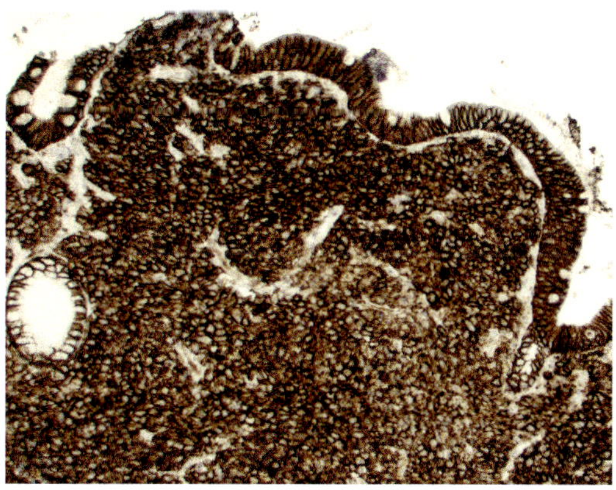

Fig. 7.30 IPSID positive reaction with CD138

Immunoproliferative Small Intestinal Disease (IPSID)/α Heavy Chain Disease (Syn. Mediterranean Lymphoma)

Is a subtype of small intestinal MALT lymphoma predominantly occurring in young adults of Middle Eastern or Mediterranean origin. IPSID is associated with *Campylobacter jejuni* infection and early stage disease may respond to antibiotic therapy [25]. Poor sanitation, concurrent parasitic infection and low socioeconomic class are risk factors for disease development.

Three stages of disease are recognised. In stage A, there is an infiltrate of essentially normal appearing lymphocytes and plasma cells in the small intestinal mucosa without disturbance of villous architecture. In stage B, nodular collections of mildly atypical lymphoid cells expand the lamina propria and cause villous blunting. Lymphoepithelial lesions and follicular colonisation can be seen. Stage C disease is a fully developed malignancy with diffuse sheets of atypical, large cells, resembling immunoblasts or plasmablasts (Fig. 7.29). Reed-Sternberg-like cells may be seen.

Immunohistochemical and molecular features are summarised in Table. The fully developed malignancy is characterised by positive staining for CD20, CD138 (Fig. 7.30) and α-heavy chain (but no light chain staining). Early in the process, the combination of villous blunting and a plasma cell-rich infiltrate in the lamina propria can resemble coeliac disease or other similar enteropathy. The absence of intraepithelial lymphocytosis and the density of the infiltrate point to the correct diagnosis. Later, the process may be mistaken for diffuse large B-cell lymphoma or plasmablastic lymphoma. Early stage disease often responds to antibiotic therapy (30–70% remission). Untreated IPSID progresses to lymphoplasmacytic and immunoblastic diffuse large cell lymphoma that invades the intestinal wall, involves mesenteric lymph nodes and may metastasize to a distant organ [26]. Later stage disease requires radiotherapy and chemotherapy.

B-Chronic Lymphocytic Leukaemia/ Small Lymphocytic Lymphoma

This lymphoma is uncommon in the small intestine and is generally only seen in advanced disease with poorer prognosis. A diffuse small cell lymphoid infiltrate is seen. There may be single cell infiltration of the epithelium.

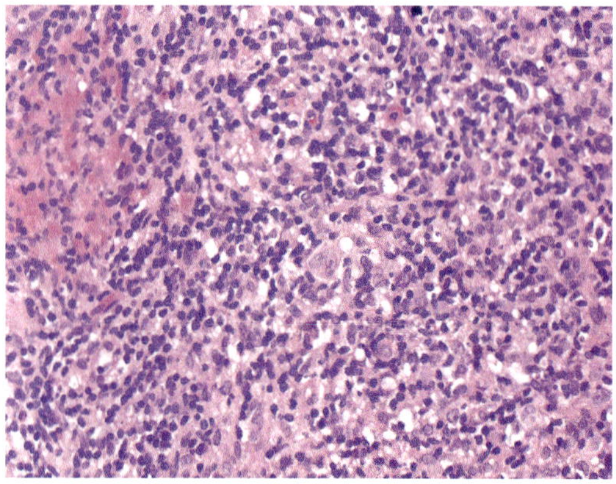

Fig. 7.31 PTLD in ileum range of cell sizes and a Reed Sternberg-like cell centrally. CMV was present in the endothelial cells

Post-transplant Lymphoproliferative Disorder

This is a lymphoproliferative disorder arising in immunosuppressed organ transplant recipients usually in association with EBV infection. Most cases are B-cell derived, although T-cell post-transplant lymphoproliferative disorder (PTLD) does exist (Fig. 7.31).

Immunosuppression required to prevent transplant rejection is the underlying cause. EBV infection is the main viral cofactor; however, it is not solely responsible for lymphomagenesis. Alterations in oncogenes and tumour suppressor genes and epigenetic changes, particularly, hypermethylation, are important. Plasmacytoid dendritic cells (PDCs) that are activated by viral infections probably play a pathogenetic role as do regulatory T cells (Treg cells), which modulate the immune reactions once incited by antigen [27].

There is a wide spectrum of histopathologic findings from B-cell (plasma cell-rich) hyperplasia to lymphoma. The attached table provides a classification scheme. The lymphoma is most often polymorphic characterised by an admixture of small lymphocytes, plasmacytoid cells, large immunoblastic cells and occasional multilobulated cells resembling Reed-Sternberg cells. Monomorphic lymphoma is usually a diffuse process with large immunoblastic or plasmoblastic cells. Geographic necrosis may be seen (Table 7.8).

Immunohistochemical and molecular features are tumour cells immunoreactive with pan B-cell

Table 7.8 Classification of PTLD [28]

(1) Early lesions
(a) Reactive plasmacytic hyperplasia
(b) Infectious mononucleosis-like lesions
(2) Polymorphic PTLD
(3) Monomorphic PTLD (classified according to lymphoma they resemble)
B-cell neoplasms
(a) Diffuse large B-cell lymphoma (DLBCL)
(b) Burkitt's lymphoma
(c) Plasma cell myeloma
(d) Plasmacytoma-like lesions
(e) Others
T-cell neoplasms
(a) Peripheral T-cell lymphoma not otherwise specified
(b) Hepatosplenic T-cell lymphoma
(c) Others
(4) Classical Hodgkin's lymphoma-type (HL-PTLD) and HL-like PTLD

PTLD = post-transplant lymphoproliferative disorder

markers CD19, CD20 and CD79a. EBV in situ hybridisation (EBV-ISH) is usually positive. Monoclonal expression of either kappa or lambda light chain is seen mostly in the monomorphic cases. PCR analysis of immunoglobulin gene rearrangement is often monoclonal. T-cell PTLD tumour cells are immunoreactive with the T-cell markers CD3 and CD5 and demonstrate clonal T-cell receptors αβ or γδ on PCR analysis. The differential diagnosis includes a broad range of B- and T-cell NHL and also Hodgkin's lymphoma, depending of the dominant morphologic pattern. In practice, the clinical setting generally provides the correct diagnosis.

T-Cell/NK-T-Cell Non-Hodgkin's Lymphoma

Ulcerative Jejunoileitis

Ulcerative jejunoileitis is a clinical syndrome of multiple intestinal ulcers, frequently complicated by haemorrhage, perforation or obstruction that is due to a coeliac disease-related clonal T-cell proliferation. This disease is infrequently sampled by routine endoscopic techniques, however, push enteroscopy may allow for biopsies to be taken. Histologically there is ulceration, acute and chronic inflammation, fibrosis and pseudopyloric gland metaplasia. Features of coeliac disease are usually evident in the adjacent small bowel mucosa. There may be collagenous sprue.

The intraepithelial lymphocytes demonstrate an aberrant immunophenotype identical to RCD2 in the majority of cases. TCR monoclonality is present.

Differential diagnosis includes other causes of multifocal ulceration:

- Drug injury, e.g. NSAIDs
- Vasculitis
- CMUSE
- Crohn's disease

These lack a history or serological evidence of coeliac disease and there are no coeliac disease enteropathy changes in non-ulcerated mucosa. Enteropathy-associated T-cell lymphoma forms a disease spectrum with UJ and separation is based on the identification of a mass lesion with ETTL.

Enteropathy-Associated T-Cell Lymphoma (Enteropathy-Type T-Cell Lymphoma, Intestinal T-cell Lymphoma)

This is a rare T-cell malignancy of the small intestine that usually, but not exclusively, arises in association with gluten-sensitive enteropathy. The association of this lymphoma with coeliac disease is based on the following evidence: (1) the presence of coeliac disease enteropathy in the adjacent mucosa, (2) history of long-standing coeliac disease in up to 10% of patients, (3) ETTL prevalence parallel coeliac disease prevalence and (4) high prevalence of HLA DQ2 haplotype in both diseases.

Two morphological variants are recognised (see Table 7.9). Prognosis is poor in both subtypes. Death is often as a result of severe malnutrition or as a complication of intestinal perforation [29, 30].

Extranodal NK-T-Cell Lymphoma, Nasal Type (ENKTL)

This is a mostly extranodal EBV infection-related lymphoma of NK-cell origin more often than T-cell origin. It is most commonly encountered in adult

Table 7.9 Two types of morphological variants

Type I or classical variant (Enteropathy associated T cell lymphoma)	Type 2 or monomorphic variant (monomorphic epitheliotropic T cell lymphoma)
• 80% to 90% of cases • Strong association with coeliac disease • Intermediate to large cells with abundant pale eosinophilic cytoplasm and round or slightly irregular central nuclei with prominent nucleoli • Associated inflammatory infiltrate of histiocytes and eosinophils • Adjacent coeliac enteropathy • CD3+, CD5−, CD7+, CD4−, CD8− (occasional +), CD103+, cytotoxic T-cell marker (TIA, granzyme, perforin) +, CD30 +/- and CD56− (rare +) • Gains 1q and 5q	• 10% to 20% • Asian populations, uncommon association with coeliac disease • Small to intermediate size cells with inconspicuous nucleoli and minimal cytoplasm (monomorphic) • No associated inflammation • Adjacent intraepithelial lymphocytosis (without villous atrophy) • CD3+, CD5−, CD8+, CD56+, CD30-, cytotoxic T-cell markers (TIA1+/−, granzyme B+, perforin+/−) • Gain 9q or deletion 16q, STAT5B mutation, MYC amplification

males of oriental or South American origin. The gastrointestinal tract is one of the more frequent sites of occurrence. The lymphoma is pleomorphic with an admixture of small and large malignant cells together with a background of eosinophils, plasma cells and histiocytes. Angioinvasive and angiodestructive growth are common leading to zones of necrosis and prominent karyorrhectic debris [31, 32]. In some tumours, there is predominance of small cells without necrosis.

Most cases have an NK-cell immunophenotype: CD2+, CD45RO+, CD43+ and CD56+. Clonality for T-cell receptor is $\alpha\beta-$ and $\gamma\delta-$. Surface CD3 is usually absent, but cytoplasmic CD3 may be detected on paraffin sections because NK cells contain an epsilon (ε) chain of the CD3 molecular that is recognised by a CD3 immunohistochemical stain. T-cell cases are characterised by surface CD3 expression and clonal T-cell receptor $\alpha\beta+$ or $\gamma\delta+$. EBV genome is demonstrable in the tumour cells (EBV-ISH+). Differential diagnosis includes:

- Reactive/infectious process associated with extensive necrosis, e.g. mycobacterium tuberculosis infection. Attention to the finding of atypia in the lymphoid cells should allow distinction.
- Other large cell lymphomas, particularly those displaying angioinvasive growth. The immunophenotypic characterisation will separate most cases.
- Vasculitic processes—The finding of an extensive and atypical lymphoid infiltrate should alert to the possibility of lymphoma.
- NK-cell enteropathy [33]—An expanding range of benign NK-cell proliferations is recognised. These may involve the gastrointestinal tract and be sufficiently dense as to cause concern for lymphoma. EBV infection may be involved in the pathogenesis of some cases.

The tumour is aggressive with high mortality. Localised disease may respond to radiotherapy.

Hodgkin's Lymphoma

Hodgkin's lymphoma is overwhelmingly a nodal disease and is very unlikely to present in the small intestine in primary form. A primary enteric lymphoma containing Reed-Sternberg-like cells is more likely to represent a form of T-cell lymphoma or PTLD than to represent Hodgkin's lymphoma.

Haemopoietic Disorders with Plasmacytic Differentiation

Extramedullary Plasmacytoma (EMP)

Primary enteric plasmacytoma is rarely encountered in the small intestine. Well-differentiated lesions may mimic a primary plasma cell-rich inflammatory process (Fig. 7.32). The near absence of other inflammatory cells is a clue to a neoplastic process. Fortunately, immunohistochemical staining for kappa and lambda light chains is usually diagnostic, showing a clear light chain restriction. Plasma cell-rich MALT lymphoma and IPSID are other diagnostic possibilities. Absence of reaction with the B-cell marker CD20 is a clue the lesion is not a form of B-cell lymphoma. The plasma cell

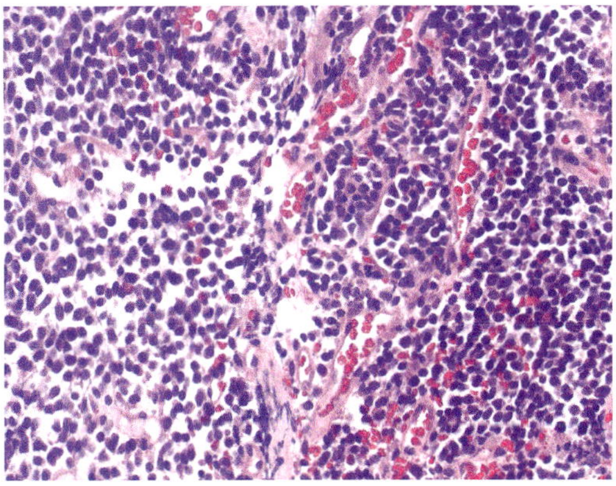

Fig. 7.32 Plasmacytoma duodenum - note the sheet like pattern of plasmacytic cells that can mimic an inflammatory process. The absence of other cell types is a clue to its neoplastic nature

nature of the tumour can be confirmed with plasma cell markers CD38 and CD138. Poorly differentiated lesions ("anaplastic plasmacytoma") have a broad differential diagnosis including high-grade lymphoma, metastatic melanoma and carcinoma. With respect to the latter, it should be remembered that some adenocarcinomas will express CD138 and many plasmacytomas express EMA.

Plasmablastic Lymphoma

Plasmablastic lymphoma (PBL) is a rare aggressive B-cell lymphoproliferative disorder that is most commonly encountered in the oral cavity of HIV-positive patients. Small intestinal location is uncommon. Cases of non-immunosuppressed, often elderly, patients are increasingly identified. Microscopically there is large cell lymphoma with plasmacytic differentiation (see Fig. 7.32). The immunophenotype is positive for CD79a (CD20 is negative), CD138, CD38, MUM-1 and CD10. EBV is often positive by in situ hybridisation. EMA may also be expressed. The Ki67 proliferation index is typically high [34].

Lymphoplasmacytic Lymphoma

Lymphoplasmacytic lymphoma is a B-cell lymphoma with plasmacytic differentiation that underlies most cases of Waldenstrom's macroglobulinaemia. The latter is characterised by deposition of IgM paraprotein producing eosinophilic, homogenous and strongly PAS+, begins within the villous lymphatics and eventually fills the lamina propria.

Other Haemopoietic Disorders

Extensive plasmacytic differentiation may be encountered in MALT lymphoma, IPSID and post-transplant lymphoproliferative disorder.

Leukaemia

Leukemic infiltration of the small intestine is rare. When present, there is generally evidence of systemic disease, although it may signal relapse of known disease. Chronic lymphocytic leukaemia, acute myeloid (myelogenous) leukaemia and acute lymphoblastic leukaemia are most commonly encountered.

Granulocytic sarcoma refers to an extramedullary tumour of myeloblasts and/or immature myeloid cells often a forerunner to the development of acute myelogenous leukaemia, but may also signal impending blast crisis in the setting of a myeloproliferative disorder or leukemic transformation in myelodysplastic syndrome. Intestinal involvement is sometimes a primary presentation of disease. The small intestine is the most common site of occurrence in the gastrointestinal tract. It tends to present as a polyp or larger ulcerated mass. Microscopically there is a diffusely infiltrating population of medium to large cells with occasional prominent nucleoli and minimal to moderate eosinophilic cytoplasm. A variable number of admixed maturing eosinophils and neutrophils are typically present in the more differentiated lesion. The immunophenotype is positive expression of CD43, in the absence of CD3 staining, lysozyme, CD34, CD117 and myeloperoxidase (MPO). Flow cytometry is also helpful. Characteristic cytogenetic abnormalities t(8;21)(q22;q22) and inv(16)(p13q22) are often found. Treatment should consist of systemic chemotherapy tailored to the treatment of AML, possibly in conjunction with surgical resection or radiation [35].

Table 7.10 Histiocytic infiltrates

Histiocytic disorders of the small intestine
Xanthogranulomatous inflammation
Infections rich in histiocytic cells, e.g. Whipple's disease, MAIC
Neoplasms, e.g. Rosai-Dorfman disease, Langerhans cell histiocytosis, juvenile xanthogranuloma, Erdheim-Chester disease, crystal storing histiocytosis, histiocytic sarcoma
Malakoplakia

Histiocytic Disorders

Xanthoma

Xanthoma is a collection of foamy histiocytes that forms single or multiple tumours. These may involve the mucosa only or the full thickness of the small intestinal wall. Multiple lesions may be present throughout the gastrointestinal tract. Hyperlipidaemia is an infrequent association in contradistinction to soft tissue xanthoma. A response to local mucosal injury is postulated as the aetiology in most cases. Confirmation of the histiocytic nature of the cells is via positive immunoreaction for histiocytic makers, e.g. CD68. The condition is benign and asymptomatic unless large. The main diagnostic considerations[2] are included in Table 7.10 [36, 37].

Malakoplakia

This is a reactive process caused by inadequate processing of bacterial products (usually derived from *E. coli*) by histiocytes. The resulting accumulation of histiocytes forms a tumour that often involves the mucosa. The terminal ileum is the most commonly involved small intestinal site. Malakoplakia is characterised by sheets of histiocytes with abundant granular eosinophilic that contain basophilic, periodic acid Schiff (PAS)-positive, diastase-resistant inclusions and diagnostic targetoid Michaelis-Gutmann bodies [38]. The latter are grey to blue with H&E and are positive for calcium von Kossa stain and iron Perls stain. The histiocytes are positive for CD68 antibody. Xanthogranulomatous inflammation is the main differential diagnosis but lacks the characteristic Michaelis-Gutmann bodies.

Langerhans Cell Histiocytosis

Gastrointestinal tract involvement by Langerhans cell histiocytosis is uncommon, and small intestinal involvement is rare. It may affect adults as well as children and mostly present as a polyp forming mucosal infiltrate measuring <10 mm diameter. Histologically, the lesion is mostly well circumscribed and contains sheets of polygonal cells with moderate pink slightly granular cytoplasm. The nuclei are characteristically grooved and are occasionally folded. An infiltrate, sometimes prominent, of eosinophils and lymphocytes may accompany the tumour. Mucosal ulceration, reactive mucosal changes, entrapped epithelial elements, focal necrosis and multinucleated giant cells can be seen [39]. By immunohistochemistry, the lesions express S-100 protein and CD1a. Adult cases are typically solitary polyps that are cured by polypectomy. In contrast, paediatric cases are usually associated with systemic disease and a poor prognosis.

Metastases to the Small Intestine Mucosa

Most originate from a remote, typically extraintestinal site. Spread is via direct invasion, transcoelomic spread or vascular/lymphatic permeation. Most small intestinal metastases are not diagnosed on endoscopic biopsies either because their complications such as obstruction, perforation or haemorrhage require emergent surgical intervention or because they are located within the deep submucosa or muscularis propria and are therefore not accessible to biopsy forceps. Mostly, metastases are readily distinguished by distinctive morphology and lack of an in situ component. Immunohistochemistry may be required to determine the site of origin.

Melanoma is the most common metastatic tumour and causes the most diagnostic difficulty because of variable morphology. The major differential diagnostic considerations include lymphoma, GIST and neuroendocrine carcinoma. Metastatic disease in the small intestine is a marker of advanced disease.

Multifocal Tumour

See Table 7.11.

Table 7.11 Multifocal tumour

Causes of multifocal tumour
Primary neoplasms—neuroendocrine, haematopoietic, e.g. lymphomatoid polyposis
Metastases
Others, e.g. infection-related tumours
Polyposis syndromes (see Chap. 1)

Spindle Cell Pattern: Benign Appearing

See Table 7.12.

Table 7.12 Spindle cell pattern: benign appearing (uniform cells with at most rare mitoses)

Leiomyoma
Schwannoma
Neurofibroma
Granular cell tumour
Solitary fibrous tumour
Inflammatory myofibroblastic tumour
Fibromatosis
Inflammatory fibroid polyp
Mastocytosis

Gastrointestinal Stromal Tumour (GIST)

GIST is a mesenchymal tumour mostly arising in the gastrointestinal tract. They are occasionally sampled in endoscopic biopsies, and establishment of the diagnosis is the most important aspect for the pathologist at this stage. GISTs originate from the interstitial cells of Cajal, a component of the gut autonomic nervous system. Most tumours harbour activating mutations of the tyrosine kinase receptors, c-KIT or platelet-derived growth factor receptor (PDGFR). Rarely mutations of exon 15 of BRAF and in genes encoding the enzyme complex of succinate dehydrogenase (SDH) have also been identified. Most GIST mutations are sporadic. Up to 5% have a hereditary basis or occur in a multi-tumour syndrome. These include (1) neurofibromatosis (NF-1)—lack both c-KIT and PDGRA mutation; (2) Carney's triad (gastric GIST, pulmonary chondroma and extraadrenal paraganglioma)—have dysfunction of SDH enzyme complex but do not have underlying gene mutation; (3) Carney-Stratakis syndrome (hereditary GIST and paraganglioma syndrome caused by germline mutations in succinate dehydrogenase (SDH)); and (4) familial GIST syndrome—have germline gain-of-function mutations in c-KIT (especially due to exon 11 mutation). PDGFRA mutation may also be found.

GISTs exhibit a wide variety of cellular and architectural patterns. (1) Cell type—this may be of spindle (70%), epithelioid (20%) or mixed (10%) type. Spindle cells range from plump smooth muscle-like cells to thin wavy neural-like cells, often with characteristic juxtanuclear vacuoles. Epithelioid cells are generally large and display cytoplasmic clearing (sometimes signet ring like). Nuclear variability and "floret"-like giant cells may be seen. (2) Architectural pattern includes short fascicles, palisading, nested (sometimes resembling neuroendocrine neoplasm), perithéliomatous, pseudovascular, pseudoglandular, haemangiopericytoma-like, linear streaming and sheeting/frankly sarcomatous patterns. (3) Stroma is also variable and includes hyalinised collagen, myxoid areas, microcystic stromal degeneration, lymphocytic infiltration and sometimes calcification and/or mature bone. Knowledge of the myriad cellular and architectural patterns is required to consider the correct diagnosis.

Routine mucosal biopsy specimens often contain little tumour submucosal-based GIST. Direct sampling of the tumour via TUNNEL or SINK procedures yields more materials.

Immunohistochemistry findings are tabulated in Table 7.13.

Gene mutation testing has potential diagnostic, prognostic and therapeutic value (see tables below) but is typically not requested on mucosal biopsy material. The differential diagnosis consists of other mesenchymal tumours of the gut. Predictive factors for progressive disease after primary resection are based on tumour size, site, mitotic activity and mutation background [40, 41]. These features are summarised in Tables 7.14, 7.15, 7.16, 7.17, and 7.18.

Table 7.13 Immunohistochemistry findings of gastrointestinal stromal tumours (GISTs)

1. CD117—positive in 95%. Pattern of reaction is at the cell membrane with a Golgi dot pattern of reaction in 45%. Negative staining may be seen in between 35% and 80% of PDGFRA mutation GIST and is more common in epithelioid tumours. Positive reaction is encountered in melanoma, seminoma and occasionally desmoid tumour
2. DOG-1—positive in >95%. Is as sensitive for c-KIT mutation spindle cell GISTs as CD117 and detects at least one third of the of the CD117 nonreactive tumours. It also reacts with a higher proportion of epithelioid and/or PDGFRA mutation GISTs
3. CD34—positive in 70%. This is more likely in gastric sites than the small intestine
4. SMA—positive in 30–40%
5. S-100—positive in 5% of all GIST but up to 1/3 of NF1-associated GIST
6. Desmin—positive in 1–2%
7. Keratin—positive in 1–2%
8. SDH subunits—SDHB is the common immunohistochemical stain used and may detect abnormalities in other subunits of the enzyme complex. There is loss of reaction in SDH mutation; hence, a good internal control (usually native gastric body mucosa) is required. SDH mutation is not expected in small intestinal GIST

Table 7.14 Risk of progressive disease in gastrointestinal stromal tumours (GISTs) according to mitotic index, size and site

Mitotic index, HPF	Size (cm)	Duodenum	Jejunum/ileum
≤5/50	≤2	None (0%)	None (0%)
≤5/50	2 to ≥5	Very low (3.8%)	Low (3.4%)
≤5/50	≥5 to >10	Insufficient data	Moderate (24%)
>5/50	>10	High (34%)	High (52%)
>5/50	≤2	Insufficient data	High (50%)
>5/50	2 to ≥5	High (50%)	High (73%)
>5/50	≥5 to >10	Insufficient data	High (85%)
>5/50	>10	High (86%)	High (90%)

Table 7.15 c-KIT

	Exon 9	Exon 11	Exon 13	Exon 17
Frequency (all GIST)	10–15%	65–70%	1%	1%
Histology	Usual pattern	Spindle > epithelioid		
Site predilection	Small intestine	Stomach	?	?
Imatinib response	++ (often requires higher dose)	+++	Variable	Variable
Progressive disease	17%	3%	?	?

GIST = gastrointestinal stromal tumours

Table 7.16 PDGFR

	Exon 12	Exon 14	Exon 18 (usually D842V)
Frequency (all GIST)	1.5%	0.5%	6%
Histopathology	Epithelioid, multinucleate giant cells, intermediate/high risk		
Site predilection	Stomach, omentum/peritoneal surface		
Imatinib response	Variable	Variable	Nil (D842V mutation is imatinib resistant)
Progressive disease	Overall less aggressive than c-kit mutant GIST		

GIST = gastrointestinal stromal tumours

Table 7.17 BRAF

	Exon 15 (V600E)
Frequency	Rare (<1%), female > male
Histopathology	Spindle cell
Site	Small intestine > stomach
Imatinib response	Nil (BRAF inhibitors may be useful in advanced disease)
Progressive disease	Insufficient data

Table 7.18 SDH deficiency

	SDHB (also SDHA, SDHC, SDHD)
Frequency	Rare (<1%), often familial, young females
Histopathology	Multinodular/plexiform; epithelioid cells
Site	Stomach only
Imatinib response	Nil (inhibition of insulin-like growth factor 1 receptor shows promise)
Progressive disease	20–25% develop liver metastases; however, long-term survival is still possible. 15% mortality (median 15 years of follow-up) Traditional risk assessment is poorly predictive of progression risk

Table 7.19 Other mesenchymal tumours encountered in mucosal biopsies of the small intestine

Mesenchymal cell of origin	Tumour type	Immunohisto-chemistry
Smooth muscle	Leiomyoma (rarely leiomyosarcoma)	SMA, Desmin
Neural	Schwannoma, neurofibroma, MPNST, perineurioma	S-100 EMA
Fibroblastic/myofibroblastic	Solitary fibrous tumour, inflammatory myofibroblastic tumour, fibromatosis	CD34, STAT 6
Vascular	Glomus tumour, angiosarcoma	SMA CD31
Adipose	Lipoma, liposarcoma	CD34
Unknown	Synovial sarcoma, clear cell sarcoma, PEComa	EMA HMB-45

Inflammatory Fibroid Polyp

See terminal ileum chapter.

Other Mesenchymal Tumours

Other mesenchymal tumours that may be encountered in mucosal biopsies of the small intestine are included in Table 7.19.

Spindle Cell Pattern: Malignant Appearing (Hypercellular with cytological atypia and readily identified mitoses) (Box 7.4)

Box 7.4 Spindle Cell Pattern—Malignant Appearing

- Inflammatory myofibroblastic tumour
- Angiosarcoma
- Sarcomatoid carcinoma
- Follicular dendritic cell tumour
- Dedifferentiated liposarcoma
- GIST
- Leiomyosarcoma
- Kaposi sarcoma
- Synovial sarcoma

Lymphoid Hyperplasia

Small reactive lymphoid follicles may also be seen in the proximal small intestine mainly as a response to food allergy in children or in primary immunodeficiency disorder (e.g. CVID, IgA deficiency).

Non-neoplastic Vascular Lesions

Pyogenic Granuloma

Pyogenic granuloma is benign proliferation of capillary vessels originating from a feeding vessel. The aetiology is often unclear. Trauma is responsible for at least some cases. Medications such as retinoids, the protease inhibitor indinavir, 5-fluorouracil, capecitabine and some EGF receptor inhibitors have been implicated [42]. This lesion is also known as lobulated capillary haemangioma befitting its morphology. Typically, it is a raised, frequently ulcerated benign proliferation of capillary sized vessels in an oedematous stroma. Variable numbers of acute and chronic inflammatory cells may be present. The vessels show a branching pattern leading off a feeding vessel at the base. The major differential diagnoses are exuberant granulation tissue and

Kaposi sarcoma. Inflammatory fibroid polyp and inflammatory myofibroblastic tumour may sometimes enter the differential diagnosis. Attention to the clinical setting will aid the differential diagnosis.

Vascular Abnormalities

- These are non-neoplastic abnormalities in the vascular architecture or vessel anatomy. They often present as gastrointestinal tract bleeding.
  - Angiectasia [43]—This is characterised by dilated, thin-walled veins lacking an elastic lamina that results from a regional or generalised increase in venous pressure.
  - Haemodialysis-associated telangiectasia [43]—This is a generalised angiectasia of the gastrointestinal tract developing in patients on long-term haemodialysis. Changes in circulatory fluid volume may be a causative factor.
  - Portal hypertensive enteropathy [44, 45]—This is a form of generalised angiectasia resulting from portal hypertension. Thick-walled dilated vessels along with oedema of the lamina propria, fibromuscular proliferation, a decreased villous/crypt ratio and thickened muscularis mucosae form a characteristic picture of portal hypertensive enteropathy. Occasionally polyp formation or ulceration may occur.
  - Dieulafoy's lesion—This is a "calibre persistent" submucosal vein that projects in the overlying mucosa.
  - Arteriovenous malformation—This is characterised by an abnormal, frequently transmural collection of vessels displaying variable thickness of their vessel walls. An internal elastic lamina can be identified in some of the vessels.
  - Lymphangioma or acquired lymphangiectasia - contains proteinaceous fluid rather than blood within the vascular lumina (Fig. 7.33).

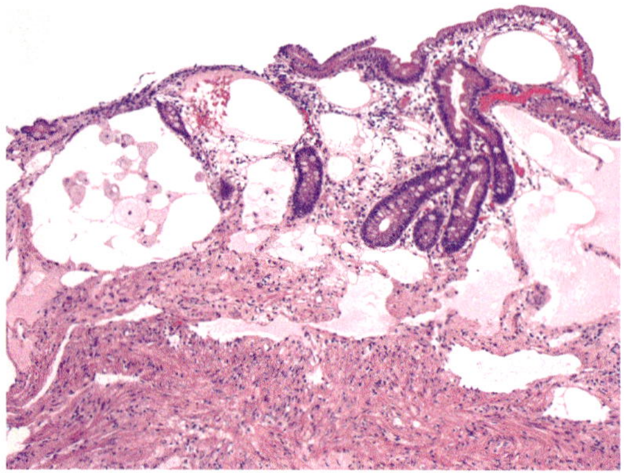

Fig. 7.33 Lymphangioma of duodenum - note proteinaceous content within dilated vascular spaces

Primary Lymphangiectasia

Primary lymphangiectasia is a rare condition of dilated intestinal lymphatics/lacteals with leakage of protein-rich material into the gut lumen leading to protein losing enteropathy and malabsorption. Dilated lymphatics appear through all layers of the intestine wall. They can appear empty or contain proteinaceous material with free floating histiocytes. There is no associated inflammation [46–48]. The main diagnostic considerations are lymphangioma, Whipple's disease, MAIC and pneumatosis intestinalis.

References

1. Genta RM, Kinsey S, Singhal A, Suterwala S. Gastric foveolar metaplasia and gastric heterotopia in the duodenum: no evidence of an etiologic role for Helicobacter pylori. Hum Pathol. 2010;41:1593–600.
2. Hoedemaeker PJ. Heterotopic gastric mucosa in the duodenum. Digestion. 1970;3:165–73.
3. Lessells AM, Martin DF. Heterotopic gastric mucosa in the duodenum. J Clin Pathol. 1982;35:591–5.
4. Yuan Z, Chen J, Zheng Q, Huang XY, Yang Z, Tang J. Heterotopic pancreas in the gastrointestinal tract. World J Gastroenterol. 2009;15(29):3701–3.
5. Bromberg SH, Camilo Neto C, Borges AF, Franco MI, França LC, Yamaguchi N. Pancreatic heterotopias: clinicopathological analysis of 18 patients. Rev Col Bras Cir. 2010;37(6):413–9.
6. Tan CL, Tan SH, So JB, Petersson F. Muco-submucosal elongated polyps of the gastrointesti-

nal tract: a case series and a review of the literature. World J Gastroenterol. 2013;19(11):1845–9.
7. de Sanctis S, Qureshi T, Stebbing JF. Clinical and pathological overlap in nonsteroidal anti-inflammatory drug-related small bowel diaphragm disease and the neuromuscular and vascular hamartoma of the small bowel. Am J Surg Pathol. 2001;25(4):539–41.
8. Shepherd NA, Jass JR. Neuromuscular and vascular hamartoma of the small intestine: is it Crohn's disease? Gut. 1987;28(12):1663–8.
9. Powers M, Sayuk GS, Wang HL. Brunner gland cyst: report of three cases. Int J Clin Exp Pathol. 2008;1(6):536–8.
10. Levine JA, Burgart LJ, Batts KP, Wang KK. Brunner's gland hamartomas: clinical presentation and pathological features of 27 cases. Am J Gastroenterol. 1995;90:290–4.
11. Gao YP, Zhu JS, Zheng WJ. Brunner's gland adenoma of duodenum: a case report and literature review. World J Gastroenterol. 2004;10(17):2616–7.
12. Vieth M, Kushima R, Borchard F, Stolte M. Pyloric gland adenoma: a clinico-pathological analysis of 90 cases. Virchows Arch. 2003;442(4):317–21.
13. Chen ZM, Scudiere JR, Abraham SC, Montgomery E. Pyloric gland adenoma: an entity distinct from gastric foveolar type adenoma. Am J Surg Pathol. 2009;33(2):186–93.
14. Khor TS, Brown I, Kattampallil J, Yusoff I, Kumarasinghe MP. Duodenal adenocarcinoma arising from a pyloric gland adenoma with a brief review of the literature. BMJ Case Rep. 2010;29.
15. Rosty C, Buchanan DD, Walters RJ, Carr NJ, Bothman JW, Young JP, Brown IS. Hyperplastic polyp of the duodenum: a report of 9 cases with immunohistochemical and molecular findings. Hum Pathol. 2011;42(12):1953–9.
16. Rubio CA. Serrated adenoma of the duodenum. J Clin Pathol. 2004;57(11):1219–21.
17. Rosty C, Campbell C, Clendenning M, Bettington M, Buchanan DD, Brown IS. Do serrated neoplasms of the small intestine represent a distinctive entity? Pathological findings and molecular alterations in a series of 13 cases. Histopathology. 2015;66:333.
18. Chu PG, Schwarz RE, Lau SK, Yen Y, Weiss LM. Immunohistochemical staining of pancreatobiliary and ampulla of Vater adenocarcinoma: application of CDX2, CK17, MUC1, and MUC2. Am J Surg Pathol. 2005;29(3):359–67.
19. Klöppel G, Rindi G, Anlauf M, Perren A, Komminoth P. Site-specific biology and pathology of gastroenteropancreatic neuroendocrine tumors. Virchows Arch. 2007;451(Suppl 1):S9–27.
20. Rindi G, Kloppel G, Alhman H, et al. TNM staging of foregut (neuro)endocrine tumors: a consensus proposal including a grading system. Virchows Arch. 2006;449:395–401.
21. Sundararajan V, Robinson-Smith TM, Lowy AM. Duodenal gangliocytic paraganglioma with lymph node metastasis: a case report and review of the literature. Arch Pathol Lab Med. 2003;127(3):139–41.
22. O'Malley DP, Goldstein NS, Banks PM. The recognition and classification of lymphoproliferative disorders of the gut. Hum Pathol. 2014;45(5):899–916.
23. Misdraji J, Harris NL, Hasserjian RP, Lauwers GY, Ferry JA. Primary follicular lymphoma of the gastrointestinal tract. Am J Surg Pathol. 2011;35(9):1255–63.
24. Takata K, Sato Y, Nakamura N, Tokunaka M, Miki Y, Yukie Kikuti Y, Igarashi K, Ito E, Harigae H, Kato S, Hayashi E, Oka T, Hoshii Y, Tari A, Okada H, Al-Kader LA, Maeda Y, Tanimoto M, Kinoshita T, Yoshino T. Duodenal follicular lymphoma lacks AID but expresses BACH2 and has memory B-cell characteristics. Mod Pathol. 2013;26(1):22–31.
25. Lecuit M, Abachin E, Martin A, Poyart C, Pochart P, Suarez F, Bengoufa D, Feuillard J, Lavergne A, Gordon JI, Berche P, Guillevin L, Lortholary O. Immunoproliferative small intestinal disease associated with Campylobacter jejuni. N Engl J Med. 2004;350(3):239–48.
26. Al-Saleem T, Al-Mondhiry H. Immunoproliferative small intestinal disease (IPSID): a model for mature B-cell neoplasms. Blood. 2005;105(6):2274–80.
27. Ibrahim HA, Naresh KN. Post-transplant lymphoproliferative disorders. Adv Hematol. 2012;2012:230173.
28. Ho-Yen C, Chang F, van der Walt J, Mitchell T, Ciclitira P. Recent advances in refractory celiac disease: a review. Histopathology. 2009;54(7):783–95.
29. Arps DP, Smith LB. Classic versus type II enteropathy-associated T-cell lymphoma: diagnostic considerations. Arch Pathol Lab Med. 2013;137(9):1227–31.
30. Shroff S, Ganapathi KA. Enteropathy associated T cell lymphoma: a review of diagnostic findings and therapeutic strategies. Diagn Histopathol. 2014;20:151–5.
31. Ferry JA. Extranodal Lymphoma. Arch Pathol Lab Med. 2008;132:565–78.
32. Mansoor A, Pittaluga S, Beck PL, Wilson WH, Ferry JA, Jaffe ES. NK-cell enteropathy: a benign NK-cell lymphoproliferative disease mimicking intestinal lymphoma: clinicopathologic features and follow-up in a unique case series. Blood. 2011;117(5):1447–52.
33. Banks PM. Gastrointestinal lymphoproliferative disorders. Histopathology. 2007;50(1):42–54.
34. Wang HW, Yang W, Sun JZ, Lu JY, Li M, Sun L. Plasmablastic lymphoma of the small intestine: case report and literature review. World J Gastroenterol. 2012;18(45):6677–81.
35. Kohl SK, Aoun P. Granulocytic sarcoma of the small intestine. Arch Pathol Lab Med. 2006;130(10):1570–4.
36. Nielsen SL, Ingeholm P, Holck S, Talbot I. Xanthomatosis of the gastrointestinal tract with focus on small bowel involvement. J Clin Pathol. 2007;60(10):1164–6.
37. Detlefsen S, Fagerberg CR, Ousager LB, Lindebjerg J, Marcussen N, Nathan T, Sørensen FB. Histiocytic disorders of the gastrointestinal tract. Hum Pathol. 2013;44(5):683–96.

38. De Petris G, Leung ST. Pseudoneoplasms of the gastrointestinal tract. Arch Pathol Lab Med. 2010;134(3):378–92.
39. Singhi AD, Montgomery EA. Gastrointestinal tract langerhans cell histiocytosis: a clinicopathologic study of 12 patients. Am J Surg Pathol. 2011;35(2):305–10.
40. Miettinen M, Lasota J. Gastrointestinal stromal tumors. Gastroenterol Clin North Am. 2013;42(2):399–415.
41. Doyle LA, Hornick JL. Gastrointestinal stromal tumors: from KIT to succinate dehydrogenase. Histopathology. 2014;64(1):53–67.
42. Shirakawa K, Nakamura T, Endo M, Suzuki K, Fujimori T, Terano A. Pyogenic granuloma of the small intestine. Gastrointest Endosc. 2007;66(4):827–8.
43. Yano T, Yamamoto H. Vascular, polypoid, and other lesions of the small bowel. Best Pract Res Clin Gastroenterol. 2009;23(1):61–74.
44. Rondonotti E, Villa F, Signorelli C, de Franchis R. Portal hypertensive enteropathy. Gastrointest Endosc Clin N Am. 2006;16(2):277–86.
45. Misra V, Misra SP, Dwivedi M, Gupta SC. Histomorphometric study of portal hypertensive enteropathy. Am J Clin Pathol. 1997;108(6):652–7.
46. Abramowsky C, Hupertz V, Kilbridge P, et al. Intestinal lymphangiectasia in children: a study of upper gastrointestinal endoscopic biopsies. Pediatr Pathol. 1989;9:289.
47. Aoyagi K, Iida M, Yao T, et al. Characteristic endoscopic features of intestinal lymphangiectasia: correlation with histological findings. Hepatogastroenterology. 1997;44:133.
48. Riemann JF, Schmidt H. Synopsis of endoscopic and other morphological findings in intestinal lymphangiectasia. Endoscopy. 1981;13:60.

Terminal Ileum: Inflammatory Patterns

8

Ian Brown

Contents

I. Brown
Envoi Pathology, Kelvin Grove, QLD, Australia
e-mail: ianbrown@envoi.com.au

Acute Inflammation (and/or Erosion)

Nonsteroidal Anti-Inflammatory Drugs (NSAIDS) Enteropathy

Nonsteroidal anti-inflammatory drugs (NSAIDs) cause injury of the small intestine mediated by microvascular changes. In addition to acute inflammation and erosion, there may be diaphragm-like strictures [1, 2]. Histologically, villous blunting, is usual, sometimes leading to a flat mucosa. Acute and chronic inflammation is often only mild. Conspicuous eosinophils are sometimes found. Erosion and gastric metaplasia of antral or pseudopyloric gland type can occur with chronic injury. A sometimes encountered pattern is prominent lipid-induced cytoplasmic vacuolation of the surface epithelium associated with epithelial serration. Hyalinisation of the lamina propria, reflecting ischaemic injury, may be appreciated in some cases.

In the terminal ileum, NSAID injury needs to be separated from Crohn's disease. Clinical history and investigations are relevant. The histological finding of granulomata and a fissuring rather than broad-based pattern of ulceration are typical of Crohn's disease, while prominent lymphangiectasia and very marked active chronic inflammation are supportive features of Crohn's disease. Extensive chronic inflammation associated with diffuse architectural disturbance is also

M. P. Kumarasinghe, I. Brown (eds.), *Endoscopic Biopsy Interpretation*,
https://doi.org/10.1007/978-3-319-79117-3_8

more typical of Crohn's disease [3]. Less common causes of ileitis are discussed below.

Isolated Ileitis/Erosion

It is common to encounter inflammation and/or ulceration limited to the distal terminal ileum and detected by ileoscopy. Causes are listed in Table 8.1.

In the most commonly encountered cases, a cause is not established, and the process follows a benign outcome. The major feature is acute inflammation with neutrophilic cryptitis with or without crypt abscess formation (Fig. 8.1). There may be associated superficial erosion, often, only identified on multiple levels [4, 5]. This may overlie reactive lymphoid tissue (aphthous-type erosion). Eosinophils are often present and may be numerous. Lymphocytes and plasma cells are increased, particularly when erosion is present. Features of chronicity including crypt architectural disarray (crypt branching and shortening), villous blunting, basal plasmacytosis and pseudopyloric gland metaplasia may be encountered.

Table 8.1 Causes of isolated ileal erosion

Crohn's disease limited to the ileum
Infection—*Yersinia*, *Mycobacterium tuberculosis*, *Campylobacter*, *Salmonella*; rarely viral, e.g. CMV, and fungal, e.g. histoplasma and streptococcal
Medications—NSAIDs, calcium channel blockers (nicorandil), chemotherapy agents (5-FU), potassium
Spondyloarthropathy—ankylosing and non-ankylosing type
Backwash ileitis in ulcerative colitis
Behcet's disease and other vasculitis
Focal ischaemia
Acute radiation injury
Idiopathic

Behcet's Disease

Behcet's disease is a multisystem vasculitic disorder of unknown aetiology involving both small and large vessels. Infection and genetic predisposition have been proposed as possible causes. There is an increased prevalence in countries that straddle the Silk Road, with the highest incidence in Turkey. HLA B51 has been associated. Hence the ethnicity of the patient is a useful diagnostic clue, although it is important to know that all populations can be affected.

The disease manifests throughout the gastrointestinal tract with the ileocaecal region being most commonly affected. Mucosal involvement varies from non-specific focal active inflammation to extensive and deep mucosal ulceration [6]. An aphthous pattern of erosion is commonly encountered. The vasculitis affects vessels of the submucosa or deeper in the intestinal wall and is therefore rarely encountered in endoscopic biopsies.

Cryptogenic Multifocal Ulcerating and Stenosing Enteritis (CMUSE)

This is an uncommon disorder characterised by multifocal ulceration and stenosis of the small intestine [7, 8]. At present the aetiology is uncer-

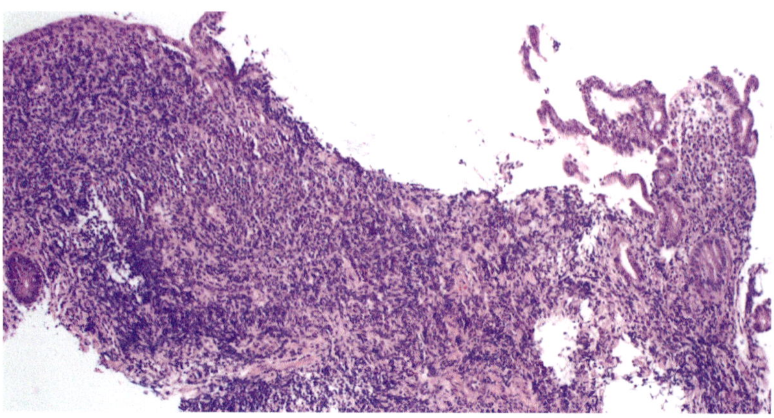

Fig. 8.1 Isolated ileal erosion. No features of chronicity

tain. Associations with complement 2 deficiency and polyarteritis nodosa [8] have been reported, and a genetic defect in the prostacyclin pathway has been reported in one family. The latter may explain the close morphological appearance to NSAID enteropathy.

Despite the name, not all cases are associated with a well developed stenosing process. Ulceration involving mucosa or superficial submucosa is consistently present and is associated with a mild mixed inflammatory infiltrate including some eosinophils. The intestine away from the ulcers is histologically normal.

Active Chronic inflammation

Causes of active chronic inflammation ± ulceration in the terminal ileum are listed in Table 8.2.

Table 8.2 Causes of active chronic inflammation and ulceration in the terminal ileum

Crohn's disease
Infection—*Yersinia* and *Mycobacterium* infection
Medication injury, e.g. NSAID
Vasculitis
CMUSE
"Backwash" ileitis in ulcerative colitis

Crohn's Disease

Crohn's disease affects all regions of the gastrointestinal tract with the terminal ileum being the most commonly affected site [9, 10]. It is characterised endoscopically by discontinuous inflammation, ulceration, sinus/fistula formation and fibrosis-related stenosis.

Mucosal biopsies display patchy variable intensity active chronic inflammation with architectural disturbance and pseudopyloric gland metaplasia (Fig. 8.2). Ulceration is frequent, and granuloma formation is seen in about one quarter of biopsies. Eosinophils may be frequent, although not numerous enough to suggest eosinophilic enteritis. The finding of granulomas represents a good marker of Crohn's disease outside of areas with a high prevalence of mycobacterium tuberculosis infection.

Intraepithelial Lymphocytosis

The causes include all those discussed for the proximal small bowel. In addition, terminal ileal lymphocytosis can be associated with lymphocytic colitis [11, 12].

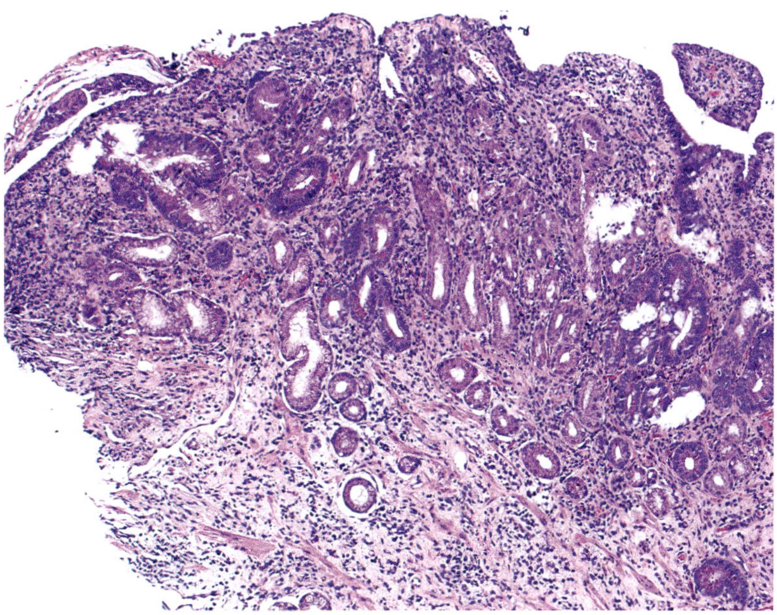

Fig. 8.2 Ileal Crohn's disease. Note superficial erosion, pseudopyloric gland metaplasia, architectural disturbance and fibrosis

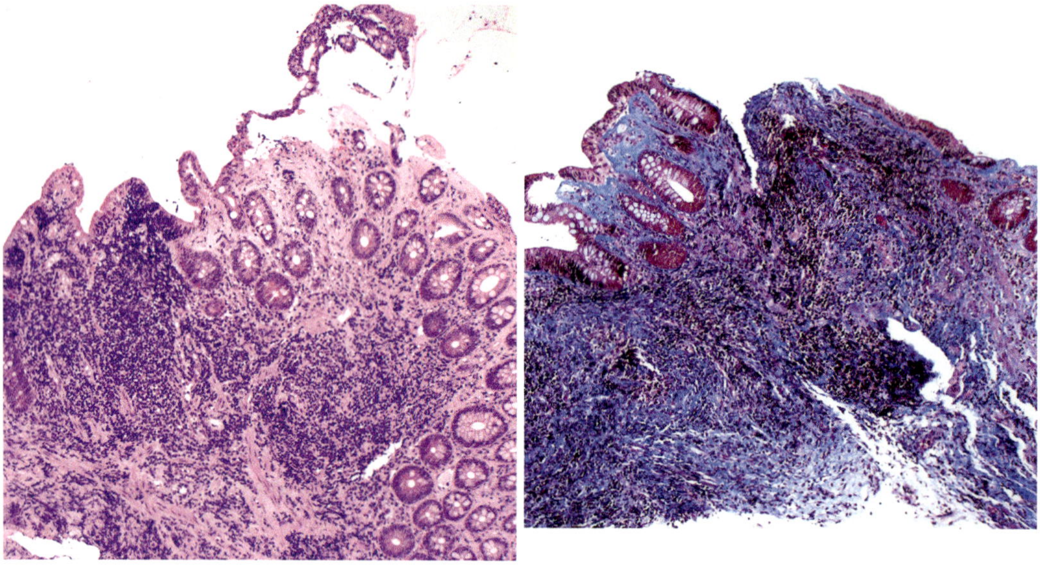

Fig. 8.3 Collagenous ileitis displaying marked thickening of the subepithelial collagen layer and sloughing of the surface epithelium (H&E and trichrome stains)

Subepithelial Collagen

Collagenous Ileitis (Fig. 8.3)

The ileum is the least common site for subepithelial collagen deposition in the gastrointestinal tract. There is a well-established association with collagenous colitis. Sartan family medications are an increasingly recognised association. NSAIDs are likely responsible for some cases. There exist a significant number of examples where the cause is never established. Associated inflammation in the lamina propria is typical [13].

Eosinophil Infiltration

Eosinophilic Enteritis

Eosinophilic enteritis is a symptomatic eosinophil-rich inflammatory disorder either limited to the small intestine or involving the small intestine as part of more extensive gastrointestinal disease. It is more extensively discussed in the proximal small intestine chapter.

Disorders associated with eosinophilic enteritis presenting mainly in the ileum include [14] parasitic infection (especially Ancylostoma caninum) and Crohn's disease after treatment. Other causes include food allergy and certain drugs, e.g. NSAIDs, gold, tacrolimus, clozapine, connective tissue disease (such as SLE), vasculitis (particularly eosinophilic granulomatosis with polyangiitis = Churg Stauss granulomatosis), hypereosinophilic syndrome, organ transplantation, chronic granulomatous disease and neoplastic disorders (such as Inflammatory fibroid polyp, Langerhans cell histiocytosis, mastocytosis, lymphoma and leukaemia). Some cases are idiopathic.

The normal mean enteric eosinophil count is <10/HPF with peak eosinophil counts in paediatric ileum being 28/HPF [15]. Diagnosis is established by diffuse mucosal involvement by eosinophils >30/HPF accompanied by villous blunting of variable degree, eosinophil infiltration of epithelium, eosinophilic crypt abscess formation and infiltration of muscularis mucosae [14, 15]. Mucosal oedema may be prominent in some case. Focal intense eosinophil infiltrates are particularly suggestive of parasitic infection. Special tests are infrequently required for ileal eosinophil infiltrates. CD117 and CD25 stains can establish underlying mastocytosis, and c-kit mutation testing can subsequently be performed. CD34 can help confirm an underlying inflammatory fibroid polyp.

Table 8.3 Histiocytic/granulomatous infiltrates

Histiocytes	• Xanthoma • Malakoplakia • Infections, e.g. Whipple's disease, MAIC • Lipid storage disorders • Muciphages
Granulomata	• Foreign body granuloma • Sarcoidosis • Crohn's disease • Pneumatosis • CVID • Chronic granulomatous disease • Infections, e.g. *Mycobacterium tuberculosis*

Where no specific cause is identified, pathologist should report mucosal eosinophilia as a reaction pattern with multiple possible causes. Potential causes may be evident in the histological sections, and their presence or absence should be specifically stated in the report. A comment to the effect that "mucosal eosinophilia is not specific but common causes include allergic reaction to food or drugs, and parasitic infection" is useful when no cause is evident in the tissue sections.

Histiocytic/Granulomatous Infiltrates

See Table 8.3.

Ischaemic Injury

Causes of intestinal ischaemia are discussed in Chap. 1. In general small intestine ischaemia results from large vessel occlusion as the good collateral blood supply of the small intestine overcomes most small vessel occlusion.

Ischaemic Enteritis

The earliest change is epithelial cell apoptosis followed by crypt atrophy and villous blunting (Fig. 8.4). Oedema and red cell extravasation will be prominent if venous obstruction is the cause. Later, hyalinisation of the lamina propria, a useful diagnostic sign, may develop. Inflammation is generally absent, but focal acute inflammation may develop, particularly when the blood supply is restored. The muscularis mucosa may be atrophic or at least focally disappear.

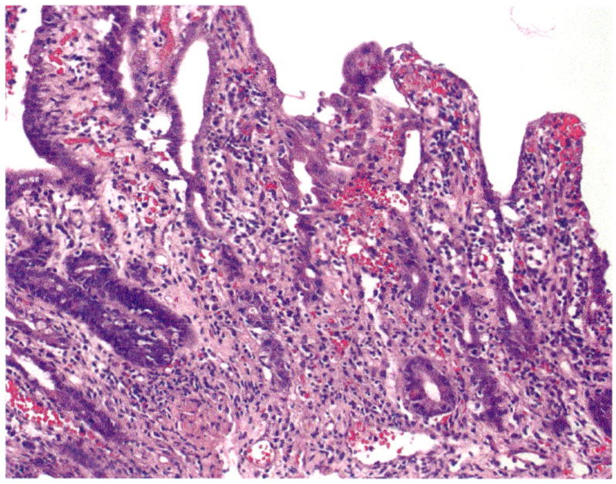

Fig. 8.4 Ileal ischaemic injury pattern

Table 8.4 Apoptosis

• Medication including chemotherapy and immunomodulatory agents, e.g. ipilimumab, mycophenolate
• Immune mediated—GVHD, CVID, thymoma-associated colitis, autoimmune enteropathy
• Infection—HIV, other virus

Apoptosis

See Table 8.4.

Toxic Injury Pattern

This is most commonly seen when there is abrupt severe injury to the epithelium leading to obvious epithelial injury. The general causes are discussed in Chap. 1.

Radiation Enteritis

Radiation enteritis occurs as a complication of pelvic or abdominal radiation [16]. Histological changes occur throughout the intestinal wall and can be acute or chronic. Acute mucosal changes range from oedema to frank mucosal ulceration or necrosis. Villous blunting and a mild increase in chronic inflammatory cells can be seen. Acute inflammation, crypt apoptosis and crypt loss occur with more severe injury. Atypical stellate cells ("radiation" fibroblasts) may be seen in the granulation tissue of an ulcer. Chronic radiation enteritis is characterised by crypt architectural irregularity with pyloric gland metaplasia in the ileum and fibrosis in the lamina propria.

Mixed Injury Pattern

In the terminal ileum, medications, such as NSAIDS and new biological agents, and Crohn's disease are the most common cause for a mixed pattern of injury.

Depositions

Pigment Depositions

Carbon

Exogenous pigmented material is a common finding in the terminal ileum within the Peyer's patches. It is believed to have an origin from ingested atmospheric pollution [17, 18].

Pseudomelanosis Ilei

This is a deposition of brown pigment, usually within the villous stroma. The pigment contains variable amounts of iron, ceroid, sulphur and melanin. A Perls' stain will highlight the iron.

True melanosis may be associated with metastatic melanoma in the local area.

Special Patterns

Infections

Yersinia

These are gram-negative coccoid bacteria affecting the small and large intestine. The most common human infections are caused by *Yersinia enterocolitica* and *pseudotuberculosis* species.

Infection is acquired from contaminated water, dairy and meat products. The ileum, right colon and appendix are typically affected. The characteristic findings are large geographic granulomata with central microabscess formation. These are often centred on reactive Peyer's patches in the ileum. Ulceration is common. Very few organisms are usually found on gram stain.

PCR performed on paraffin shavings from the tissue block is useful in confirming infection.

Exclusion of mycobacterial infection, Crohn's disease and other bacterial infections associated with ileitis, in particular *Salmonella* and *Campylobacter*, is required.

References

1. De Petris G, López JI. Histopathology of diaphragm disease of the small intestine. Am J Clin Pathol. 2008;130:518–25.
2. Isaacs PE, Sladen GE, Filipe I. Mefenamic acid Enteropathy. J Clin Pathol. 1987;40(10):1221–7.
3. Brown IS, Miller GC, Bettington ML, Rosty C. Histopathological findings of extra-ileal manifestations at initial diagnosis of Crohn's disease-related ileitis. Virchows Arch. 2016;469:515.
4. Courville EL, Siegel CA, Vay T, Wilcox AR, Suriawinata AA, Srivastava A. Isolated asymptomatic ileitis does not progress to overt Crohn's disease on long-term follow-up despite features of chronicity in ileal biopsies. Am J Surg Pathol. 2009;33(9):1341–7.
5. Goldstein NS. Isolated ileal erosions in patients with mildly altered bowel habits. A follow-up study of 28 patients. Am J Clin Pathol. 2006;125:838–46.
6. Ebert EC. Gastrointestinal manifestations of Behçet's disease. Dig Dis Sci. 2009;54(2):201–7.
7. Freeman HJ. Multifocal stenosing ulceration of the small intestine. World J Gastroenterol. 2009;15(39):4883–5.
8. Perlemuter G, Chaussade S, Soubrane O, Degoy A, Louvel A, Barbet P, Legman P, Kahan A, Weiss L, Couturier D. Multifocal stenosing ulcerations of the small intestine revealing vasculitis associated with C2 deficiency. Gastroenterology. 1996;110:1628–32.
9. Satsangi J, Silverberg MS, Vermeire S, Colombel JF. The Montreal classification of inflammatory bowel disease: controversies, consensus, and implications. Gut. 2006;55(6):749–53.
10. Padmanabhan V, Callas PW, Li SC, Trainer TD. Histopathological features of the terminal ileum in lymphocytic and collagenous colitis: a study of 32 cases and review of literature. Mod Pathol. 2003;16(2):115–9.
11. Sapp H, Ithamukkala S, Brien TP, Ayata G, Shaz B, Dorfman DM, Wang HH, Antonioli DA, Farraye FA, Odze RD. The terminal ileum is affected in patients

with lymphocytic or collagenous colitis. Am J Surg Pathol. 2002;26(11):1484–92.
12. Paerregaard A. What does the IBD patient hide in the upper gastrointestinal tract? Inflamm Bowel Dis. 2009;15(7):1101–4.
13. O'Brien BH, McClymont K, Brown I. Collagenous ileitis: a study of 13 cases. Am J Surg Pathol. 2011;35(8):1151–7.
14. DeBrosse CW, Case JW, Putnam PE, et al. Quantity and distribution of eosinophils in the gastrointestinal tract of children. Pediatr Dev Pathol. 2006;9(3):210–8.
15. Lucendo AJ, Arias A. Eosinophilic gastroenteritis: an update. Expert Rev Gastroenterol Hepatol. 2012;6(5):591–601.
16. Tankel HI, Clark DH, Lee FD. Radiation enteritis with malabsorption. Gut. 1965;6:560–9.
17. Shepherd NA, Crocker PR, Smith AP, Levison DA. Exogenous pigment in Peyer's patches. Hum Pathol. 1987;18(1):50–4.
18. Urbanski SJ, Arsenault AL, Green FH, Haber G. Pigment resembling atmospheric dust in Peyer's patches. Mod Pathol. 1989;2(3):222–6.

Terminal Ileum: Neoplastic Pattern and Mimics

9

Ian Brown

Contents

I. Brown
Envoi Pathology, Kelvin Grove, QLD, Australia
e-mail: ianbrown@envoi.com.au

Benign Tumours and Mass-Forming Lesions

Endometriosis

Endometriosis is the presence of endometrial glands and stroma outside of the endometrial cavity. Gastrointestinal tract involvement is encountered in 4–37% of patients with pelvic endometriosis [1]. The ileum is the most common site of small intestinal involvement but is overall less frequent than sigmoid or rectal location [1]. The mucosa is involved in about one third of cases with intestinal wall endometriosis [2]. The disease most often presents as a mural mass with stricture formation. Mucosal polyps may occur in this setting or sometimes without evident mural disease.

The classic diagnostic triad is (1) endometrial glands, (2) endometrial stromal and (3) evidence of haemorrhage. At least two of these elements are required for a confident diagnosis. Endometrial glands may be admixed with native intestinal glands and can be easily missed. Mucosal prolapse changes of lamina propria fibrosis, smooth muscle proliferation and crypt elongation may be seen. Acute and chronic inflammation and sometimes ulceration with mucosal distortion are possible and can be a mimic for Crohn's disease [2]. The combination of chronic ulceroinflammatory changes and stricture can be mistaken for Crohn's disease

M. P. Kumarasinghe, I. Brown (eds.), *Endoscopic Biopsy Interpretation*,
https://doi.org/10.1007/978-3-319-79117-3_9

A panel of CK7 (+), CK20 (−), CDX-2 (−) and PAX-8 (+) immunohistochemical stains can distinguish endometriotic glands from native intestinal glands.

Pseudopolyp (Benign Mucosal Polyp, Inflammatory Pseudopolyp)

This is a generic term for a benign polypoidal mucosal lesion characterised by stromal and epithelial expansion without evidence of a neoplastic process. Several different processes are included under this generic designation. Local trauma or inflammation is most common. Inflammation may be related to Crohn's disease [3], or to medications, e.g. NSAIDs. Local mucosal ischaemia is a rare cause in the small intestine.

There is expansion of the lamina propria by fibrosis and/or a fibroblastic proliferation, and inflammation is often present. Smooth muscle and neural hyperplasia and lymphangiectasia may occur, particularly in Crohn's disease-associated pseudopolyps [3]. The crypt epithelium is frequently hyperplastic and may be dilated. Villi tend to be shortened. In some cases, there is ulceration, and variable amounts of granulation tissue may comprise the polyp. Occasionally there is only granulation tissue, and in this circumstance the lesion can be designated a "granulation tissue polyp".

Lymphoid Hyperplasia

Lymphoid hyperplasia is a hyperplasia of preexisting lymphoid tissue in the Peyer's patches of the terminal ileum due to a local or systemic activation of the immune system. The most common reasons for this include viral infection, recent vaccination and medication reaction [4, 5].

The normal ileal lymphoid tissue undergoes enlargement characterised by development of irregular reactive germinal centres and expansion of the mantle/marginal zone region. Follicle lysis may be seen when the process is marked. In pure form, there is no associated acute inflammation, ulceration or granuloma formation.

Lymphoma, particularly of follicular type, always needs to be considered. Features that raise concern for lymphoma include:

1. Finding of lymphoepithelial lesions or lymphocytes with destructive invasion of the epithelium with disappearance of glands.
2. Sheets of large lymphoid cells or any population of markedly atypical or enlarged lymphoid cells
3. Atypical follicle architecture (i.e. lack of polarisation, no tingible body macrophages, mantle/marginal zones absent or poorly seen, mantle/marginal zones that are markedly enlarged, uniform cellular appearance)

Pneumatosis Intestinalis

Pneumatosis intestinalis is a condition characterised by the development of gas-filled cysts in the wall of the small intestine or colon. These may produce a polypoidal appearance to the mucosa [6, 7]. Two main theories of pathogenesis exist: (1) the mechanical theory, implicating mucosal disruption and increased intraluminal pressure, and (2) the microbiological theory, implicating gas-forming bacteria.

The gas cysts may be single or multiple and vary from the size of adipocytes up to several centimetres. Cysts tend to be located in the submucosa or subserosa. The roof of submucosal cysts may be appreciated in mucosal biopsies. They often have no lining appearing as a clear space surrounded by compressed or fibrotic tissue. Sometimes multinucleate giant cells surround the cysts and rarely an apparent single cell lining by histiocytes is seen [6]. Neutrophils, eosinophils, lymphocytes and plasma cells may infiltrate the stroma around the cysts. Progressive fibrosis leads to involution of the cyst over time.

The differential diagnosis can be broad and includes lymphangioma, fat necrosis, granulomatous inflammatory conditions (when multinucleate giant cells are present), infections due to gas-forming bacteria and artefactual pseudolipomatosis.

Non-neoplastic Vascular Lesions

Vascular Abnormalities

These are non-neoplastic abnormalities in vascular architecture or vessel anatomy. They often present as gastrointestinal tract bleeding. These are discussed in more detail in the small intestine chapter. Lesions seen in the ileum include angiectasia, lymphangioma/lymphangiectasia and arteriovenous malformation [8].

Benign Epithelial Tumours

Adenoma

Intestinal-type adenoma is quite rare in the terminal ileum. The possibility of genetic predisposition syndrome (e.g. familial adenomatous polyposis) should always be considered when encountered. Gastric-type adenomas are not described at this site.

Malignant Epithelial Tumours

Adenocarcinoma: Intestinal Type

This is a malignant neoplasm arising from the glandular epithelium of the small intestine. It is morphologically similar to its colonic counterpart. There is an increased risk in familial adenomatous polyposis, Lynch syndrome, juvenile polyposis syndrome, Peutz-Jeghers syndrome and neurofibromatosis type 1. The diagnosis is usually straight forward.

Neuroendocrine Neoplasm

Neuroendocrine neoplasm of the small intestine are more extensively covered in Chapter 7. Features of these tumours occurring in the terminal ileum are summarised in Table 9.1 [9].

Table 9.1 Neuroendocrine neoplasm of the terminal ileum

Ileum
• 25% of all GIT NENs • 1/3–1/2 of all small intestinal neoplasms • M:F = 1.5:1 • Sixth/seventh decade • Non-syndromic • 95% non-functional • 5% functional (carcinoid syndrome) • Midgut pattern—insular nests in a fibro vascular stroma. Tumour cells are uniform and intermediate size with high nuclear to cytoplasmic ratio. The vast majority are grade 1. Despite this they are fully malignant lesions • Multiple tumours—20–50% • Prognosis: 5-year survival
I. If no metastasis ~100% II. if lymph node metastases ~75% III. if distant metastases ~50%
• Metastasis to lymph nodes develop in 10–40% of tumours <10 mm diameter

Mesenchymal Tumours

Gastrointestinal Stromal Tumour (GIST)

This is uncommon in the terminal ileum. Features are identical to those discussed above for the proximal small intestine.

Inflammatory Fibroid Polyp

Inflammatory fibroid polyp is a distinctive benign neoplasm limited to the luminal gastrointestinal tract and characterised by a spindle cell and small vessel proliferation typically accompanied by eosinophil-rich inflammation. In biopsies it is evident at the base as a spindle cell proliferation that varies from paucicellular with fibromyxoid stroma to moderately cellular with onionskin-like patterns around vessels and glands (see Fig. 9.1). The spindle cells may be thin and wavy, to plump and almost stellate. Occasionally multinucleate cells are seen (see Fig. 9.2). Mitotic figures are generally rare. Numerous eosinophils and mast cells are

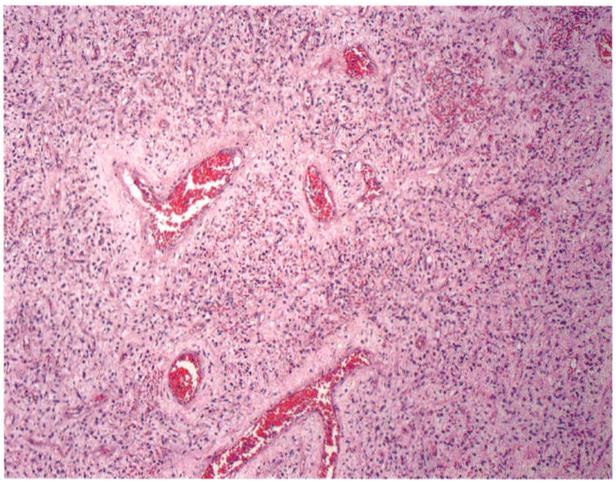

Fig. 9.1 Inflammatory fibroid polyp of ileum ×40 - perivascular oedema, prominent vessels and prominent eosinophil infiltration

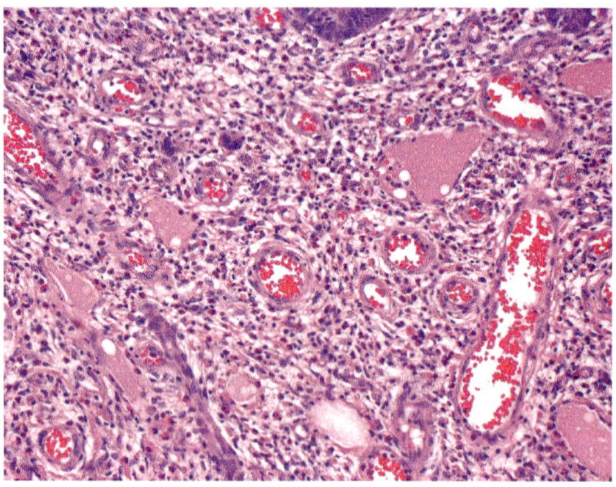

Fig. 9.2 Inflammatory fibroid polyp of ileum ×200 - note the multinucleate cells which are an occasional finding

usually present. Variable numbers of lymphocytes, plasma cells and histiocytes are also present. Zones of stromal hyalinisation devoid of inflammatory cells also occur but are infrequent in mucosal biopsy specimens. Immunohistochemistry reveals reaction with CD34 (Fig. 9.3) and PDGFR. Occasional cells may react with SMA, desmin, cyclin D1, CD68 and factor XIIIa. Non-reactive stains are CD117, DOG-1, S-100, EMA and keratin (e.g. AEI/AE3). Mutations in the gene transcribing the α subunit of platelet-derived growth factor receptor (a surface tyrosine kinase receptor) have been identified and confirm that the lesion is a true neoplasm and not a reactive inflammatory process. Mutations at exon 12 and 18 are most frequent and produce constitutive activation of the cell surface receptor (PDGFR). Exon 12

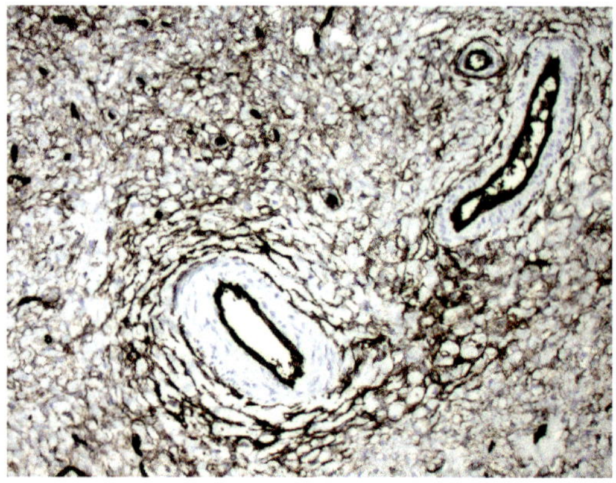

Fig. 9.3 Inflammatory fibroid polyp of ileum - typical pattern of CD34 expression

mutations are more commonly associated with small intestinal site. The differential diagnosis includes inflammatory myofibroblastic tumour, exuberant healing ulcer site, granulation tissue and eosinophil-rich neoplastic process, e.g. Langerhans cell histiocytosis and neoplasms with often prominent inflammation such as schwannoma [10–13].

Other Mesenchymal Tumours

These are uncommonly encountered in terminal ileal biopsies. The general approach to these lesions is discussed in Chapter 1.

Haematopoietic Tumours

Mantle Cell

An aggressive form of B-cell lymphoma that has a predilection for the gut (facilitated by α-4-β-7 integrin expression) where it frequently presents as multiple polyps. In the intestine, mantle cell lymphoma most commonly exhibits diffuse architecture with sheets of small to intermediate (and occasionally large "blastic") cells destroying native glands without lymphoepithelial lesion formation (Fig. 9.4). Occasionally, a nodular pattern or a mantle zone pattern around reactive germinal centres may be seen. The presence of epithelioid histiocytes and perivascular sclerosis may be clues to the diagnosis (Figs. 9.5 and 9.6).

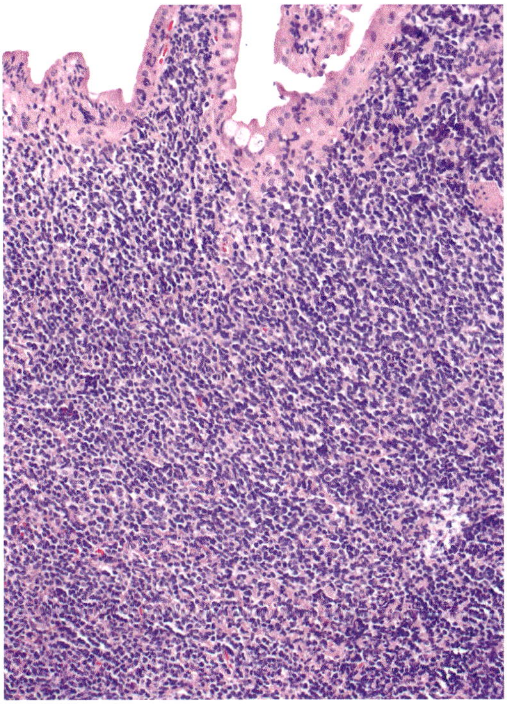

Fig. 9.4 Mantle cell lymphoma ileum high power. Sheets of irregular small to intermediate sized cells

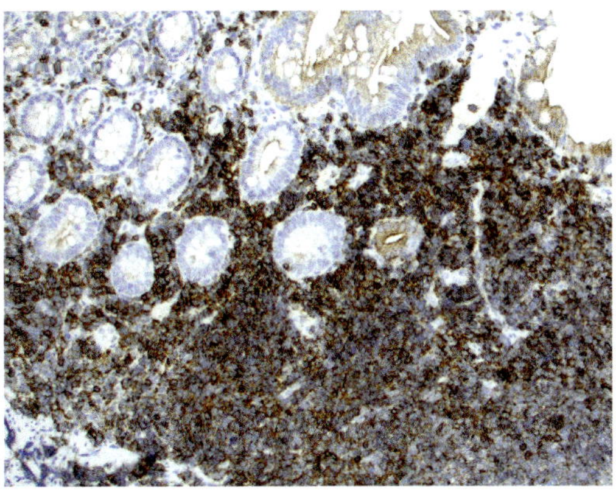

Fig. 9.5 Mantle cell lymphoma ileum CD5 reaction

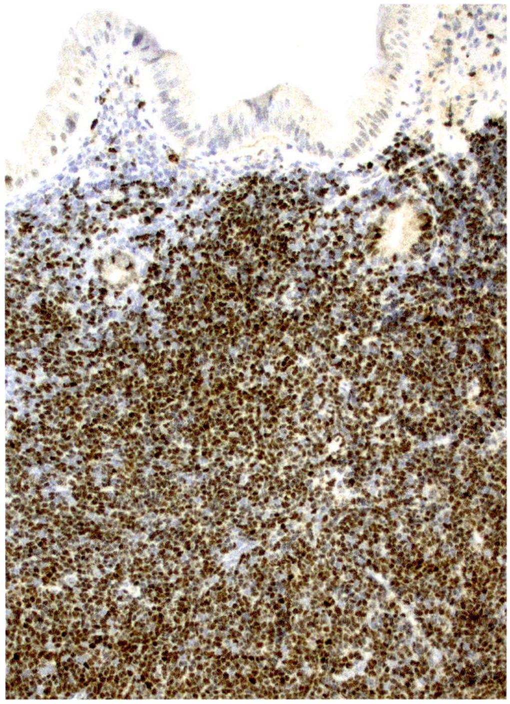

Fig. 9.6 Mantle cell lymphoma ileum nuclear cyclin D1 reaction

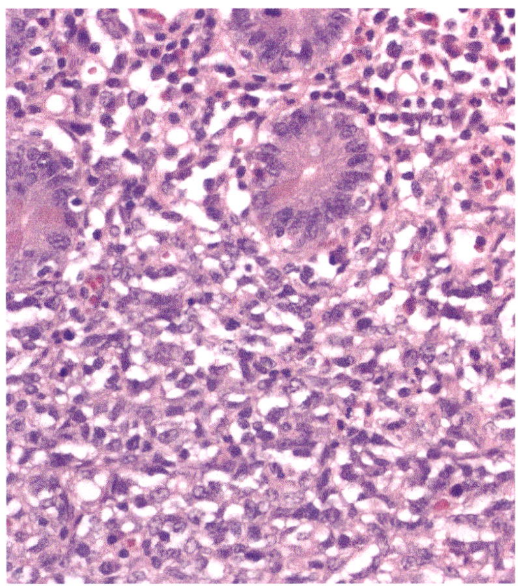

Fig. 9.7 Ileum diffuse large B-cell lymphoma high power

Diffuse Large B-Cell Lymphoma

As with other sites in the gastrointestinal tract, diffuse large B-cell lymphoma may present as a solitary mass in the ileum (Fig. 9.7). It may arise de novo or as a result of transformation from another B-cell lymphoma, e.g. MALT. CD20 expression is typical unless the patient is undertaking treatment with anti-CD20 medication. CD10 expression is associated with a better prognosis than cases showing no expression. Mutations in Bcl-2 and Bcl-6 genes may be found. At least 10% of cases display a high proliferation index (>95%) by Ki67 stain. This is usually the result of additional mutations involving c-myc gene - a "double-hit lymphoma". Rarely mutations of Bcl-2, Bcl-6 and c-myc occur, and these "triple-hit" lymphomas are particularly aggressive.

Burkitt Lymphoma Ileum

Burkitt lymphoma is an aggressive lymphoma occurring in both endemic (EBV infection associated) and sporadic forms. In both forms, gastrointestinal tract involvement has a predilection for the ileocaecal region.

The endemic form is strongly associated with EBV infection. Endemic areas are in Africa and the Middle East, with the latter region showing an increased predilection for intestinal disease. There is an increased risk for Burkitt lymphoma development in HIV-infected individuals.

Classical Burkitt lymphoma is characterised by a diffuse infiltrate of intermediate-sized cells with squared-off cell borders, round nuclei and 2–5 small to medium-sized paracentral nucleoli. Cytoplasmic vacuoles may be seen [14]. Reflecting the high proliferation rate of this tumour is numerous mitoses and apoptotic bodies, the latter being engulfed by histiocytes and imparting the characteristic "starry sky" appearance (Fig. 9.8).

Other high-grade non-Hodgkins lymphoma of both B- and T-cell types can mimic Burkitt lymphoma. Immunohistochemistry is of assistance in excluding T-cell lymphoma. In practice the most difficult separation is with DLBCL with c-myc-related double- or triple-hit mutation. Attention to the clinical setting, site of occurrence and cell morphology is the most helpful feature. Expression of EBV (EBER-ISH) is helpful in confirming endemic and immunodeficiency-related cases.

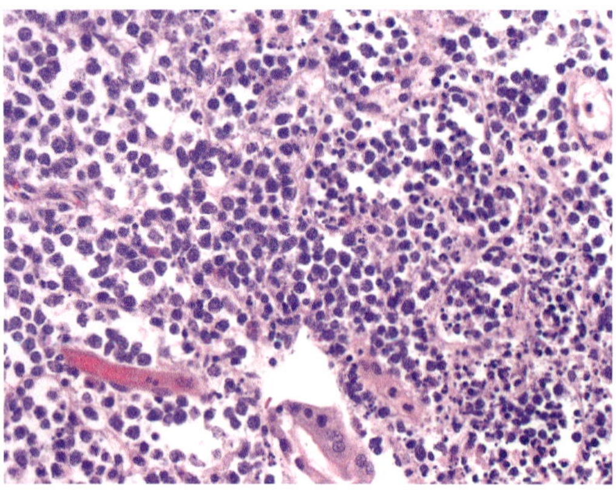

Fig. 9.8 Burkitt lymphoma ileum. Note the prominent apoptosis

Mastocytosis

Mastocytosis affecting the intestine is said to be part of a systemic process although cases confined to the gastrointestinal tract are often encountered and may be the initial site of presentation of disease. The colon and terminal ileum are most commonly involved. Tumour may be single and present as a polyp or multifocal and plaque like or indistinct and is composed of round to spindle-shaped cells expanding the lamina propria. The round cells frequently display cytoplasmic clearing leading to a "fried egg"-like appearance (Fig. 9.9, 9.10, 9.11, and 9.12). The cells show a tendency to collect around the glands and to form a dense superficial band. The process may be patchy. An associated eosinophil infiltrate is usual and can overwhelm the background mast cells, suggesting a diagnosis of eosinophilic enteritis. A rare pleomorphic tumour variant (mast cell sarcoma) has been described in the gastrointestinal tract [15, 16]. Toluidine blue histochemical stains usually highlight the cells but have been superseded by immunochemistry for c-kit and mast cell tryptase. CD25 reaction is highly specific for neoplastic mast cells and confirms the diagnosis of systemic mastocytosis. Consensus criteria for the diagnosis have been established and are presented in Table 9.2. Systemic mastocytosis is the result of a mutation of the gene encoding for the c-kit (tyrosine kinase) receptor. Mutation analysis of the c-kit gene may be beneficial as some mutations (except the common codon 816 mutation) are associated with a favourable response to tyrosine kinase receptor antagonists.

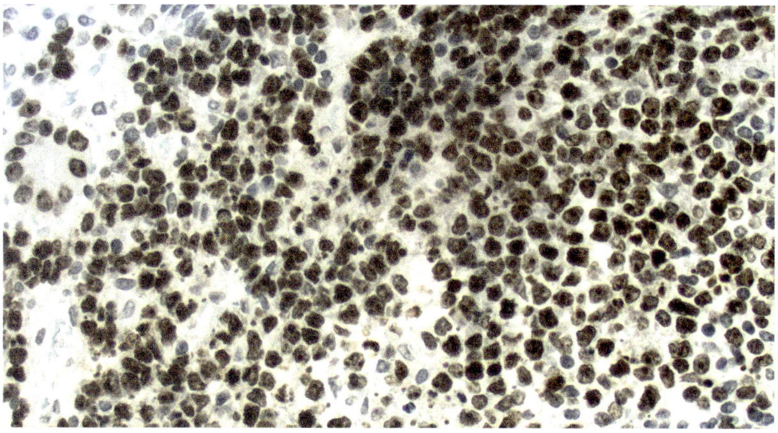

Fig. 9.9 Burkitt lymphoma ileum Ki67 index. Expression in essentially all tumour cells

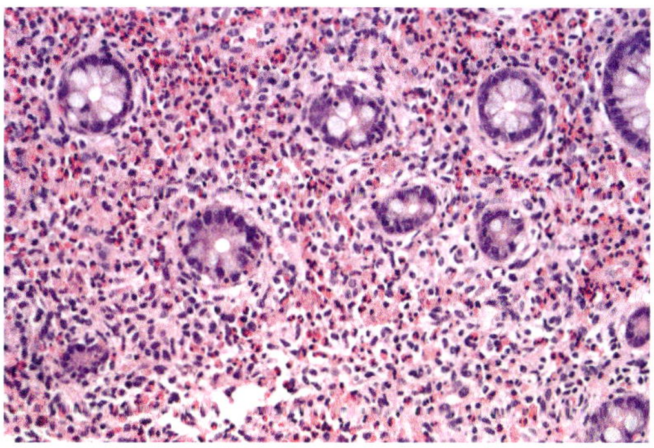

Fig. 9.10 Mastocytosis characterised by oval cells with clear cytoplasm and background rich in eosinophils. H & E stain

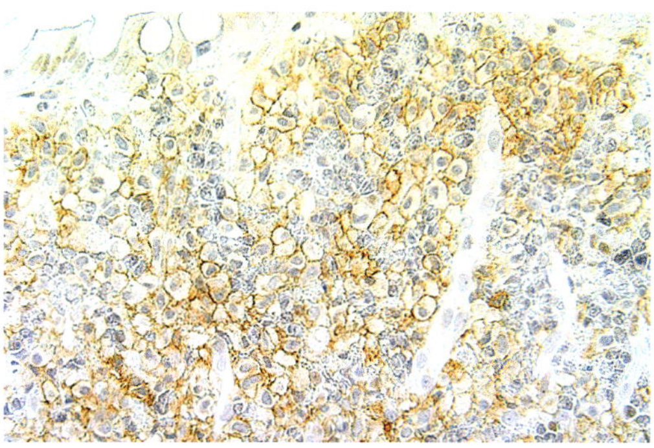

Fig. 9.11 CD25 stain mastocytosis

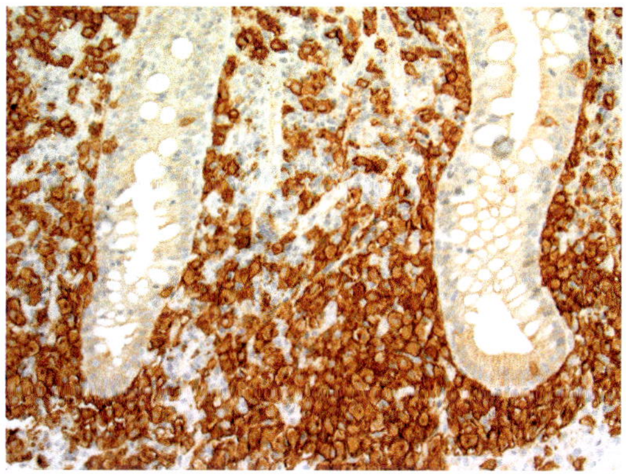

Fig. 9.12 CD117 mastocytosis

Table 9.2 Diagnostic criteria for systemic mastocytosis

Major
Multifocal dense aggregates of mast cells with more than 15 cells per aggregate in an extracutaneous tissue
Minor
1. >25% of mast cells have morphologic abnormalities, e.g. spindle shape, irregular outline
2. Expression of CD25 with or without CD2 by mast cells
3. Detection of a codon 816 c-kit mutation by a sensitive technique in lesional tissue or peripheral blood
4. Serum baseline tryptase >20 ng/mL
Diagnosis = 1 major and 1 minor criterion or 3 minor criteria

References

1. Jiang W, Roma AA, Lai K, Carver P, Xiao SY, Liu X. Endometriosis involving the mucosa of the intestinal tract: a clinicopathologic study of 15 cases. Mod Pathol. 2013;26(9):1270–8.
2. Yantiss RK, Clement PB, Young RH. Endometriosis of the intestinal tract: a study of 44 cases of a disease that may cause diverse challenges in clinical and pathologic evaluation. Am J Surg Pathol. 2001;25(4):445–54.
3. Kahn E, Daum F. Pseudopolyps of the small intestine in Crohn's disease. Hum Pathol. 1984;15(1):84–6.
4. Mukhopadhyay S, Harbol T, Floyd FD, Sidhu JS. Polypoid nodular lymphoid hyperplasia of the terminal ileum. Arch Pathol Lab Med. 2004;128(10):1186–7.
5. Krauss E, Konturek P, Maiss J, Kressel J, Schulz U, Hahn EG, Neurath MF, Raithel M. Clinical significance of lymphoid hyperplasia of the lower gastrointestinal tract. Endoscopy. 2010;42(4):334–7.
6. Koreishi A, Lauwers GY, Misdraji J. Pneumatosis intestinalis: a challenging biopsy diagnosis. Am J Surg Pathol. 2007;31(10):1469–75.
7. Di Giorgio A, Sofo L, Ridolfini MP, Alfieri S, Doglietto GB. Pneumatosis cystoides intestinalis. Lancet. 2007;369(9563):766.
8. Yano T, Yamamoto H. Vascular, polypoid, and other lesions of the small bowel. Best Pract Res Clin Gastroenterol. 2009;23(1):61–74.
9. Walsh JC, Schaeffer DF, Kirsch R, Pollett A, Manzoni M, Riddell RH, Albarello L. Ileal "carcinoid" tumors-small size belies deadly intent: high rate of nodal metastasis in tumors ≤1 cm in size. Hum Pathol. 2016;56:123–7.
10. Daum O, Hatlova J, Mandys V, et al. Comparison of morphological, immunohistochemical, and molecular genetic features of inflammatory fibroid polyps (Vanek's tumors). Virchows Arch. 2010;456:491–7.
11. Liu TC, Lin MT, Montgomery EA, Singhi AD. Inflammatory fibroid polyps of the gastrointestinal tract: spectrum of clinical, morphologic, and immunohistochemistry features. Am J Surg Pathol. 2013;37(4):586–92.
12. Schildhaus HU, Caviar T, Binot E, Buttner R, Wardelmann E, Merkelbach-Bruse S. Inflammatory fibroid polyps harbour mutations in the platelet-derived growth factor receptor alpha (PDGFRA) gene. J Pathol. 2008;216(2):176–82.
13. Lasota J, Wang ZF, Sobin LH, Miettinen M. Gain of function PDGFRA mutations, earlier reported in gastrointestinal stromal tumors, are common in small intestinal inflammatory fibroid polyps. A study of 60 cases. Mod Pathol. 2009;22(8):1049–56.
14. Said J, Lones M, Yea S. Burkitt lymphoma and MYC: what else is new? Adv Anat Pathol. 2014;21(3):160–5.
15. Doyle LA, Hornick JL. Pathology of extramedullary mastocytosis. Immunol Allergy Clin North Am. 2014;34(2):323–39.
16. Akin C, Valent P. Diagnostic criteria and classification of mastocytosis in 2014. Immunol Allergy Clin North Am. 2014;34(2):207–18.

Part V

Large Intestine

Large Intestine: Inflammatory Patterns

10

Ian Brown and Gregory C. Miller

Contents

I. Brown (✉)
Envoi Pathology, Kelvin Grove, QLD, Australia
e-mail: ianbrown@envoi.com.au

G. C. Miller
Envoi Pathology, Kelvin Grove, QLD, Australia

Faculty of Medicine, University of Queensland, Brisbane, QLD, Australia

Acute Inflammation (and/or Erosion)

Acute inflammation pattern (also known as active inflammation) is characterised by neutrophil infiltration in the mucosa. The normal lamina propria inflammatory cell infiltrate consists of lymphocytes, plasma cells and histiocytes. Collections of neutrophils in the lamina propria are abnormal; however in most cases, the finding of neutrophil infiltration of the crypt epithelium "cryptitis" with or without extension into the crypt lumen "crypt abscess formation" is required to define this pattern. Active inflammation in the colon is further classified as focal or diffuse, depending on the extent of neutrophil infiltration. Focal active inflammation involves only a single or at most a few adjacent

M. P. Kumarasinghe, I. Brown (eds.), *Endoscopic Biopsy Interpretation*,
https://doi.org/10.1007/978-3-319-79117-3_10

crypts, often in a multifocal fashion, with normal intervening mucosa (Fig. 10.1; focal active colitis (FAC) due to *C. difficile*). Diffuse active inflammation is characterised by neutrophil infiltration of the majority of the crypts in the biopsy material. Most causes of severe active inflammation also can produce surface erosion. A defining feature of the active inflammation pattern is the absence of changes suggesting chronicity (see later).

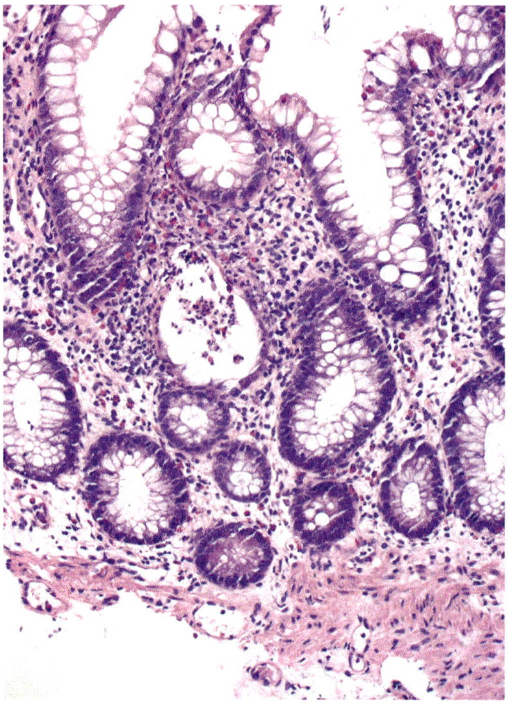

Fig. 10.1 Focal active colitis secondary to *C. difficile* infection

Focal Active Colitis

Several studies have identified the causes of focal active colitis pattern, and there are distinct differences between adult and paediatric cases (see Table 10.1). In both adults and children, an infective or presumed infective cause (on the basis of symptoms and self-limited behaviour) is most common. Other associations in adults are medications, in particular NSAIDs, and irritable bowel syndrome. Our experience is that the use of sodium phosphate bowel preparation is also an important contributor. Importantly, inflammatory bowel disease, in particular Crohn's disease, is not commonly associated with the pattern of inflammation in adults, but it often manifests with this pattern in children.

Knowledge of these associations is important for reporting. Text containing the following comments can be added to the pathology report when focal active colitis pattern is identified.

In adults: "focal active colitis pattern is most commonly associated with infection, medication effect, or a non-specific finding. It is only rarely associated with inflammatory bowel disease at first presentation". In children: "focal active colitis pattern is most commonly associated with infection or represents an early phase in the development of inflammatory bowel disease. In approximately one quarter of patients a cause is not established" [1–6].

Diffuse Active Colitis

Clinically, a diffuse active colitis presents with an abrupt onset of diarrhoea sometimes with per

Table 10.1 Associations of focal active colitis pattern in adults and children

	Greenson et al. 1997 [2]	Volk et al.1998 [3]	Shetty et al.2011 [1]	Xin et al. 2003 [4]
Cause	Adult($N = 42$)	Adult($N = 31$)	Adult ($N = 90$)	Paediatric ($N = 31$)
Self-limited (probable or proven infection)	39%	48%	19%	31%
Drugs	39%	–	24%	0%
Irritable bowel syndrome	14%	–	33%	0%
Inflammatory bowel disease(Crohn's disease usually)	0%	13%	16%	31%
Ischaemia	4%	10%	–	–
Allergy	–	–	–	6.5%
Hirschsprung's disease	–	–	–	3.2%
Idiopathic/asymptomatic	22%	29%	8%	27.6%

rectal bleeding. It is often accompanied by fever and abdominal pain.

The major causes of diffuse active colitis are listed below.

- Infection (see below)
- Topical injury
  - Chemical (including medications)
  - Physical trauma
- Early ulcerative colitis
- Medication
  - methyl-DOPA, immune modulatory medications.

Of the causes listed, the most important is infection. Most cases of diffuse active colitis run a self-limited clinical course, and it is believed that infective processes are responsible for the majority of these cases even if an organism is unable to be identified. The term **acute self-limited colitis** is applied for such situations and is defined by the absence of recurrence of colitis in follow-up of at least 2 years. In the 30–40% of cases where an organism is identified, the most common pathogens are *Campylobacter jejuni*, *Salmonella* and *Shigella*. Other associations include *C. difficile*, *Chlamydia*, *Yersinia enterocolitica*, *E. coli* 0157:H7 and *Aeromonas* species.

The histological features of diffuse active colitis vary with the duration of the disease. The maximum activity stage occurs between 0 and 4 days after the onset of bloody diarrhoea. There is usually prominent mucosal oedema accompanied by an impression of crypt elongation. Cryptitis and crypt abscesses are numerous, and the abscesses may appear to involve the colonic crypts in a beaded fashion, which has been referred to as a "string of pearls" appearance (Figs. 10.2 and 10.3) (infective colitis low power and infective colitis high power). Resolution usually begins within 6–9 days of onset of bloody diarrhoea and is characterised by regenerative features in the crypts, which contain residual focal neutrophilic cryptitis and degenerating neutrophils in the lumen. In the latter stages of resolution, along with some regenerative features, occasional crypts with transmigrating lymphocytes may be present. Chronic inflammatory cells may increase over time; however the development of crypt distortion and basal plasmacytosis suggests an active chronic colitis such as ulcerative colitis rather than an acute self-limited colitis with diffuse active inflammation. Repeat endoscopy at 2–3 months following the onset of symptoms can help differentiate equivocal cases [7, 8].

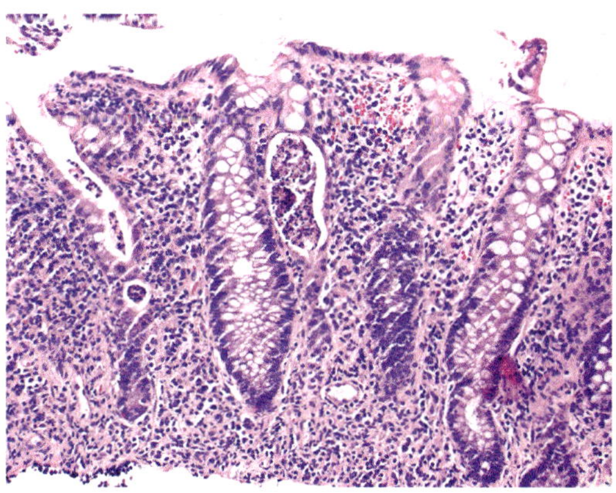

Fig. 10.3 Diffuse active colitis seen in infective colitis 20×

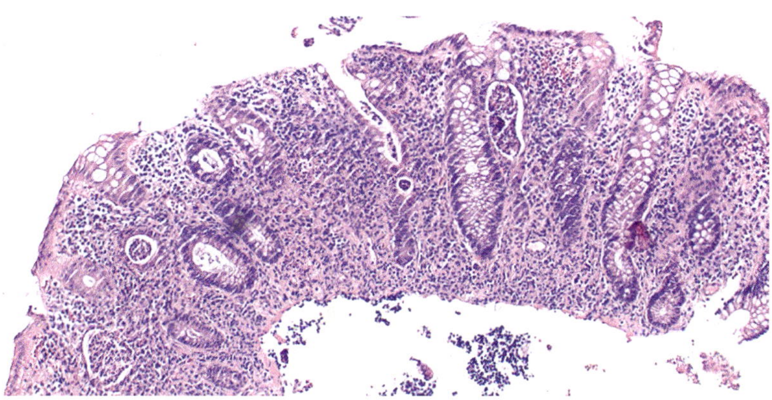

Fig. 10.2 Diffuse active colitis seen in infective colitis 4×

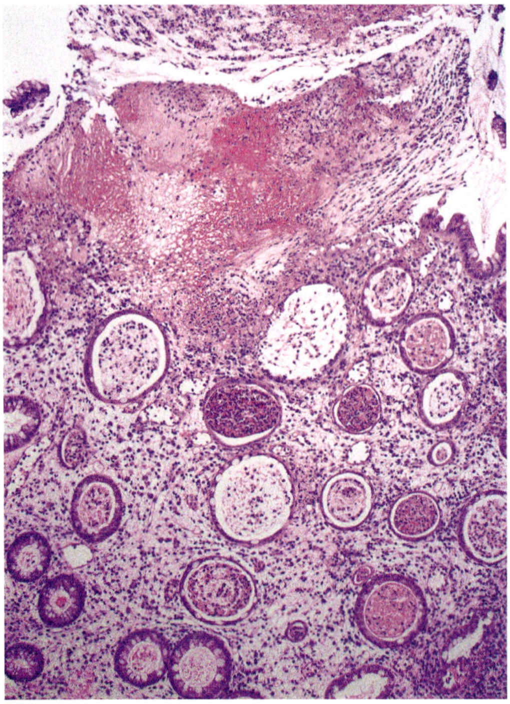

Fig. 10.4 Pseudomembranous colitis - low power demonstrating characteristic pseudomembrane

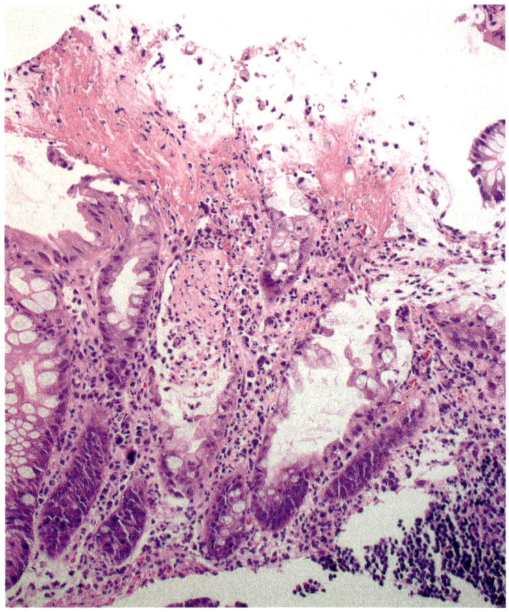

Fig. 10.5 Pseudomembranous colitis - high power of typical "volcano like" exudate forming the pseudomembrane

Acute Colitis with "Pseudomembranous Colitis"

Occasionally a diffuse, or sometimes focal, active colitis is accompanied by areas of superficial mucosal erosion with a distinctive fibrinous exudate within which are variable numbers of neutrophils—pseudomembranes (Figs. 10.4 and 10.5). A number of causes for pseudomembrane formation are recognised [9–15]. These are listed below.

- *C. difficile toxin (post antibiotic)*:
- Other infections: *Shigella*, *E. coli* 0157:H7, CMV and *Klebsiella oxytoca, amoebiasis*
- Drug/toxin:
  - Chlorpropamide, mercuric compounds, NSAIDs, chemotherapy e.g. 5-FU and gold
- Superimposed on lesions/mass:
  - Solitary rectal ulcer syndrome and cap polyposis
- Ischaemia
- Collagenous colitis

The most common association is *with C. difficile* infection. *C. difficile* is a nosocomial infection that is epidemic or endemic in hospitals or nursing homes. *C. difficile* is a gram-positive obligate anaerobic rod-shaped bacterium that colonises the intestine when the native microflora has been altered. Pseudomembranous colitis is a toxin-mediated disease, and there are two toxins produced by *C. difficile* organisms. Toxin A is an enterotoxin, whereas toxin B is a cytotoxin. Although many laboratories assay for only one of these toxins in stool, both are present in every case, and testing for both increases sensitivity of the diagnosis. Pseudomembranous colitis usually occurs as a complication of antibiotic therapy but is also associated with abdominal surgery, colonic obstruction, uraemia or prolonged hypotension or hypoperfusion of bowel and in the setting of immunosuppression. Increasingly *C. difficile* colitis is being recognised to complicate the course of inflammatory bowel disease.

Of the two exotoxins, toxin A (enterotoxin) plays the more significant role and is responsible for inflammation and inflammatory exudate. Stool cytotoxin assay is positive in 95% of patients. Not all patients with *C. difficile* infection develop pseudomembranous colitis. Pseudomembranous colitis may progress to toxic megacolon with secondary perforation and peritonitis.

Erosion

Causes of colonic mucosal erosion:

- Inflammatory bowel disease
- Infection—*C. difficile*, cytomegalovirus (CMV), *Campylobacter*, *Yersinia*, amoeba, helminths (hookworm), tuberculosis (TB) and others
- Ischaemia
- Diverticulum related
- Stercoral
- Vasculitis—Behcet's disease and others
- Medications—NSAID, OCP, nicorandil, chemotherapy (5-FU), potassium chloride and resins
- Neoplasms
- Radiotherapy related
- Idiopathic

Active Chronic Colitis

Active chronic inflammation differs from acute inflammation in showing signs of chronicity.

> The features of chronicity are:
>
> 1. Crypt architectural irregularity—crypt shortening, crypt branching, irregular size and placement of crypts
> 2. Chronic inflammation in the basal aspect of the mucosa—more than one basal lymphoid aggregate per biopsy piece, collections of plasma cells sitting just above the muscularis mucosae and chronic inflammatory cells as numerous in the basal half as in the superficial half of the mucosa
> 3. Evidence of epithelial metaplasia—Paneth cell metaplasia and pyloric gland metaplasia

As with active inflammation, this process may be focal or diffuse.

Focal Active Chronic Colitis

This is characterised by active and chronic inflammation involving only parts of the submitted biopsies from the large intestine with relatively normal mucosa elsewhere. Typically chronic inflammation is the predominant process.

The causes of this pattern include:

- Crohn's disease
- Medications—NSAID and biological agents
- Diverticular disease-associated colitis
- Ongoing ischaemic injury
- Partially treated ulcerative colitis
- Chronic infection—*Yersinia* and TB

Diffuse Active Chronic Colitis

Diffuse active chronic inflammation is characterised by involvement of all parts of the submitted biopsies. Generally the inflammation is uniform with minimal variability in intensity.

Causes

- Ulcerative colitis—most common cause
- Chronic infection—*Campylobacter* and *Salmonella*
- Drug reaction - mycophenolate, immune modulatory medications
- Diverticular disease-associated colitis
- Diversion colitis
- Obstructive colitis - proximal to an obstructing mass lesion
- Crohn's disease—occasional cases of paediatric-onset disease

Inflammatory Bowel Disease

Inflammatory bowel disease is a chronic immunologically driven inflammation of the intestine. Two major forms are currently recognised, ulcerative colitis and Crohn's disease. Clinical and histological differences exist between these two forms, and in the classic presentation, diagnostic separation is easy (see Table 10.2); however there exist variant forms (discussed below) where the distinction is difficult.

Currently the aetiology and pathogenesis of both forms of inflammatory bowel disease is believed to represent an unregulated and exaggerated local immune response to commensal microbes (or bacterial products) in the gut, in genetically susceptible

Table 10.2 Features of ulcerative colitis and Crohn's disease

Ulcerative colitis	Crohn's disease
Clinical M = F Age peaks 15–25 and 60–70 years Incidence: 5–18/100,000/year 25% affected relatives High twin concordance More common away from equator Extraintestinal lesions[a] Appendectomy protective Atypical pANCA	*Clinical* M = F Age peaks 20–30 and 60–70 Incidence: <1–10/100,000/year 10% affected relatives High twin concordance More common away from equator Extraintestinal lesions[a] Increased risk with smoking ASCA
Endoscopic Continuous involvement from rectum for a variable distance proximally into colon Hyperaemic (non-ulcerated) mucosa	*Endoscopic* Discontinuous involvement, entire GIT can be affected Ulceration (longitudinal) with intervening preserved mucosa
Histopathology Mucosa/submucosa Uniform inflammation No granulomata No fissuring ulceration No fibrosis or neural hyperplasia	*Histopathology* Transmural (not appreciable in biopsy specimens) Discontinuous and variable inflammation Granulomata (25%) Fissuring ulceration Fibrosis and neural hyperplasia

[a]Extraintestinal manifestations: Joints - arthritis, sacroiliitis; Skin: erythema nodosum, pyoderma gangrenosum; Liver: primary sclerosing cholangitis; Eyes: uveitis

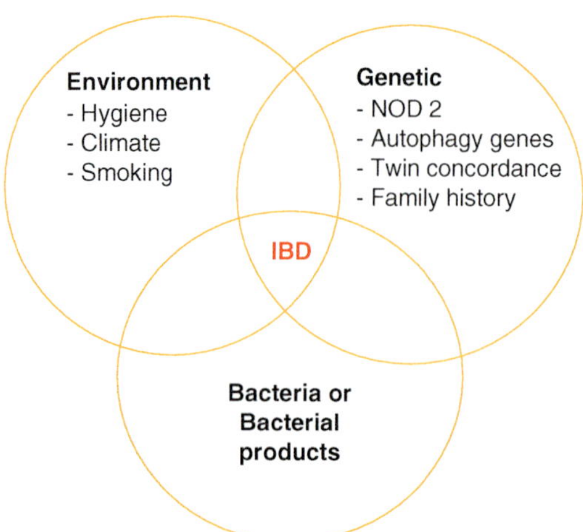

Fig. 10.6 Interaction of factors in the aetiology of inflammatory bowel disease

individuals (see Fig. 10.6). A breakdown of the mucosal barrier (both physical and immunological) is a necessary initial step. The subsequent inappropriate immune response is responsible for the pathological features that develop.

Ulcerative Colitis

The classical histology is of uniform diffuse active chronic inflammation beginning at the rectum and extending for a variable distance proximally in the colon. Skip lesions are absent and the ileum and upper gastrointestinal tract should be spared. It is increasingly recognised that variant histological features do occur. These are summarised below.

Atypical Presentation of Ulcerative Colitis

Paediatric Pattern

Paediatric ulcerative colitis is more likely to present with inflammation, which may be variable in location, intensity and rectal involvement. This is particularly true in patients presenting in preteenage years. There may be relative rectal sparing, that is, less inflammation in the rectum than elsewhere in the colon, in up to 34% of paediatric patients. Absolute rectal sparing is seen in 3%. Apparent skip lesions may be observed in up to 23%. In addition, paediatric patients are more likely to present with subtotal or pan colitis than adults (42% versus 11%) [16–18].

Upper Gastrointestinal Tract Involvement

Two patterns of upper gastrointestinal tract involvement are seen with ulcerative colitis. Firstly, a diffuse duodenitis or panenteritis is a rare manifestation of ulcerative colitis, almost always in the setting of recent colectomy for severe pancolitis. Inflammation is characterised by active chronic inflammation closely resembling colonic ulcerative colitis. The cause for this is unknown, but it is probably secondary to an immunological process. Infection, in particular *C. difficile*, needs to be excluded. Secondly, a focally enhanced gastritis, which is more commonly seen with Crohn's disease, does develop in a small subset of ulcerative colitis patients, particularly in the paediatric age group [19–24].

Rectal Sparing

Ulcerative colitis is typically defined by inflammation that involves the rectum and extends for a variable distance proximally. Hence, if the rectum appears to be uninvolved or minimally involved, the diagnosis may be called into question except in the clinical settings highlighted below. Rectal sparing may be relative, with less inflammation than elsewhere in the large intestine, or absolute, where no inflammatory changes are seen. This can occur in the following clinical scenarios:

Initial presentation—Relative rectal sparing has been reported at initial presentation at the 34% of paediatric patients and up to 5% of adults. Absolute sparing is reported in approximately 1–2% of ulcerative colitis at first presentation.

Burnt-out (long-standing) disease—This is a relative process where the disease resolves more in the rectum than elsewhere.

Effect of therapy—This is seen in up to 40% of patients treated with topical steroid enemas.

Patchy Distribution (Skip Lesions)

Patchiness in the distribution of inflammation has been reported in between 30% and 38% of all cases in endoscopic biopsy series for ulcerative colitis. This is typically enhanced by medications used to treat the disease. A characteristic skip lesion is the so-called caecal patch, which is inflammation limited to the region of the appendiceal orifice but sometimes involving the entire cecum and even proximal ascending colon. This usually occurs concurrently with active inflammation in the rectum; however it may be an isolated finding [25–29]. This right-sided inflammation is seen in up to 75% of endoscopic examinations.

Ileitis in UC

Ileitis, which may be acute, or active chronic in nature may be encountered in patients with ulcerative colitis. Potential causes for this are listed below.

- Bowel preparation effects
- Drugs (NSAIDs)
- Bacterial overgrowth
- Ischaemia
- Infection (CMV, *Yersinia*, TB)
- Backwash ileitis in 20% of ulcerative colitis cases

It is important to remember that ileitis does not always equate to Crohn's disease, and if the large intestine inflammatory pattern is typical of ulcerative colitis by being superficial, uniform and diffuse, and lacking granulomata, then the ileitis may be due to one of the processes listed above rather than Crohn's disease [30].

Ulcerative Colitis Without Chronicity (Early Ulcerative Colitis)

As with any chronic inflammatory process in the large intestine, there is a period of time required before the chronic architectural and inflammatory changes become apparent. Before this the exclusion of another process in particular is problematic. Table 10.3 summarises data from a prospective study of patients presenting with acute colitis. The important message is that it may take up to 1 month before the chronic changes become apparent and up to 4 months before they are well established. Hence, within the first 4 weeks of symptoms, a definitive diagnosis of ulcerative colitis may not be possible, and the patient would be advised to have biopsies at a later time when characteristic chronic

Table 10.3 Changes in colon biopsies over time in patients presenting with acute colitis

Time course since symptoms began	Crypt distortion	Vertical crypt branching >2	Villous mucosa	Mucosal atrophy	Focal/diffuse basal lymphoplasmacytosis	Upper half inflammation
1–15 days	0%	0%	0%	0%	38%	25%
16–30 days	23%	23%	23%	31%	54%	23%
1–4 months	20%	24%	33%	43%	81%	0%
4–10 months	78%	44%	33%	44%	89%	0%
1 year	29%	29%	0%	31%	42%	15%
First biopsy of infective colitis	3%	0%	0%	6%	3%	28%
1 year biopsy of infective colitis	0%	0%	0%	0–4%	4%	19%

changes should be better developed. As discussed above, paediatric ulcerative colitis may not show chronic architectural change and hence can be an exception to the data presented below [31–33].

Ulcerative Colitis with Granulomata

Not infrequently, active ulcerative colitis and the associated crypt inflammation lead to crypt rupture. This can elicit a local histiocytic and granulomatous reaction. If single crypts are involved, the diagnosis is generally apparent. When several crypts undergo rupture and form granulomata, this causes a diagnostic issue in excluding Crohn's disease. The finding of the granulomata at the site of the ruptured crypt or immediately adjacent to the point of rupture are important clues. Often there is a neutrophilic and eosinophilic infiltrate associated with the crypt rupture granuloma and there may be some extravasated mucin. The granuloma may appear to extend into the crypt lumen. The presence of diffuse uniform inflammation throughout the large intestine and the absence of ileal inflammation favour ulcerative colitis. If granulamata are numerous then Crohn's disease is more likely, even, if there is evidence of crypt rupture as the immediate cause.

Crohn's Disease

Isolated Crohn's disease accounts for no more than 20% of cases of chronic colitis and is characterised by very active chronic inflammation usually accompanied by ulceration. Granulomas may be encountered in up to 25% of cases. A characteristic pattern is the presence of stromal oedema and crypt elongation without crypt branching in non-ulcerated mucosa. Goblet cell mucin is typically well preserved. Lymphocytes and histiocytes are the dominant inflammatory cells present. Plasma cells are uncommon aside from areas of ulceration.

Cancer Risk Associated with Inflammatory Bowel Disease

There is an increased risk of developing dysplasia and adenocarcinoma in both ulcerative colitis and Crohn's disease. The risk appears to be similar for both ulcerative colitis and Crohn's disease. A small increased risk for lymphoproliferative disorders is also known. In terms of the risk for adenocarcinoma in ulcerative colitis, the following factors are established. Firstly the risk increases with duration of disease with an overall incidence of 0.5–1.0% per year. The risk is greatest in patients who have had the disease for 10 years or more and those who have inflammation affecting the whole or a large proportion of the colon (total or subtotal colitis). Patients who develop ulcerative colitis as children (0–14 years old) have a higher risk of eventually developing cancer than those whose first attack of UC occurs as adults (15–39 years old). A number of other risk factors are recognised including severe colitis, a family history of colorectal adenocarcinoma and concurrent primary sclerosing cholangitis (PSC) [34, 35].

Reporting Scheme for Inflammatory Bowel Disease Biopsies

The acronym "PAID" has been suggested as a scheme for reporting all inflammatory bowel disease biopsies.

P—Pattern of chronic changes: presence, distribution and extent.

A—Activity: cryptitis, crypt abscess formation and surface ulceration.

I—Interpretation: whether the process represents inflammatory bowel disease and if so whether it is ulcerative colitis or Crohn's disease. The term inflammatory bowel disease, unclassified, can be applied to biopsies where there is certainty about the chronic nature of the process but uncertainty as to its exact type.

D—Dysplasia: location and severity.

Grading of the histological changes is becoming increasingly important to assess for disease response to treatment and as a predictor of relapse following treatment. A reproducible system is the Geboes score for assessment of ulcerative colitis histologic disease activity, which is listed below [35, 36].

Geboes Scoring Scheme for Ulcerative Colitis

Grade 0 Structural (architectural changes)

0.0—No abnormality

0.1—Mild abnormality

0.2—Mild or moderate diffuse or multifocal abnormalities
0.3—Severe diffuse or multifocal abnormalities
Grade 1 Chronic inflammatory infiltrate
1.0—No increase
1.1—Mild but unequivocal increase
1.2—Moderate increase
1.3—Marked increase
Grade 2 Lamina propria neutrophils and eosinophils
2A—Eosinophils
2A.0—No increase
2A.1—Mild but unequivocal increase
2A.2—Moderate increase
2A.3—Marked increase
2B—Neutrophils
2B.0—No increase
2B.1—Mild but unequivocal increase
2B.2—Moderate increase
2B.3—Marked increase
Grade 3 Neutrophils in epithelium
3.0—None
3.1—< % crypts involved
3.2—<50% crypts involved
3.3—>50% crypts involved
Grade 4 Crypt destruction
4.0—None
4.1—Probable—local excess of neutrophils in part of crypt
4.2—Probable—marked attenuation
4.3—Unequivocal crypt destruction
Grade 5 Erosion or ulceration
5.0—No erosion, ulceration or granulation tissue
5.1—Recovering epithelium + adjacent inflammation
5.2—Probable erosion focally stripped
5.3—Unequivocal erosion
5.4—Ulcer or granulation tissue

Diversion Colitis

Diversion colitis arises in colonic segments excluded from the faecal stream usually because of a surgical procedure (e.g. Hartmann's procedure). It is found in 50–100% of patients with a diverted segment and is reversible by restoration of the normal faecal stream. The aetiology of the inflammation is believed to be a lack of faecal butyrate and other fatty acids that are required for normal cell proliferation and maturation. This places the colonic enterocytes under metabolic stress. Subsequent release of cytokines and other chemicals induces the inflammatory process.

The histological pattern is dominated by reactive lymphoid follicles in the base of the mucosa. There is an associated increased chronic inflammatory cell infiltrate in the mucosa with mild acute inflammation characterised by cryptitis and crypt abscess formation with only minimal crypt architectural disturbance. Surface erosion may be present, and granulomas can be encountered in up to 25% of cases. The diagnosis is straightforward in patients known to have a diverted faecal stream. However, it may be more challenging in patients with a previous history of inflammatory bowel disease.

Two issues arise in assessing a diverted segment of colon; firstly, is the inflammation due to recurrence of active inflammatory bowel disease or purely due to diversion colitis? The dominance of reactive lymphoid follicles combined with minimal crypt architectural disturbance and relatively mild plasma cell infiltration are features in favour of diversion as the cause. Secondly, does the pattern of inflammation represent Crohn's disease in a patient previously diagnosed with ulcerative colitis? When the clinical history is of a diverted segment, the diagnosis of ulcerative colitis should not be changed unless there is evidence on pre-diversion biopsy material to suggest otherwise [37, 38].

Diverticular Disease-Associated Colitis

A wide variety of inflammatory changes can be associated with diverticular disease. They vary from mild/moderate non-specific inflammation to florid inflammatory changes associated with crypt architectural distortion mimicking inflammatory bowel disease. In most cases, the changes are restricted to the segment affected by diverticular disease and are most prominent at the neck of the diverticula. This should be distinguished from diverticulitis, which is active inflammation occurring primarily in the diverticula themselves.

In some cases, an intense inflammatory response to the diverticula with the formation of granulomatous inflammation and fissuring ulceration can be observed. However, the changes are usually restricted to the segment of colon involved. This is almost always the sigmoid colon and generally in patients older than 50 years of age with acquired diverticulosis. An important feature is that inflammation is absent in other segments of the large intestine.

A general rule of thumb is to never diagnose inflammatory bowel disease in chronically inflamed biopsies limited to/taken only from the sigmoid colon region, since inflammation limited to this region can be diverticular disease-associated colitis, particularly in older patients [39–42].

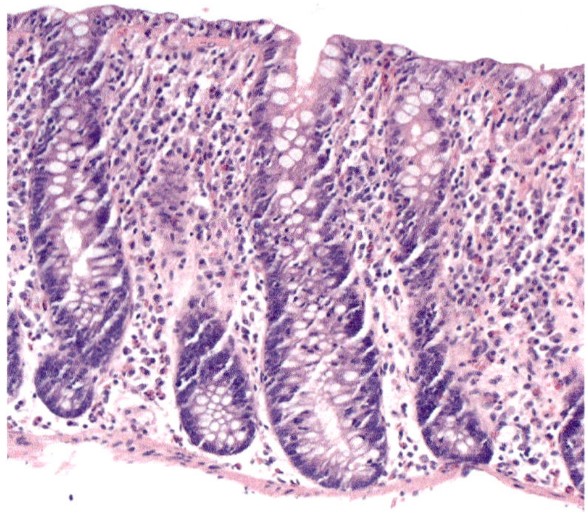

Fig. 10.7 Lymphocytic colitis - milder end of the histological spectrum with inflammation limited to the upper half of the mucosa

Intraepithelial Lymphocytosis

In the normal large intestine, intraepithelial lymphocytes number ≤10/100 enterocytes. Lymphocytosis >20/100 enterocytes is regarded as abnormal. This abnormality was first appreciated in colonic biopsies taken from patients with a history of chronic diarrhoea but with normal endoscopic appearance. Hence the term microscopic colitis was applied. The initial description of microscopic colitis corresponds to what is now known as lymphocytic colitis. The concept of microscopic colitis (normal endoscopic appearance with histological inflammation) has broadened to include four processes: lymphocytic colitis, collagenous colitis, granulomatous microscopic colitis and microscopic colitis, unclassified (or incomplete). It is increasingly recognised by higher-resolution endoscopy that at least some cases of lymphocytic or collagenous colitis show subtle endoscopic abnormalities; hence the term microscopic colitis may become a historical designation [43].

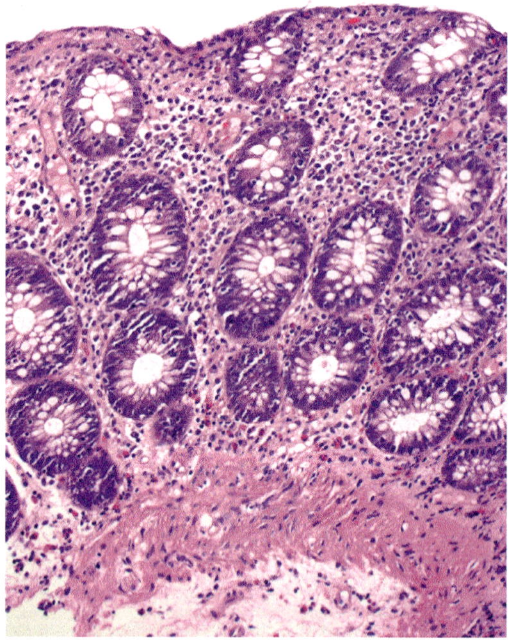

Fig. 10.8 Lymphocytic colitis - more marked inflammation extending to the base of the mucosa

Lymphocytic Colitis

This condition presents with chronic watery diarrhoea. The female-to-male ratio is 2.5:1. It may occur in all ages but is more common in patients older than 60 years of age. The major diagnostic feature is intraepithelial lymphocytosis of >20 lymphocytes/100 enterocytes. Lymphocytes typically involve the surface epithelium with relative sparing of the crypts (Figs. 10.7, 10.8, and 10.9). They are CD3/CD8-positive T lymphocytes. By definition the subepithelial collagen band is <10 μm thick. Inflammation in the lamina propria is present to a variable degree. Several histological patterns are appreciated as discussed below.

It is useful to consider this pattern in terms of the potential aetiologies and in terms of the histological variants.

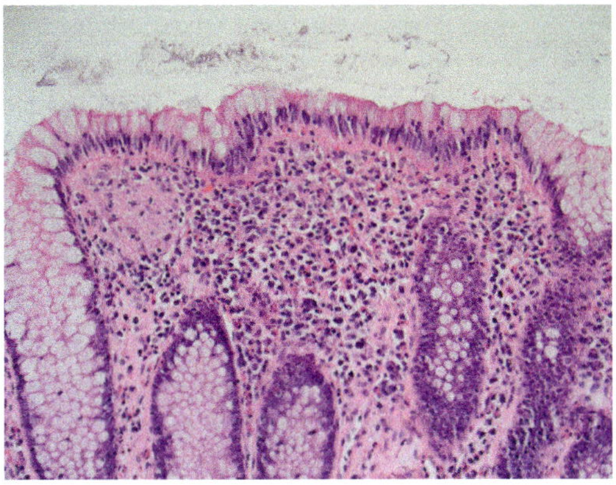

Fig. 10.9 Lymphocytic colitis with giant cells

Clinical Classification (Etiological)

- Idiopathic (~75%)
- Secondary (~25%)
- Coeliac disease (~5%, usually mild lympho cytosis only)
- Drugs (~10%)
  - NSAIDs, PPIs, SSRIs, herbal remedies, ticlopidine and carbamazepine
- Autoimmune disease
  - Hashimoto's thyroiditis and autoimmune enteropathy
- Other immune dysfunctions, e.g. CVID (common variable immunodeficiency) and SCID (severe combined immunodeficiency)
- Infection
  - Brainerd diarrhoea and resolving infective colitis
- Malignancy
  - Infiltrate—lymphoma/leukaemia
  - Immune reaction, e.g. MSI high CRC and melanoma

Histological Classification (See Table 10.4)

Reporting Colonic Lymphocytosis Paucicellular Patterns

Because these histological subtypes are more often associated with an identifiable cause for the lymphocytosis, we find it useful to add the following comment to the histological report.

"This pattern may be associated with coeliac disease, medications (e.g. NSAID's, PPI's, SSRI's), systemic autoimmune disease or colonic infection" [44–52].

Table 10.4 Lymphocytic colitis patterns

Pattern	Histological feature
Conventional (usual)	Inflammation in the lamina propria Superficial or full thickness may include eosinophils and neutrophils (Figs. 10.7 and 10.8)
Colonic lymphocytosis	No lamina propria inflammation
Paucicellular	Minimal lymphocytosis >7 to <20 IEL/100 enterocytes or patchy, but otherwise conventional, lymphocytosis. Must exclude: Cecum only site, mucosa overlying lymphoid follicle, Crohn's disease.
Variant forms	Giant cells; see below (Fig. 10.9) Inflammatory bowel disease-like; see below Cryptal—involving predominantly the crypts

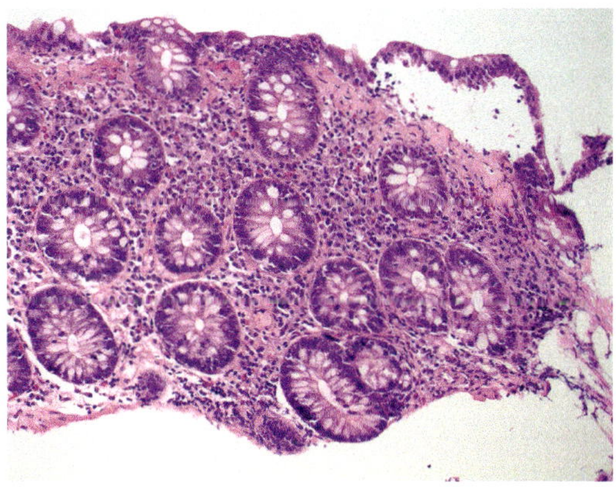

Fig. 10.10 Collagenous colitis - thickened subepithelial collagen plate, epithelial sloughing and lamina propria inflammation

Subepithelial Collagen

Collagenous Colitis

This condition presents with chronic watery diarrhoea. The female-to-male ratio is at least 3:1. It is more common in patients older than 60 years of age. Paediatric cases are rare. The diagnostic feature is irregular thickening to >10 μm of the subepithelial collagen layer (Figs. 10.10 and 10.11). This is predominantly collagen types 1 and 3. Surface epithelial detachment accompanies the thickened collagen. Collagen band thickness varies throughout the large intestine, being maximal

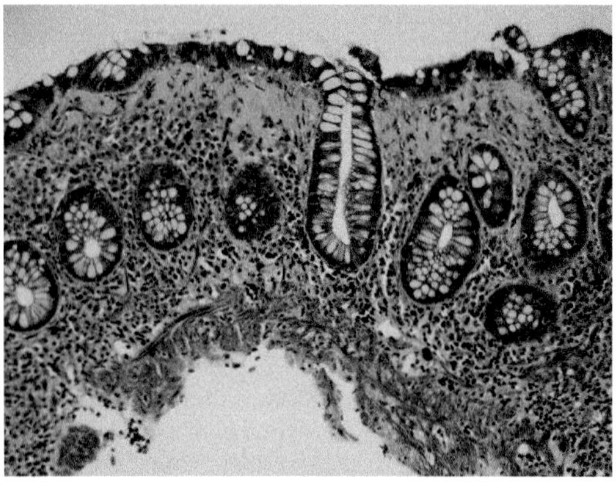

Fig. 10.11 Collagenous colitis (trichrome histochemical stain highlighting the thickened collagen table)

in the transverse colon and minimal and sometimes non-existent in the rectum. Hence the diagnosis of collagenous colitis cannot be excluded on a rectum-only biopsy. Increased intraepithelial lymphocytes are always seen but may be mild. Inflammation in the lamina propria involves the full thickness of the mucosa and comprises lymphocytes, plasma cells and eosinophils, often conspicuous, and occasionally neutrophils. In the absence of obvious lamina propria inflammation and intraepithelial lymphocytosis, the diagnosis of collagenous colitis should be reconsidered. Variant histological forms are discussed below.

Most cases of collagenous colitis are idiopathic. Some cases are associated with the following diseases.

- Drugs
  - NSAIDs, sartan family medications, and immune modulatory medications and new biological therapies e.g. idelalisib
- Autoimmune conditions
  - Autoimmune thyroid disease/rheumatoid arthritis
- Immune dysregulation
  - Common variable immunodeficiency
- Coeliac disease

The Differential Diagnosis

- Lymphocytic Colitis
  - This is an issue when limited biopsy sampling is undertaken; for instance, the rectum only is biopsied and collagen deposition seen elsewhere in the colon is not present. There is also a situation where all biopsies show patchy minimal subepithelial collagen thickening which may only focally reach the threshold of >10 μm thickness. There is data to suggest that these cases behave more like typical collagenous colitis than lymphocytic colitis, and our practical approach is to regard all cases with >10 μm thickness of collagen in at least 10% of the biopsy material as representing collagenous colitis.
- Ischaemic Colitis
  - This issue typically arises when there is segmental ischaemic injury such as at the splenic flexure. Hyaline collagen deposition due to ischaemia may involve the superficial aspect of the mucosa and hence resemble collagenous colitis. The absence of lamina propria inflammation and intraepithelial lymphocytosis helps rule out collagenous colitis.
- Subepithelial Collagen Thickening
  - This may be seen in hyperplastic polyps, in areas of radiation injury and at the site of healed erosion.
- Amyloidosis
  - A collagen stain should be performed in all cases to confirm that the subepithelial pink material is indeed collagen. If not, a Congo red stained for amyloid should be performed.
- Basement Membrane Thickening in Diabetes
  - This seldom reaches the threshold thickness for collagenous colitis. Furthermore it is not associated with inflammation.
- Tangential Sectioning
  - Care should always be taken to ensure that the collagen thickness is not the result of tangential sectioning, as many inflammatory processes are associated with a minimal subepithelial collagen deposition that will be magnified by a tangential section, most particularly lymphocytic colitis.

Variant Histological Forms of Microscopic Colitis

Microscopic Colitis with Giant Cells

The finding of multinucleate giant cells is present in 1–2% of cases of lymphocytic colitis or collagenous colitis. The giant cells occur in the superficial mucosa either immediately beneath the surface epithelium or beneath the thickened collagen layer. The cause of these giant cells is uncertain. A heightened immune response has been proposed on the basis of the more frequent association with autoimmune conditions than typical microscopic colitis in these patients. Intimate association of the giant cells with the thickened collagen layer has also led to speculation that they represent an attempt at collagen regression in collagenous colitis cases. Overall, their presence does not appear to be of any clinical significance [49].

Inflammatory Bowel Disease-Like Feature

Not unexpectedly, the chronic inflammatory process of both lymphocytic colitis and collagenous colitis may produce chronic architectural abnormality and metaplasia (Fig. 10.12). This is seldom a prominent feature; however care should be taken not to overdiagnose these changes as representing inflammatory bowel disease. The following table (Table 10.5) highlights the spectrum of chronic epithelial and inflammatory changes that are reported in microscopic colitis cases [53].

Pseudomembranous Collagenous Colitis

Rarely pseudomembranes characterised by fibrin and neutrophil exudate can be seen in collagenous colitis. These are not associated with *C. difficile* infection. Because many patients with collagenous colitis are elderly and potentially have coexistent vascular disease, the possibility of superimposed ischaemia as the mechanism of pseudomembrane formation has been proposed [13].

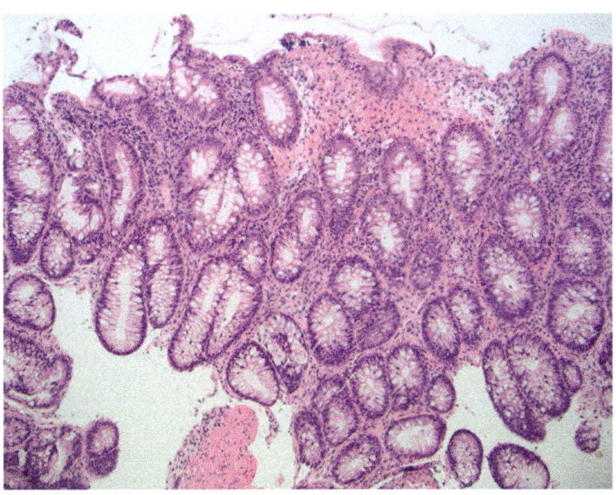

Fig. 10.12 Microscopic colitis with crypt architectural changes

Table 10.5 Chronic features in lymphocytic and collagenous colitis

Features	Collagenous colitis (%)	Lymphocytic colitis (%)
Surface ulceration	2.5	0
Active crypt inflammation	30	38
Paneth cell metaplasia	44	14
Crypt atrophy or irregularity	7.6	4.2
Lymphoid nodules	65	69

Granulomatous Microscopic Colitis

Rarely, patients with a history of chronic watery diarrhoea and normal endoscopic appearance are found to have isolated epithelioid granulomata in the lamina propria in biopsies. There may be mild associate inflammation, however the typical pattern of either lymphocytic colitis or collagenous colitis is lacking. These patients do not prove to have Crohn's disease or an infective process on long-term follow-up. Some almost certainly represent a medication reaction based upon the resolution of changes on cessation of particular medications. However the process remains poorly defined [54].

Eosinophil Infiltration

Eosinophilic Colitis/Colonic Eosinophilia

Eosinophils are a normal component of the lamina propria of the large intestine. The number of eosinophils per HPF ranges in published studies from 3 to 68 in adults. Defining the normal number of eosinophils, and therefore what is abnormal, has proven difficult for a number of reasons. Firstly, there is variation in number throughout the large intestine, with the highest density being reported in the cecum with progressively less numbers on moving distally towards the rectum. Secondly there is a recognised geographical variation with higher numbers of eosinophils found in patients who live closer to the equator. For example, there is a 35-fold increase in the mean colonic eosinophil count between Boston and New Orleans. There also exist racial differences and importantly environmental factors play a role. In particular patients with an allergic diagnosis will show increased numbers of eosinophils in springtime when they are typically exposed to more allergens.

At present a density of >30 eosinophils/HPF is considered abnormal and represents "colonic eosinophilia". Ideally this eosinophilia would be present beyond the caecal region and is definitely abnormal in the left colon or rectum. The diagnosis of "eosinophilic colitis" requires additional morphologic features (Figs. 10.13 and 10.14). These features include:

- Accumulation of eosinophils within the superficial lamina propria.
- Clustering of eosinophils suggests an abnormal eosinophil infiltrate is present, since the cells usually reside in a single fashion within the lamina propria.
- Identification of eosinophils infiltrating muscularis mucosae, within Peyer's patches or extending into superficial submucosa.
- Significant numbers of intraepithelial (surface) and crypt (cryptitis and crypt abscesses) eosinophils, particularly, if clustered in these locations.
- Evidence of eosinophil activation by identification of degranulation (extracellular granules). Care must be taken to exclude degranulation secondary to biopsy trauma, which is normally seen at the edge of the biopsy fragment.
- Evidence of epithelial or tissue injury due to inflammation such as mucin depletion.
- Enlargement/hyperchromatism, nucleoli and mitoses are abnormal. Tissue remodelling/stromal fibrosis may be seen with prolonged and sustained eosinophilic inflammation.

Mucosal eosinophilia is also likely to be significant if there is a clinical association. Typical clinical presentations of eosinophilic colitis include the following:

- Diarrhoea (±nausea/vomiting)
- Abdominal pain
- Tumour effect (obstruction, intussusception)
- Gastrointestinal tract bleeding
- Protein-losing state (hypoalbuminemia)
- Peripheral blood eosinophilia
- Increased serum IgE level
- Colonoscopy finding of oedema with or without punctate erythema or rarely a mass lesion

The causes of colonic eosinophilia are listed in Table 10.6. Pathologists potentially play an important role in identifying the cause of colonic eosinophilia. It is therefore not sufficient to sim-

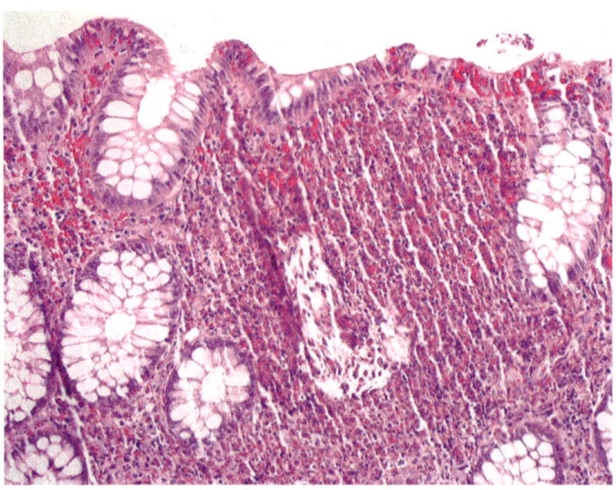

Fig. 10.13 Eosinophilic colitis - dense eosinophil infiltration in the lamina propria involving the surface and crypt epithelium

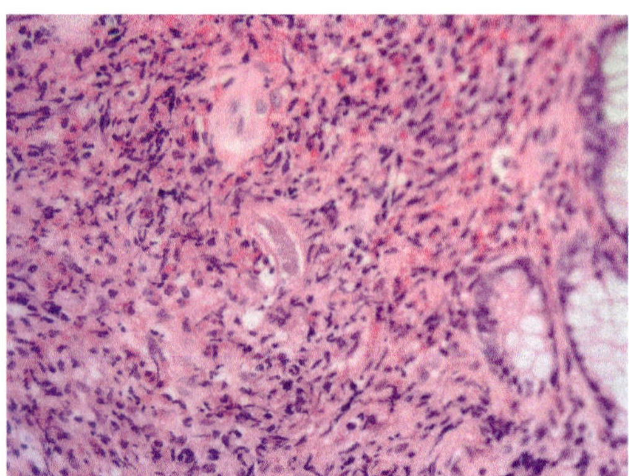

Fig. 10.14 Eosinophilic colitis secondary to *Strongyloides (organism central)*

Table 10.6 Causes of colonic eosinophilia

Cause	Clinical or histological clue
Common	
Idiopathic	History of allergic diathesis; peripheral blood eosinophilia; increased serum IgE level
Parasitic infection (e.g. *Enterobius*, *Strongyloides*, hookworms)	Focal intense eosinophil infiltration sometimes erosion; identification of parasite (Fig. 10.14)
Allergy—food, cow's milk, soy protein, allergic proctocolitis	History of specific food allergy (Fig. 10.17)
Drugs—NSAIDs, gold, L-tryptophan, carbamazepine, methotrexate, tacrolimus, azathioprine, rifampicin, clozapine, enalapril immune modulatory medications	History of medication use
Inflammatory bowel disease	History of ulcerative colitis or Crohn's disease recently treated
Occasional	
Connective tissue disorders	Known connective tissue disorder
Vasculitis—Churg-Strauss syndrome	History of asthma
Neoplasia—Lymphoma, Langerhans cell histiocytosis, systemic mastocytosis, myeloid neoplasms	Neoplastic cells in the background of the eosinophilic infiltrate (Figs. 10.15, 10.16, 10.18, and 10.19)
Inflammatory fibroid polyp	Spindle cell and vascular proliferation, perivascular oedema and spindle cell cuffing, polyp or mass identified at colonoscopy
Solid organ and bone marrow transplantation	History of transplantation
Hypereosinophilic syndrome	Marked peripheral blood eosinophilia

ply establish the diagnosis of increased eosinophils in the mucosa. Pathologists should look for evidence of an underlying condition. Based on the causes listed in the table, we suggest that pathologists should consider the undertake the following structured approach: 1) examine deeper levels to look for a causative parasite; 2) look carefully in the background mucosa for a neoplastic process, which may be obscured by an intense eosinophil infiltrate (e.g. mastocytosis (Figs. 10.15 and 10.16), leukaemia, lymphoma, or inflammatory fibroid polyp); 3) Examine for evidence of chronic architectural disturbance which may indicate treated inflammatory bowel disease; 4) Examine for the following additional histological clues - vasculitis in the superficial submucosa (e.g. Churg-Strauss syndrome), granulomas (e.g. Crohn's disease) and lymphoid follicles and red cell extravasation [allergic proctocolitis (Fig. 10.15)]; and 5) Consider that mild colonic eosinophilia confined to the left colon may represent a medication reaction [55–58].

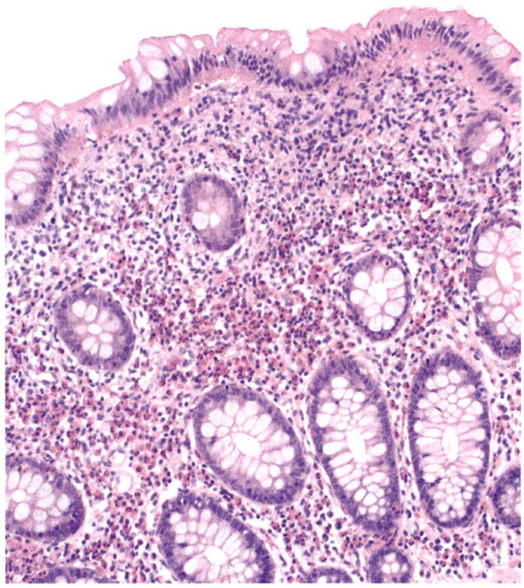

Fig. 10.15 Mastocytosis - demonstrating an eosinophil rich infiltrate

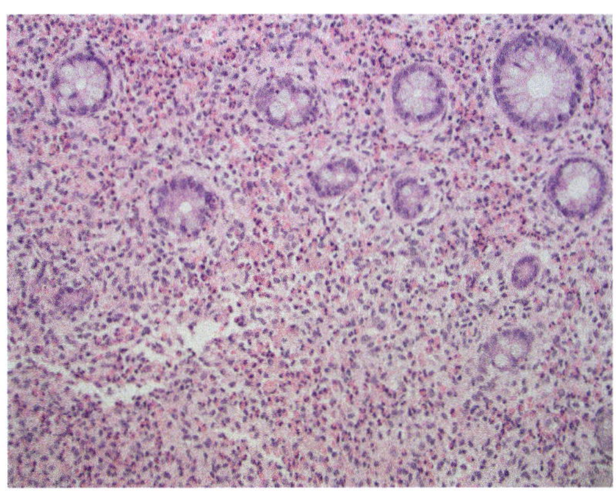

Fig. 10.16 Mastocytosis - eosinophils and background spindle to oval cells with clear cytoplasm

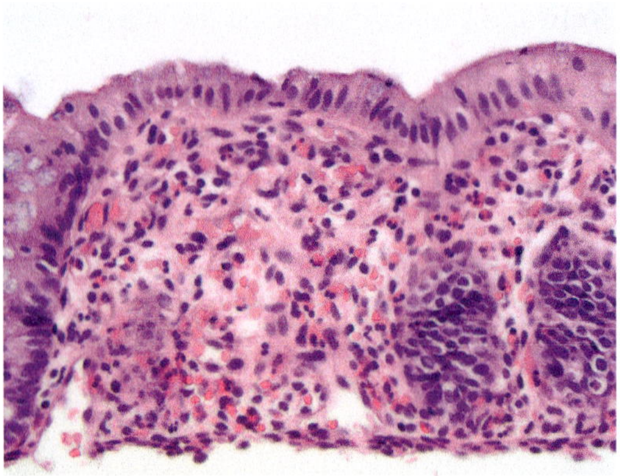

Fig. 10.17 Allergic proctitis

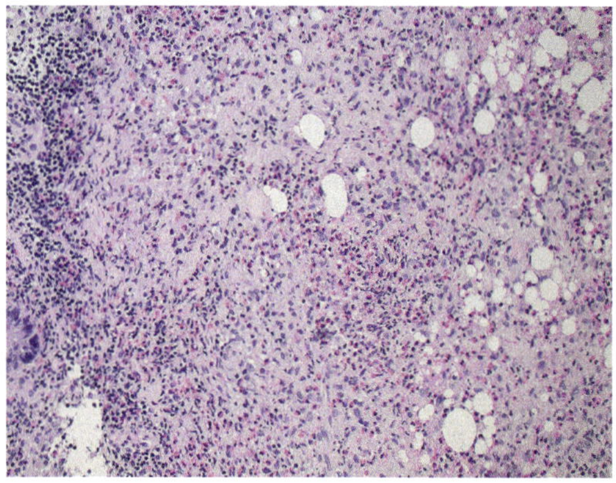

Fig. 10.18 Langerhans cell histiocytosis - collections of spindle to oval shaped cells and background eosinophils

Histiocytic/Granulomatous Infiltrates

Potential causes of histiocytic collections or true granulomas, a circumscribed organised collection of histiocytes, (Figs. 10.18 and 10.19)] in the large intestine are as follows:

- Crohn's disease
- Infection
  - Systemic (TB, histoplasmosis)
  - Gastrointestinal infections (*Salmonella*, *Yersinia*, *Campylobacter*, parasites)
  - Venereal infections (syphilis, lymphogranuloma venereum)
- Drugs (e.g. NSAID—diclofenac)
- Foreign body (talc, starch, barium, faecal material)
- Ulcerative colitis (mucin granuloma)
- Sarcoidosis
- Inherited (chronic granulomatous disease, Hermansky-Pudlak syndrome)
- Other—diverticular disease-associated colitis, pneumatosis coli and neoplasia related

The pattern of histiocytic infiltration or morphology of the granuloma may provide a clue as to the diagnosis.

General forms of granuloma include:

1. *Foreign body type* characterised by multinucleate cells with eccentrically or haphazardly arranged nuclei.
   Cause—foreign material

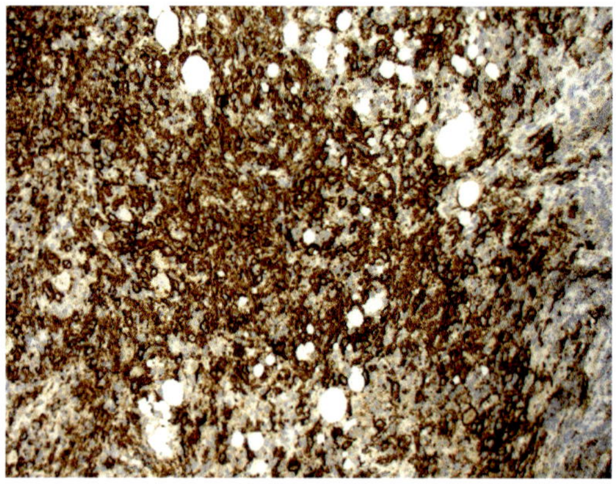

Fig. 10.19 CD1a stain confirming the diagnosis of Langerhans cell histiocytosis

2. *Epithelioid* characterised by single or multinucleate collections of histiocytes with abundant eosinophilic cytoplasm and "foot print"-like nuclei.
   Cause—Crohn's disease
3. *Sarcoidal*, a form of epithelioid granuloma devoid of other inflammatory cells and often containing calcified bodies (Schaumann bodies and/or asteroid bodies).
   Cause—Crohn's disease, sarcoidosis and medication reaction
4. *Necrobiotic* characterised by a central zone of eosinophilic degeneration of associated collagen.
   Cause—rarely seen in the large intestine
5. *Xanthogranulomatous* characterised by collections of lipid-laden macrophages and multinucleate cells.

Cause—follows longstanding chronic inflammation

6. *Suppurative* with a central zone of neutrophils and necrotising, with central necrosis that may retain the structure of the underlying necrotic tissue or may be devoid of any structure (*caseous* type).
   Cause—infection

While the morphological pattern may give some clues, additional investigations and procedures should be carried out in all cases where the cause of the granuloma is not clinically apparent. These include:

Studying the background histology. For instance, look for foreign material, parasites or pigments (e.g. chronic granulomatous disease). The tissue should be polarised, as some birefringent foreign material may not be visible on the haematoxylin and eosin stain. *Organism stains (Gram, PAS, ZN, Wade-Fite) should be performed.* If necessary, additional studies to look for an infective aetiology can be performed, e.g. PCR from the paraffin material examining for evidence of tuberculosis, fungi, parasites or *Yersinia*. Additional clinical investigations may be required to look for evidence of infection or sarcoidosis. Knowledge of the findings in previous biopsies of the gastrointestinal tract or outside of the gastrointestinal tract may also be useful in formulating a likely diagnosis.

If the histological appearance does not allow for a specific cause to be established, there is great use in discussing the case with the referring clinician. For instance, the following features can help narrow down the likely diagnosis and direct further pathological or clinical investigations.

- Past history
- Age
- Endoscopic appearance
- Upper gastrointestinal tract disease
- Extra-intestinal disease
- Immunocompetence
- Recent medication/travel
- Response to any treatment

Ischaemic Injury

Ischaemic injury pattern results whenever there is insufficient blood flow to the colonic mucosa. The mucosa is the most susceptible portion of the large intestine wall with the arcade-like pattern of vascular supply to the mucosa leading to the most superficial aspects of the mucosa being the most susceptible. It is worthwhile being aware of the various clinical patterns of ischaemia. These include the following:

- Reversible/transient (50%)
- Persistent/chronic (20%)
- Stricture inducing (20%)
- Fulminant (with gangrene +/− perforation) (10%)
- Mass forming—may mimic malignancy

The left colon is most frequently involved (75%), in particular the watershed zone at the junction of the superior mesenteric artery and inferior mesenteric artery in the splenic flexure region. While the right colon is less frequently involved (25%), ischaemia at this site is associated with higher morbidity and mortality. Endoscopy is the initial investigation of choice.

Aetiology

- Vascular obstruction
  - *External compression*
    Adhesions
    Volvulus
    Incarceration in hernia sac
    Iatrogenic, e.g. surgical ligation
  - *Vessel wall abnormality*
    Atherosclerosis
    Vasculitis—Polyarteritis nodosa, Churg-Strauss, Takayasu's, Wegener's granulomatosis, connective tissue disorder-related, Behcet's
    Radiotherapy-related intimal hyperplasia
    Amyloidosis
    Arterial dissection
    Scleroderma

Fibromuscular hyperplasia
HUS/TTP thrombotic microangiopathies
- *Vascular lumen*
Thrombosis
Hypercoagulable state, e.g. embolus
Thromboembolus
Cholesterol
Tumour
Foreign body
- Intestinal hypoperfusion
  - Hypovolemia
  - Cardiac failure
  - Excessive exercise
- Drugs
  - Digoxin
  - Cocaine
  - NSAIDs
  - Pseudoephedrine
  - Vasopressor agents
  - OCP/oestrogenic compounds
- Colonic luminal obstruction with backpressure
  - Tumours
  - Hirschsprung's disease
  - Faecal impaction
- Infection
  - *C. difficile*
  - Shiga toxin-producing bacteria, e.g. *E. coli* (O157:H7)
- Miscellaneous
  - Mucosal prolapse associated
  - Colonoscopy prep related

From a clinical point of view, it is useful to consider the causes of ischaemic colitis in terms of the age of the affected patient. This will direct investigations for the cause.

Young age:

- Thrombus—coagulation screen required
- OCP
- NSAID
- Exercise
- Infection

Elderly:

- Atherosclerosis
- Embolus
- Drugs
- Colonoscopy preparation related

Microscopic Pathology (Typical)

The typical pathological changes begin with mucosal oedema, congestion and in some cases red cell extravasation. This is followed by a combination of superficial mucosal coagulative necrosis and crypt "withering". Abundant apoptosis may be observed. There is typically minimal inflammation in the mucosa until the vascular supply is re-established, at which stage neutrophils and some eosinophils become apparent. A characteristic feature of ischaemia is hyalinisation of the lamina propria whereby the stromal collagen acquires a light pink-staining homogenous appearance (Fig. 10.20; ischaemic colitis).

Other features that may exist include pseudomembrane formation, erosion or ulceration and haemosiderin deposition demonstrable on Perls' stain. If the ischaemia is persistent, there may be loss of muscularis mucosae and features of chronicity in the epithelium particularly crypt architectural disturbance and Paneth cell metaplasia. Lamina propria fibrosis may become prominent. Atypical patterns of ischaemia are occasionally encountered. Table 10.7 discusses the differential diagnosis [59, 60].

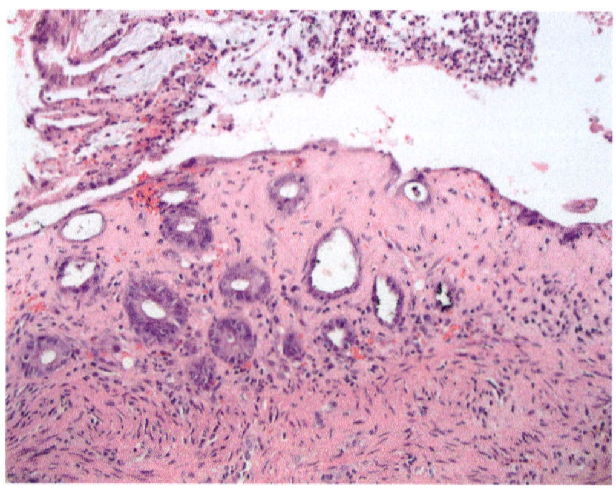

Fig. 10.20 Ischaemic colitis with lamina propria hyalinisation and crypt withering

Table 10.7 Atypical patterns of ischaemic colitis

Pattern mimic	Clue
Focal active colitis	Ischaemia responsible in 0% [1], 5% [2] and 10% [3] Hyalinisation of lamina propria is the most important clue
Focal active chronic colitis	This most commonly mimics Crohn's disease. The clinical setting is the most important factor in this differential diagnosis
Pseudomembranous colitis	Hyalinisation of the lamina propria is the feature indicating ischaemia
Chronic quiescent colitis	The clinical setting is the most important factor in this differential diagnosis
Collagenous colitis	Ischaemia is typically focal while collagenous colitis is a diffuse process
Neoplasia	Mass-forming or stricturing disease may mimic malignancy. Regenerative epithelium after an episode of ischaemia may mimic dysplasia

Apoptosis

This pattern is characterised by prominent apoptosis leading to gland loss in the setting of minimal or no inflammation (Figs. 10.21 and 10.22; apoptosis due to 5-FU; apoptosis due to taxanes). Aetiology is listed below:

- Medications
  - Chemotherapy
  - Immunomodulatory agents
  - Mycophenolate
  - NSAIDs
- Immune mediated
  - GvHD
  - CVID
  - Thymoma-associated colitis
  - Autoimmune enteropathy
  - HIV or other viruses
- Ischaemia

In most cases the clinical setting is the most important factor in establishing the aetiology, so a discussion with the referring clinician is essential in all cases where this pattern is identified [61, 62].

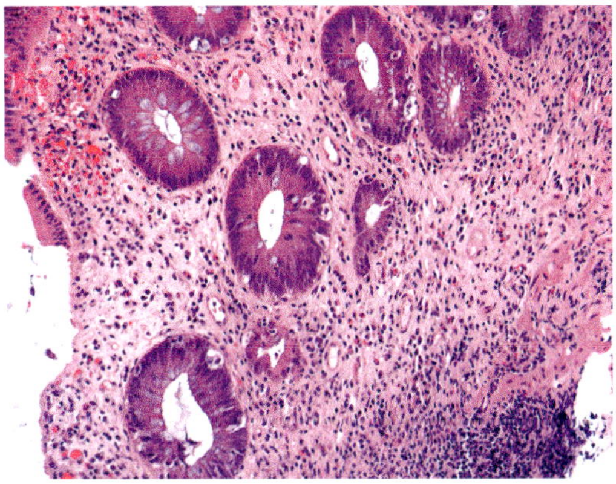

Fig. 10.21 Apoptosis in crypts secondary to 5-FU

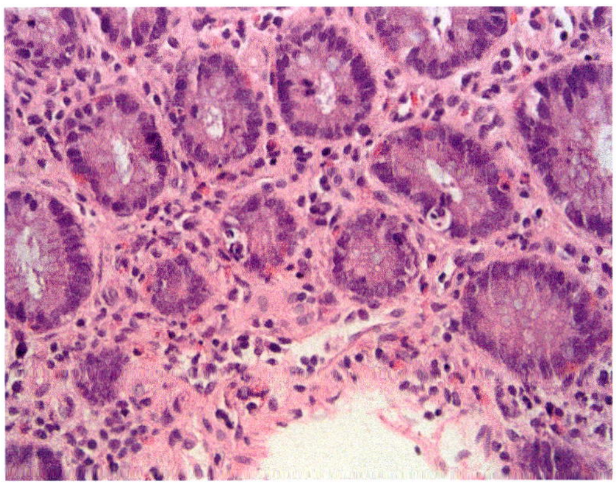

Fig. 10.22 Apoptosis in crypts secondary to taxane chemotherapy

Toxic Injury Pattern

This pattern is increasingly being recognised, particularly in the setting of new biological medications and chemotherapeutic drugs. The most important histological features are crypt destruction (by apoptosis or directly as a result of inflammation) together with mixed inflammation in the lamina propria. The process is often of variable intensity and extent of crypt injury.

Causes:

- Biological/immunomodulatory medications
- Chemotherapy
- Other medications

Table 10.8 Biological drugs in the colon

Drug	Target	Action	GIT sites	Injury pattern(s)
Idelalisib	PI3 kinase inhibitor	Lymphocyte apoptosis and immunomodulation	Small intestine, colon	Intraepithelial lymphocytes + apoptosis + cryptitis +/− eosinophils
Ipilimumab Tremelimumab	Anti-CTLA4	Immune checkpoint inhibitor; immunomodulatory	Stomach, small intestine, colon	Intraepithelial lymphocytes + apoptosis + cryptitis +/− eosinophils
Pembrolizumab Nivolumab Atezolizumab	Anti-PD-1 or Anti-PD-L1	Immune checkpoint inhibitor, immunomodulatory	Stomach, small intestine, colon	Apoptosis + neutrophils + cryptitis +/− eosinophils +/-intraepithelial lymphocytes
Etanercept Infliximab Adalimumab	Anti-TNF-alpha	Anti-inflammatory	Small intestine, colon	New onset or exacerbation of inflammatory bowel disease; Crohn's disease; apoptotic enteropathy
Rituximab	Anti-CD20	Anti-B lymphocyte	Colon	Diffuse colitis—new onset of inflammatory bowel disease
Bevacizumab	Anti-VEGF	Vascular inhibitor	Colon, anastomoses	Ischaemia; perforation
Sorafenib Sunitinib	VEGF tyrosine kinase inhibitor	Vascular inhibitor	Colon	Pneumatosis coli

Mixed Injury Pattern

The mixed injury pattern comprises at least two of the patterns described above. Most commonly this is either a combination of intraepithelial lymphocytosis and apoptosis or a combination of acute and chronic inflammation of the lamina propria. The potential causes are listed below [63–75]:

- Medications
  - Olmesartan
  - immunomodulatory medications (see Table 10.8 and Figs. 10.23 and 10.24)
- Autoimmune enteropathy
- Immune dysregulation/immunodeficiency
- CVID
- Infection (uncommon)
- Crohn's disease

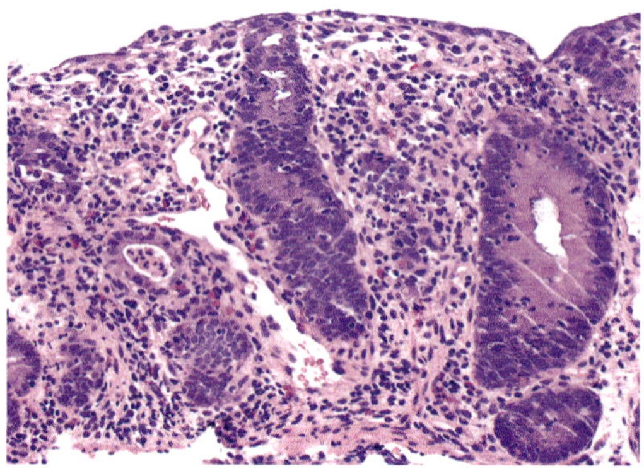

Fig. 10.23 Idelalisib colitis - acute inflammation and eosinophil infiltration

Depositions

Lipofuscin

Lipofuscin "melanosis coli" accumulation in the lamina propria of the colorectum is common. It results from undigested cellular material that results from epithelial apoptosis. Laxative use was an initial association however, lipofuscin accumulation may follow any chronic inflammatory disorder or epithelial injury such as graft-versus-host disease or medication use. Lipofuscin is PAS positive but Perls stain negative. Melanosis coli typically spares adenomas and other neoplastic processes of the colon.

Resins (Table 10.9)

Resins are non-absorbable in compounds that are used to bind elements or compounds within the lumen of the gastrointestinal tract to prevent reabsorption of this material and additionally remove the material in the faeces (Table 10.9). Most commonly encountered are the potassium sequestrant sodium polystyrene sulphonate (Kayexalate™) and the phosphate sequestrant sevelamer (Renagel™). Kayexalate is given either orally or as an enema and is most likely to be associated with severe injury such as ulceration and perforation. An inflammatory pseudotumour-mimicking malignancy can also develop. Sevelamer can cause gastrointestinal tract ulceration and chronic crypt changes, but necrosis appears to be rare. Other resins occasionally encountered include the bile acid sequestrants, cholestyramine (Questran™) and colesevelam (Welchol™), which may be associated with mild mucosal changes, but we do not believe that they are the direct cause of this injury.

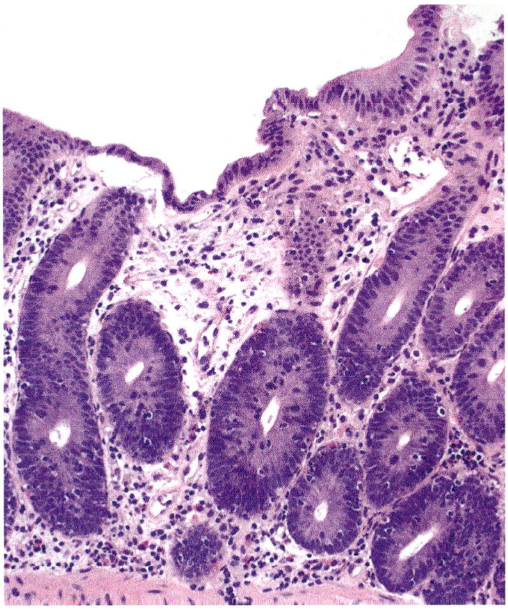

Fig. 10.24 Idelalisib colitis - intraepithelial lymphocytes

Heavy Metals

Patients with chronic renal failure may also be treated with lanthanum carbonate, a heavy metal used as a phosphate binder. Weakly soluble in an acid environment, it may be taken up by macrophages in the stomach, appearing as enlarged eosinophilic histiocytes within the lamina propria, some of which contain grey-brown crystalline foreign material [76–84].

Table 10.9 Non-absorbable resins seen in gastrointestinal biopsies

Resin	Binds	Colour—H&E	Colour—ZN	Internal structure
Kayexalate	Potassium	Purple	Black	Fish scales
Sevelamer	Phosphate	Yellow and pink	Magenta	Fish scales (curved)
Cholestyramine Colesevelam	Bile acids	Orange-pink	Yellow	Homogenous

References

1. Shetty S, Anjarwalla SM, Gupta J, Foy CJW, Shaw IS, Valori RM, Shepherd NA. Focal active colitis: a prospective study of clinicopathological correlations in 90 patients. Histopathology. 2011;59:850–6.
2. Greenson JK, Stern RA, Carpenter SL, Barnett JL. The clinical significance of focal active colitis. Hum Pathol. 1997;28:729–33.
3. Volk E, Shapiro BD, Easley KA, Goldblum JR. The clinical significance of a biopsy-based diagnosis of focal active colitis: a clinicopathologic study of 31 cases. Mod Pathol. 1998;11:789–94.
4. Xin W, Brown PI, Greenson JK. The clinical significance of focal active colitis in paediatric patients. Am J Surg Pathol. 2003;27:1134–8.
5. Lamps LW, Schneider EN, Havens JM, et al. Molecular diagnosis of Campylobacter jejuni infection in cases of focal active colitis. Am J Surg Pathol. 2006;30:782–5.
6. Wang NACS, Penman ID, Campbell S, et al. Microscopic focal cryptitis associated with oral sodium phosphate preparations. Histopathology. 2003;36:476–8.
7. Kumar NB, Nostrant TT, Appelman HD. The histopathologic spectrum of acute self-limited colitis (acute infectious-type colitis). Am J Surg Pathol. 1982;6(6):523–9.
8. Surawicz CM, Belic L. Rectal biopsy helps to distinguish acute self-limited colitis from idiopathic inflammatory bowel disease. Gastroenterology. 1984;86(1):104–13.
9. Romero-Gómez M, Suárez García E, Castro Fernández M. Pseudomembranous colitis induced by diclofenac. J Clin Gastroenterol. 1998;26:228.
10. Uc A, Mitros FA, Kao SC, Sanders KD. Pseudomembranous colitis with *Escherichia coli* O157:H7. J Pediatr Gastroenterol Nutr. 1997;24:590–3.
11. Olofinlade O, Chiang C. Cytomegalovirus infection as a cause of pseudomembrane colitis: a report of four cases. J Clin Gastroenterol. 2001;32:82–4.
12. Högenauer C, Langner C, Beubler E, et al. *Klebsiella oxytoca* as a causative organism of antibiotic-associated hemorrhagic colitis. N Engl J Med. 2006;355:2418–26.
13. Yuan S, Reyes V, Bronner MP. Pseudomembranous collagenous colitis. Am J Surg Pathol. 2003;27:1375–9.
14. Bartlett JG. Clinical practice. Antibiotic-associated diarrhea. N Engl J Med. 2002;346:334–9.
15. Surawicz CM, Brandt LJ, Binion DG, et al. Guidelines for diagnosis, treatment, and prevention of *Clostridium difficile* infections. Am J Gastroenterol. 2013;108:478–98.
16. Glickman JN, Bousvaros A, Farraye FA, Zholudev A, Friedman S, Wang HH, Leichtner AM, Odze RD. Pediatric patients with untreated ulcerative colitis may present initially with unusual morphologic findings. Am J Surg Pathol. 2004;28(2):190–7.
17. Washington K, Greenson JK, Montgomery E, et al. Histopathology of ulcerative colitis in initial rectal biopsy in children. Am J Surg Pathol. 2002;26:1441–9.
18. Robert ME, Tang L, Hao LM, et al. Patterns of inflammation in mucosal biopsies of ulcerative colitis: perceived differences in pediatric populations are limited to children younger than 10 years. Am J Surg Pathol. 2004;28:183–9.
19. Wright CL, Riddell RH. Histology of the stomach and duodenum in Crohn's disease. Am J Surg Pathol. 1998;22:383–90.
20. Lin J, McKenna BJ, Appelman HD. Morphologic findings in upper gastrointestinal biopsies of patients with ulcerative colitis: a controlled study. Am J Surg Pathol. 2010;34:1672–7.
21. Tobin JM, Sinha B, Ramani P, et al. Upper gastrointestinal mucosal disease in pediatric Crohn disease and ulcerative colitis: a blinded, controlled study. J Pediatr Gastroenterol Nutr. 2001;32:443–8.
22. Valdez R, Appelman HD, Bronner MP, et al. Diffuse duodenitis associated with ulcerative colitis. Am J Surg Pathol. 2000;24:1407–13.
23. Oberhuber G, Puspok A, Oesterreicher C, et al. Focally enhanced gastritis: a frequent type of gastritis in patients with Crohn's disease. Gastroenterology. 1997;112:698–706.
24. Ushiku T, Moran CJ, Lauwers GY. Focally enhanced gastritis in newly diagnosed pediatric inflammatory bowel disease. Am J Surg Pathol. 2013;37(12):1882–8.
25. Kim B, Barnett JL, Kleer CG, et al. Endoscopic and histological patchiness in treated ulcerative colitis. Am J Gastroenterol. 1999;94:3258–62.
26. Kleer CG, Appelman HD. Ulcerative colitis: patterns of involvement in colorectal biopsies and changes with time. Am J Surg Pathol. 1998;22:983–9.
27. Joo M, Odze RD. Rectal sparing and skip lesions in ulcerative colitis: a comparative study of endoscopic and histologic findings in patients who underwent proctocolectomy. Am J Surg Pathol. 2010;34:689–96.
28. D'Haens G, Geboes K, Peeters M, et al. Patchy cecal inflammation associated with distal ulcerative colitis: a prospective endoscopic study. Am J Gastroenterol. 1997;92(8):1275–9.
29. Mutinga ML, Odze RD, Wang HH, Hornick JL, Farraye FA. The clinical significance of right-sided colonic inflammation in patients with left-sided chronic ulcerative colitis. Inflamm Bowel Dis. 2004;10(3):215–9.
30. Haskell H, Andrews CW Jr, Reddy SI, et al. Pathologic features and clinical significance of "backwash" ileitis in ulcerative colitis. Am J Surg Pathol. 2005;29:1472–81.
31. Schumacher G. First attack of inflammatory bowel disease and infectious colitis. A clinical, histological and microbiological study with special reference to early diagnosis. Scand J Gastroenterol Suppl. 1993;198:1–24.
32. Schumacher G, Kollberg B, Sandstedt B. A prospective study of first attacks of inflammatory bowel disease and infectious colitis. Histologic course during

the 1st year after presentation. Scand J Gastroenterol. 1994;29(4):318–32.
33. Allison MC, Hamilton-Dutoit SJ, Dhillon AP, Pounder RE. The value of rectal biopsy in distinguishing self-limited colitis from early inflammatory bowel disease. Q J Med. 1987;65(248):985–95.
34. Gillen CD, Walmsley RS, Prior P, Andrews HA, Allan RN. Ulcerative colitis and Crohn's disease: a comparison of the colorectal cancer risk in extensive colitis. Gut. 1994;35:1590–2.
35. Feakins RM. Inflammatory bowel disease biopsies: updated British Society of Gastroenterology reporting guidelines. J Clin Pathol. 2013;66(12):1005–26.
36. Geboes K, Riddell R, Öst A, et al. A reproducible grading scale for histological assessment of inflammation in ulcerative colitis. Gut. 2000;47:404–9.
37. Geraghty JM, Talbot IC. Diversion colitis: histological features in the colon and rectum after defunctioning colostomy. Gut. 1991;32:1020–3.
38. Edwards CM, George B, Warren B. Diversion colitis: new light through old windows. Histopathology. 1999;34:1–5.
39. Gore S, Shepherd NA, Wilkinson SP. Endoscopic crescentic fold disease of the sigmoid colon: the clinical and histopathological spectrum of a distinctive endoscopic appearance. Int J Colorectal Dis. 1992;7:76–81.
40. Makapugay LM, Dean PJ. Diverticular disease-associated chronic colitis. Am J Surg Pathol. 1996;20:94–102.
41. Shepherd NA. Diverticular disease and chronic idiopathic inflammatory bowel disease: associations and masquerades. Gut. 1996;38:801–2.
42. Mulhall AM, Mahid SS, Petras RE, Galandiuk S. Diverticular disease associated with inflammatory bowel disease-like colitis. A systematic review. Dis Colon Rectum. 2009;52:1072–9.
43. Read NW, Krejs GJ, Read MG, Santa Ana CA, Morawski SG, Fordtran JS. Chronic diarrhea of unknown origin. Gastroenterology. 1980;78(2):264–71.
44. Carmack SW, Lash RH, Gulizia JM, Genta RM. Lymphocytic disorders of the gastrointestinal tract: a review for the practicing pathologist. Adv Anat Pathol. 2009;16:290–306.
45. Langner C, Aust D, Ensari A, Villanacci V, Becheanu G, Miehlke S, Geboes K, Münch A. Histology of microscopic colitis-review with a practical approach for pathologists. Histopathology. 2015;66:613–26.
46. Wang N, Dumot JA, Achkar E, Easley KA, Petras RE, Goldblum JR. Colonic epithelial lymphocytosis without a thickened subepithelial collagen table: a clinicopathologic study of 40 cases supporting a heterogeneous entity. Am J Surg Pathol. 1999;23:1068–74.
47. Fernández-Bañares F, Casalots J, Salas A, Esteve M, Rosinach M, Forné M, Loras C, Santaolalla R, Espinós J, Viver JM. Paucicellular lymphocytic colitis: is it a minor form of lymphocytic colitis? A clinical pathological and immunological study. Am J Gastroenterol. 2009;104:1189–98.
48. Goldstein NS, Bhanot P. Paucicellular and asymptomatic lymphocytic colitis: expanding the clinicopathologic spectrum of lymphocytic colitis. Am J Clin Pathol. 2004;122:405.
49. Brown IS, Lambie DL. Microscopic colitis with giant cells: a clinico-pathological review of 11 cases and comparison with microscopic colitis without giant cells. Pathology. 2008;40:671–5.
50. Mahajan D, Goldblum JR, Xiao SY, Shen B, Liu X. Lymphocytic colitis and collagenous colitis: a review of clinicopathologic features and immunologic abnormalities. Adv Anat Pathol. 2012;19:28–38.
51. Rubio CA, Lindholm J. Cryptal lymphocytic coloproctitis: a new phenotype of lymphocytic colitis? J Clin Pathol. 2002;55:138–40.
52. Beaugerie L, Pardi DS. Review article: drug-induced microscopic colitis - proposal for a scoring system and review of the literature. Aliment Pharmacol Ther. 2005;22:277–84.
53. Ayata G, Ithamukkala S, Sapp H, et al. Prevalence and significance of inflammatory bowel disease-like morphologic features in collagenous and lymphocytic colitis. Am J Surg Pathol. 2002;26:1414–23.
54. Saurine TJ, Brewer JM, Eckstein RP. Microscopic colitis with granulomatous inflammation. Histopathology. 2004;45(1):82–6.
55. Pascal RR, Gramlich TL, Parker KM, et al. Geographic variations in eosinophil concentration in normal colonic mucosa. Mod Pathol. 1997;10:363–5.
56. Matsushita T, Maruyama R, Ishikawa N, Harada Y, Araki A, Chen D, Tauchi-Nishi P, Yuki T, Kinoshita Y. The number and distribution of eosinophils in the adult human gastrointestinal tract: a study and comparison of racial and environmental factors. Am J Surg Pathol. 2015;39:521.
57. Hurrell JM, Genta RM, Melton SD. Histopathologic diagnosis of eosinophilic conditions in the gastrointestinal tract. Adv Anat Pathol. 2011;18:335–48.
58. Casella G, Villanacci V, Fisogni S, Cambareri AR, Di Bella C, Corazzi N, Gorla S, Baldini V, Bassotti G. Colonic left-side increase of eosinophils: a clue to drug-related colitis in adults. Aliment Pharmacol Ther. 2009;29:535–41.
59. Carpenter HA, Talley NJ. The importance of clinicopathological correlation in the diagnosis of inflammatory conditions of the colon: histological patterns with clinical implications. Am J Gastroenterol. 2000;95:878–96.
60. Cappell MS. Colonic toxicity of administered drugs and chemicals. Am J Gastroenterol. 2004;99:1175.
61. Lee FD. Importance of apoptosis in the histopathology of drug related lesions in the large intestine. J Clin Pathol. 1993;46:118–22.
62. Parfitt JR, Jayakumar S, Driman DK. Mycophenolate mofetil-related gastrointestinal mucosal injury: variable injury patterns, including graft-versus-host disease-like changes. Am J Surg Pathol. 2008;32:1367–72.

63. Weidner AS, Panarelli NC, Geyer JT, et al. Idelalisib-associated colitis: histologic findings in 14 patients. Am J Surg Pathol. 2015;39:1661–7.
64. Louie CY, DiMaio MA, Matsukuma KE, et al. Idelalisib-associated enterocolitis: clinicopathologic features and distinction from other enterocolitides. Am J Surg Pathol. 2015;39:1653–60.
65. Oble DA, Mino-Kenudson M, Goldsmith J, et al. Anti-CTLA-4 mAb-associated panenteritis: a histologic and immunohistochemical analysis. Am J Surg Pathol. 2008;32:1130–7.
66. Freeman HJ. Colitis associated with biological agents. World J Gastroenterol. 2012;18:1871–4.
67. Gonzalez RS, Salaria SN, Bohannon CD, et al. PD-1 inhibitor gastroenterocolitis: case series and appraisal of 'immunomodulatory gastroenterocolitis'. Histopathology. 2017;70:558.
68. Toussirot E, Houvenagel E, Goeb V, et al. Development of inflammatory bowel disease during anti-TNF-alpha therapy for inflammatory rheumatic disease: a nationwide series. Joint Bone Spine. 2012;79:457–63.
69. Soldini D, Gaspert A, Montani M, et al. Apoptotic enteropathy caused by antimetabolites and TNF-alpha antagonists. J Clin Pathol. 2014;67:582–6.
70. Prescott K, Costner M, Cohen S, et al. Tumor necrosis factor-alpha inhibitor associated ulcerative colitis. Am J Med Sci. 2007;333:137–9.
71. Ardelean DS, Gonska T, Wires S, et al. Severe ulcerative colitis after rituximab therapy. Pediatrics. 2010;126:e243–6.
72. El Fassi D, Nielsen CH, Kjeldsen J, et al. Ulcerative colitis following B lymphocyte depletion with rituximab in a patient with Graves' disease. Gut. 2008;57(5):714.
73. Adenis A, Vanseymortier L, Foissey D, et al. Bevacizumab and postponed suture leakages after surgery for ulcerative colitis and rectal cancer. Gut. 2007;56:734.
74. Schellhaas E, Loddenkemper C, Schmittel A, et al. Bowel perforation in non-small cell lung cancer after bevacizumab therapy. Invest New Drugs. 2009;27:184–7.
75. Coriat R, Ropert S, Mir O, et al. Pneumatosis intestinalis associated with treatment of cancer patients with the vascular growth factor receptor tyrosine kinase inhibitors sorafenib and sunitinib. Invest New Drugs. 2011;29:1090–3.
76. Abraham SC, Bhagavan BS, Lee LA, et al. Upper gastrointestinal tract injury in patients receiving kayexalate (sodium polystyrene sulfonate) in sorbitol: clinical, endoscopic, and histopathologic findings. Am J Surg Pathol. 2001;25:637–44.
77. Harel Z, Harel S, Shah PS, et al. Gastrointestinal adverse events with sodium polystyrene sulfonate (Kayexalate) use: a systematic review. Am J Med. 2013;126:264.e9–24.
78. Rashid A, Hamilton SR. Necrosis of the gastrointestinal tract in uremic patients as a result of sodium polystyrene sulfonate (Kayexalate) in sorbitol: an underrecognized condition. Am J Surg Pathol. 1997;21:60–9.
79. Swanson BJ, Limketkai BN, Liu TC, et al. Sevelamer crystals in the gastrointestinal tract (GIT): a new entity associated with mucosal injury. Am J Surg Pathol. 2013;37:1686–93.
80. Seminerio J, McGrath K, Arnold CA, et al. Medication-associated lesions of the GI tract. Gastrointest Endosc. 2014;79:140–50.
81. Arnold MA, Swanson BJ, Crowder CD, et al. Colesevelam and colestipol: novel medication resins in the gastrointestinal tract. Am J Surg Pathol. 2014;38:1530–7.
82. Bui M, Chou SY, Faubert P, et al. Resin-induced colonic pseudotumor: rare complication from chronic use of potassium binders in a hemodialysis patient. Case Rep Nephrol. 2016;2016:3692086.
83. Okwara C, Choi C, Park JY. Sevelamer-induced colitis presenting as a pseudotumor. Clin Gastroenterol Hepatol. 2015;13:A39–40.
84. Haratake J, Yasunaga C, Ootani A, et al. Peculiar histiocytic lesions with massive lanthanum deposition in dialysis patients treated with lanthanum carbonate. Am J Surg Pathol. 2015;39:767–71.

Large Intestine: Neoplastic Patterns and Mimics

11

Ian Brown and Gregory C. Miller

Contents

I. Brown (✉)
Envoi Pathology, Kelvin Grove, QLD, Australia
e-mail: ianbrown@envoi.com.au

G. C. Miller
Envoi Pathology, Kelvin Grove, QLD, Australia

Faculty of Medicine, University of Queensland, Brisbane, QLD, Australia

Normal Tissue in the Wrong Site

Heterotopias

Gastric Heterotopia

Heterotopic gastric mucosa is a rare finding in the rectum. It usually presents with painless rectal bleeding, and a polypoid lesion is often seen on the posterolateral rectum, 5–8 cm from the anal verge. The lining mucosa is almost always of pure specialised oxyntic or antral type. A variable admixture of colorectal epithelium is sometimes seen. *Helicobacter* organisms have rarely been identified. Some cases are associated with a duplication. Gastric heterotopia is regarded as a benign lesion; however, there is a case report of gastric pyloric-type heterotopia associated with invasive adenocarcinoma [1].

M. P. Kumarasinghe, I. Brown (eds.), *Endoscopic Biopsy Interpretation*,
https://doi.org/10.1007/978-3-319-79117-3_11

Non-neoplastic Glandular Proliferations

Hamartomas

Hamartomatous polyps are most commonly identified in children and will often be a manifestation of a hamartomatous polyposis syndrome, usually juvenile polyposis, Peutz-Jeghers syndrome or Cowden syndrome. Juvenile polyps and Peutz-Jeghers polyps often present with rectal bleeding but can be incidental findings on a colonoscopy performed for another indication. The histological features and molecular changes seen in various hamartomatous polyposis syndromes are outlined in Chapter 2 (Fig. 11.1). In all hamartomatous polyps of the colon, dysplastic and malignant transformation is a rare but well-documented phenomenon. In adults, polyps with a morphology identical to a hamartomatous polyp are sometimes encountered. While they may represent a true hamartomatous polyp, these are much more likely to be a manifestation of a mucosal prolapse-type polyp.

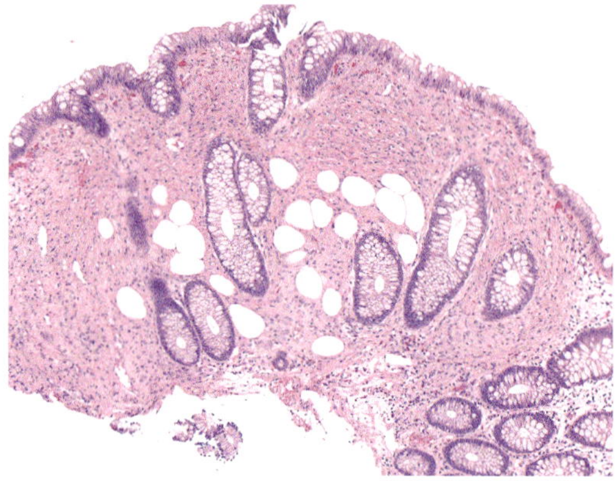

Fig. 11.1 Cowden hamartoma - note the adipose tissue within a spindle cell stroma

Glandular Tumours with No Stromal Invasion

Pathological Features of Intestinal Polyps

Intestinal-Type Adenoma

Intestinal-type adenoma, also known as conventional adenoma, is the most common neoplastic overgrowth of the colonic epithelium. It is characterised by variable cytological dysplasia (low or high grade) and different architectural patterns (tubular, tubulovillous or villous). Tubular adenomas are defined by the presence of more than 75% tubular structures in the polyp. The villous component of a conventional adenoma is significant if it comprises at least 25% of the polyp: if between 25% and 75% of the polyp, this is termed as tubulovillous adenoma; if >75% of the polyp, this is termed as villous adenoma. The latter is very uncommon outside of the rectum.

Adenomas with a villous component, high-grade dysplasia or diameter >10 mm are regarded as advanced adenomas, and these warrant follow-up endoscopic surveillance at a shorter interval (typically 3 years).

The majority of adenomas are sporadic and have risk factors for their development similar to sporadic colorectal carcinoma. A small percentage arise in the setting of inherited cancer syndromes such as familial adenomatous polyposis (FAP), MUTYH-associated polyposis (MAP) or Lynch syndrome. Clues to inherited origin include young age at onset and multiple cumulative adenomas (>10). Adenomas arising in Lynch syndrome are often high grade and have a villous component.

Histological Features

Adenomas show variable cytological and glandular abnormality (Fig. 11.2). In adenomas with low-grade dysplasia, the gland architecture is regular, and the lining epithelium is typically composed of multilayered, hyperchromatic, penicillate cells. In high-grade dysplasia, glandular architectural derangement occurs which is characterised by closely packed glands, back-to-back configuration, complex budding, cribriform patterns and glands with papillary infolding. Cytological changes include loss of perpendicular nuclear polarity with respect to the basement membrane, nuclear pleomorphism and prominent nucleoli.

Differential Diagnosis

The diagnosis of adenoma is usually straightforward. Occasionally regenerative atypia following ulceration or ischaemic injury, particularly of mass-forming type, may mimic adenoma. The comparison with invasive adenocarcinoma is discussed below.

Ancillary Investigations

These are not typically warranted with conventional adenoma. Loss of staining for mismatch repair proteins in an adenoma may indicate Lynch syndrome; however, adenomas in patients with proven Lynch syndrome may show preserved staining, making testing in this setting of limited use.

Serrated Lesions

Serrated polyps have a characteristic gland architecture characterised by serration or sawtooth pattern of the luminal border. The serration occurs as a result of asymmetrical proliferation throughout the crypt. Nearly half of all polyps detected at colonoscopy are of serrated type. There are three subgroups of serrated polyps: hyperplastic polyp (HP), sessile serrated adenoma/polyp (SSA/P) and traditional serrated adenoma (TSA).

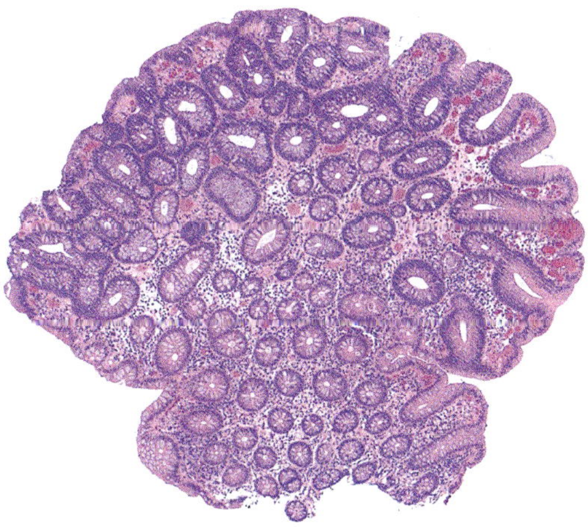

Fig. 11.2 Tubular adenoma with low-grade dysplasia

Hyperplastic Polyp

This is the most commonly encountered form. It is typically a small lesion in the distal colon or rectum. It is believed to be in an innocuous lesion with no risk for malignant transformation.

In hyperplastic polyps, the crypt base is narrow with serration being most marked in the upper half of the crypt (Fig. 11.3). Epithelial cells should contain clear cytoplasm corresponding to a micro-vesicular pattern of mucin in the epithelium. Cytological atypia is absent and apoptotic bodies are infrequent. Rarely a goblet cell rich type is identified. Occasionally, distal hyperplastic polyps may undergo mucosal prolapse which can produce basal crypt dilatation. The finding a muscle proliferation in the lamina propria is a clue that this the situation.

Sessile Serrated Adenoma/Polyp

This lesion comprises up to 15% of all polyps detected at colonoscopy. Unlike hyperplastic polyps, serrated adenomas are recognised to be a precursor lesion for the development of colorectal adenocarcinomas demonstrating BRAF mutations and CpG island hypermethylation phenotype (CIMP) high status. These lesions are more commonly encountered in the proximal colon.

Characteristic histological features are serrations extending to the base of the crypts, leading

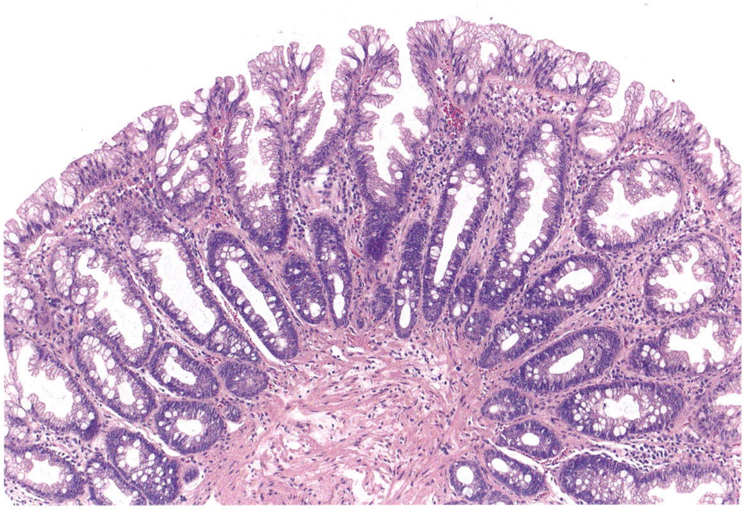

Fig. 11.3 Hyperplastic polyp - usual microvesicular type. Note the narrow crypt base

to basal crypt dilatation and crypts that run parallel to be muscularis mucosae (Fig. 11.4). The lining epithelium shows clear to eosinophilic-staining cytoplasm without evidence of cytological atypia unless dysplasia develops within the polyp. Cytological dysplasia is characterised by the development of closely packed glands with nuclear atypia and stratification. This may maintain a serrated architecture or resemble a conventional adenoma. Development of dysplasia represents progression to a more advanced lesion with potential for rapid development of adenocarcinoma. Traditional serrated adenoma (see below) may also develop from a sessile serrated adenoma.

Ancillary investigations are infrequently required; however, 80% of cases with dysplasia will show loss of MLH1 protein by immunohistochemistry in the dysplastic area, which can be useful in identifying cases with subtle dysplastic features [2, 3].

Traditional Serrated Adenoma

This is the least common serrated polyp. It is a precursor lesion for development of colorectal adenocarcinoma through both BRAF and KRAS mutation pathways.

Most lesions are exophytic and characterised by a tubulovillous architecture, but sometimes, especially in the distal rectum, the lesions are flat but with characteristic cytology. The lining epithelium has elongated columnar cells with eosinophilic cytoplasm and centrally placed small penicillate nuclei (Fig. 11.5). Ectopic crypt foci and slit-like epithelial serrations are characteristic features. In proximal lesions, an adjacent component of SSA is occasionally seen and these lesions harbour a BRAF mutation rather than a KRAS mutation seen in more typical distally located examples. Conventional cytological dysplasia developing in a traditional serrated adenoma represents an advanced molecular abnormality with increased risk for subsequent development of adenocarcinoma, typically with aggressive clinical behaviour. This may mimic conventional tubulovillous adenoma. A component of at least 25% typical traditional serrated adenoma is needed for the diagnosis of TSA [4].

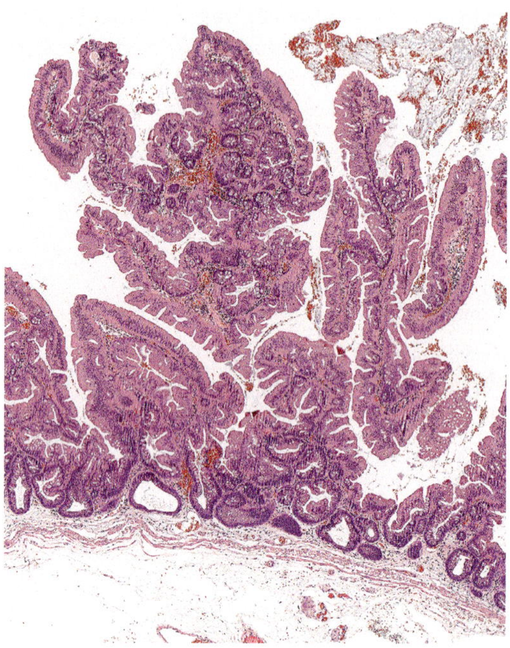

Fig. 11.5 Traditional serrated adenoma

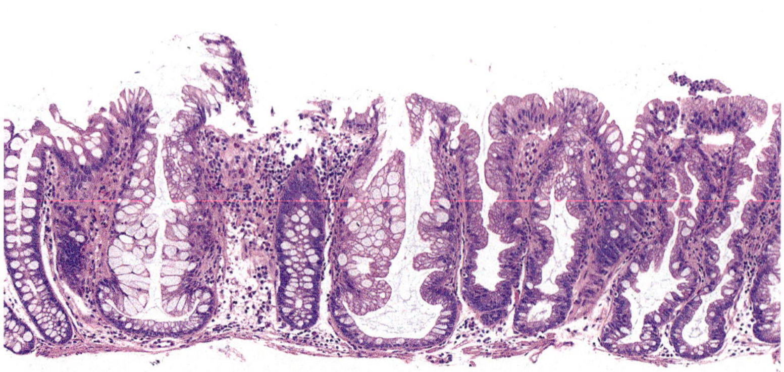

Fig. 11.4 Sessile serrated adenoma - note the basal crypt dilatation and asymmetrical crypt proliferation

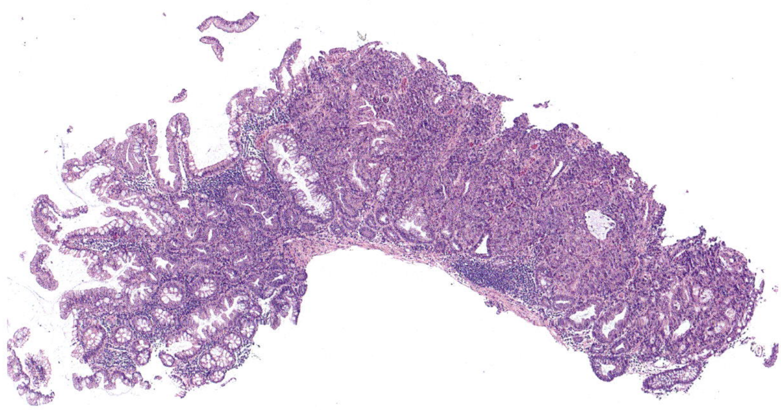

Fig. 11.6 Sessile serrated adenoma with cytological dysplasia

Sessile Serrated Adenoma with Dysplasia (SSAD)

The SSAD is the progressed form of the SSA. Endoscopically, the dysplastic component of the SSAD can be either protuberant or, more commonly, sessile making distinction from an SSA problematic.

Histologically, SSAD is characterised by two important features. Firstly, there should be overt cytological dysplasia, although the pattern of dysplasia can be variable ranging from conventional adenoma-like to a subtle serrated appearance. Secondly, the dysplasia should arise abruptly from the adjacent ordinary SSA. For diagnostic purposes this should generally occur within the same tissue fragment.

Mismatch repair deficiency (MMRD) in SSADs is more common than mismatch repair-proficient (MMRP) cases, and the mismatch repair enzyme status underlies important differences in the clinicopathological and molecular features of these polyps. Since most cases show a loss of the mismatch repair enzyme, MLH1, immunohistochemistry for this enzyme can be useful in confirming SSAD. Mismatch repair-proficient (MMRP) SSAs often display abnormal overexpression of p53.

The dysplastic component of a true SSAD is overtly atypical and, depending on the exact pattern, will display a combination of loss of maturation, cellular crowding, enlarged nuclei, irregular nuclei, prominent nucleoli, frequent mitoses and atypical mitoses (Fig. 11.6). Even in the most subtle serrated-type dysplasia, cellular maturation is lost, and the nuclei are enlarged, irregular and vesicular with a prominent nucleolus. Mitoses are frequent and can be atypical. In comparison, the cytology of TSA-type change is bland. The cells have abundant pink cytoplasm. The penicillate nuclei are arranged in an orderly manner in the centre of the cells with even chromatin distribution. Mitoses are rarely seen. A TSA arising from an SSA essentially never loses staining for MLH1; thus, loss of MLH1 staining (in the setting of an SSA) is strong evidence of conventional dysplasia. It is increasingly recognised that TSAs can arise from SSAs, and this finding should not be interpreted as serrated dysplasia arising from an SSA. The terminology for these lesions is evolving, and at present, we favour calling these lesions traditional serrated adenoma even when the majority of the lesion has a sessile serrated adenoma morphology.

Traditional Serrated Adenoma with Dysplasia

Most authors consider traditional serrated adenoma itself to be a dysplastic lesion, based on cell multilayering producing apparent epithelial proliferation. However, there are reasons to suggest that this may not be the case. These include an absence of cellular atypia, minimal mitotic activity and lack of any of the usual molecular alterations typically seen in dysplasia. A subset of traditional serrated adenomas contain definite areas of conventional dysplasia. Similar to the SSAD, these foci are char-

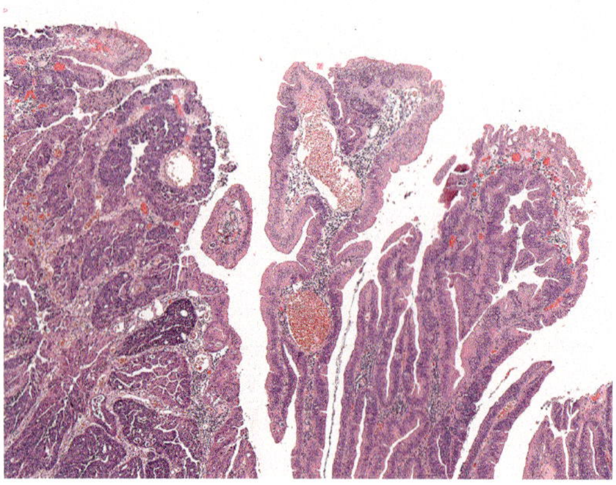

Fig. 11.7 Traditional serrated adenoma with high-grade dysplasia

acterised by an abrupt transition to areas showing cytological and architectural atypia identical to conventional dysplasia seen in intestinal-type adenoma (Fig. 11.7). A serrated architectural pattern may persist in these foci with significant cytological atypia. Significant molecular alterations can be identified in these dysplastic areas.

Differential Diagnosis

The major differential diagnosis is the tubulovillous adenoma. There is a subset of tubulovillous adenoma whereby significant parts of the lesion show serrated morphology and ectopic crypt foci. Varying amounts of eosinophilic cytoplasm may be seen in the tumour cells. The high frequency of KRAS mutation has been identified similar to typical traditional serrated adenoma. To date it is not clear how these two processes interrelate, but conceivably the "serrated" tubulovillous adenoma may represent a progressed form of traditional serrated adenoma.

Serrated polyposis syndrome (SPS)

Diagnostic Criteria

Serrated polyposis syndrome remains a clinicopathological diagnosis. The current WHO diagnostic criteria are arbitrary. They are any of:

1. At least five serrated polyps proximal to the sigmoid colon at least two of which are >10 mm
2. Any serrated polyp in a first-degree relative of an SPS patient (often omitted)
3. >20 serrated polyps of any size throughout the large bowel

For the diagnosis of SPS, a serrated polyp can include an HP, SSA or TSA, and polyp counts are cumulative over time. The mean age of cancer diagnosis in SPS is around 50.4 years. Most of the cancers arise in the proximal colon. Although serrated polyps dominate in most patients, there is a definite increase in conventional adenomas in many of these patients as well. The combination of serrated and conventional polyps raises the possibility of *MUTYH*-associated polyposis in some of these patients, and in fact 18% of patients meeting the criteria for SPS in one series were found to have *MAP*. Interestingly, the cancers that arise in SPS do not appear to always arise from serrated pathway lesions. In the series of Rosty et al., only 46% had a *BRAF* mutation and only 38% were MMRD [5].

Cancer Risk and Surveillance Guidelines in SPS

The risk of developing colorectal carcinoma in SPS is not clear. In one study the lifetime risk was >50%, but this is likely to be an overestimate. There does not appear to be any increased incidence of cancers outside of the large bowel. Surveillance guidelines are based mostly on expert opinion, but colonoscopy every 1–3 years (depending on polyp burden) is advocated by most centres. In some patients, the polyp burden becomes impractical to manage by colonoscopy, and prophylactic colectomy can be offered to these patients. First-degree relatives of patients with SPS appear to have an increased risk of carcinoma (up to fivefold), but screening recommendations for these patients are not uniform. The current consensus appears to suggest commencing screening at the age of SPS diagnosis in the affected relative or at 40 years of age, whichever is earlier.

Genetics of SPS

Despite years of intensive research, the genetic basis of SPS remains elusive. This fact alone suggests that no one gene is likely to be responsible for the syndrome. Instead a complex genetic basis is favoured and variable penetrance is likely.

Dysplastic Lesions Arising in Inflammatory Bowel Disease

These may resemble conventional intestinal-type adenoma or show a serrated morphology often resembling traditional serrated adenoma. In the former situation, distinction from conventional adenoma may be difficult. This is generally of limited clinical importance since the main decision rests on whether the lesion is endoscopically resectable or not. Certain clinical and histological clues may point to the lesion being a sporadic intestinal-type adenoma. These are detailed in Table 11.1.

Table 11.1 Clinical and histological clues to sporadic intestinal-type adenoma

Feature	Conventional adenoma	Polypoidal inflammatory bowel disease dysplasia
Age	Older (>50 years)	Younger (<50)
Duration of disease	Short (<10 years)	Long (>10 years)
Resectability	Yes	+/−
Dysplastic glands	Present throughout the lesion, regular architecture	Interspersed with normal glands, irregular architecture
Cytology	Polarity is retained unless high grade. Dystrophic goblet cells are uncommon	Haphazard, nuclear rounding and loss of polarity is more frequent; dystrophic goblet cells are common
Stroma	Minimal	Often prominent and containing prominent inflammation
Demarcation from surrounding mucosa	Sharp	Less clear
Dysplasia in adjacent flat mucosa	Absent	Often present
p53	Negative	Positive
Beta catenin	Positive nuclear staining	Cell membrane staining

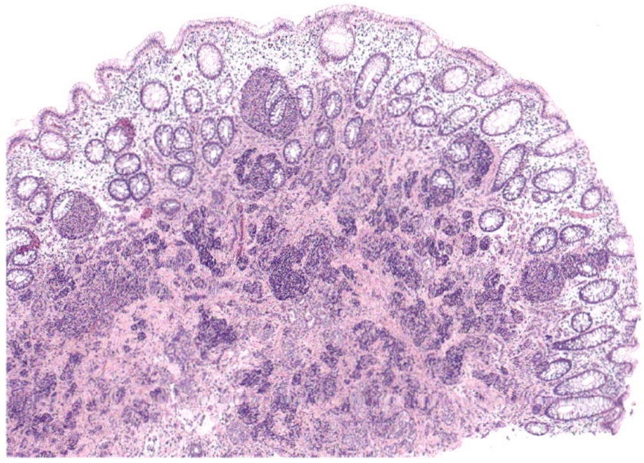

Fig. 11.8 Rectal neuroendocrine neoplasm (Grade 1)

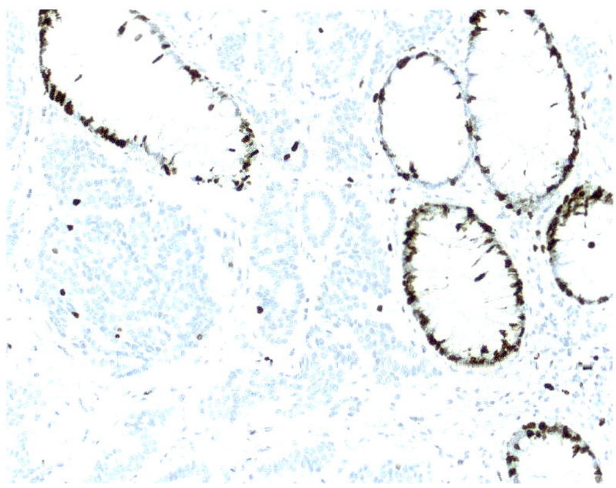

Fig. 11.9 Rectal neuroendocrine neoplasm (Ki67 <3%)

Neuroendocrine Neoplasm (NEN)

Rectal "Carcinoid" Tumour

The rectum is the most common site for neuroendocrine neoplasm to arise in the large intestine. Rarely they are seen elsewhere, particularly in the sigmoid. They are usually smaller than 10 mm in diameter and are confined to the mucosa and superficial submucosa. Most lesions are Grade 1 NEN and show a typical neuroendocrine trabecular or nested pattern or growth and bland cytology and have a low mitotic rate/Ki67 proliferation index (<3%) (Figs. 11.8 and 11.9). Almost all rectal NENs smaller than 10 mm in size behave in a benign fashion. Current recommendations are to re-examine the resection site several months after resection to ensure the lesion has been completely removed. Tumours

Table 11.2 WHO types of adenocarcinoma

Type	Diagnostic criteria
Adenocarcinoma (conventional)	(Fig. 11.10—adenocarcinoma)
Mucinous adenocarcinoma	When >50% of the lesion is composed of pools of extracellular mucin that contains malignant cells
Signet-ring cell carcinoma	>50% of the cells in a lesion contain prominent intracytoplasmic mucin with displacement and moulding of the nucleus
Medullary carcinoma	Sheets of malignant cells with vesicular nuclei, prominent nucleoli and eosinophilic cytoplasm with a prominent intraepithelial lymphocytosis
High-grade neuroendocrine carcinoma	
Large cell neuroendocrine carcinoma	Tumours with organoid, nesting, trabecular, rosette-like or palisading growth; cells with abundant cytoplasm, prominent nucleoli and vesicular nuclei; the tumour must show neuroendocrine differentiation on IHC
Small cell neuroendocrine carcinoma	Diffuse or nested growth pattern; small cells with minimal cytoplasm and nuclei with granular chromatin and inconspicuous nucleoli; mitotic activity is very high
Squamous cell carcinoma	Carcinoma with only squamous differentiation
Adenosquamous carcinoma	Features of both squamous cell carcinoma and adenocarcinoma, either as separate or intermixed components of a carcinoma
Micropapillary carcinoma	Clusters of tumour cells within stromal spaces mimicking vascular channels
Serrated adenocarcinoma	Serrated architecture
Spindle cell carcinoma	Spindle cell sarcomatoid component that is at least focally positive for cytokeratins
Mixed adenoneuroendocrine carcinoma	A carcinoma with morphologically recognisable neuroendocrine and adenocarcinomatous components where both comprise at least 30% of the tumour
Undifferentiated carcinoma	Carcinomas without morphological, immunohistochemical or molecular evidence of more than epithelial differentiation
Carcinoma, type cannot be determined	

that are >20 mm in diameter, those that invade the muscularis propria and those that have lymphovascular invasion and/or higher proliferation (Grade 2 or 3 NEN) are at risk for adverse outcomes.

Tumours with Stromal Invasion

Carcinoma

These are malignant tumours invading at least the submucosa. Most represent tumours of glandular differentiation. The subclassification is provided by the WHO (see table 11.2).

The Malignant Colorectal Polyp

This is carcinoma (almost always adenocarcinoma) found in an endoscopically resected polypoidal tumour (Fig. 11.10). It is either a

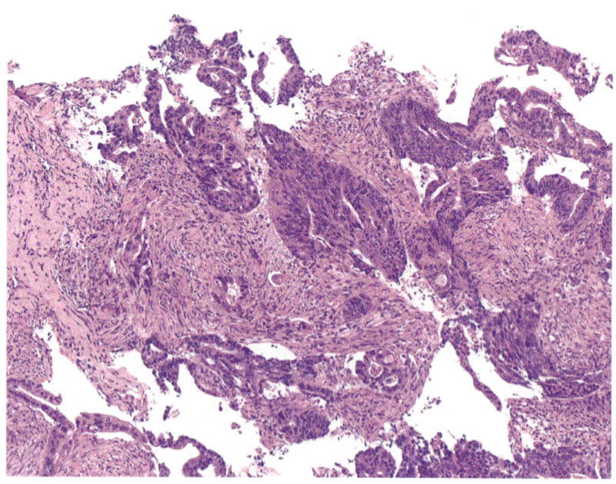

Fig. 11.10 Adenocarcinoma

submucosal invasive adenocarcinoma developing from a pre-existing adenoma (conventional or serrated) (Fig. 11.11) or a polypoidal carcinoma. Identification of adenocarcinoma is important for the following potential adverse outcomes:

1. Residual disease, either adenoma or adenocarcinoma at the polypectomy site

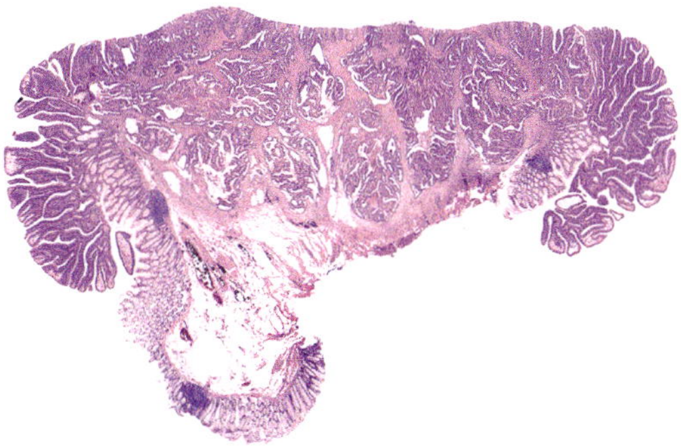

Fig. 11.11 Malignant colorectal polyp - submucosal invasive adenocarcinoma arising from a tubulovillous adenoma

2. Lymph node metastases
3. Haematogenous metastases
4. Risk of synchronous or metachronous tumour

This is more likely in patients with serrated polyposis, Lynch syndrome, familial adenomatous polyposis or inflammatory bowel disease. Overall, the risk of any malignant colorectal polyp developing lymph node metastases is approximately 4%. The risk for haematogenous metastases is approximately 1%. A number of histological features can help predict which lesions are high risk for developing adverse outcomes and may benefit from surgical resection. Carcinomas with adverse features have a lymph node metastasis rate between 7% and 9%. When adenocarcinoma is close to (<1 mm from) or at the polypectomy resection margin, the risk of residual adenoma or carcinoma at the polypectomy site is reported to be around 10–15%.

The pathologist's role assessing malignant colorectal polyps is to provide this risk assessment for a high-risk lesion. The following pathological features can help predict which lesions will develop lymph node metastases or show residual disease at the polypectomy site.

Two main groups of pathological risk factors exist:

1. Qualitative—poor tumour differentiation, high level of tumour budding, vascular invasion, positive margin status, and possibly rectal site

Table 11.3 Features that should be recorded in the pathology report of a malignant colorectal polyp

Site in the large intestine
Size
Depth of invasion (mm)
Width of invasion (mm)
Haggitt (pedunculated) or Kikuchi (sessile) level
Differentiation/grade (based on least differentiated area)
Tumour budding
Lymphatic invasion
Venous invasion
Margin status
Mismatch repair immunohistochemistry status

2. Quantitative—large invasive tumour size, depth of invasion (>2mm) and tumour width (>4mm); Haggitt level (pedunculated polyps) and Kikuchi level (sessile polyps)

It is important to note that the risk factors are summative. If no risk factors exist, then there is essentially no risk for residual disease in the bowel wall. By contrast if ≥2 adverse factors are identified, this is associated with >10% risk of residual disease in subsequent resection specimens. Positive margin status is a risk for residual disease at the polypectomy site but not lymph node spread.

Table 11.3 lists features that should be recorded in the pathology report of a malignant colorectal polyp [6, 7].

Metastasis (Foreign Appearance for Site)

Metastases to the colon are rare. The most common tumours seen which metastasise (or spread directly) to the colon and rectum are gastric adenocarcinoma, breast (particularly lobular) carcinoma and prostatic adenocarcinoma. Other rare types include ovarian, cervical, renal and lung adenocarcinoma. Metastasis should be suspected when there is a history of another carcinoma or an atypical histologic pattern such as normal mucosa overlying the carcinoma or intralymphatic spread. Immunohistochemistry is useful to differentiate these from primary colorectal adenocarcinoma (see chapter 1).

Diffuse Round Cell (Epithelioid-Like) Pattern

The differential diagnosis of diffuse round cell lesions is broad and generally requires immunohistochemistry to confirm the diagnosis (see Chapter 2 for further details).

Most cases seen in the colon are non-malignant diffuse round cell lesions (see Box 11.1) [8].

Box 11.1 Non-invasive Round Cell Lesions in the Colon

PEComa
Epithelioid GIST
Histiocytic collections and neoplasms
Xanthoma
Glomus tumour
Mastocytosis
Granular cell tumour

Xanthoma

Xanthoma is identified almost exclusively in the sigmoid colon/rectum and presents as a red/yellow nodule. In addition to the characteristic sheets of foamy histiocytes, there may be evidence of mucosal injury. It is proposed that xanthomas represent areas of regeneration following mucosal injury [9].

Spindle Cell Pattern

Spindle Cell Tumours

See Box 11.2.

Box 11.2 Spindle Cell Tumours

Granular cell tumour
Langerhans cell histiocytosis
Leiomyoma
Perineurioma
Schwannoma
Schwann cell hamartoma
Neurofibroma
Inflammatory fibroid polyp
GIST
Ganglioneuroma
Mastocytosis
Follicular dendritic cell tumour
Kaposi sarcoma
Elastofibroma

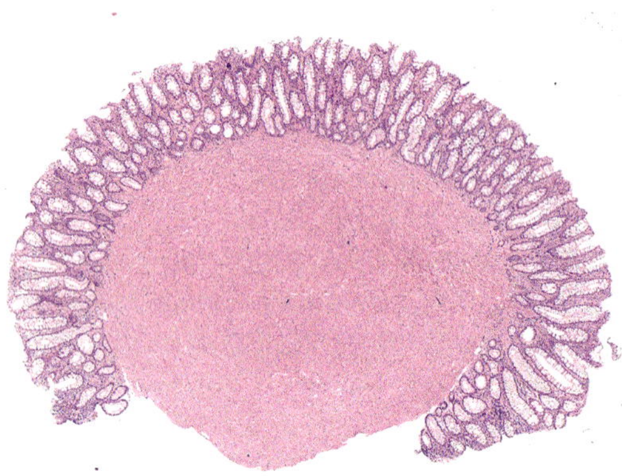

Fig. 11.12 Leiomyoma of muscularis mucosae

Leiomyoma of Muscularis Mucosae

This is the most common mesenchymal tumour identified in the large intestine. It can be seen throughout the colon but is most common in the sigmoid or rectum. These are typically small lesions with a median size of 4 mm. They closely resemble the adjacent muscularis mucosae from which they arise (Fig. 11.12).

The haphazardly arranged smooth muscle cells typically lack atypia or mitotic activity. Cytoplasm is abundant and eosinophilic. The overlying mucosa may be normal, attenuated or mildly inflamed. The histological appearance is usually so typical as to not require any further investigation or immunohistochemical stain before rendering the diagnosis. A rare "symplastic" variant is characterised by significant cytological atypia and an increased mitotic activity but has no clinical significance [10].

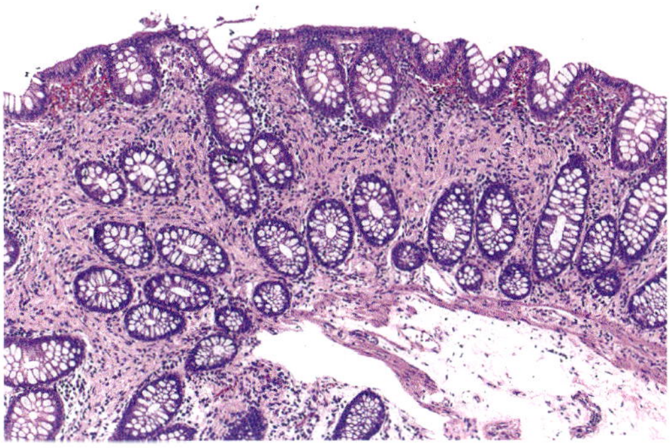

Fig. 11.13 Schwann cell hamartoma HE

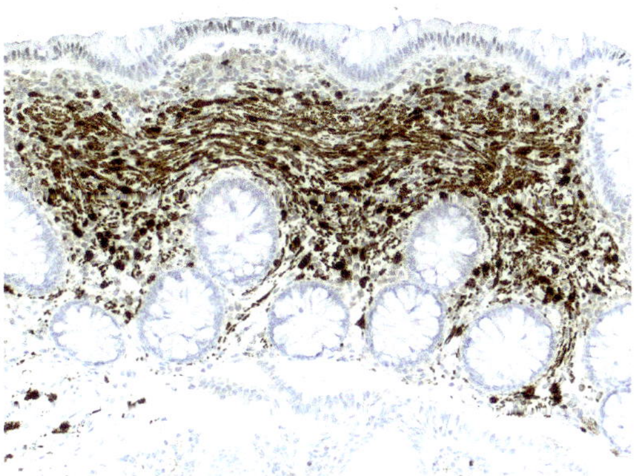

Fig. 11.14 Schwann cell hamartoma (S100)

Mucosal Schwann Cell Hamartoma

This is a benign proliferation of Schwann cells typically localised to the mucosa. Most cases occur in the distal large intestine. The spindle-shaped Schwann cells may show a tendency to grouping of their nuclei. Sometimes the cells acquire an epithelioid morphology, and the term epithelioid nerve sheath lesion is used. There is also a subtype that resembles tactile corpuscle bodies. All lesions are benign and are not associated with an underlying syndrome. The diagnosis of mucosal Schwann cell hamartoma can be confirmed by positive staining with S100 immunohistochemistry (Figs. 11.13 and 11.14) [11].

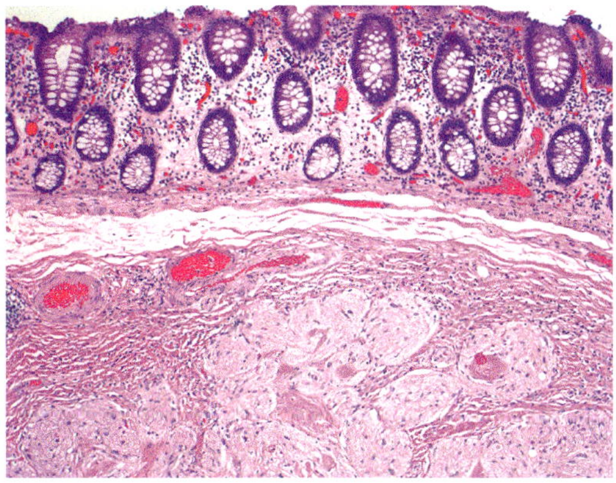

Fig. 11.15 Granular cell tumour

Granular Cell Tumour

This tumour is composed of spindle to oval cells with eosinophilic granular cytoplasm (Fig. 11.15). PAS positive eosinophilic globules may be seen. When larger, a sparse lymphocyte cuff can be appreciated surrounding the lesion. Granular cell tumours show positive staining with S100 by immunohistochemistry [12].

Other Neural Tumours

Table 11.4 summarises the neural tumours of the large intestine.

Fibroblastic Polyp

These are also known as perineurioma since perineural differentiation has been documented in these lesions. They are usually small, intramucosal and located in the distal large intestine. Some cases are associated with a serrated lesion, the cells of which demonstrate BRAF mutation. The spindle cells resemble fibrocytes or perineural cells in having elongate nuclei long tapering cytoplasmic processes (Fig. 11.17). Cells are arranged parallel to the epithelial surface and associated with variable

Table 11.4 Summary of neural tumours of the large intestine

Tumour type	Associated syndrome	Distinctive feature
Schwann cell hamartoma		See above
Granular cell tumour		See above
Ganglioneuroma	Mostly sporadic; may occur in MEN3,neurofibromatosis type I, familial adenomatous polyposis and Cowden syndrome	Ganglion cells in a background spindle cell proliferation (Fig. 11.16)
Neurofibroma	Neurofibromatosis type I	Elongate wavy spindle cell nuclei in a prominent collagenous background
Schwannoma		Cellular spindle cell tumour with background lymphoid cuff. Usually in the submucosa
Fibroblastic polyp/perineurioma		See below
Mucosal neuroma		Spindle cell proliferation. An epithelioid variant is recognised

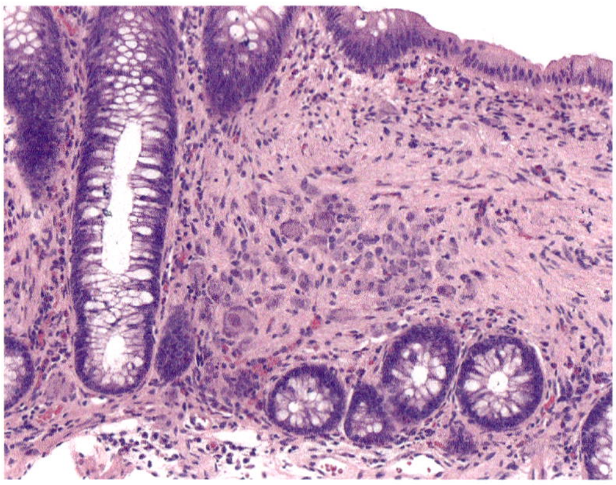

Fig. 11.16 Ganglioneuroma - ganglion cell collections and a spindle cell neural proliferation

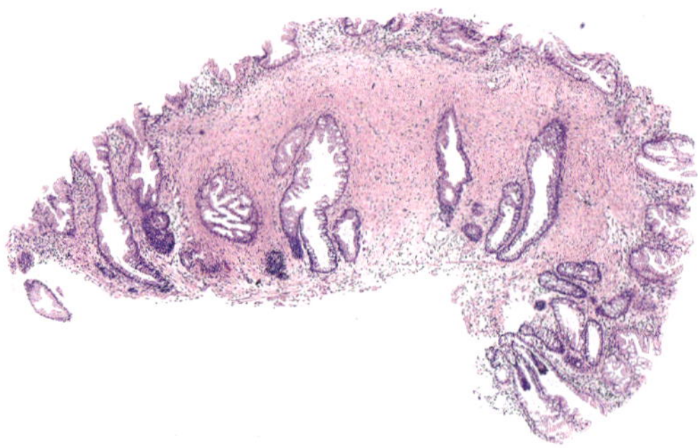

Fig. 11.17 Fibroblastic polyp

amounts of collagen. Uncommonly collagen may be the predominant component. Collections of adipocytes may also be observed within the lesion [13, 14].

Non-invasive Round Cell Tumours

Vascular Lesions

Vascular Proliferations

Vessel dilation:

1. Lymphatic—lymphangiectasia and lymphangioma
2. Venous—venous bleb
3. Capillary—ectasia

Vessel proliferation:

4. Pyogenic granuloma
5. AV malformation
6. Portal hypertensive colonopathy (severe)
7. Angiodysplasia
8. Haemangioma
9. Kaposi's sarcoma
10. Angiosarcoma

Adipose Tissue (Like)

Lipoma

Lipoma is the most common submucosal mesenchymal tumour in the large intestine. It is usually an incidental finding. Larger lesions may present with obstruction or intussusception. It is occasionally sampled in biopsies particularly when the overlying mucosa has been peeled away and the underlying protruding fat is separately sampled. The overlying mucosa is generally normal but may display inflammation, erosion, reactive change or mucosal prolapse-related change. Lipoma is typically composed of uniform mature adipocytes lacking nuclear atypia. Variable amounts of collagen and vessels may occur. Sometimes adipose tissue is encountered in the mucosa. This may be in the setting of a fibroblastic polyp as discussed above. Adipose tissue collections in the mucosa may also represent hamartomas of Cowden syndrome, particularly if more than one is encountered.

The differential diagnosis includes:

1. Pseudolipomatosis—resulting from air insufflation during colonoscopy. The small variable size of the gas pockets contrasts with the uniform larger appearance of typical adipocytes. Additionally, pseudolipomatosis is often irregular in outline and the cells do not express S100 protein, unlike true adipocytes.
2. Everted diverticulum—most commonly occurring in the sigmoid colon, this may present as a rounded protuberant mass composed of adipose tissue. The endoscopic appearance is important in the distinction. The adjacent ostium of a diverticulum may be seen.

Liposarcoma

Liposarcoma of the colon is documented but is extremely rare and is most commonly local/recurrent growth from a retroperitoneal liposarcoma. The key histological features are variably sized adipocytes, atypical nuclei and blast cells.

Biphasic Pattern: Glandular and Stromal Proliferation

Endometriosis is typically seen in the rectum of young women but can occur anywhere in the colon. It typically presents as a mass lesion. Histologically, the lesion is usually centred in the deep tissues with normal overlying mucosa, but endometriosis can infiltrate into the mucosa. The

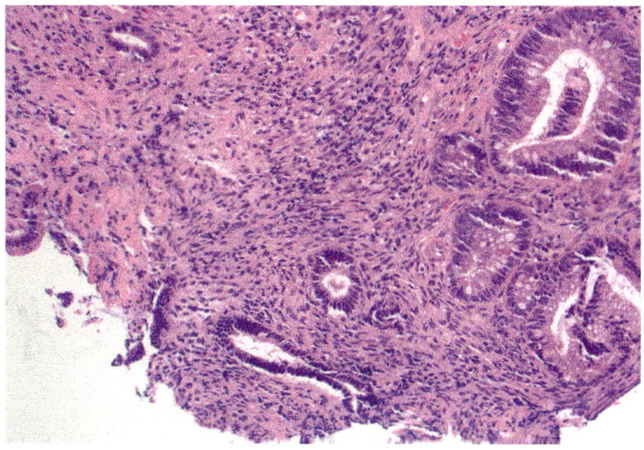

Fig. 11.18 Endometriosis in the colonic mucosa - endometriotic glands and stroma at the base of the mucosa

histological features are of endometriosis anywhere in the abdominal cavity. There are endometrial glands, endometrial stoma and haemosiderin deposition (Fig. 11.18). It is important not to overdiagnose endometriosis as carcinoma.

Other very rare lesions with a biphasic glandular and stromal proliferation are synovial sarcoma and rare metastatic lesions.

Stromal Expansion with Stromal Inflammation

- Mucosal prolapse
- Inflammatory fibroid polyp
- Juvenile polyp
- Cronkhite-Canada syndrome
- Inflammatory pseudopolyp

Mucosal Prolapse Polyp

This may occur anywhere in the large intestine but has the predilection for the sigmoid colon and distal rectum. A number of terms have been used for this process including:

- Inflammatory cap polyp—when there is surface ulceration with a cap of granulation tissue and inflammatory exudate
- Inflammatory cloacogenic polyp—when located in the distal rectum
- Solitary rectal ulcer syndrome—when located in the anterior rectum approximately 2 cm above the dentate line

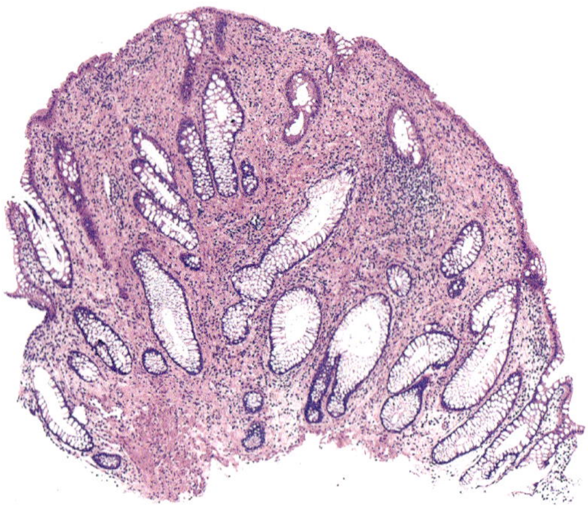

Fig. 11.19 Mucosal prolapse polyp - crypt elongation and an expanded inflamed stroma

- Inflammatory myoglandular polyp—when smooth muscle proliferation is prominent and associated with glandular dilatation

A rare syndrome of inflammatory cap polyposis exists which is characterised by multiple inflammatory cap-type polyps giving rise to profuse diarrhoea and protein-losing enteropathy.

Common histological features of these polyps include (Fig. 11.19):

- Expanded lamina propria with solidification by fibromuscular proliferation
- Variable inflammation and haemorrhage, sometimes with haemosiderin deposition in the stroma
- Architectural disturbance of colonic crypts with branching, elongation, dilatation and serration
- Superficial erosion with reactive cytological changes

There are a number of secondary changes that occur in prolapse-type inflammatory polyps that may cause diagnostic issues. These include:

- Prominent regenerative or reactive changes secondary to ulceration that may mimic dysplasia or conventional adenoma.
- Serration in expanded crypt epithelium may mimic serrated polyps. This is compounded by the problem that true serrated polyps may undergo secondary prolapse.
- Difficulty in distinguishing some forms of prolapse-type polyps from hamartomatous polyps as both lesions are characterised by epithelial and stromal expansion.

Careful attention to the clinical setting in the presence of secondary changes in the stroma such as haemorrhage is important in separating these possibilities. A rare variant of mucosal prolapse is the colonic muco-submucosal elongated polyp, which is characterised by expansion of the submucosa with a relatively normal overlying mucosa. A traction prolapse aetiology has been proposed. The majority of these tumours occur in the sigmoid colon and are usually solitary lesions [15–19].

Inflammatory Pseudopolyp

These may occur in the setting of inflammatory bowel disease or as isolated lesions presumably arising secondary to a local inflammatory focus. Lesions in inflammatory bowel disease may be multiple, often involving a segment of the large intestine. The polyps may be elongated and produce an appearance of filiform polyposis. Histologically the degree of inflammation is variable. When inflammation is prominent, there may be associated erosion and reactive epithelial atypia, which may be difficult to separate from true dysplasia. In cases where inflammation is minimal, there is often stromal fibrosis, proliferation of ganglion cells and smooth muscle proliferation. At times this may overlap with mucosal prolapse polyps or with a hamartomatous polyp.

Inflammatory pseudopolyp not arising in the setting of inflammatory bowel disease may show a variety of inflammatory patterns including being eosinophil-rich. The cecum is a favoured site of origin. Often the initiating inflammatory process is not identified.

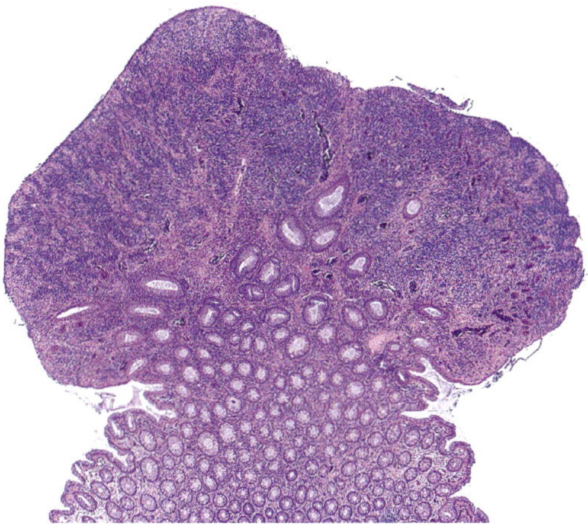

Fig. 11.20 Granulation tissue polyp - erosion of the surface with an underlying vascular proliferation and numerous plasma cells

Cystic Lesions

Gas: Pneumatosis

Discussed in the small intestine chapter.

Tumour-Like Inflammatory Lesions

The most commonly mass-forming inflammatory lesions are part of mucosal prolapse-associated polyps and inflammatory pseudopolyps (see above). Other polypoidal inflammatory lesions include polypoid granulation tissue (Fig. 11.20), which is typically seen adjacent to colonic anastomoses, polypectomy sites or diverticula and inflammatory polyps that occur following ischaemia.

References

1. Devereaux CE, Devereaux RG. Heterotopic gastric mucosa of the rectum with a review of the literature. J Clin Gastroenterol. 1994;19(1):41–5.
2. Bettington M, Walker N, Rosty C, et al. Critical appraisal of the diagnosis of the sessile serrated adenoma. Am J Surg Pathol. 2014;38:158–66.
3. Rex DK, Ahnen DJ, Baron JA, et al. Serrated lesions of the colorectum: review and recommendations from an expert panel. Am J Gastroenterol. 2012;107:1315–29.
4. Bettington ML, Walker NI, Rosty C, et al. A clinicopathological and molecular analysis of 200 traditional serrated adenomas. Mod Pathol. 2015; Mar;28(3):414–27.
5. Rosty C, Bettington M. Serrated colorectal polyps and polyposis. Diagn Histopathol. 2014;20:30–7.
6. Brown I, et al. Adverse histological features in malignant colorectal polyps: a contemporary series of 239 cases. J Clin Pathol. 2016;69(4):292–9.
7. Ueno H, et al. Risk factors for an adverse outcome in early invasive colorectal carcinoma. Gastroenterology. 2004;127:385–94.
8. Doyle LA, Hornick JL, Fletcher CD. PEComa of the gastrointestinal tract: clinicopathologic study of 35 cases with evaluation of prognostic parameters. Am J Surg Pathol. 2013;37(12):1769–82.
9. Nakasono M, Hirokawa M, Muguruma N, Okahisa T, Okamura S, Ito S, Miyamoto H, Wada S, Fukuda T, Sano T. Colorectal xanthomas with polypoid lesion: report of 25 cases. APMIS. 2004;112(1):3–10. Review
10. Miettinen M, Sarlomo-Rikala M, Sobin LH. Mesenchymal tumors of muscularis mucosae of colon and rectum are benign leiomyomas that should be separated from gastrointestinal stromal tumors--a clinicopathologic and immunohistochemical study of eighty-eight cases. Mod Pathol. 2001;14:950–6.
11. Gibson JA, Hornick JL. Mucosal schwann cell "hamartoma": clinicopathologic study of 26 neural colorectal polyps distinct from neurofibromas and mucosal neuromas. Am J Surg Pathol. 2009;33(5):781–7.
12. An S, Jang J, Min K, Kim MS, Park H, Park YS, Kim J, Lee JH, Song HJ, Kim KJ, Yu E, Hong SM. Granular cell tumor of the gastrointestinal tract: histologic and immunohistochemical analysis of 98 cases. Hum Pathol. 2015;46(6):813–9.
13. Groisman GM, Polak-Charcon S. Fibroblastic polyp of the colon and colonic perineurioma: 2 names for a single entity? Am J Surg Pathol. 2008;32(7):1088–94.
14. Huber AR, Shikle JF. Benign fibroblastic polyps of the colon. Arch Pathol Lab Med. 2009;133(11):1872–6.
15. Williams GT, Bussey HJR, Morson BC. Inflammatory cap polyps of the large intestine. Br J Surg. 1985;72(Suppl):133.
16. Lobert PF, Appelman HD. Inflammatory cloacogenic polyp. A unique inflammatory lesion of the anal transitional zone. Am J Surg Pathol. 1981;5:761–6.
17. Nakamura S, Kino I, Akagi T. Inflammatory myoglandular polyps of the colon and rectum. A clinicopathological study of 32 pedunculated polyps, distinct from other types of polyps. Am J Surg Pathol. 1992;16:772–9.
18. Kelly JK. Polypoid prolapsing mucosal folds in diverticular disease. Am J Surg Pathol. 1991;15:871–8.
19. Alizart MM, Rosty C, Brown IS. Colonic mucosubmucosal elongated polyp: a clinicopathologic study of 13 cases and review of the literature. Am J Surg Pathol. 2011;35(12):1818–22.

Molecular Testing in Colorectal Carcinoma

12

Connull Leslie, M. Priyanthi Kumarasinghe, and Ian Brown

Contents

While the molecular biology underlying colorectal carcinoma (CRC) has been extensively investigated and distinct molecular pathways described, a comprehensive molecular classification system allowing diagnostic and therapeutic subgroups continues to evolve [1–3]. Tumours with a hypermutated phenotype are a population consistently identified by all classification systems, with specific diagnostic and predictive attributes [4].

While molecular features may be associated with tumour site and morphology [5, 6], there is sufficient overlap that molecular testing should reflect consensus recommendations as applied to all colorectal carcinomas rather than those with particular pathological features [7]. With this caveat, microsatellite instability (MSI-H) and BRAF mutation are more often seen in mucinous or medullary histology, and colorectal carcinoma NOS tends to have a lower overall mutation count [8].

Molecular testing may be performed in a colorectal carcinoma specimen for three general reasons:

1. Diagnosis
   - Suggest further testing for hereditary conditions
     - Demonstration of MSI-H with absence of BRAF mutation suggests Lynch syndrome.
   - Confirm classification and grading [9]
     - Medullary carcinoma (appropriate morphology, MSI-H)

C. Leslie (✉)
Anatomical Pathology, PathWest Laboratory Medicine, QEII Medical Centre, Nedlands, WA, Australia
e-mail: connull.leslie@health.wa.gov.au

M. P. Kumarasinghe
Department of Anatomical Pathology, PathWest Laboratory Medicine, QEII Medical Centre and University of Western Australia, Perth, WA, Australia
e-mail: priyanthi.kumarasinghe@health.wa.gov.au

I. Brown
Envoi Pathology, Kelvin Grove, QLD, Australia

M. P. Kumarasinghe, I. Brown (eds.), *Endoscopic Biopsy Interpretation*,
https://doi.org/10.1007/978-3-319-79117-3_12

- Mucinous/signet ring carcinoma—low grade if MSI-H, high grade if MSS (microsatellite stable), as per WHO 2010.
2. Predictive of response to therapy (generally in stage III or IV disease)
   - The presence of RAS mutation (either KRAS or NRAS) predicts lack of response to anti-EGFR therapy [10].
3. Prognosis
   - BRAF mutation and MSS phenotype are suggested to have worse prognosis although evidence remains mixed [11, 12].

There will be future evolution in recommended biomarkers or genes of relevance, and practising pathologists should refer to up-to-date consensus statements by national or international organisations [7].

MSI-H Identification

All colorectal carcinomas should be tested for microsatellite instability or mismatch repair protein deficiency. Mismatch repair (MMR) protein deficiency results in microsatellite instability (MSI) and a hypermutated tumour phenotype; hence, these tests are complementary and assess different expressions of the same molecular mechanisms. Approximately 15% of CRCs are MSI phenotype, and this phenotype is more commonly present in right-sided tumours [13]. MSI status is essential in screening for Lynch syndrome, required for WHO grading in the case of mucinous or signet ring morphology, and in conjunction with BRAF mutation status has prognostic implications.

Lynch syndrome, also known as hereditary nonpolyposis colorectal carcinoma cancer (HNPCC), is a disorder caused by germline mutation in one copy of one of the MMR genes. Carriers have a high lifetime risk of CRC, as well as endometrial carcinoma and other cancers [14]. Detection of Lynch syndrome is important as carriers benefit from intensive screening programmes. Although the most common form of hereditary CRC, Lynch syndrome cases only account for approximately 2–7% of CRC cases [2]. The remaining MSI-high CRC cases are sporadic and due to epigenetic silencing of the MLH1 gene by hypermethylation. These sporadic cases are almost always associated with mutation in the BRAF gene (V600E hotspot) [15], which should be assessed in conjunction with MSI testing (see below).

Immunohistochemical Assessment of MMR Proteins

Immunohistochemical staining for the most important MMR proteins (MLH1, MSH2, PMS2 and MSH6) is generally used in diagnostic laboratories rather than molecular testing for MSI. The mismatch repair machinery in human cells comprises five heteroduplex complexes formed by combinations of seven proteins, which recognise and correct errors in the newly synthesised DNA strand [16]. Normal tissue (adjacent colonic epithelium, lymphocytes, stromal cells) expresses all MMR proteins in a nuclear staining pattern, although expression pattern may be patchy and weak. Loss of function of any one of the MMR proteins will result in MSI status. Nuclear expression in tumour cells is considered to indicate an intact and functional protein (Fig. 12.1a, b). As there is degradation of the smaller component of MMR heterodimer complexes, resulting in absence of staining for PMS2 if MLH1 is lost and absence of staining for MLH6 if MSH2 is lost, some centres suggest a two-panel antibody screening (PMS2 and MLH6) rather than testing for all four proteins [17]. Although this is a reasonable screening approach, at our institute we prefer four-panel testing. The loss of PMS2 in a two-panel approach then requires reflex testing for MLH1, and loss of MSH6 requires reflex testing of MSH2, in order to determine which MMR protein has a possible germline mutation. Known

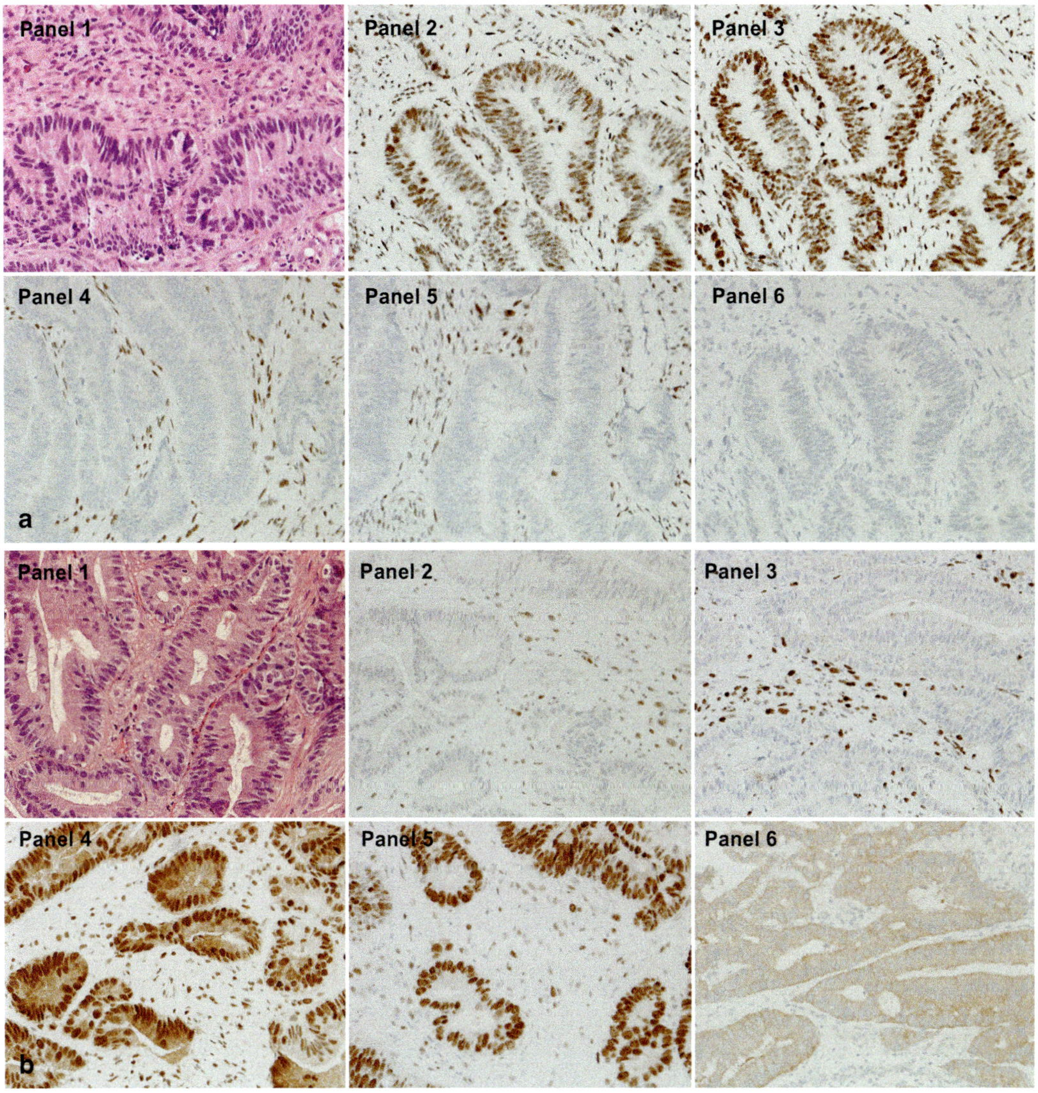

Fig. 12.1 (**a**) Panel 1: CRC H+E (×60). Panel 2: MLH1 intact. Panel 3: PMS2 intact. Panel 4: MSH2 loss (note stromal cell internal control). Panel 5: MSH6 loss. Panel 6: BRAF VE1 negative. This immunoprofile suggests loss of MMR protein MSH2, in conjunction with absence of BRAF mutation highly suggestive of MSI-H in context of Lynch syndrome. (**b**) Panel 1: CRC H+E (×60). Panel 2: MLH1 loss (note stromal cell internal control). Panel 3: PMS2 loss. Panel 4: MSH2 intact. Panel 5: MSH6 intact. Panel 6: BRAF VE1 positive (diffuse, cytoplasmic). This immunoprofile suggests loss of expression of MMR protein MLH1, in conjunction with presence of BRAF mutation highly suggestive of MSI-H with sporadic promotor methylation of MLH1 promotor and downregulation of gene expression

Lynch syndrome-associated gene mutations are predominant in MLH1 (50%), MSH2 (40%) or MSH6 (10%), with few in PMS2 (<5%) [18]. In addition to avoiding a need to perform additional immunohistochemical staining, a four-panel approach assists in determining technical deficiencies in immunohistochemical staining and interpretation, well recognised with these clones and likely associated with fixation variability [19, 20]. Ideally each MMR protein should show staining in the nuclei of background benign colonic epithelium, stromal cells and lymphocytes, generally stronger in proliferating cells such as lymphoid follicle germinal centres or the base of colonic mucosa crypts, which serve as internal controls. The tumour should ideally show either complete retention of staining or complete loss. Aberrant staining patterns (cytoplasmic, extremely patchy or weak, dot-like nuclear) are common and in the first instance require internal laboratory optimisation [21]. The use of the initial diagnostic biopsy for immunohistochemical assessment of MMR proteins may reduce fixation-related technical problems as well as facilitate earlier assessment of MMR status at time of endoscopic biopsy [22]. Importantly, as discussed further below, silencing of MLH1 by hypermethylation results in an MSI colorectal carcinoma in the absence of germline mutation; hence, loss of expression of MSH1 in particular requires further investigation before suggesting Lynch syndrome. It should be noted also that intact expression of all four MMR proteins does not entirely exclude Lynch syndrome as proteins may be present with retained epitope although non-functional due to a missense mutation [21, 23].

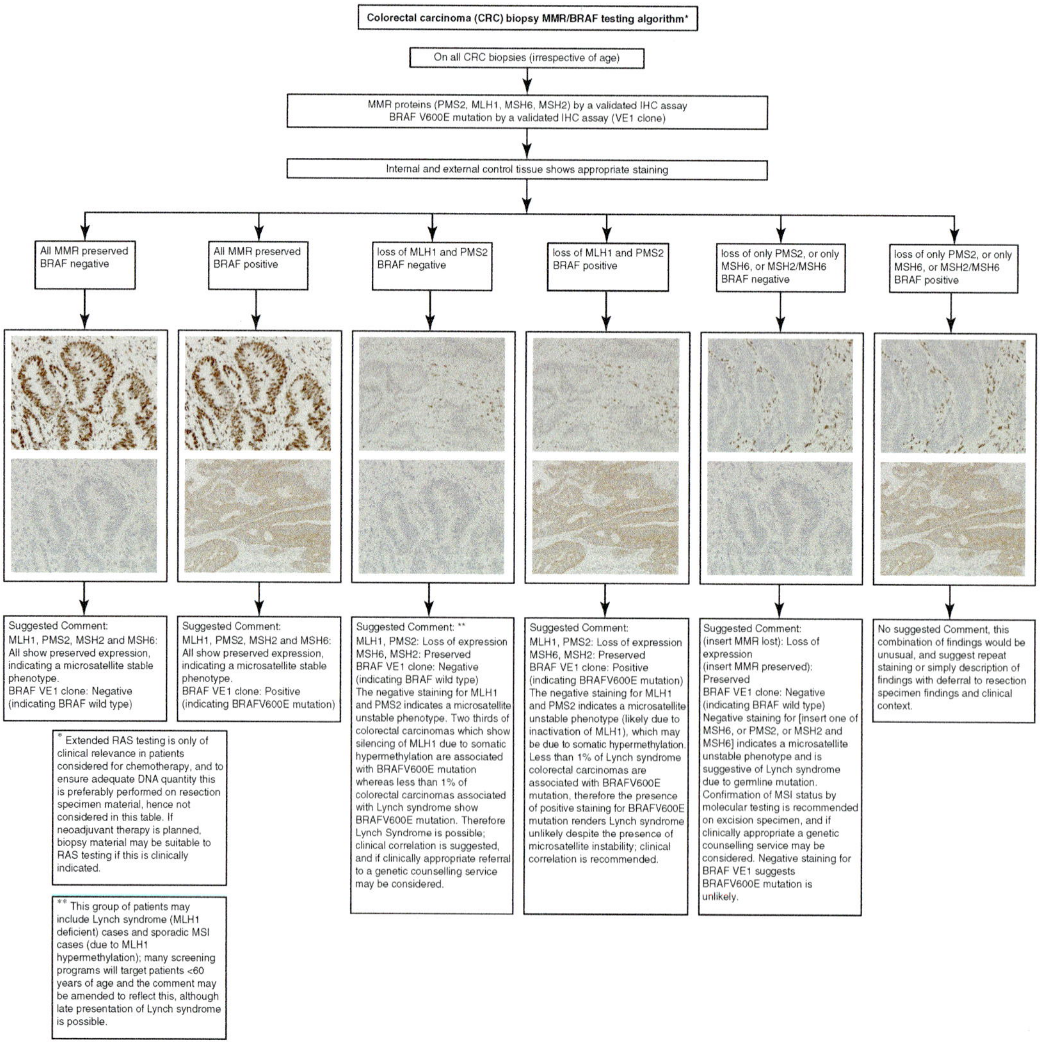

Interpretation of MMR protein immunohistochemistry and suggested comment

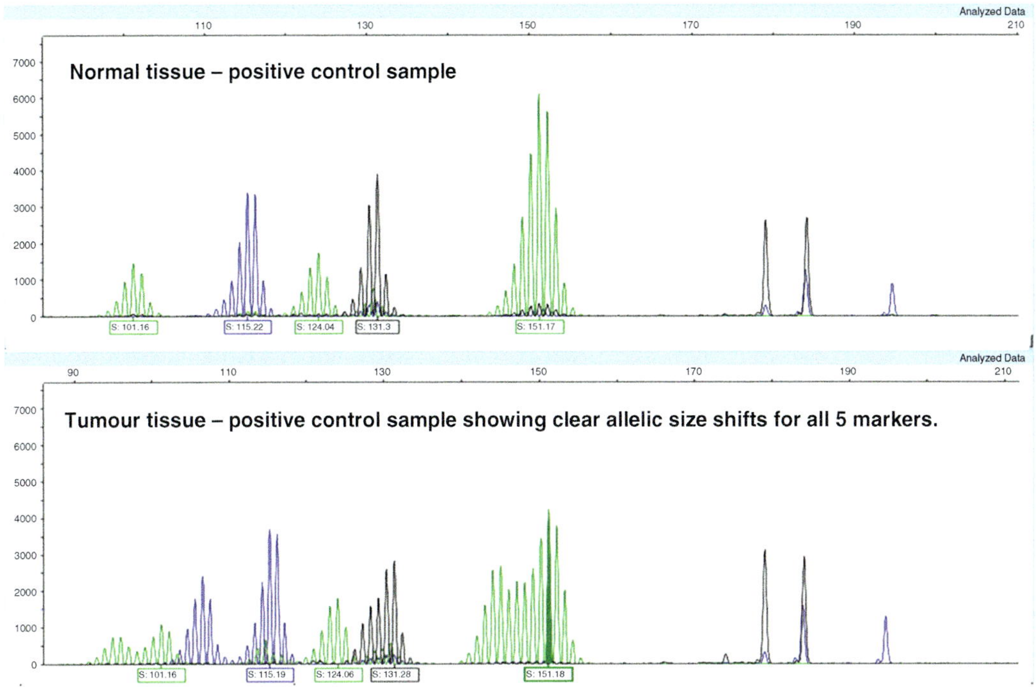

Fig. 12.2 This example demonstrates microsatellite instability in a colorectal carcinoma, using the pentaplex panel of mononucleotide markers BAT-25, BAT-26, NR-21, NR-24 and NR-27. Each peak represents the size of an amplified mononucleotide repeat, with "stuttered" appearance due to "slippage" of DNA polymerase during amplification. The upper panel represents the patient's normal tissue and the lower panel the patient's tumour. In addition to the mononucleotide markers, there are on the right two pentanucleotide markers which are highly polymorphic and act as an identification control. Note there are two peaks for each mononucleotide marker in the tumour panel representing the altered length of the mononucleotide repeat in the neoplastic cells, with background stromal tissue retaining the identical length as control normal tissue

Molecular Assessment of Microsatellite Instability

Microsatellite instability (MSI) is defined by detection of an alteration in the length of microsatellite markers, traditionally requiring mutation in two or more markers from a panel of five (the specific markers tested have evolved with time). Initial panels included dinucleotide markers and occasionally resulted in alterations only in a minority of markers. These cases were designated MSI-L, although are not clearly a distinct subset of colorectal carcinoma [24]. The revised Bethesda guidelines recommend using a panel of mononucleotide markers, which has improved sensitivity, and to include MSI-L tumours with MSS tumours [25]. A commercially available kit includes the five mononucleotide markers BAT25, BAT-26, MONO27, NR-21 and NR-24 (Promega, Madison, WI).

Comparison of microsatellite markers does not always require separate analysis of normal tissue and tumour samples, as tumour samples will include a significant amount of background parenchymal tissue; however, we recommend including separate analysis of normal tissue to ensure accurate assessment of product size differences. This may include a pretreatment biopsy sample and an unrelated previous sample (e.g. a skin excision from which normal tissue can be microdissected) if required (Fig. 12.2).

Following recent evidence that immune checkpoint blockade is of clinical benefit in treatment refractory mismatch-repair deficient tumours [26], there is increased interest in MSI status as a biomarker predicting response to PD-1-pathway blockade in many tumour types including colorectal carcinoma [27]. In other tumours, in particular lung carcinoma, confirmation that tumour cells show expression of PD-L1 predicts response to anti-PD-1 therapy. There is early evidence that MSI-H CRC are higher expressors of PD-L1, however high expression of PD-L1 was present in only 5% of assessed tumours and association with prognosis required correlation with PD-1 expression in tumour infiltrating lymphocytes [28]. Further studies are required to determine whether these biomarkers add value beyond assessment of MSI status in selecting patients for immunotherapy.

BRAF: Prognostic Biomarker

In conjunction with assessment of MSI status (by either molecular or immunohistochemistry), BRAF mutation status should also be assessed. The presence of BRAF mutation in a microsatellite stable tumour appears to be associated with poorer overall survival regardless of tumour stage [29]. In the context of MSI tumours, the presence of BRAF mutation essentially excludes Lynch syndrome-associated colorectal carcinoma [30], and in advanced (stage III) colon carcinoma, the proficiency or deficiency in DNA mismatch repair appears to have greater prognostic significance than the presence of BRAF mutation [31]. Although there is some evidence that presence of BRAF mutation remains a poor prognostic indicator in metastatic CRC treated with chemotherapy and anti-EGFR therapy [11, 12, 32], BRAF mutation testing is not currently considered a predictive biomarker in response to anti-EGFR inhibitors [33].

BRAF is a serine/threonine protein kinase, an effector in the MAPK signalling pathway, and in colorectal carcinoma, the activating mutation is almost exclusively c.1799T>A, p.Val600Glu (often stated as V600E). There is a commercially available antibody to BRAF protein with p. Val600Glu mutation (clone VE1, Ventana, Tucson, AZ), with mixed literature regarding the sensitivity and specificity of immunohistochemistry in assessing BRAF mutation in colorectal carcinoma [30, 34–37]. We find that interpretation of BRAF VE1 immunohistochemistry is especially difficult in poorly fixed resection specimens and mucinous/signet ring carcinomas (Fig. 12.3) and recommend the use of biopsy samples preferentially with prudence in interpretation of poor-quality staining). Given that both MMR and BRAF IHC staining patterns are better interpreted on biopsy specimens, we routinely perform a combination of BRAF VE1, MLH1, PMS2, MSH2 and MSH6 immunohistochemical stains on the initial biopsy of CRC, if the tissue is representative and adequate.

If the presence of BRAF mutation will have therapeutic consequences in advanced CRC, mutation status should be verified by molecular studies. The V600E mutation is common in melanoma, and there are highly sensitive allele-specific commercial systems (e.g. Roche Cobas® BRAF V600 Mutation Test) marketed in that context. PCR amplification for Sanger sequencing remains less sensitive although will detect rare alternative mutations.

RAS: Predictive Biomarker

Testing for RAS mutations (KRAS and NRAS) should be performed in all patients considered for anti-EGFR therapy, as recognised by most clinical and pathology guidelines [38]. Whether testing is performed as a reflex test on all colorectal carcinomas or after clinician request depends on the practice setting. At our institute all patients likely to require adjuvant therapy (AJCC stage III or IV or pT4) are tested immediately to avoid delay. Only patients with wild-type RAS show response to anti-EGFR therapy, with data showing that RAS mutations beyond the common KRAS codons 12 and 13 in exon 2 also indicate unlikely benefit from anti-EGFR therapy [39].

Both histology and cytology specimens can reliably be used to detect KRAS mutation [40], with a high level of concordance (estimated 80%) between primary and metastatic tumours [41]. There is evidence of intratumour heterogeneity in colorectal carcinoma although RAS mutations are usually present in the majority of neoplastic

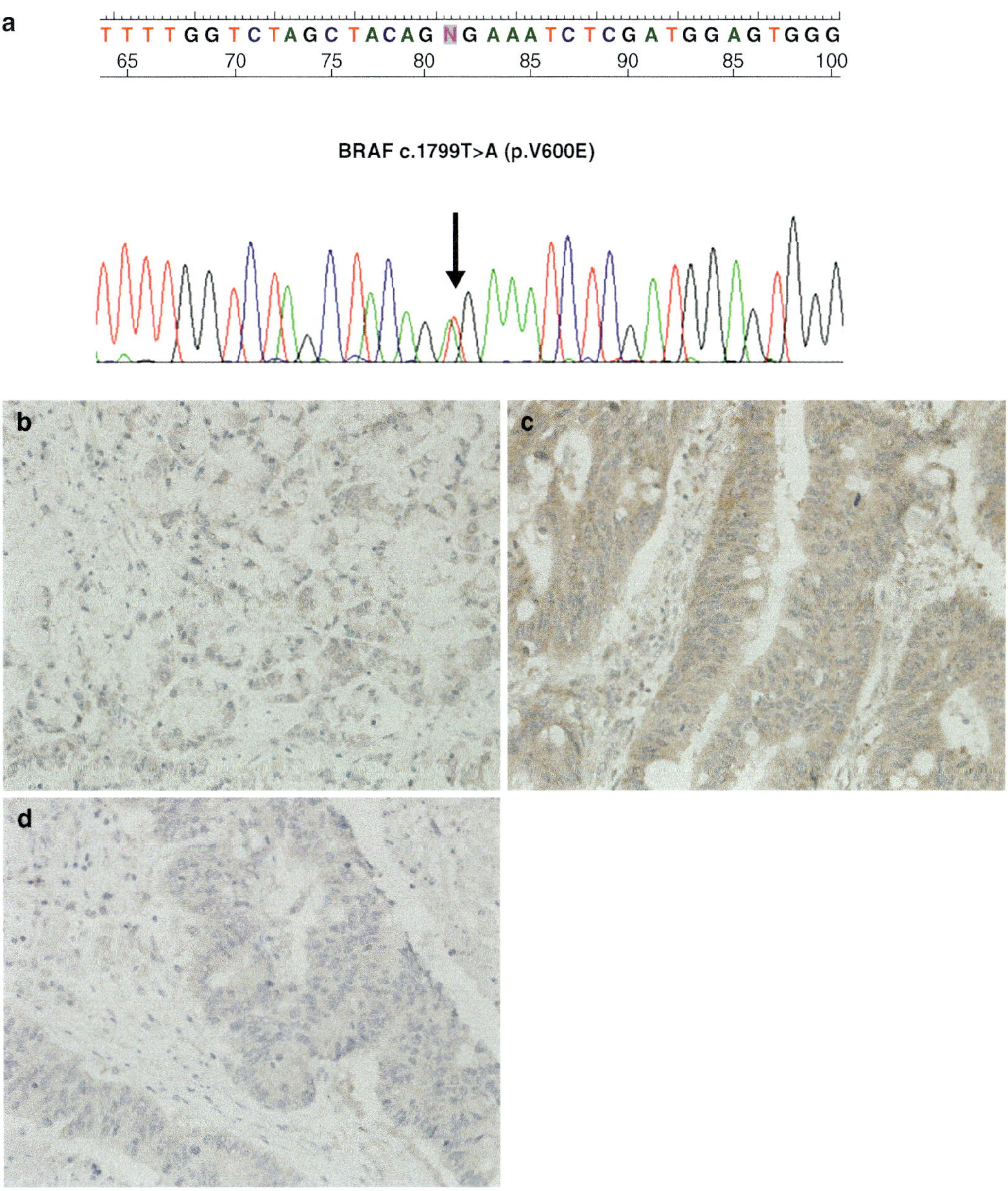

Fig. 12.3 (**a**) Sanger sequencing demonstrates point mutation c.1799T>A, resulting in p.Val600Glu alteration. (**b**) Same case (colectomy sample) shows very weak cytoplasmic staining with BRAF variable VE1 immunohistochemical staining. (**c**, **d**) Different areas of a CRC from a colectomy specimen with variable BRAF VE1 immunohistochemical staining, in a case with confirmed BRAF c.1799T>A by molecular testing. The difference in staining strength probably reflects fixation artefact

cells [42]. As with all molecular samples, if significant (generally >50%) non-neoplastic or necrotic tissue is present, then test tissue should be macrodissected from serial unstained slides to enrich for neoplastic DNA content.

There are numerous assay platforms available to detect RAS mutations including Sanger sequencing, pyrosequencing and HRM analysis, as well as proprietary Cobas and Therascreen platforms. Laboratory choice will depend on

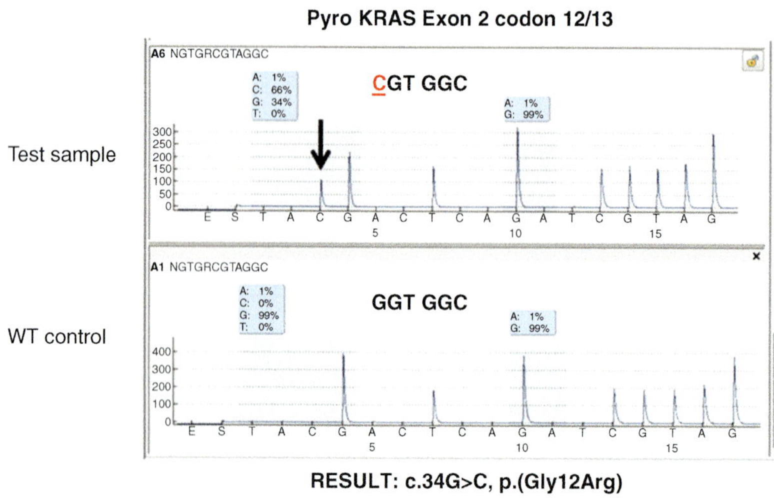

Fig. 12.4 Pyrosequencing relies on detection of pyrophosphate release on nucleotide incorporation, determining the order of nucleotides as the sequence is synthesised. The presence of a peak indicates nucleotide incorporation, with the height reflecting number of incorporated nucleotides (two nucleotides will be twice the height of one nucleotide). The sequenced region is very short and specific to the region of interest (as opposed to Sanger sequencing which reads amplified regions of hundreds of bases); hence, multiplex platforms are required to detect other mutations of interest. The nucleotides are dispensed in an order optimised to the region of interest; hence, pyrosequencing reads are best interpreted with concurrent wild-type control. In this example the lower wild-type read (GGT GGC—note height of peaks) differs from the tumour sample in which a proportion of tissue reads **C**GT GGC, reflecting the KRAS exon 2 c.34G>C mutation resulting in codon 12 alteration p.Gly12Arg

cost, degree of automation and expected turn-around-time. Due consideration should be given to the evidence that an extended RAS panel appears to have clinical relevance and importance (coverage should include KRAS exons 2, 3 and 4 and NRAS exons 1, 2, 3 and 4) (Fig. 12.4), and validation should document limit of detection by dilution studies. An approach to validation of KRAS mutation analysis and development of a reporting template has been described [43].

When extended RAS mutation testing is performed, an estimated 53% of colorectal carcinomas will be RAS mutated (as opposed to 42% when only the most common KRAS exon 2 mutation is tested), and all tumours harbouring RAS mutations are unlikely to significantly benefit from anti-EGFR therapy [39].

PI3K Signalling Pathway and Other Evolving Gene Alterations

In colorectal carcinoma as well as other malignancies there has been interest in abnormalities in the PI3K signalling pathway, with mutations present in the PIK3CA, PTEN or AKT genes among others [44]. Although there have been studies suggesting both prognostic [45] and predictive [46] significance in some components of the pathway, other studies show no predictive value in the context of anti-EGFR therapy [11]. There is not currently considered sufficient evidence to recommend mutational testing for components of the PI3K pathway in routine diagnostic practice, although this may change as abnormalities in these pathways potentially predict resistance to anti-EGFR therapy. Referral to current local guidelines is essential as recommendations will change as evidence accumulates.

Next-generation sequencing platforms, with the ability to simultaneously assess a large number of gene mutations albeit with less sensitivity than targeted platforms, may potentially improve prognostication and treatment selection. There is evidence that NGS platforms correlate with expected outcome in patients treated with anti-EGFR therapy [47] in addition to suggesting other actionable targets.

Which Tissue Specimen Should Be Used for Biomarker Testing?

The clinical expectation of both reflex and specifically requested molecular testing in CRC should be anticipated by the anatomical pathology laboratory. Tissue should be preserved during microtomy and also by retaining unstained sections during levelling into tissue block. Laboratory technicians should be informed and aware of the need to preserve tissue especially in the case of minimal tissue specimens. Predictive marker results should be available promptly. Discussion with colleagues in Medical Oncology and other recipients on how best to facilitate reporting of results in a timely manner is recommended.

There is high concordance between primary tumours and corresponding metastasis in KRAS and BRAF mutations [48] (pooled rate 92% and 96%, respectively), although in this meta-analysis an estimated 11% of patients with mutant KRAS primary tumours has wild-type KRAS in metastasis and may have potentially benefited from anti-EGFR therapy, while 9% of patients with wild-type KRAS in primary tumour who received anti-EGFR therapy had mutant KRAS in metastasis. If tissue from a metastatic lesion is available and adequate, this would be preferable as is likely to represent the most aggressive clone.

Adequate endoscopic biopsy material is acceptable if resection specimens are unavailable. Material in which predominantly adenoma rather than invasive malignancy is present represents more controversial material. RAS/RAF mutations are generally early events and hence likely to be present in precursor adenoma, with diagnostic biopsy material appearing representative of driver mutations [11, 49], however ideally material representative of invasive malignancy would be preferred.

Summary

Molecular testing expected in CRC has evolved from detecting Lynch syndrome and limited KRAS exon 2 mutation testing to an expectation that extended RAS testing will occur to assess benefit from anti-EGFR therapy, and there are recognised prognostic implications in MSI status and BRAF mutation. Expanded mutation analysis of the EGFR signalling pathway may become standard of care in the near future. The large variety of commercially available assays requires tissue pathology laboratories to closely evaluate the mutation coverage these tests provide, with awareness of the limits of detection, sensitivity and specificity. Test reporting should include tissue block reference number, neoplastic cell content, analytical method, usage of HGVS nomenclature of nucleotide and predicted amino acid changes and clinical interpretation of the result [38]. Any laboratory offering molecular testing should be involved in an external quality assurance scheme.

References

1. Jass JR. Classification of colorectal cancer based on correlation of clinical, morphological and molecular features. Histopathology. 2007;50:113–30.
2. Shi C, Washington K. Molecular testing in colorectal cancer. Am J Clin Pathol. 2012;137(6):847–59.
3. Guinney J, Dienstmann R, Wang X, et al. The consensus molecular subtypes of colorectal cancer. Nat Med. 2015;21(11):1350–6.
4. Müller MF, Ibrahim AE, Arends MJ. Molecular pathological classification of colorectal cancer. Virchows Arch. 2016;469:125–34.
5. Rosty C, Young JP, Walsh MD, et al. Colorectal carcinomas with KRAS mutation are associated with distinctive morphological and molecular features. Mod Pathol. 2013;26(6):825–34.
6. Jass JR. HNPCC and sporadic MSI-H colorectal cancer: a review of the morphological similarities and differences. Fam Cancer. 2004;3(2):93–100.
7. Sepulveda AR, Hamilton SR, Allegra CJ, Grody W, et al. Molecular biomarkers for the evaluation of colorectal cancer: guideline from the American Society for Clinical Pathology, College of American Pathologists, Association for Molecular Pathology, and American Society of Clinical Oncology. Am J Clin Pathol. 2017;147(3):221–60.
8. Shia J, Schultz N, Kuk D, et al. Morphological characterization of colorectal cancers in The Cancer Genome Atlas reveals distinct morphology–molecular associations: clinical and biological implications. Mod Pathol. 2017;30:599–609.
9. Hamilton SR, Bosman FT, Boffetta P, Ilyas M, et al. WHO classification of tumours of the digestive sys-

tem. In: Bosman FT, Carneiro F, Hruban RH, Theise ND, editors. Carcinoma of the colon and rectum. 4th ed. Lyon: IARC Press; 2010. p. 134–46.

10. Douillard JY, Oliner KS, Siena S, Tabernero J, et al. Panitumumab–FOLFOX4 treatment and RAS mutations in colorectal cancer. N Engl J Med. 2013;369(11):1023–34.
11. Karapetis CS, Jonker D, Daneshmand M, et al. PIK3CA, BRAF, and PTEN status and benefit from cetuximab in the treatment of advanced colorectal cancer—results from NCIC CTG/AGITG CO. 17. Clin Cancer Res. 2014;20(3):744–53.
12. Yuan ZX, Wang XY, Qin QY, et al. The prognostic role of BRAF mutation in metastatic colorectal cancer receiving anti-EGFR monoclonal antibodies: a meta-analysis. PLoS One. 2013;8(6):e65995.
13. Yamauchi M, Morikawa T, Kuchiba A, et al. Assessment of colorectal cancer molecular features along bowel subsites challenges the conception of distinct dichotomy of proximal versus distal colorectum. Gut. 2012;61(6):847–54.
14. Peltomaki P, Offerhaus GJA, HFA V. WHO classification of tumours of the digestive system. In: Bosman FT, Carneiro F, Hruban RH, Theise ND, editors. Lynch syndrome. 4th ed. Lyon: IARC Press; 2010. p. 152–5.
15. Domingo E, Niessen RC, Oliveira C, et al. BRAF-V600E is not involved in the colorectal tumorigenesis of HNPCC in patients with functional MLH1 and MSH2 genes. Oncogene. 2005;24(24):3995–8.
16. Jiricny J. The multifaceted mismatch-repair system. Nat Rev Mol Cell Biol. 2006;7(5):335–46.
17. Hall G, Clarkson A, Shi A, Langford E, Leung H, Eckstein RP, Gill AJ. Immunohistochemistry for PMS2 and MSH6 alone can replace a four antibody panel for mismatch repair deficiency screening in colorectal adenocarcinoma. Pathology. 2010;42(5):409–13.
18. Peltomäki P. Lynch syndrome genes. Fam Cancer. 2005;4(3):227–32.
19. Müller A, Giuffre G, Edmonston TB, Mathiak M, et al. Challenges and pitfalls in HNPCC screening by microsatellite analysis and immunohistochemistry. J Mol Diagn. 2004;6(4):308–15.
20. Overbeek LI, Ligtenberg MJ, Willems RW, Hermens RP, et al. Interpretation of immunohistochemistry for mismatch repair proteins is only reliable in a specialized setting. Am J Surg Pathol. 2008;32(8):1246–51.
21. Shia J, Holck S, DePetris G, Greenson JK, Klimstra DS. Lynch syndrome-associated neoplasms: a discussion on histopathology and immunohistochemistry. Fam Cancer. 2013;12(2):241–60.
22. Kumarasinghe AP, de Boer B, Bateman AC, Kumarasinghe MP. DNA mismatch repair enzyme immunohistochemistry in colorectal cancer: a comparison of biopsy and resection material. Pathology. 2010;42(5):414–20.
23. van Riel E, Ausems MG, Hogervorst FB, Kluijt I, et al. A novel pathogenic MLH1 missense mutation, c. 112A> C, p. Asn38His, in six families with Lynch syndrome. Hereditary Cancer Clin Pract. 2010;8(1):1.
24. Pawlik TM, Raut CP, Rodriguez-Bigas MA. Colorectal carcinogenesis: MSI-H versus MSI-L. Dis Markers. 2004;20(4-5):199–206.
25. Umar A, Boland CR, Terdiman JP, Syngal S, et al. Revised Bethesda Guidelines for hereditary nonpolyposis colorectal cancer (Lynch syndrome) and microsatellite instability. J Natl Cancer Inst. 2004;96(4):261–8.
26. Le DT, Uram JN, Wang H, Bartlett BR et al. PD-1 blockade in tumors with mismatch-repair deficiency. New England Journal of Medicine. 2015;372(26):2509-20.
27. Dudley JC, Lin MT, Le DT, Eshleman JR. Microsatellite instability as a biomarker for PD-1 blockade. Clinical Cancer Research. 2016;22(4):813-20.
28. Lee LH, Cavalcanti MS, Segal NH, Hechtman JF, et al. Patterns and prognostic relevance of PD-1 and PD-L1 expression in colorectal carcinoma. Modern Pathology. 2016;29(11):1433.
29. Samowitz WS, Sweeney C, Herrick J, Albertsen H, et al. Poor survival associated with the BRAF V600E mutation in microsatellite-stable colon cancers. Cancer Res. 2005;65(14):6063–9.
30. Toon CW, Walsh MJ, Chou A, Capper D, et al. BRAFV600E immunohistochemistry facilitates universal screening of colorectal cancers for Lynch syndrome. Am J Surg Pathol. 2013;37(10):1592.
31. Sinicrope FA, Shi Q, Smyrk TC, Thibodeau SN, et al. Molecular markers identify subtypes of stage III colon cancer associated with patient outcomes. Gastroenterology. 2015;148(1):88–99.
32. Kaczirek K, Ciuleanu TE, Vrbanec D, Marton E, et al. FOLFOX4 plus cetuximab for patients with previously untreated metastatic colorectal cancer according to tumor RAS and BRAF mutation status: updated analysis of the CECOG/CORE 1.2. 002 Study. Clin Colorectal Cancer. 2015;14(2):91–8.
33. Calonge N, Fisher NL, Berg AO, Campos-Outcalt D, et al. Recommendations from the EGAPP Working Group: can testing of tumor tissue for mutations in EGFR pathway downstream effector genes in patients with metastatic colorectal cancer improve health outcomes by guiding decisions regarding anti-EGFR therapy? Genet Med. 2013;15(7):517–27.
34. Adackapara CA, Sholl LM, Barletta JA, Hornick JL. Immunohistochemistry using the BRAF V600E mutation-specific monoclonal antibody VE1 is not a useful surrogate for genotyping in colorectal adenocarcinoma. Histopathology. 2013;63(2):187–93.
35. Loes IM, Immervoll H, Angelsen JH, Horn A, et al. Performance comparison of three BRAF V600E detection methods in malignant melanoma and colorectal cancer specimens. Tumor Biol. 2015;36(2):1003–13.
36. Vakiani E, Yaeger R, Brooke S, Zhou Y, et al. Immunohistochemical detection of the BRAF V600E mutant protein in colorectal neoplasms. Appl Immunohistochem Mol Morphol. 2015;23(6):438–43.

37. Lasota J, Kowalik A, Wasag B, Wang ZF, et al. Detection of the BRAF v600e mutation in colon carcinoma–critical evaluation of the imunohistochemical approach. Am J Surg Pathol. 2014;38(9):1235.
38. Wong NA, Gonzalez D, Salto-Tellez M, Butler R, Diaz-Cano SJ, Ilyas M, Newman W, Shaw E, Taniere P, Walsh SV. RAS testing of colorectal carcinoma—a guidance document from the Association of Clinical Pathologists Molecular Pathology and Diagnostics Group. J Clin Pathol. 2014;67:751.
39. Sorich MJ, Wiese MD, Rowland A, Kichenadasse G, et al. Extended RAS mutations and anti-EGFR monoclonal antibody survival benefit in metastatic colorectal cancer: a meta-analysis of randomized, controlled trials. Ann Oncol. 2015;26(1):13–21.
40. Pang NK, Nga ME, Chin SY, Ismail TM, et al. KRAS and BRAF mutation analysis can be reliably performed on aspirated cytological specimens of metastatic colorectal carcinoma. Cytopathology. 2011;22(6):358–64.
41. Han CB, Li F, Ma JT, Zou HW. Concordant KRAS mutations in primary and metastatic colorectal cancer tissue specimens: a meta-analysis and systematic review. Cancer Invest. 2012;30(10):741–7.
42. Normanno N, Rachiglio AM, Lambiase M, Martinelli E, et al. Heterogeneity of KRAS, NRAS, BRAF and PIK3CA mutations in metastatic colorectal cancer and potential effects on therapy in the CAPRI GOIM trial. Ann Oncol. 2015;26:1710.
43. Kamel-Reid S, Zhang T, Persons DL, et al. Molecular Oncology Resource Committee of the College of American Pathologists. Validation of KRAS testing for anti-EGFR therapeutic decisions for patients with metastatic colorectal carcinoma. Arch Pathol Lab Med. 2012;136(1):26–32.
44. Danielsen SA, Eide PW, Nesbakken A, Guren T, Leithe E, Lothe RA. Portrait of the PI3K/AKT pathway in colorectal cancer. Biochim Biophys Acta. 2015;1855(1):104–21.
45. Rosty C, Young JP, Walsh MD, Clendenning M, Sanderson K, Walters RJ, et al. PIK3CA activating mutation in colorectal carcinoma: associations with molecular features and survival. PLoS One. 2013;8(6):e65479.
46. Therkildsen C, Bergmann TK, Henrichsen-Schnack T, Ladelund S, Nilbert M. The predictive value of KRAS, NRAS, BRAF, PIK3CA and PTEN for anti-EGFR treatment in metastatic colorectal cancer: a systematic review and meta-analysis. Acta Oncol. 2014;53(7):852–64.
47. Ciardiello F, Normanno N, Maiello E, Martinelli E, Troiani T, Pisconti S, Giuliani F, Barone C, Cartenì G, Rachiglio AM, Montesarchio V. Clinical activity of FOLFIRI plus cetuximab according to extended gene mutation status by next-generation sequencing: findings from the CAPRI-GOIM trial. Ann Oncol. 2014;25(9):1756–61.
48. Mao C, Wu XY, Yang ZY, Threapleton DE, Yuan JQ, Yu YY, Tang JL. Concordant analysis of KRAS, BRAF, PIK3CA mutations, and PTEN expression between primary colorectal cancer and matched metastases. Sci Rep. 2015;5:8065.
49. Fadhil W, Ibrahem S, Seth R, AbuAli G, Ragunath K, Kaye P, Ilyas M. The utility of diagnostic biopsy specimens for predictive molecular testing in colorectal cancer. Histopathology. 2012;61(6):1117–24.

Overview of Endoscopic Features of Gastrointestinal Pathology (Colon)

13

Ammar O. Kheir, Nicholas J. Tutticci, and David G. Hewett

Contents

A. O. Kheir · N. J. Tutticci · D. G. Hewett (✉)
Faculty of Medicine, University of Queensland, Brisbane, QLD, Australia

Department of Endoscopy, Queen Elizabeth II Jubilee Hospital, Brisbane, QLD, Australia
e-mail: d.hewett@uq.edu.au

Endoscopic Anatomy

- Appreciation of endoscopic anatomical landmarks by the endoscopist is important for accurate localisation and documentation, especially for management of colorectal neoplasia.
- The colon is broadly divided into:
  - Proximal—proximal to the splenic flexure
  - Distal—distal to the splenic flexure
- In the absence of colonoscopic instrument looping, anatomical landmarks that can be identified during colonoscopy are (Fig. 13.1):
  - Rectum
  - Sigmoid colon
  - Descending colon
  - Splenic flexure
  - Transverse colon
  - Hepatic Flexure
  - Ascending colon
  - Cecum
  - Appendiceal orifice
  - Ileocaecal valve
  - Terminal ileum

Colitides

Inflammatory Bowel Disease

Ulcerative Colitis

- Ulcerative colitis (UC) is endoscopically characterised by confluent colonic inflammation

M. P. Kumarasinghe, I. Brown (eds.), *Endoscopic Biopsy Interpretation*,
https://doi.org/10.1007/978-3-319-79117-3_13

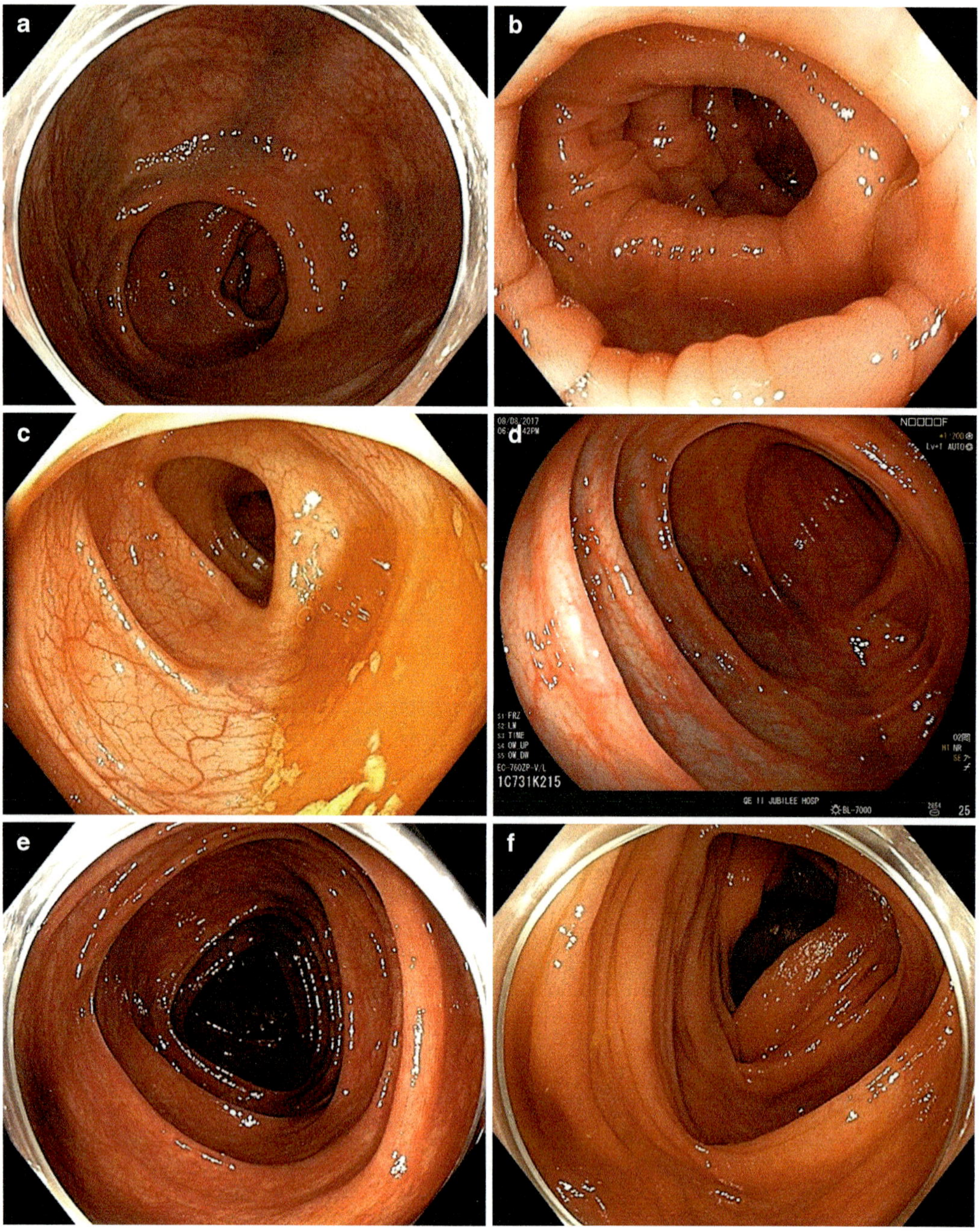

Fig. 13.1 (**a**) Rectum with view of the semilunar rectal folds, also known as "valves of Houston". (**b**) Sigmoid colon at 25 cm from the anal verge characterised by a concentric circular luminal appearance. (**c**) Descending colon at 40 cm from the anal verge characterised by the presence of fluid level when the patient is in the left lateral decubitus position. (**d**) Blue splenic flexure discolouration through the lumen of the proximal descending colon. (**e**) Transverse colon at 55 cm from the anal verge characterised by a triangular-shaped lumen. The image also shows a transparent distal cap attachment on the instrument, which is used to assist in maintaining visualisation while inspecting proximal aspects of colonic folds. (**f**) Ascending colon, with the ileocaecal valve in the distance (top). (**g**) Distal ascending colon and hepatic flexure with the colonoscope tip in retroflexion, to assist visualisation of blind spots on the proximal surfaces of colonic folds and flexures. (**h**) Ileocaecal valve (left) appearing as a semilunar thickened fold. (**i**) Appendiceal orifice. (**j**) Terminal ileum. (**k**) Taenia coli (muscularis externa) can be seen extending longitudinally in the direction of the lumen (bottom)

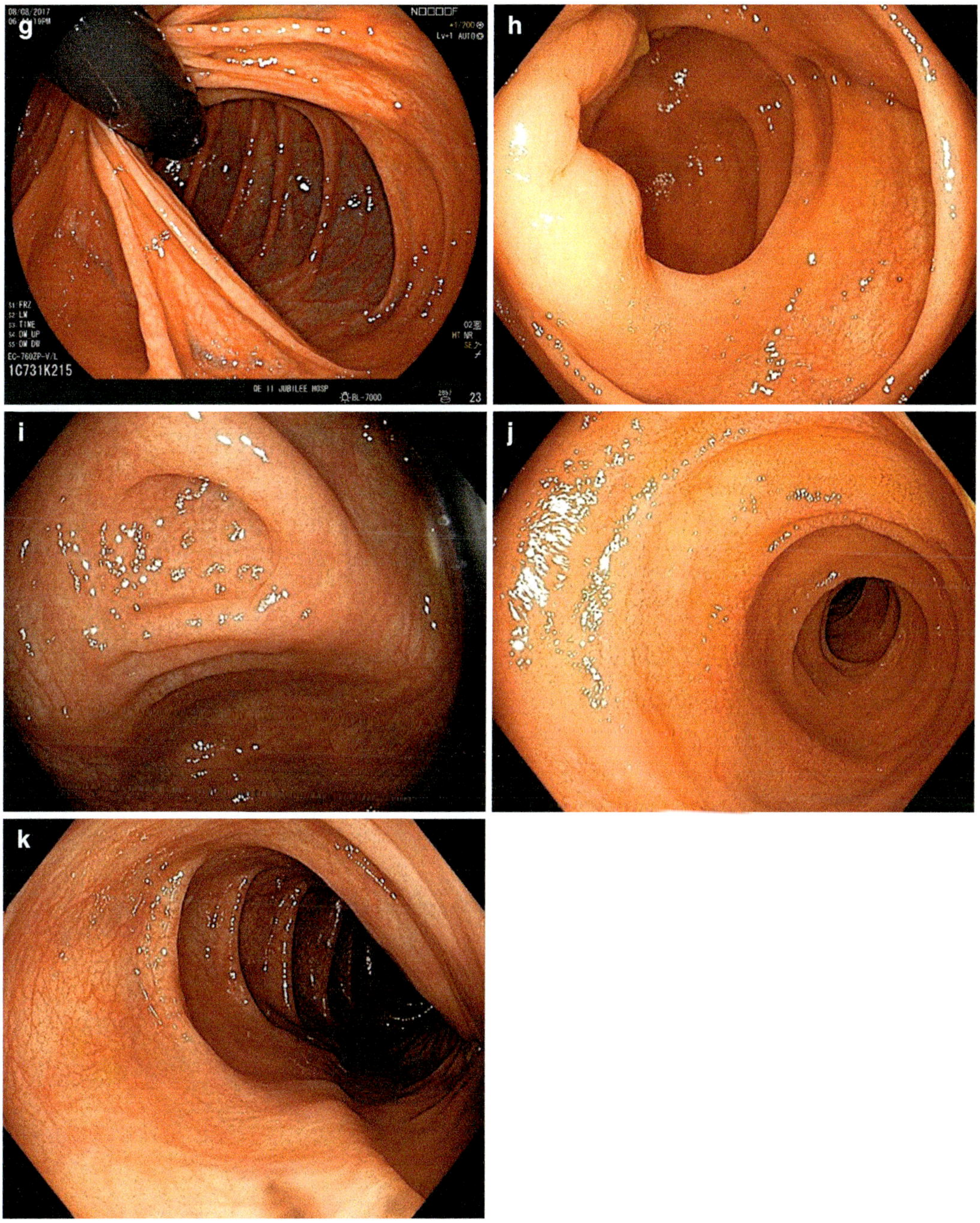

Fig. 13.1 (continued)

starting at the rectum and extending proximally (Fig. 13.3).

- Phenotypically, UC can be classified based on the anatomical extent of colonic inflammation (Table 13.1). The Montreal classification is used during colonoscopy to categorise UC into [1]:
  - **E1**, ulcerative proctitis—inflammation is limited to the rectum.
  - **E2**, left-sided ulcerative colitis (distal UC)—inflammation does not extend proximally beyond the splenic flexure.
  - **E3**, extensive ulcerative colitis (pancolitis)—inflammation extends proximally beyond the splenic flexure.

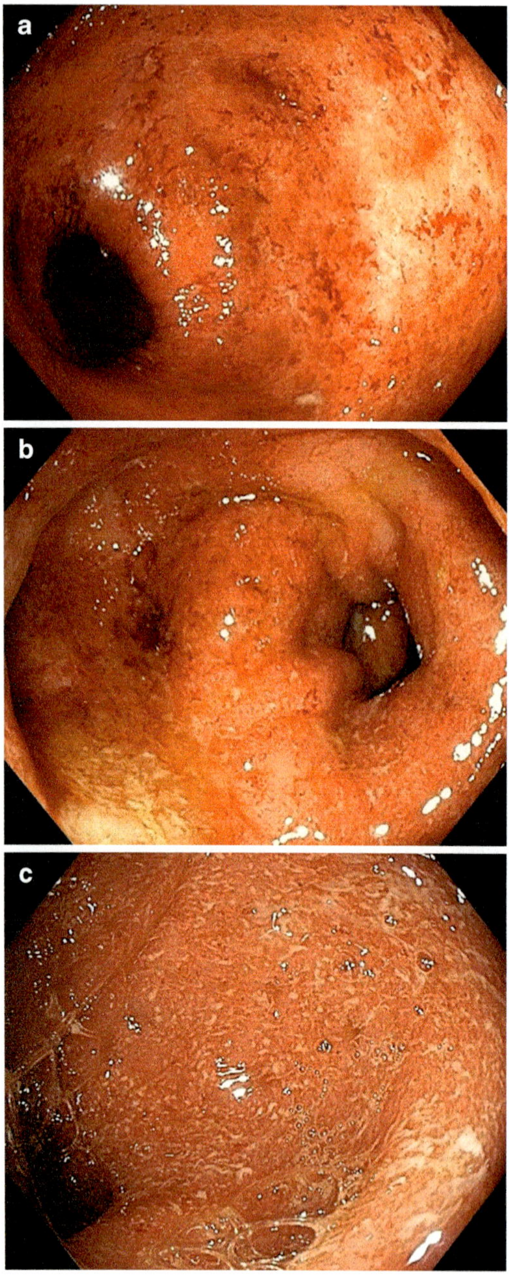

Fig. 13.2 (**a**–**c**) Moderately active ulcerative colitis with diffuse mucosal granularity, oedema, absent vascular markings, erythema, exudates, spontaneous bleeding, and luminal narrowing

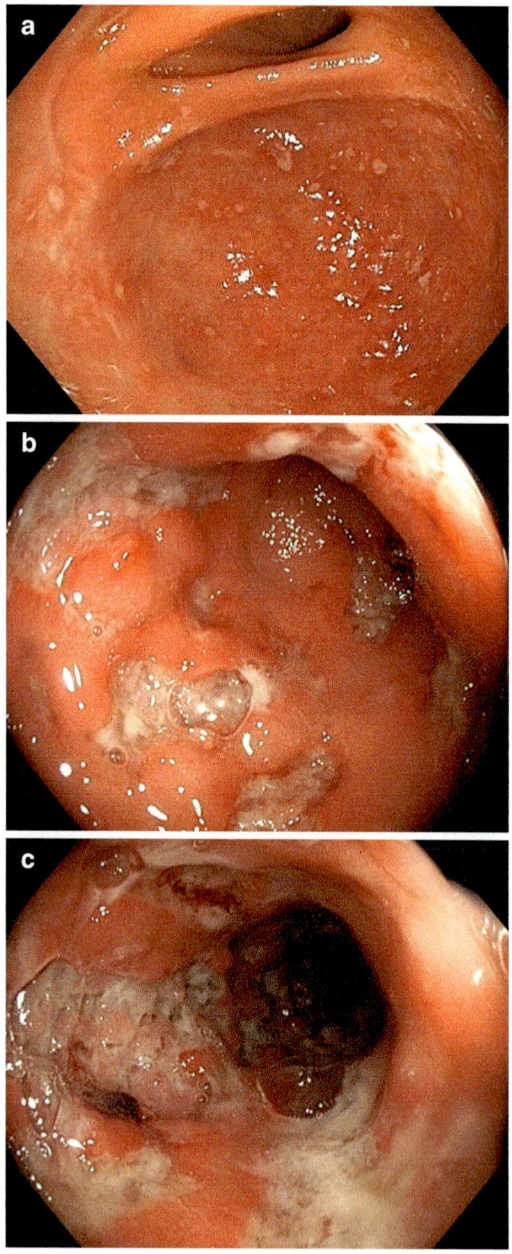

Fig. 13.3 (**a**–**c**) Severe active Crohn's colitis with deep linear ulcers, oedema, absent vascular markings, erythema, and luminal narrowing. A guide wire was passed through the stricture prior to balloon dilatation. The stricture was successfully traversed after dilatation

- Additionally, the severity of colonic inflammation is classified clinically as:
  - **S0**, clinical remission—asymptomatic
  - **S1**, mild UC—≤4 bloody or non-bloody stools daily, no systemic illness, and normal ESR
  - **S2**, moderate UC—>4 bloody stools daily with minimal sign of systemic illness or toxicity (Fig. 13.2)
  - **S3**, severe UC—≥6 bloody stools daily, tachycardia (≥90 bpm), temperature ≥37.5 °C, anaemia (Hb < 105 g/L), and ESR ≥30 mm/h

Table 13.1 Mayo Endoscopic score for ulcerative colitis

Score	Severity	Description
0	Normal	Normal or inactive disease
1	Mild	Erythema, reduced mucosal vascular pattern
2	Moderate	Marked erythema, absent mucosal vascular pattern, mucosal friability, erosions
3	Severe	Spontaneous bleeding, ulceration

- Fulminant UC is characterised by >10 bloody stools daily, toxicity, abdominal distention and tenderness, severe anaemia requiring blood transfusion, and colonic dilatation on imaging.
- The severity of colonic inflammation is scored endoscopically using the Mayo endoscopic core as:
  - Normal or inactive disease
  - Mild (erythema, reduced mucosal vascular pattern)
  - Moderate (marked erythema, absent mucosal vascular pattern, mucosal friability, erosions)
  - Severe (spontaneous bleeding, ulceration)

Crohn's Disease

- Crohn's disease (CD) is endoscopically characterised by transmural inflammation (erythema, erosions, deep ulceration, strictures) of the terminal ileum with or without patchy inflammatory areas in the colon with intervening normal colonic mucosa (Figs. 13.4 and 13.5).
- Can affect the any part of the luminal gastrointestinal tract.
- Patients often present with abdominal pain and anaemia.
- The Vienna and Montreal classification is used during colonoscopy to categorise CD (Table 13.2) [1].
- The endoscopic recurrence severity score is used to assess the ileocolonic anastomosis and ileum (Table 13.3).

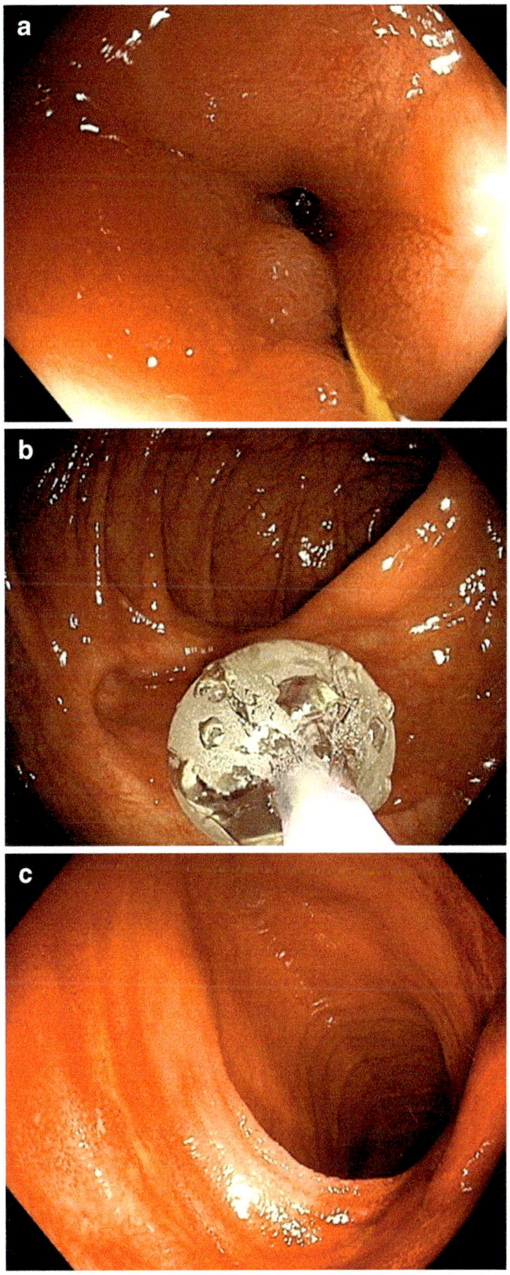

Fig. 13.4 (a–c) Severe neo-terminal ileal fibrotic anastomotic stricture in a Crohn's patient following ileocolonic resection. A guide wire was passed through the stricture prior to balloon dilatation. The stricture was successfully traversed after dilatation

SCENIC and DALM

In 2015, an international expert multidisciplinary panel including gastrointestinal pathologists developed the International Consensus Statement on Surveillance and Management of Dysplasia in Inflammatory Bowel Disease (SCENIC) [2, 3]. Some of their key recommendations included:

- To abandon the use of less accurate endoscopic terminology including "dysplasia-associated lesion or mass (DALM)",

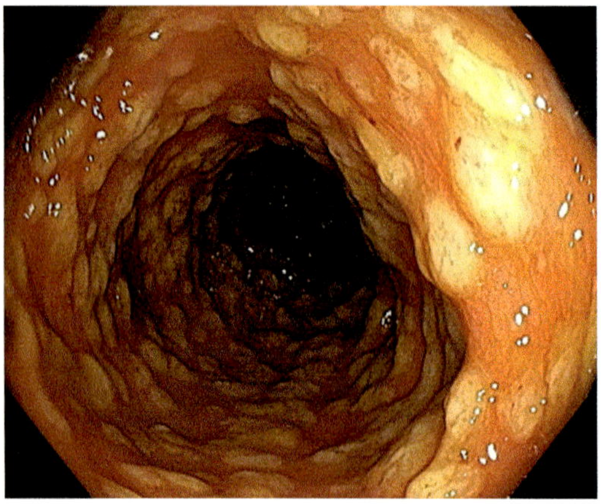

Fig. 13.5 Pseudomembranous colitis with typical yellow-white pseudomembranes

Table 13.2 Vienna and Montreal classification for categorising Crohn's disease

	Vienna	Montreal
Age at diagnosis	A1 below 40 years	A1 under 16 years
	A2 above 40 years	A2 between 17 and 40 years
		A3 above 40 years
Location	L1 ileal	L1 ileal
	L2 colonic	L2 colonic
	L3 ileocolonic	L3 ileocolonic
	L4 upper	L4 isolated upper disease
Behaviour	B1 non-stricturing, non-penetrating	B1 non-stricturing, non-penetrating
	B2 stricturing	B2 stricturing
	B3 penetrating	B3 penetrating
		P perianal disease

Table 13.3 Endoscopic recurrence severity score for assessing ileocolonic anastomosis in Crohn's disease

Score	Lesions	Endoscopic diagnosis
0	No lesions	No recurrence
1	<5 aphthous ulcers	
2	≥5 aphthous ulcers confined to the ileocolonic anastomosis or 2–5 larger lesions >5 mm	Recurrence
3	Diffuse aphthous ileitis	
4	Diffuse inflammation with larger ulcers or anastomotic narrowing	

"adenoma-like", or "non-adenoma-like" and use "endoscopically resectable" or "nonendoscopically resectable".

Table 13.4 Common bacterial pathogens causing infectious colitis

Clostridium difficile
Shigella
Escherichia coli
Yersinia enterocolitica
Salmonella
Campylobacter jejuni
Clostridium perfringens
Staphylococcus aureus
Vibrio cholerae
Plesiomonas shigelloides
Aeromonas

- Using chromoendoscopy with targeted biopsy is superior to white-light colonoscopy with random biopsy.
- Confirmation of dysplasia by a specialised gastrointestinal pathologist.

Infectious Colitis

- Infectious colitis is diagnosed by the combination of:
  - Characteristic histologic inflammatory changes on colonic biopsies positive microbiological testing for the culprit organism (Table 13.4) [4].
  - Colonoscopic findings in early disease (within 4–5 days) usually show distal colitis with relative sparing of the rectum. Th e rectum can be severely affected later in the disease course, which causes endoscopic and histologic confusion for differentiating infectious colitis from ulcerative colitis.
- Colitis due to *Clostridium difficile* shows characteristic yellow-white pseudomembranes known as "pseudomembranous colitis" (Fig. 13.5).

Microscopic Colitis

- Colonoscopic examination is usually normal.
- Occasionally mild mucosal erythema, oedema, or reduced mucosal vascularity can be noted.
- Patients usually present with chronic diarrhoea.

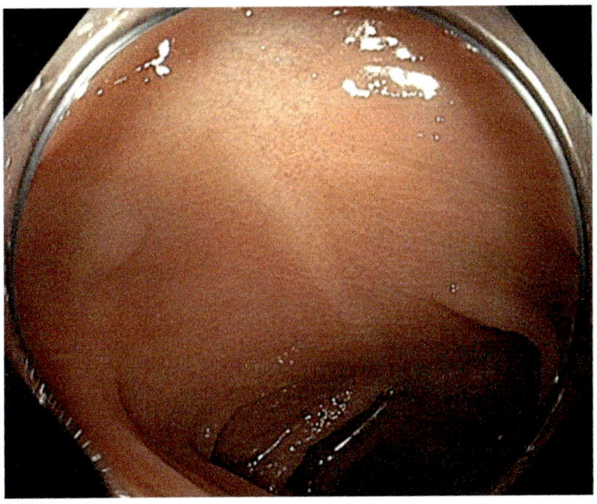

Fig. 13.6 A resolved tram-track sign in a patient with healed ischaemic colitis

Ischaemic Colitis

- Ischaemic colitis often referred to as mesenteric ischaemia can be acute or chronic.
- Endoscopic and histologic features vary according to the phase, severity, and duration of ischaemic injury.
- Anatomical involvement corresponds to the affected vascular territory but commonly affect the splenic flexure and rectosigmoid junction, also known as "watershed areas".
- These features are usually segmental in distribution with an abrupt transition between injured and non-injured colonic mucosa. Endoscopic features can include:
  - Confluent necrosis of colonic wall
  - Colonic wall and colonic folds oedema
  - Mucosal friability, ulceration, and petechial haemorrhage
  - Intraluminal bleeding and clots
  - Segmental distribution with an abrupt transition between injured and non-injured
  - "Colon-stripe" sign (longitudinal ulcer along watershed area) or "double colon-stripe" sign, also known as a "tram-track" sign (Fig. 13.6).
  - Follow-up colonoscopy after resolution of ischaemic injury often shows complete resolution of colitis with healed mucosal scarring.

Radiation Colitis

- Diffuse mucosal changes caused by radiotherapy.

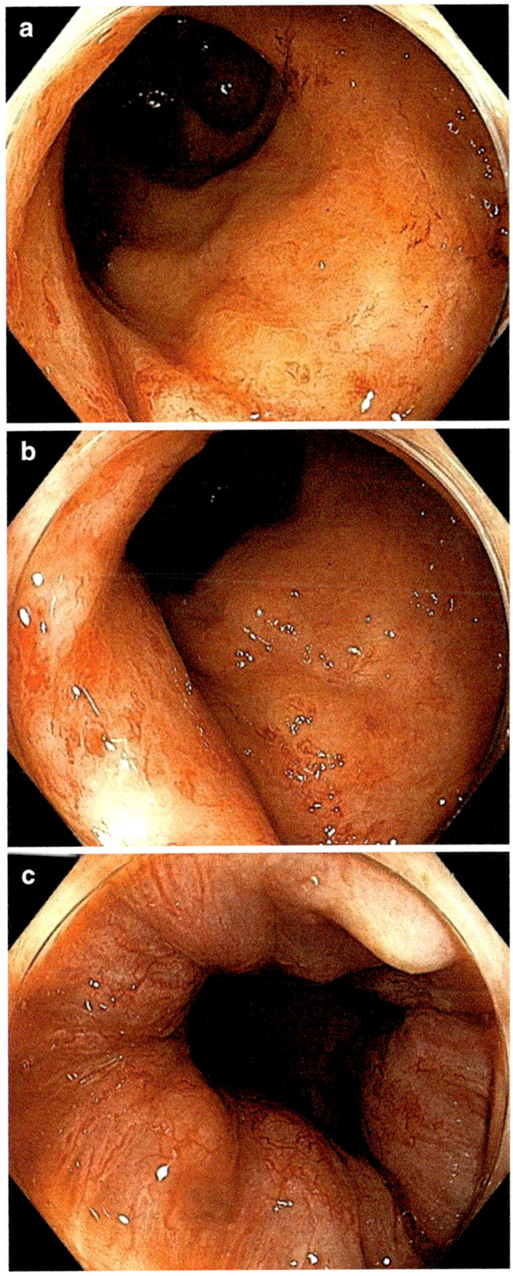

Fig. 13.7 (**a**–**c**) Chronic radiation proctitis characterised by neovascularisation with telangiectatic mucosal capillaries, loss of normal vascular background, patchy erythema, and mucosal oedema

- Radiation proctitis can be frequently seen in men following radiation therapy for prostate cancer.
- They appear as an acquired angioectasias and can frequently cause bleeding (Fig. 13.7).
- Treatment with argon plasma coagulation is effective.

Table 13.5 NBI International Colorectal Endoscopic (NICE) classification

	Type 1	Type 2	Type 3
Colour	Same or lighter than background	Browner relative to background colour arising from vessels	Brown to dark brown relative to background sometimes patchy whiter areas
Vessel	None or isolated lacy vessels coursing across the lesion	Brown vessels surrounding white structures	Has area(s) of disrupted or missing vessels
Surface pattern	Dark or white spots of uniform size or homogenous absence of surface pattern	Oval, tubular, or branched white structures surrounded by brown vessels	Amorphous or absent surface pattern
Most likely pathology	Serrated polyp (hyperplastic or sessile serrated polyp)	Adenoma	Deep submucosal invasive cancer

Colorectal Neoplasia

The latest-generation, high-definition endoscope systems all have built-in electronic image-enhancement technologies that can be used for optical diagnosis of colorectal polyps [5–7]. The most widely used technology is narrow-band imaging (NBI) for differentiating serrated from adenomatous colorectal polyps. Endoscopic imaging has revolutionised real-time management of colorectal polyps during colonoscopy. Historically, large polyps were biopsied initially to exclude the presence of carcinoma before being removed endoscopically. Modern therapeutic approaches advocate avoiding tissue biopsy, which can induce submucosal fibrosis and may compromise the technical success of complete and safe endoscopic removal of colorectal polyps.

The NBI International Colorectal Endoscopic (NICE) classification is a simple and validated classification that can be used in real time to optically diagnose colorectal polyps into serrated, adenomatous, or carcinoma with deep submucosal invasion (Table 13.5) [8–10]. Increasingly, expert colonoscopists can detect focal areas within polyps that may contain invasive cancer. This allows the selection of an appropriate en bloc endoscopic therapy, such as endoscopic submucosal dissection, or piecemeal endoscopic mucosal resection with targeted sampling of potentially invasive regions and submission for separate histologic assessment.

Colorectal Cancer

- Colorectal cancers range in endoscopic morphology from large, fungating, and firm luminal masses to subtle, flat or depressed lesions (Fig. 13.8). The endoscopic surface and vascular pattern correlates with the depth of submucosal invasive cancer. Deep (1000μm or greater) submucosally invasive cancers are characterised by a NICE type 3 appearance with disruption or absence of mucosal surface and vascular pattern (Fig. 13.9).
- When large and circumferential, cancers can cause luminal obstruction with inability of the colonoscope to traverse the lesion.

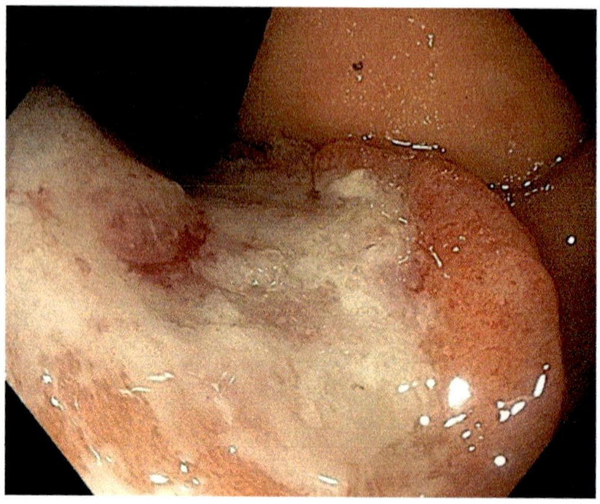

Fig. 13.8 Colorectal cancer

Colorectal Polyps

- The endoscopic morphology of colorectal polyps should be described using the Paris classification (Table 13.6) [11].
- Optical diagnosis using the Kudo pit pattern classification (Table 13.7) requires topical dye spray together with magnifying endoscopy to accurately and reliably differentiate between normal, nonneoplastic, neoplastic, and cancer-

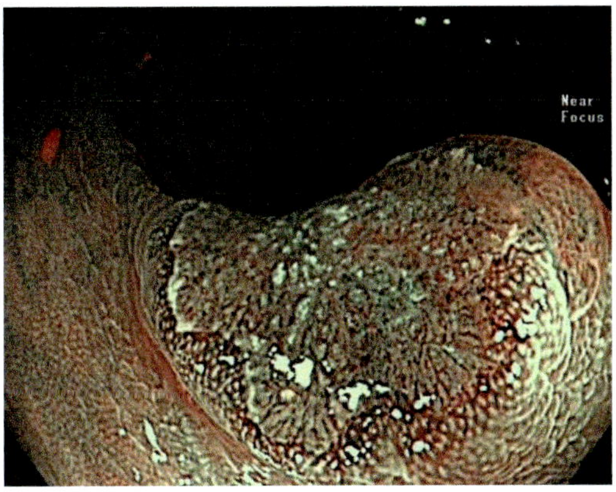

Fig. 13.9 A small malignant polyp (with deep submucosal invasion) showing NICE type 3 under NBI

Table 13.6 Paris classification

Endoscopic appearance	Paris class	Description
Protruded Lesions (>2.5 mm)	Ip	Pedunculated polyp
	Is	Sessile polyp
Flat elevated Lesions (≤2.5 mm)	IIa	Flat elevation of mucosa
	IIb	Flat mucosal change
	IIc	Mucosal depression
Excavated lesions	III	Excavated ulcer

Table 13.7 Kudo pit pattern classification

Kudo type	Endoscopic feature	Most likely diagnosis
Type I	Round	Normal
Type II	Papillary or stellar	Hyperplastic
Type III_s	Small round or tubular	Tubular adenoma
Type III_L	Large round or tubular	Tubular adenoma
Type IV	Gyrus-like	Villous adenoma
Type V	Nonstructural or amorphous	Submucosal cancer

ous lesions [12]. Electronic imaging using the NICE classification offers a quicker and more convenient approach to optical diagnosis.

- Colorectal polyps have characteristic endoscopic features that are highly predictive of the pathological diagnosis (Fig. 13.10) [8, 13].

Diverticular Disease

- Diverticular disease appears endoscopically as outpouchings of the colonic wall that vary in size and number (Fig. 13.11).
- Occurs most commonly in the sigmoid colon but can be seen throughout the colon.
- Diverticular disease spectrum includes:
  - Asymptomatic diverticular disease
  - Symptomatic uncomplicated diverticular disease
  - Complicated diverticular disease which can manifest as:

    Diverticulitis (acute or chronic)—Microscopic perforation results in localised inflammatory response caused by bacterial overgrowth.

    Diverticular disease-associated colitis—Rare and usually associated with diverticulitis.

    Diverticular bleeding (Fig. 13.12).

    Diverticular perforation (Table 13.8).

The majority of diverticular disease is simple without complications. Complicated diverticular disease can develop peritonitis, sepsis, abscesses, fistula, and bowel obstruction (Table 13.8).

Anorectal

Anorectal Junction

Retroflexion in the rectum conveniently shows the dentate line demarcating transition from colonic mucosa to anal squamous mucosa (Fig. 13.13).

Anal Intraepithelial Neoplasia (Condyloma Accuminata)

- Raised verrucous-like lesions within the dentate line (Figs. 13.14 and 13.15)

Anal Squamous Cell Carcinoma (SCC)

- Endoscopic features vary by stage:
  - Early SCC can be small and appear similar to condyloma acumulatuma
  - Advanced lesions can be large, ulcerated, or fungating.
  - They can be differentiated endoscopically from distal rectal carcinoma by their verrucous appearance, and that they arise from the anal squamous mucosa at or beyond the dentate line (Fig. 13.16).

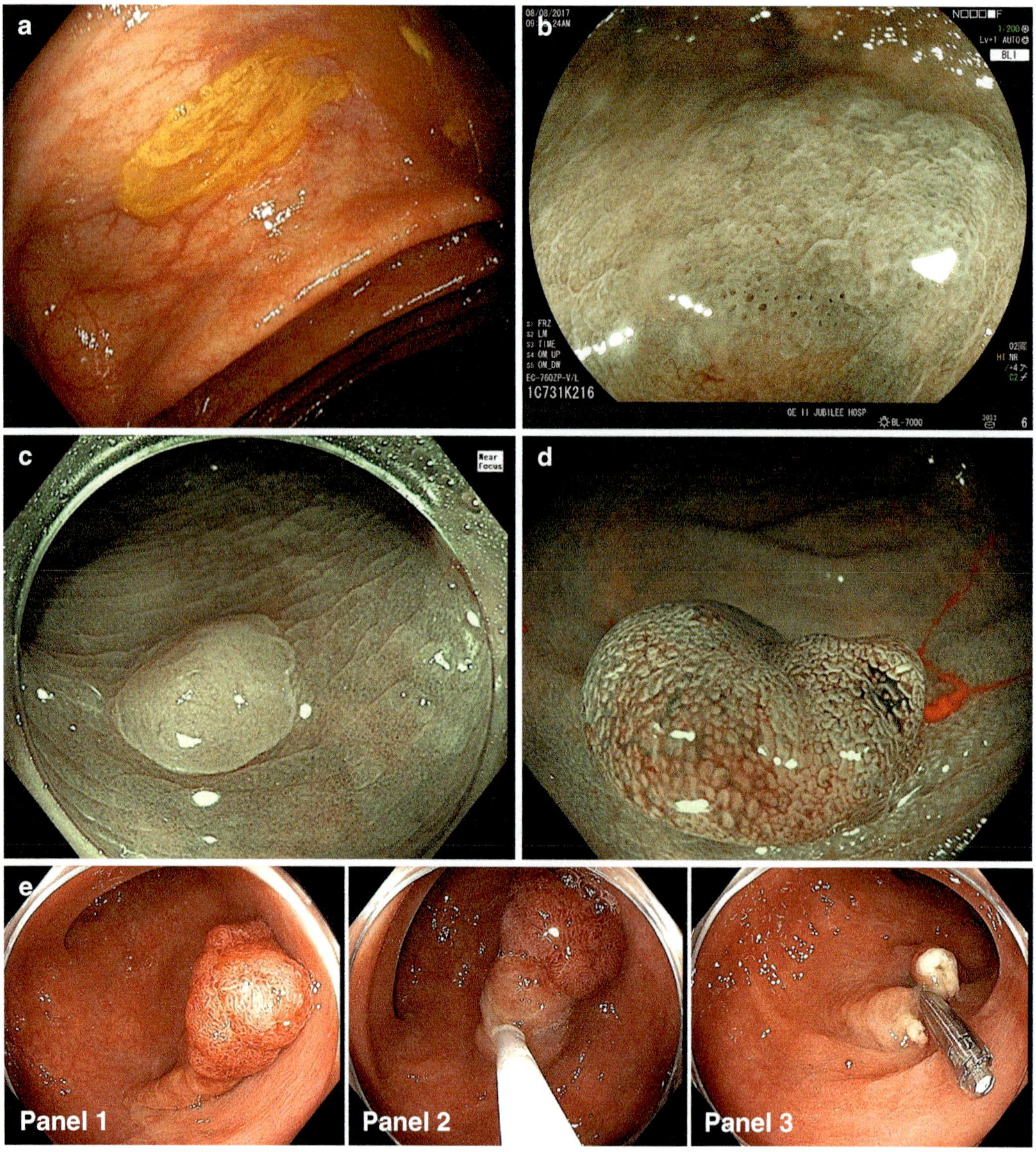

Fig. 13.10 (**a**) Characteristic endoscopic appearance of a sessile serrated adenoma/polyp in the ascending colon. Endoscopic features including flat morphology, indistinct margins, and yellow mucus cap. (**b**) Characteristic endoscopic appearance of a sessile serrated adenoma/polyp with NICE type 1 and open crypts that correlate histologically with dilated mucin filled crypts. (**c**) Hyperplastic polyp under NBI. (**d**) Tubular adenoma under NBI. (**e**) Panels 1–3: A pedunculated polyp in the proximal sigmoid colon removed by snare polypectomy with electrocautery. Resection yields a clear margin of normal tissue; a haemostatic clip was applied to prevent delayed haemorrhage. (**f**) Panels 1–3: A large rectal tubulovillous adenoma removed using endoscopic mucosal resection (EMR). Panel 4: The EMR scar on endoscopic surveillance at 4 months showing no endoscopic evidence of residual adenoma

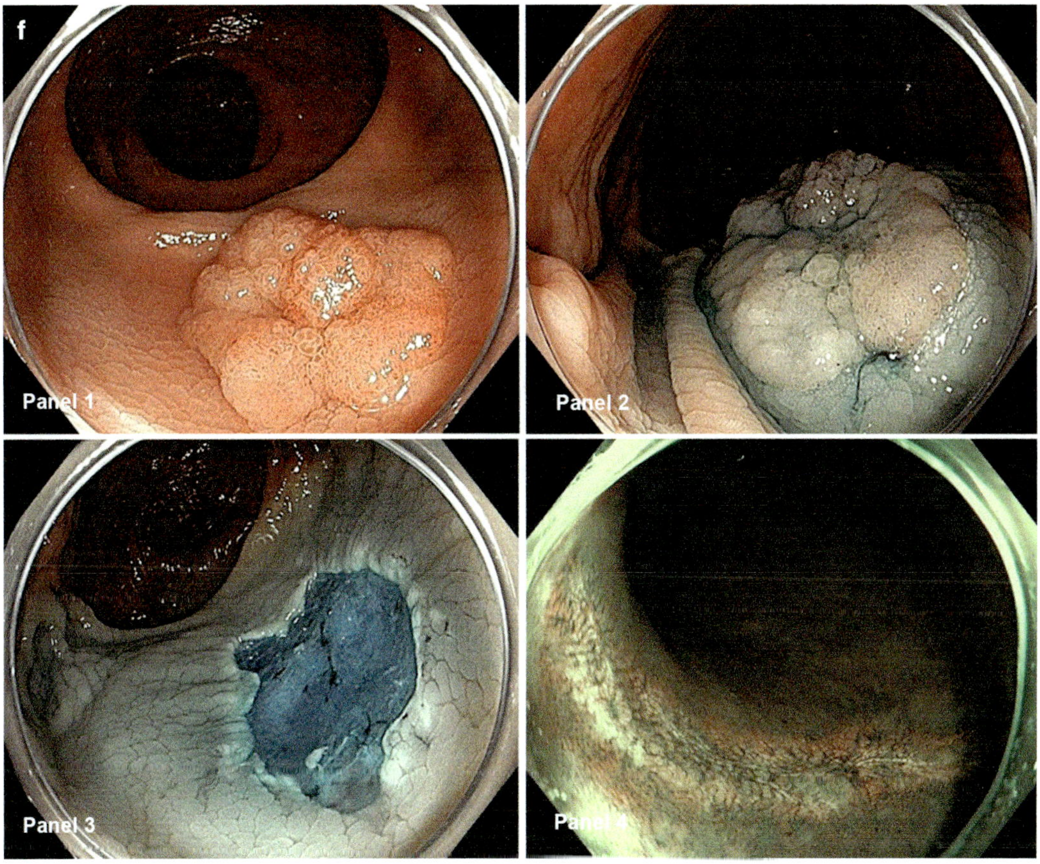

Fig. 13.10 (continued)

Haemorrhoids

They appear as protruded or polypoid vessels in the distal rectum (Fig. 13.17).

Miscellaneous

Melanosis Coli

- Reversible mucosal brown pigmentation of the colon (Fig. 13.18).
- Caused by use of anthraquinone laxatives (Table 13.9).
- Adenomas do not take up the lipofuscin pigment and can be easier to detect in melanosis coli during colonoscopy (Fig. 13.19).

Mucosal Prolapse (Solitary Rectal Ulcer Syndrome)

- Erythematous and/or ulcerated mucosa of the most distal rectum
- Can present with rectal bleeding

Angiodysplasia

- Flat red vascular lesions.
- Under NBI they appear brown or darker in colour than surrounding normal mucosa (Fig. 13.20).
- Often a feeding vessel can be seen.
- Mostly found in the ascending colon and cecum.

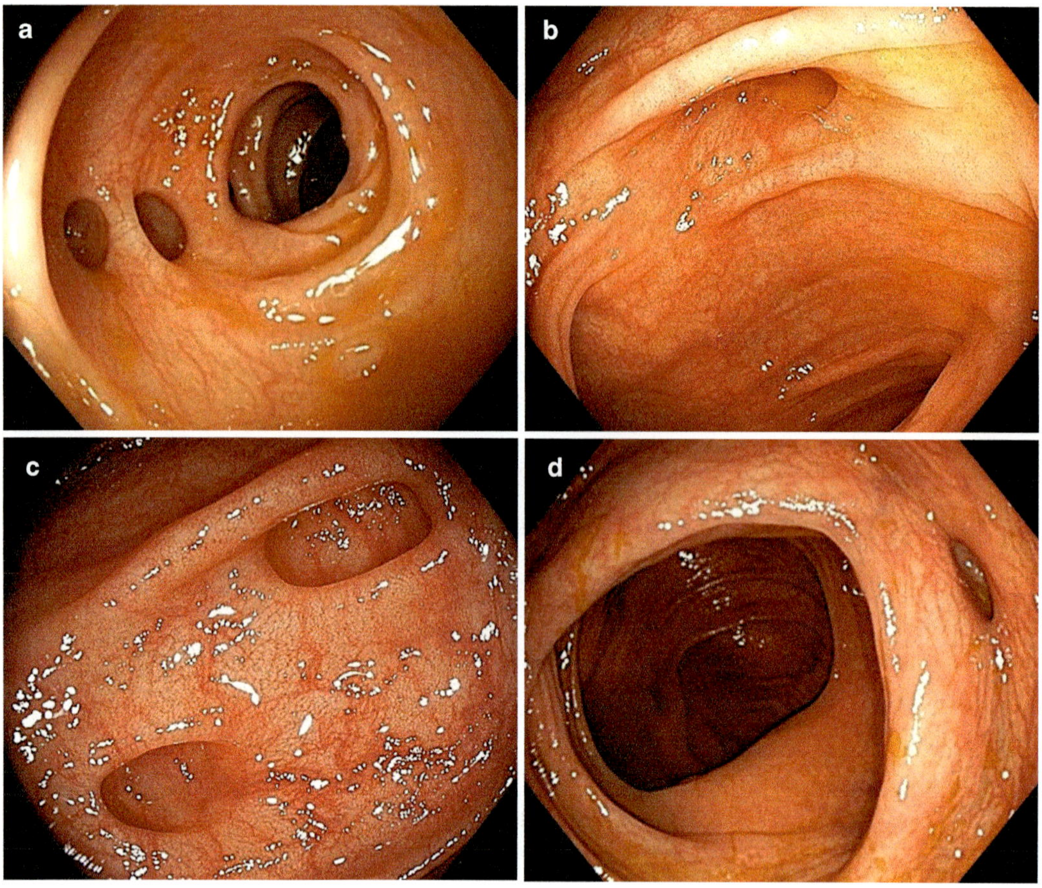

Fig. 13.11 (a–d) Diverticular disease

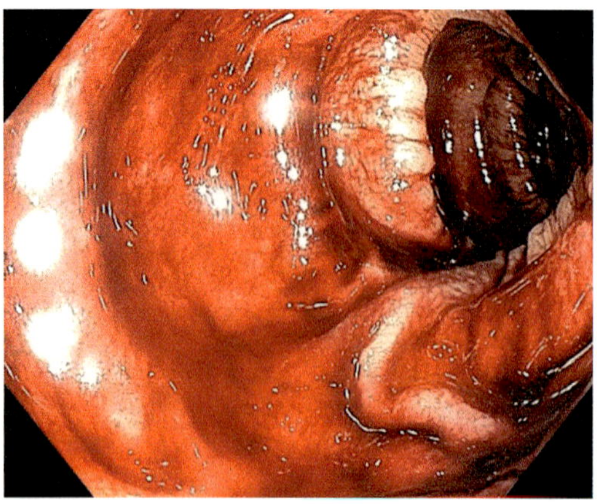

Fig. 13.12 Diverticular bleeding

Table 13.8 Complications of diverticular perforation

Peritonitis
Sepsis
Abscess
Fistula
Bowel obstruction

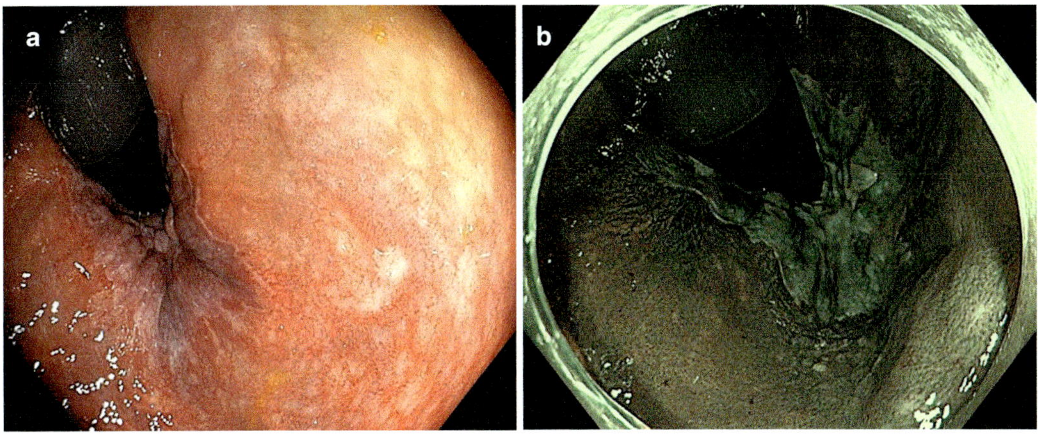

Fig. 13.13 (**a**, **b**) Rectal retroflexion under white light and NBI showing anorectal junction

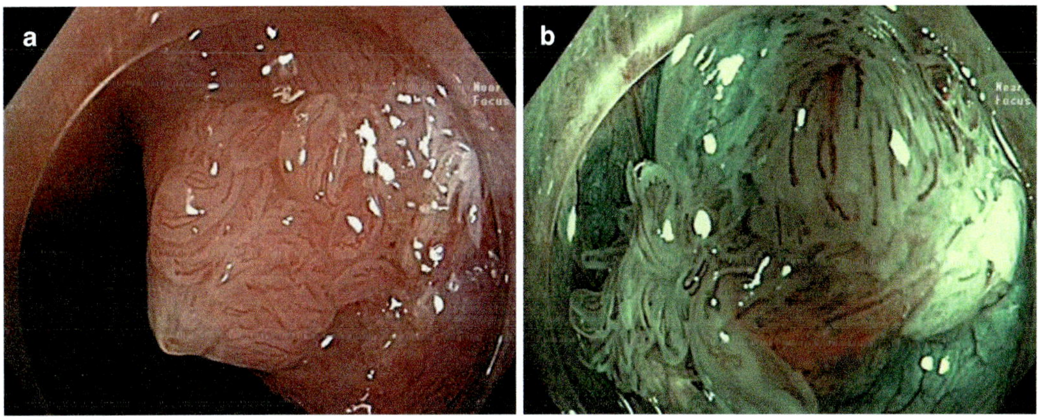

Fig. 13.14 (**a**, **b**) AIN under white-light and narrow-band imaging

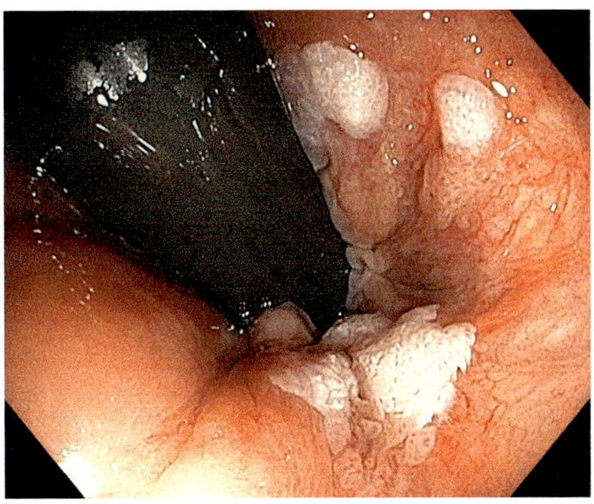

Fig. 13.15 Patient on immunosuppression with clusters of AIN

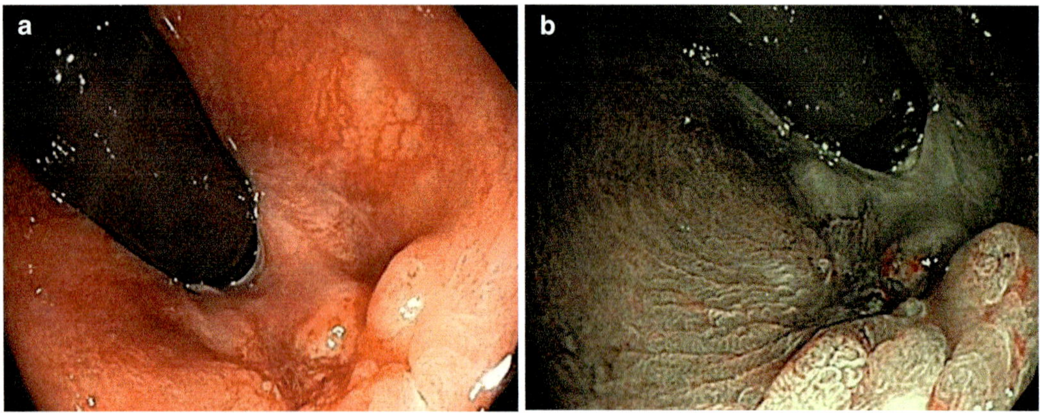

Fig. 13.16 (**a**, **b**) Ulcerated squamous cell carcinoma in a 79-year-old lady presenting with rectal bleeding seen on rectal retroflexion. The lesion was arising from the anorectal junction and invading the rectal mucosa

Fig. 13.17 Non-bleeding internal and external haemorrhoids seen on retroflexion view

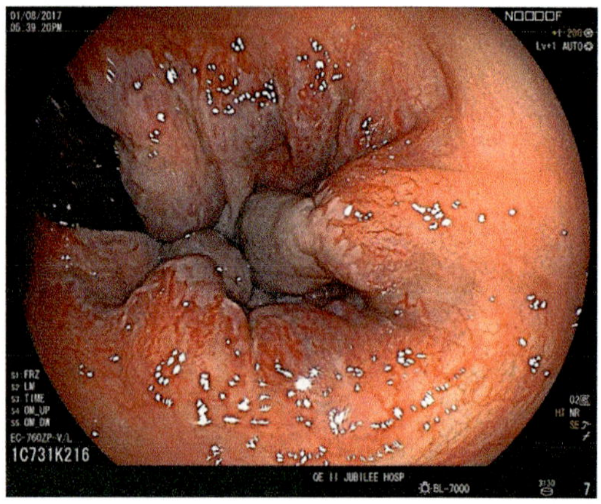

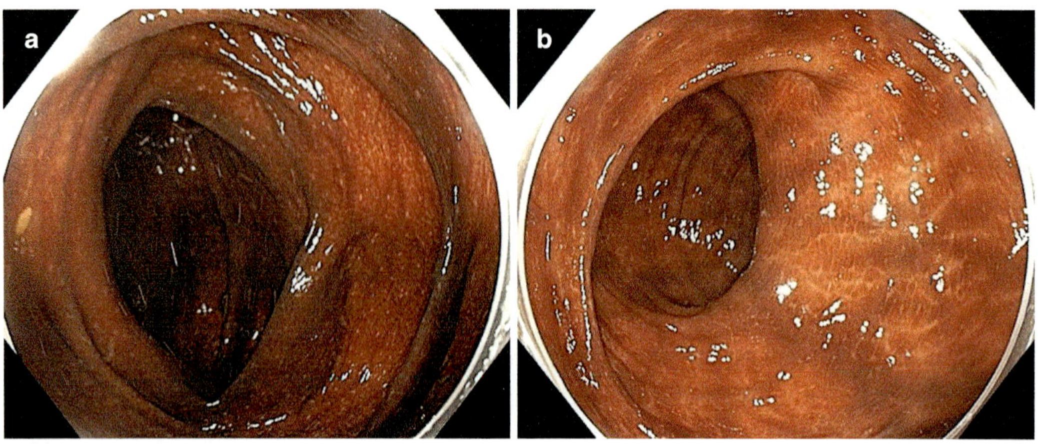

Fig. 13.18 (**a**, **b**) Melanosis coli

Table 13.9 Anthraquinone laxatives

Senna
Cascara
Aloe
Rhubarb
Frangula

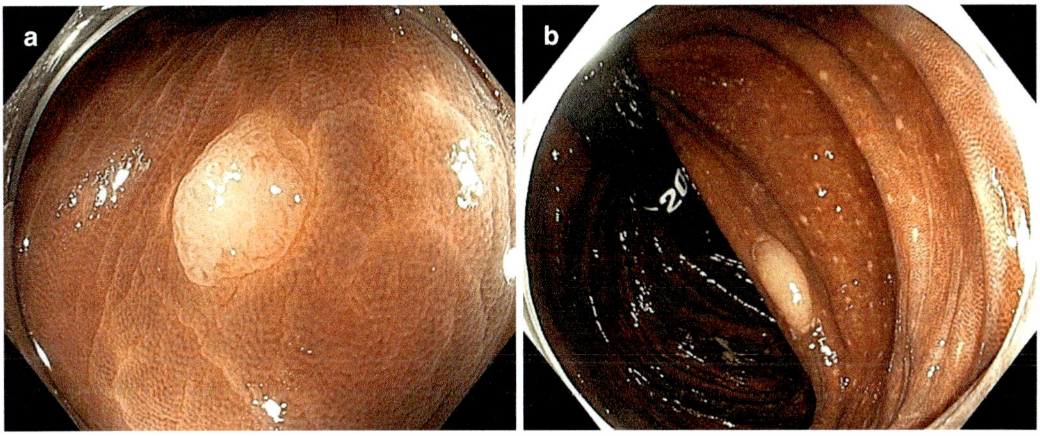

Fig. 13.19 (**a**, **b**) Adenomas can be easier to detect when melanosis coli is present

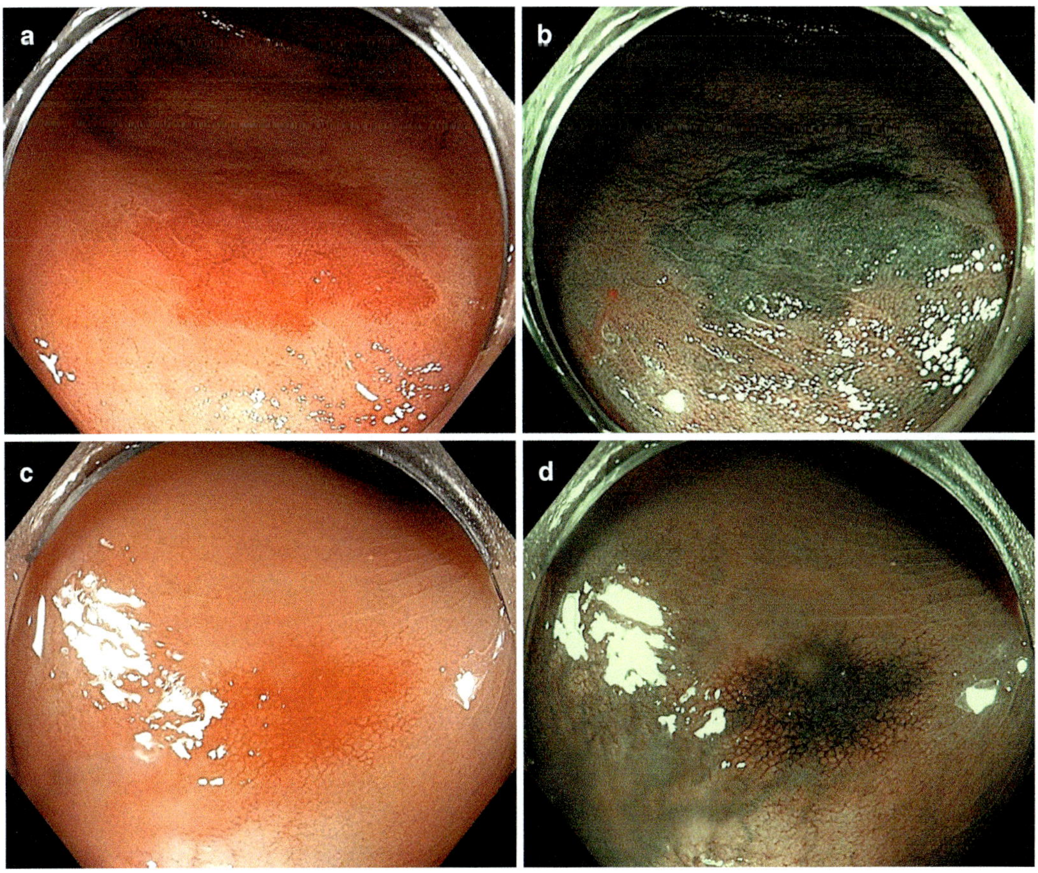

Fig. 13.20 (**a**–**d**) Non-bleeding angiodysplastic lesions of the colon (under white light and NBI)

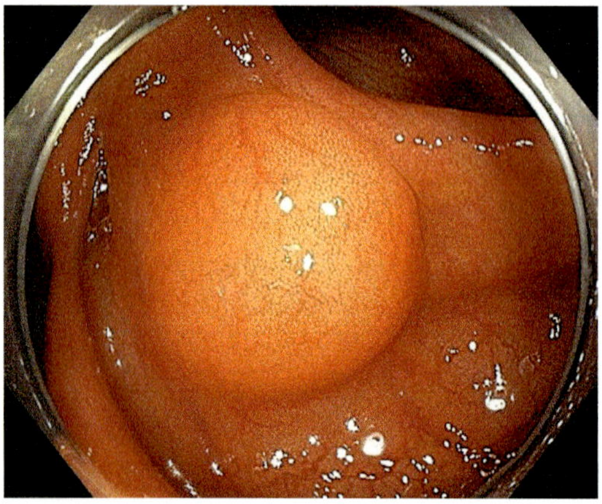

Fig. 13.21 Lipoma of the ascending colon with smooth surface and yellow discolouration

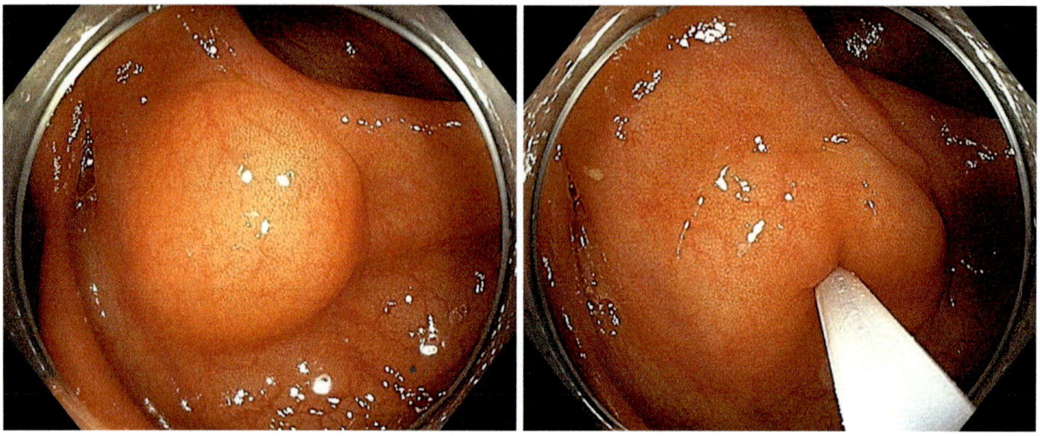

Fig. 13.22 Lipoma "cushion" or "pillow" sign

- Can be an incidental finding during colonoscopy, or patients may present with history of painless intermittent rectal bleeding, haematochezia, or anaemia
- If symptomatic, they can be treated with argon plasma coagulation (APC).

Lipoma

- Smooth sessile lesions
- Normal underlying mucosa with a tinge of yellow discolouration (Fig. 13.21)
- Soft when palpated using endoscopic accessory device, also known as "pillow sign" (Fig. 13.22)

Bowel Preparation-Related Mucosal Changes

- Non-specific
  - Normal
  - Mild patch erythema
  - Mild oedema
  - Small haemorrhages
- Commonly seen in the distal rectum but can be seen throughout the colon

Summary

Effective communication between gastroenterologists and pathologists is important for high-quality patient care. Advances in endoscopic imaging have improved the endoscopic detection, characterisation, and therapy of gastrointestinal pathology.

References

1. American Society for Gastrointestinal Endoscopy Standards of Practice C, Shergill AK, Lightdale JR, Bruining DH, Acosta RD, Chandrasekhara V, et al. The role of endoscopy in inflammatory bowel disease. Gastrointest Endosc. 2015;81(5):1101-21.e1–13.
2. Laine L, Kaltenbach T, Barkun A, McQuaid KR, Subramanian V, Soetikno R, et al. SCENIC international consensus statement on surveillance and management of dysplasia in inflammatory bowel disease. Gastroenterology. 2015;148(3):639–51.e28.
3. Laine L, Kaltenbach T, Barkun A, McQuaid KR, Subramanian V, Soetikno R, et al. SCENIC international consensus statement on surveillance and management of dysplasia in inflammatory bowel disease. Gastrointest Endosc. 2015;81(3):489–501.e26.
4. DuPont HL. Bacterial diarrhea. N Engl J Med. 2009;361(16):1560–9.
5. Kheir AO, Kaltenbach T, Soetikno R. Chromoendoscopy. In: Vani KJA, Waxman I, editors. Endoscopic imaging techniques and tools. New York, NY: Springer International Publishing; 2016. p. 29–48.
6. Kaltenbach T, Sano Y, Friedland S, Soetikno R, American Gastroenterological A American Gastroenterological Association (AGA) Institute technology assessment on image-enhanced endoscopy. Gastroenterology. 2008;134(1):327–40.
7. Committee AT, Abu Dayyeh BK, Thosani N, Konda V, Wallace MB, Rex DK, et al. ASGE Technology Committee systematic review and meta-analysis assessing the ASGE PIVI thresholds for adopting real-time endoscopic assessment of the histology of diminutive colorectal polyps. Gastrointest Endosc. 2015;81(3):502.e1–e16.
8. Hewett DG, Kaltenbach T, Sano Y, Tanaka S, Saunders BP, Ponchon T, et al. Validation of a simple classification system for endoscopic diagnosis of small colorectal polyps using narrow-band imaging. Gastroenterology. 2012;143(3):599–607.e1.
9. Sakata S, Kheir AO, Hewett DG. Optical diagnosis of colorectal neoplasia: a western perspective. Dig Endosc. 2016;28(3):281–8.
10. Hayashi N, Tanaka S, Hewett DG, Kaltenbach TR, Sano Y, Ponchon T, et al. Endoscopic prediction of deep submucosal invasive carcinoma: validation of the narrow-band imaging international colorectal endoscopic (NICE) classification. Gastrointest Endosc. 2013;78(4):625–32.
11. The Paris classification of superficial neoplastic lesions: esophagus, stomach, and colon. Gastrointest Endosc. 2003;58(Supp):S3–S43.
12. Kudo S, Tamura S, Nakajima T, et al. Diagnosis of colorectal tumorous lesions by magnifying endoscopy. Gastrointest Endosc. 1996;44:8–14.
13. IJspeert JE, Bastiaansen BA, van Leerdam ME, Meijer GA, van Eeden S, Sanduleanu S, et al. Development and validation of the WASP classification system for optical diagnosis of adenomas, hyperplastic polyps and sessile serrated adenomas/polyps. Gut. 2016;65:963.

Index

M. P. Kumarasinghe, I. Brown (eds.), *Endoscopic Biopsy Interpretation*,
https://doi.org/10.1007/978-3-319-79117-3

O

Printed by Printforce, the Netherlands